List of activities

ESSA Student Manual for **Health, Exercise** and **Sport Assessment**

Second Edition

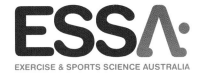

EXERCISE & SPORTS SCIENCE AUSTRALIA

ESSA Student Manual for Health, Exercise and Sport Assessment

Second Edition

Jeff S Coombes

BEd (Hons), BAppSc, MEd, PhD, ESSAM, AES, AEP, FACSM, FESSA
Professor of Clinical Exercise Physiology
School of Human Movement and Nutrition Sciences
The University of Queensland, Brisbane, QLD, Australia

Tina L Skinner

BAppSc (Hons), PhD, ESSAM, AES, AEP
Associate Professor of Clinical Exercise Physiology
School of Human Movement and Nutrition Sciences
The University of Queensland, Brisbane, QLD, Australia

ELSEVIER

ELSEVIER

Elsevier Australia. ACN 001 002 357
(a division of Reed International Books Australia Pty Ltd)
Tower 1, 475 Victoria Avenue, Chatswood, NSW 2067

ISBN: 978-0-7295-4269-2

Notice

Practitioners and researchers must always rely on their own experience and knowledge in evaluating and using any information, methods, compounds or experiments described herein. Because of rapid advances in the medical sciences, in particular, independent verification of diagnoses and drug dosages should be made. To the fullest extent of the law, no responsibility is assumed by Elsevier, authors, editors or contributors for any injury and/or damage to persons or property as a matter of products liability, negligence or otherwise, or from any use or operation of any methods, products, instructions, or ideas contained in the material herein.

National Library of Australia Cataloguing-in-Publication Data

A catalogue record for this book is available from the National Library of Australia

Senior Content Strategist: Melinda McEvoy
Content Project Manager: Kritika Kaushik
Copy edited by Chris Wyard
Proofread by Tim Learner
Cover and internal design by Georgette Hall
Index by SPi Global
Typeset by GW Tech
Printed in Singapore by Morkono Printing media pte limited

Last digit is the print number: 9   8   7   6   5   4   3   2   1

Contents

Contents *(continued)*

Foreword

Exercise science in Australia is a rapidly growing profession. Exercise Scientists are professionals equipped with the knowledge and skills to apply the science of exercise when developing interventions that improve health and fitness, wellbeing and performance, and that assist in the prevention of injury and chronic conditions.

Accredited Exercise Scientists teach, coach and motivate clients to facilitate self-management of physical activity, exercise and healthy lifestyles, using models of behaviour change, scientific evidence and critical thinking, while accounting for individual factors and social determinants of health. An Accredited Exercise Scientist practises in a culturally safe and inclusive manner and according to the principles of client-centred care.

The assessment of health, fitness and sports is an important aspect of exercise and sports science and should be one of the most important skills a graduate from an exercise science program has developed. Assessments not only help to develop an appropriate, individualised program, they also provide an imperative function of screening for risk of heart disease, other chronic diseases and injuries.

This text is a unique book in the Australian setting, providing the theoretical understanding and procedures to allow Australian students and graduates to work competently within the health, exercise and sport industry. It is also the first text available in Australia that has considered Exercise & Sports Science Australia's (ESSA's) exercise science accreditation framework.

ESSA's Student Manual for Health, Fitness and Sports Assessments 2e is a beneficial text for any student undertaking an exercise and sports science degree, providing content related to the knowledge and skills required to undertake an assessment, no matter the setting.

The editors of this text are expert educators and researchers who have structured this text based on years of experience teaching the content to cover commonly performed health, fitness and sports assessments.

Exercise & Sports Science Australia is the peak organisation in Australia representing and advocating for university-trained exercise and sports science professionals, including the allied health profession of exercise physiology. As the peak professional body representing exercise and sports science in Australia, ESSA provides national and international leadership and advocacy on key issues, and supports its members and the community by fostering excellence in professional practice, education and training, and research.

One of the association's key roles is to promote professional standards by providing high-quality education, accreditation and management of standards. For this reason, ESSA is pleased to support this text as one way we look to ensure consistent and high standards within our professions.

In my opinion, the most important element of this textbook is the easy-to-read style and strong use of imagery, which will help readers to understand complex and vital information.

Anita Hobson-Powell
Executive Officer
Exercise & Sports Science Australia

Preface

This second edition of the *ESSA Student Manual for Health, Exercise and Sport Assessment* continues the editors' efforts to provide a user-friendly resource for exercise science students. There have been numerous additions since the first edition, including a new practical on the assessment of static and dynamic posture, as well as significant changes to many of the previous practicals. Feedback from users of the manual has led to an increased discussion on the reliability and validity of the tests, and the objectives of different practicals are mapped against ESSA's Exercise Science Standards for Health, Exercise and Sport Assessment. We hope that this will be useful for university courses seeking or re-applying for accreditation.

In keeping with the first edition, this manual contains the basic theory and detailed step-by-step protocols to enable students develop the competencies to safely conduct health and fitness evaluations and perform common health-, exercise- and sport-related assessments. The manual identifies and explains the common processes and equipment required to conduct assessments across various aspects of health, exercise and sport. The safety of the tester and the participant is addressed throughout the manual, with an appendix describing cleaning and disinfection from a contemporary occupational health and safety perspective. Emphasis is placed on the need for accurate measuring devices, with a separate practical covering test accuracy, reliability and validity with the rationale and fundamentals of calibration and verification. The scientific rationale, purpose, assumptions and validity of procedures are described, along with the limitations, contraindications and additional considerations where appropriate. The manual focuses on the analysis, interpretation and communication (e.g. feedback and discussion) of test results to the participant. Practicals contain case study questions and examples that show how these important steps can be conducted and provide advice for common scenarios.

The content of this manual has been developed by the editors and authors over many years of teaching this material. It is the editors' observations, while teaching these skills, that the subject(s) containing this content is one of the most challenging, enjoyable and rewarding that a student will complete during their degree. An important reason for this, we believe, is because it requires and allows students to develop individual skill competency. We have witnessed that the successful completion of a subject(s) that teaches and assesses technical skill competency gives students more confidence during their practicum placements and within the industry. It may also lead students to seek placements and work in areas of exercise and sport science that they may not have previously considered (e.g. as a cardiac technician or sports scientist).

About the editors

Jeff S Coombes

Jeff is a Professor of Clinical Exercise Physiology in the School of Human Movement and Nutrition Sciences at The University of Queensland and Chair of the Exercise is Medicine Australia initiative. He obtained an undergraduate education degree and a research Master's in education from the University of Tasmania before completing a PhD at the University of Florida in 1998. Since 2000 he has been coordinating and teaching exercise science technical skills courses at The University of Queensland. These experiences are the basis for the majority of the activities and pedagogical approaches used in this book. He was national president of ESSA from 2006 to 2011 and has been on committees that have reviewed the professional standards for Exercise Science, Sport Science and Clinical Exercise Physiology. His practical experience includes over 15 years working in health and fitness and conducting exercise and sport science research. He is an Accredited Exercise Scientist and has been an Accredited Exercise Physiologist since 2006.

Tina L Skinner

Tina is an Associate Professor in Clinical Exercise Physiology in the School of Human Movement and Nutrition Sciences at The University of Queensland. She graduated with honours from an undergraduate exercise science degree before completing a PhD in sports science at The University of Queensland. She completed her Graduate Certificate in Higher Education in 2009 and since then has undertaken numerous scholarly activities designed to encourage independent and reflective learning. Tina has taught across all year levels, from large first year classes to specialist clinical postgraduate courses that are central to the accreditation of the programs at The University of Queensland. She has been an Accredited Exercise Physiologist since 2007.

Acknowledgements

Given the work that went into our first edition, a second edition seemed like a fairly straightforward and simpler process. Five years and thousands of hours later, we realise how wrong we were. A team of people, both personal and professional, made this textbook possible.

To have Australia and New Zealand's leading teachers and researchers in our field co-author the practicals within this textbook has been extraordinary and truly humbling. Your expertise and contributions have made this textbook what it is today. We cannot thank you enough.

To all our supportive colleagues within and beyond the School of Human Movement and Nutrition Sciences at The University of Queensland – thank you. We are indebted to you all, especially Simon Austen, Megan King, Stephanie Hannan, Mia Schaumberg, Kirsten Adlard, Chloe Salisbury and Kylie Maguire, who have contributed to the practical content which underpins this textbook. Without your invaluable roles in the evolution of the course material since the year 2000, this textbook would not exist. Further, to all the 'Exercise Science Technical Skills' and 'Advanced Exercise Physiology' practical coordinators, tutors and students, both past and present, we thank you for the thousands of hours of practicals, open labs and exams which have formed the foundations of this textbook.

To Exercise and Sports Science Australia (ESSA): thank you for your support and endorsement of this textbook. Special thanks go to the Chief Executive Officer, Anita Hobson-Powell and the National Board for their support.

We greatly appreciate the many reviewers who provided detailed feedback on each of the practicals.

Thank you to all the companies and their representatives who assisted with approval of the numerous protocols, tables and figures used throughout this textbook.

Without the team at Elsevier, this resource would not exist. Thank you for your patience – lots of patience.

And finally, to our families and friends who have supported us through this lengthy and tiring process, thank you for your unwavering support. We dedicate this textbook to you.

Contributors

Tania Louise Brancato Best BScAppHMS (ExSc) (Hons), GC (Higher Ed), GD (Ex Rehab), AEP, AES
Lecturer in Clinical Exercise Physiology
School of Exercise and Nutrition Sciences
Queensland University of Technology
Brisbane, QLD, Australia

Martyn John Binnie BSc (Hons), PhD
Performance Scientist (Rowing)
High Performance Service Centre
Western Australian Institute of Sport
Perth, WA, Australia

David Bishop BHMS (Hons), PhD
Professor in Exercise Physiology
Institute for Health and Sport
Victoria University
Melbourne, VIC, Australia

Jeff Coombes BAppSc, BEd (Hons), MEd, PhD, ESSAM, AES, AEP, FACSM, FESSA
Professor of Clinical Exercise Physiology
School of Human Movement and Nutrition
Sciences
The University of Queensland
Brisbane, QLD, Australia

Troy J Cross BExSc (Hons), PhD
Senior Lecturer in Exercise and Sport Science
Sydney School of Health Sciences
Faculty of Medicine and Health
The University of Sydney
Sydney, NSW, Australia

Sjaan Gomersall BPhysio (Hons), PhD
Senior Lecturer in Physiotherapy
School of Health and Rehabilitation Sciences
The University of Queensland
Brisbane, QLD, Australia

G Gregory Haff PhD, CSCS*D, FNSCA
School of Medical and Health Sciences
Edith Cowan University
Joondalup, WA, Australia

Anthony Leicht BAppSc (Hons), GD (FET), PhD, ESSAF, FECSS
Associate Professor
Sport and Exercise Science
College of Healthcare Sciences
James Cook University
Townsville, QLD, Australia

Deirdre McGhee BAppSc (Phty), PhD
Associate Professor
School of Medicine
Faculty of Science, Medicine and Health
The University of Wollongong
Wollongong, NSW, Australia

Norman Morris BAppSc (Phty), BSc, DipEd, PhD
Professor of Physiotherapy
School of Health Sciences and Social Work
The Menzies Health Institute
Griffith University
Gold Coast, QLD, Australia
and
Metro North Hospital and Health Service
The Prince Charles Hospital
Allied Health Research Collaborative
Chermside, QLD, Australia

Robert U Newton BHMS (Hons), MHMS, PhD, DSc
Professor of Exercise Medicine
School of Medical and Health Sciences
Edith Cowan University
Joondalup, WA, Australia

Kevin Norton Bed (PE) (Hons), MA, PhD
Professor of Exercise Science
Health and Human Performance
University of South Australia
Adelaide, SA, Australia

Surendran Sabapathy BExSc (Hons), PhD
Senior Lecturer, Exercise and Sport
School of Health Sciences and Social Work
Griffith University
QLD, Australia

xi

Contributors *(continued)*

Julian Sacre BAppSc, PhD
Postdoctoral Research Fellow
Clinical Diabetes and Epidemiology
Baker Heart and Diabetes Institute
Melbourne, VIC, Australia

Mia Schaumberg BExSS (Hons), GC (Higher Ed), PhD
Senior Lecturer in Physiology
School of Health and Behavioural Sciences
Sunshine Coast Health Institute
University of the Sunshine Coast
Sippy Downs, QLD, Australia

Martin Schultz BAppSc, GD (Ex Rehab), MAppSc, PhD
Senior Research Fellow
Menzies Institute for Medical Research
University of Tasmania

Tina Skinner BAppSc (Hons), PhD, ESSAM, AES, AEP
Associate Professor of Clinical Exercise
Physiology
School of Human Movement and Nutrition
Sciences
The University of Queensland
Brisbane, QLD, Australia

Gary Slater BSc, GD (Nutr Diet), MSc, PhD
Associate Professor in Nutrition and Dietetics
School of Health and Behavioural Sciences
University of the Sunshine Coast
Sippy Downs, QLD, Australia

Margaret Torode BAppSc (HM), Dip Teach, MSc, PhD, FASMF, FESSA
Adjunct Associate Professor,
School of Exercise Science, Sport and Health
Charles Sturt University
Bathurst, NSW, Australia

Andrew Williams BSc (Hons), BAppSc (Ex & Sport Sc), GCULT, PhD
Associate Professor in Clinical Exercise Science
School of Health Sciences
University of Tasmania
Launceston, TAS, Australia

Reviewers

Emily Gray BPhysio, PG Dip Sports Med, MPNZ
School of Physiotherapy
University of Otago
North Dunedin, Dunedin, New Zealand

Daniel Hackett BExSc, GradDip Ed, MHlthSc (ExSpSc) (Hon), PhD (Ex Physiol),
The University of Sydney
Sydney, NSW, Australia

Brad Wall PhD, ESSAM, AES, AEP
Senior Lecturer, Exercise Science
Murdoch University
Perth, WA, Australia

ESSA and the professions

Exercise & Sports Science Australia (ESSA) is the peak professional organisation in Australia committed to establishing, promoting and defending the career paths of university-qualified Accredited Exercise Scientists, Accredited Sports Scientists and Accredited Exercise Physiologists.

The following terms are used throughout the manual to refer to qualifications, accreditations and professions associated with applying the knowledge and skills. Although from the Australian context, defining these will assist with the use of the manual in broader contexts.

Accredited Exercise Physiologist (AEP): A university-qualified individual who has been accredited by Exercise & Sports Science Australia (ESSA) to prescribe, deliver and adapt movement, physical activity and exercise-based interventions to facilitate and optimise health status, function, recovery and independence. AEPs provide services to people across the full health spectrum: healthy individuals through to those at risk of developing a health condition, and people with health conditions, a disability and age-related illnesses and conditions, including chronic, complex conditions. The person is recognised as an allied health professional.

Accredited Exercise Scientist (AES): A university-qualified individual who has been accredited by Exercise & Sports Science Australia (ESSA) to apply the science of exercise to design and deliver physical activity and exercise-based interventions to improve health, fitness, well-being and performance and assist in the prevention of injury and chronic conditions.

Accredited Sport Scientist (ASpS): A university-qualified individual who has been accredited by Exercise & Sports Science Australia (ESSA) to specialise in the application of scientific principles and techniques to assist coaches and athletes improve their performance at an individual level or within the context of a team environment. They may also apply their knowledge and skills to relevant projects (e.g. teaching and research) within the sports industry, to corporate bodies and to the community.

Exercise Professional: A qualified and registered/accredited person who supplies exercise services to the public.

PRACTICAL 1
TEST ACCURACY, RELIABILITY AND VALIDITY

Tina Skinner, Jeff Coombes and Anthony Leicht

LEARNING OBJECTIVES

- Demonstrate an understanding of the principles, rationale, terminology, application, assumptions, limitations and protocol considerations of test accuracy, reliability and validity
- Calculate inter- and intra-tester reliability and interpret the results
- Perform verification and calibration tests on various pieces of equipment used in health, exercise and sport assessments and interpret the results to recognise when additional work (e.g. adjustments, calibration curves) is needed
- Record information from calibration and verification procedures

Equipment and other requirements

- Self-retracting, flexible metal anthropometry tape
- Masking tape
- Tape measure
- Flat base ruler (tip of rule = 0 cm)
- Inclinometer or 1 m spirit level, preferably with an adjustable lever
- Stopwatch
- Motorised treadmill
- Cycle ergometer
- Calculator
- Calibration weights (e.g. 1–4 kg)
- Allen keys
- Body mass scales
- Tissues
- Temperature, humidity and barometric pressure monitor
- Metabolic system
- Calibration gas tanks
- Calibration syringe

INTRODUCTION

Exercise professionals need to have a thorough understanding of the concepts underpinning the ability to make accurate, reliable and valid measures. This understanding is made difficult by the number of terms that are used, with some being interchanged in certain situations. For example, the terms precision,

1

reliability, reproducibility, agreement and repeatability are often used interchangeably as they are generally referring to the same overarching concept. However, there are differences in how similar terms (e.g. reproducibility, agreement and repeatability) are defined, depending on the context.[1,2] The following sections will discuss the need to define the context in which the terms accuracy, validity and reliability are used to gain a better understanding of these important concepts in exercise, health and sport assessments.

DEFINITIONS

Accuracy: the proximity of measurement results to the true value or an accepted comparator.

Agreement: the similarity between two measurement results.

Calibration: the action of adjusting and confirming the true value or accuracy of a measurement in comparison with an acceptable standard.

Cardiorespiratory fitness: the ability of the circulatory and respiratory systems to supply oxygen and support the energy demands during sustained physical activity. Also known as aerobic fitness or aerobic endurance.

Concurrent validity: the degree to which an assessment (e.g. test or measure) accurately measures what it is intended to measure. May refer to the validity of a test (e.g. physical activity is not a valid measure of cardiorespiratory fitness) or the validity of a measure (e.g. a step counter accurately measures the number of steps). Also known as **test validity**.

Face validity: the extent to which a test appears to correctly measure what it is intended to measure.

Gold standard: a benchmark or most accurate measure that is regarded as the best available.

Inter-tester reliability: also known as between-tester reliability, this is the amount of agreement (reliability) between two different testers measuring the same parameter on the same individual.

Intra-tester reliability: also known as within-tester reliability, this is the amount of agreement (reliability) from the same tester measuring the same parameter on different occasions using the same equipment.

Predictive validity: the ability of a measure to predict the effect of a therapeutic intervention on an outcome.

Prognostic validity: the ability of a measure to predict an outcome, independent of treatment.

Reference method: a thoroughly investigated method in which the reliability and accuracy are known and commensurate with the methods used for assessing the accuracy of other methods employed to obtain the same information.

Reliability: the magnitude of agreement between two measures.

True value: The value that would be obtained in an ideal measurement (with no errors).

Validity: the extent to which an assessment (e.g. test or measure) accurately predicts, measures or appears to measure what it is intended to measure. Different types of validity include prognostic, predictive, concurrent (also known as test) and face validity.

Verification: the action of checking, but not adjusting, the equipment/instrument against the calibration measure.

Accuracy

A test is accurate when it measures what it is supposed to measure (i.e. the *true value*). There are a number of related concepts to test accuracy such as reliability, validity, calibration and verification. Indeed, the large number of terms used to describe the same or similar approaches often causes confusion when understanding test accuracy. To better illustrate what accuracy entails, the following examples show the factors that may affect test accuracy:

1 Protocol selection – e.g. using a submaximal protocol to predict maximal oxygen consumption ($\dot{V}O_2$max) will *decrease* the accuracy of the measurement compared with a $\dot{V}O_2$max test.

2 Procedure selection – e.g. using equations based upon different sex and/or training status to calculate percent body fat would *decrease* the accuracy of the measurement compared with the four-compartment model.

3 Equipment selection – e.g. using a ruler where the tip doesn't start at 0 cm when completing the weight-bearing lunge test will *decrease* the accuracy of the measurement.

4 Participant preparation – e.g. consuming caffeine prior to a submaximal assessment of cardiorespiratory fitness that is based on the person's heart rate response to exercise will *decrease* the accuracy of the measurement.

5 Protocol problems – e.g. failure to correctly calibrate metabolic analysers before a $\dot{V}O_2$max test will *decrease* the accuracy of the measurement.

6 Tester skill – e.g. poor technique in taking skinfold measures will *decrease* the accuracy of the measurement.

7 Technical problems – e.g. an uncalibrated automated blood pressure monitor will *decrease* the accuracy of the measurement.

MEASURING TEST ACCURACY

Test accuracy is usually measured by comparing the assessment outcome with another measure (comparator). The best way to assess test accuracy is when the true value is known. The 'gold standard' is the most accurate measure of a true known value (e.g. body mass measured with calibrated weighing scales). Therefore, it is ideal to compare your measure against a gold standard measure to determine test accuracy. However, for many measures (e.g. body composition), the true value can be extremely difficult or impossible to measure directly. In this situation, a known assessment (including the procedure and equipment) that has been widely accepted to provide a good estimate of the measure is the reference method or criterion standard. A reference method or criterion standard is also the terminology used when there is disagreement among experts on whether a true gold standard exists for that measure. For example, skinfolds measured by an exercise professional could be compared with measures performed on the same individual from a level 3 or 4 anthropometrist (criterion standard). For some measures, the comparator may be an estimate (e.g. the reference method for determining body fat percentage is the 'four-compartment model', which includes multiple measurements, each with their own assumptions).[1]

Calibration and verification

Calibration and verification of measuring equipment are important components of the quality management process that is essential for obtaining accurate results from exercise testing. In Australia, the Australian Sports Commission established the National Sport Science Quality Assurance (NSSQA) program in 1989. The NSSQA program takes a national leadership role in overseeing quality assurance in sport science testing laboratories and standards involved in the assessment of athletes. The primary aim of the accreditation process is to achieve comparability of results of athlete testing among different laboratories. Secondary aims include developing a database of appropriate measurement error tolerances for commonly conducted tests. The NSQAA provides standards across all aspects of athlete testing, including the appropriate calibration and verification of equipment. Outside of the sport science environment, the Australia Government has created the National Measurement Institute. It promotes and monitors the use of *good practice* to ensure the accuracy of measures conducted in the biological, chemical and physical trades.

One of the first steps in the calibration and/or verification of a piece of equipment/device is to determine whether it is possible to adjust (calibrate) it. For example, some weighing scales have a dial that allows the measuring scale to be moved and this would allow for a single point calibration (e.g. zeroing), whilst other scales have no ability to be adjusted. Some equipment has to be sent back to the manufacturer to be calibrated, while others (e.g. electronically braked cycle ergometers) require special calibration/verification equipment.

Calibration is achieved by comparing the measuring device or equipment with a gold/criterion standard and adjusting accordingly. For example, to calibrate weighing scales there are certified weights available from the National Measurement Institute. Weighing scales are calibrated (if able to be adjusted) or verified (if unable to be adjusted) by comparing the value provided by the scale with the certified weight. Using a gold standard will increase the probability that the measured value will be accurate and very close to the true value (i.e. test validity). The calibration process is usually completed against gold/criterion standards that cover a range of expected values. For example, when calibrating weighing scales, it would be important to determine the accuracy across the range in which they are most likely to be used (e.g. if using with apparently healthy adults then calibrating/verifying using certified weights between 50 and 120 kg).

Verification is the process of checking but not adjusting the measuring scale. For example, after calibrating a measuring device before a test (e.g. oxygen (O_2) and carbon dioxide (CO_2) analysers before a $\dot{V}O_2max$ or $\dot{V}O_2peak$ test) the tester should also check (verify) it after the test to see whether its calibration state has changed. In devices that are not able to be calibrated, or have only the ability for a single point calibration (e.g. weighing scales), a verification curve can be established over a range of measures (see Activity 1.1).

Most manufacturers of equipment used in exercise testing (e.g. treadmills, cycle ergometers and gas analysers) provide calibration and/or verification processes that should be followed meticulously. In *good practice* a log of these processes should be kept, along with any associated data, so any problem or abnormality can be identified, corrected and monitored over time as necessary (e.g. manufacturer calibration).

Acceptable error

To quantify accuracy, the measurement result is compared with a gold standard or criterion standard measure to determine the level of agreement and/or error, e.g. percentage error or limits of agreement.[3] Although accuracy is a relative concept (i.e. not all-or-nothing), it is often used in a categorical statement (e.g. if the agreement between the assessment and the gold/criterion standard is low then it is common to say that the test is 'inaccurate'). However, there are often no clear rules for what level of agreement cut-off should be used to make these decisions. While errors >10% have been previously used to describe poor accuracy,[2] this value will depend on numerous factors (e.g. complexity of the measure, normal physiological variability). For example, the International Society for the Advancement of Kinanthropometry (ISAK) provides cut-off values for comparing the accuracy of measures with a level 3 or 4 anthropometrist. Thresholds have been set at 7.5% for skinfold readings and 1.5% for girths and breadths.[2]

In summary, all tests within health, sport and physical assessment contain inherent measurement error. Assessors should ensure that this measurement error is as small as practically possible through using correct techniques and equipment, and standardised assessment procedures (i.e. pre-assessment preparation, environment, etc.).

Validity

The word 'valid' is derived from the Latin *validus*, meaning strong. This should not be confused with notions of certainty or necessity. The extent to which an assessment (e.g. test or measure) accurately measures what it is intended to measure is known as validity. There are a number of different types of validity, including concurrent validity, prognostic validity, predictive validity and face validity. In this manual, any reference to validity is clarified depending on the context. Similar to accuracy, validity is often used with an 'all-or-none' application (e.g. this test is valid, but this one is invalid). Although the terms accuracy and validity may represent similar concepts, they fundamentally refer to different components. A test may be performed accurately by using correct techniques, calibrated equipment and standardised assessment procedures; however, the test performed may be invalid for the outcome intended to measure. Suppose, for example, you want to measure the body composition of a participant. You conduct *accurate* measures of height and body mass to calculate the participant's body mass index (BMI) using correct techniques, calibrated equipment and standardised assessment procedures; however, BMI is an *invalid* measure of body composition.

CONCURRENT VALIDITY

Concurrent validity, also known as test validity, is demonstrated when a test or measure correlates well with a test or measure that has previously been 'validated'. The validity of most of the assessments comprised within this manual will be discussed within the context of concurrent validity. With concurrent validity, it is important to understand the context. For example, is the grip strength test a 'valid' measure of overall strength? If the context was leg strength in elite track sprint cyclists, then the answer would be *'no'*. However, if the test is being used to assess the forearm strength of older individuals then it would be considered to have high concurrent validity.

PROGNOSTIC VALIDITY

Prognostic validity is similar to concurrent validity, with the difference due to the time at which the two measures are administered. Concurrent validity requires the two measures to be performed at approximately the same time, whereas prognostic validity has one of the measures performed at a later time. For example, the ability of an assessment to predict a health outcome is an example of prognostic validity. In this manual, this term will be mainly used in clinical contexts (e.g. survey to predict the onset of cardiovascular disease). Differences between the participant being assessed and the population used to establish the prognostic data will affect prognostic validity. For example, using a cardiovascular disease risk calculator that has been derived from Caucasians is going to be less valid for assessment of Aboriginal and/or Torres Strait Islander peoples.

PREDICTIVE VALIDITY

Predictive validity is a similar concept to prognostic validity, with the exception that predictive validity gives information about the effect of a therapeutic intervention on an outcome. For example, if you plan on implementing an exercise training intervention, you may be able to determine the predictive validity of the intervention on markers of insulin sensitivity based on previous literature.

FACE VALIDITY

Face validity, i.e. the extent to which a test appears to correctly measure what it is intended to measure, is the common starting point for the determination of the validity of a test. This involves a subjective assessment and covers the contextual relevance of the test to participants and its transparency. In general, face validity determines whether the assessment looks like it is measuring what it is supposed to be measuring. Face validity is increased when a person or group of people with extensive knowledge and experience using defined criteria assess face validity.

Activity 1.1 Treadmill speed and grade verification

AIM: to determine the speed and grade accuracy of a treadmill by comparing the displayed values with actual (measured) values.

Background

If a treadmill used for an exercise test has an inaccurate speed and/or grade, then the test may be inaccurate. Treadmill belts wear out and stretch over time with changes in belt length accounting for some of the speed errors. If possible, maintenance of the treadmill should involve re-tensioning the belt. Other error sources may be in the internal mechanisms or electronics of the treadmill. For the majority of treadmills, it is not possible or easy to calibrate (adjust) their speed and/or grade. Therefore, the process of checking (verifying) the speed and grade of a treadmill will clarify whether the equipment needs to be serviced/maintained or calibrated (if possible) to correct for unacceptable error. Verification should be performed over a range of speeds and grades. If there is an unacceptable error (e.g. $\geq 5\%$) and calibrating is not possible, then a calibration curve/s should be developed for that treadmill.

Protocol summary

Determine speed and grade accuracy of a treadmill, and construct calibration curves for each.

Protocol

Measuring treadmill belt length

1 Mark the start of the treadmill belt by placing a piece of masking tape on the belt. The tape should be perpendicular to the belt. Label this tape (tape #1).

2 Mark the end of the treadmill belt below by placing another piece of masking tape perpendicularly on the belt. Label this tape (tape #2).

3 Use a measuring tape to measure the distance from the bottom of tape #1 to the bottom of tape #2 (Figure 1.1) and record it in the data-recording sheet.

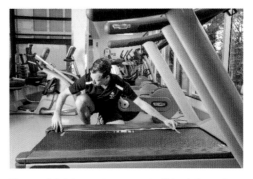

Figure 1.1 Measuring treadmill belt length
Used with permission from Technogym

4   Progress the treadmill belt forward so that tape #2 is now at the start of the belt. Mark the end of the belt with a third piece of masking tape placed perpendicularly on the belt (tape #3).

5   Use a measuring tape to measure and record the distance from the bottom of tape #2 to the bottom of tape #3.

6   Progress the treadmill belt forward to measure and record the distance from the bottom of tape #3 to the bottom of tape #1.

Assessing treadmill speed accuracy

1   Remove two of the pieces of tape that were on the treadmill belt (to measure treadmill belt length) so that only one piece of tape remains on the belt.

2   Place a piece of masking tape on the treadmill frame perpendicular to and directly beside the belt and towards the end of the belt. This will be used as a stable reference point.

3   Provide treadmill safety precautions to the participant (see Appendix D). An assessment of their ability to walk/jog safely should be conducted prior to starting the test.

4   Provide details of the test, including the protocol, hand signals the participant can use during the test, test termination and safety (see Appendix F).

5   Ask the participant to walk/run on the treadmill while it is travelling at 5 km/h.

6   Start a stopwatch when the tape on the belt aligns with the reference point.

7   Stop the stopwatch when the treadmill belt has completed 30 revolutions and the tape on the belt aligns with the reference point.

8   Record this time in the data-recording sheet (rounded to the nearest second).

9   Repeat steps #5 to #8 at 15 km/h.

10   Remove the tape from the treadmill belt.

Assessing treadmill grade accuracy

1   Start the treadmill and increase the grade to a 5% incline.

2   Once the desired grade has been achieved, stop the treadmill.

3   Place an inclinometer or 1 m long spirit level on the treadmill parallel to the belt (if the spirit level has an adjustable lever this should be towards the back of the treadmill) (Figure 1.2).

4   If using an inclinometer, the angle measured on the inclinometer needs to be converted to the grade percentage using the tangent of the measured angle and calculating the rise over 1 m.

For example, if the inclinometer is reading 5°, then:

$$\% \text{ grade} = \tan(\text{angle}) \times 100$$
$$= \tan(5) \times 100$$
$$= 8.75\%$$

5   If using a 1 m long spirit level, adjust the lever height so that the bubble in the spirit level is in the middle.

6   If using a 1 m long spirit level with an adjustable level, use a straight-edged ruler where the tip = 0 cm and measure the vertical height (in centimetres) between the bottom of the spirit level (towards the back end of the treadmill) and the treadmill surface. This height in cm is the treadmill grade percentage. Record this value in the data-recording sheet.

7   Increase the grade of the treadmill to a 15% incline and repeat steps #1 to #6

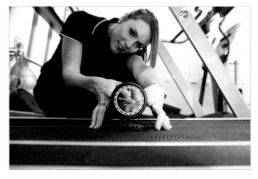

Figure 1.2 Treadmill grade verification
Used with permission from Technogym

Data analysis

Treadmill speed

To calculate the real speed of the treadmill in km/h, you first need to convert the treadmill speed from revolutions (revs)/s into revs/min. This is done by dividing the number of revolutions by the time it took to complete these revolutions, and multiplying it by 60. Then multiply the number of revs/min by the treadmill belt length to obtain the distance (in metres) covered in 1 minute. Divide this value by 1000 to get this value in km/min. Then multiply this amount by 60 to obtain your speed in km/h.

For example: if the treadmill belt is 2.4 m long and completed 30 revolutions in 42 seconds at a displayed 5 km/h:

$$= 30 \text{ revs/42 s}$$
$$(30 \div 42) = 0.71 \text{ revs/s}$$
$$(\times 60 \text{ s to convert to revs/min}) = 42.6 \text{ revs/min}$$
$$(\times \text{ the measured belt length, in this case 2.4 m}) = 102.2 \text{ m/min}$$
$$(\div 1000 \text{ to convert to km/min}) = 0.1022 \text{ km/min}$$
$$(\times 60 \text{ to convert to km/h}) = 6.13 \text{ km/h} = \text{speed}$$

For each speed, express the difference between the measured and displayed speed as a percentage error – see formula below.

> **Note:** The measured speed is the reference measure. An error between the measured and displayed speed of $\geq 5\%$ is usually deemed unacceptable.

$$\text{Absolute speed percentage error} = 100 - \left[\frac{\text{displayed speed} \times 100\%}{\text{measured speed}} \right]$$

e.g. if the displayed speed is 5 km/h but the measured speed is 6.1 km/h:

$$\text{Absolute speed percentage error} = 100 - \left[\frac{5.0 \times 100}{6.1} \right]$$
$$= 18.0\%$$

Treadmill grade

For each grade, express the difference between the measured and displayed grade as a percentage error – see formula below.

> **Note:** The measured grade is the reference measure. An error between the measured and displayed grade of $\geq 5\%$ is usually deemed unacceptable.

$$\text{Absolute grade percentage error} = 100 - \left[\frac{\text{displayed grade} \times 100\%}{\text{measured grade}} \right]$$

e.g. if the displayed grade is 5% but the measured grade is 5.8%:

$$\text{Absolute grade percentage error} = 100 - \left[\frac{5.0 \times 100}{5.8} \right]$$
$$= 13.8\%$$

Constructing a calibration curve

Calibration curves for treadmill speed and grade can be constructed from the equation of the line of best fit.

> **Note:** Constructing a calibration curve and equation of the line is usually only required when at least one of the percentage errors is not deemed to be 'acceptable' (e.g. $\geq 1\%$ in research settings or $\geq 5\%$ in community/clinic settings).

In a research setting, a calibration curve would involve multiple speeds and grades (i.e. >5); however, for the purpose of this practical we will describe a two-point calibration curve.

For example, if the treadmill displays 4 km/h but is actually travelling at 6 km/h, and then displays 15 km/h when it is moving at 18 km/h, then these points could be plotted on a graph to produce a calibration curve (Figure 1.3).

The following approach can then be used to calculate the equation of the line so that accurate speeds can be obtained with the known error of the treadmill.

Equation of the line: $y = mx + c$

where m = slope and c = y intercept.

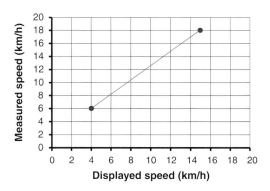

Figure 1.3 Treadmill speed calibration curve

To determine the real treadmill speed (y) from the speed displayed on the treadmill (x), the first point has coordinates $x1$ and $y1$ and the second point has coordinates $x2$ and $y2$.

1 Calculate the slope of the line (m) using:

$m = (y2 - y1)/(x2 - x1)$.

2 Calculate the y intercept (c) by substituting the slope you found in the previous step for m in $y = mx + c$. Then substitute one of the points' coordinates for y and x in the equation.

For example, a treadmill that displays 4.0 km/h is measured as running at 6.0 km/h. When you increase the treadmill display to 15.0 km/h, it is measured as running at 18.0 km/h.

Calculate the slope of the line (m) using the points: $x1 = 4.0$; $y1 = 6.0$; $x2 = 15.0$; $y2 = 18.0$:

$$m = (18.0 - 6.0)/(15.0 - 4.0)$$
$$= 1.09$$

Then substitute one of the points' coordinates for y (e.g. $y1 = 6.0$) and x (e.g. $x1 = 4.0$) in the equation:

$$6.0 = 1.09 \times 4.0 + c$$
$$c = 1.64$$

Therefore, the equation of the line is $y = 1.09x + 1.64$.

This equation can then be used to determine the real speed (y) from the displayed speed (x) at other speeds;

e.g. you want to know the real speed of the treadmill when it is displaying 7 km/h:

$$y = 1.09 \times 7 + 1.64$$
$$y = 9.3 \text{ km/h}$$

In this example, when the treadmill displays 7 km/h, the real speed is 9.3 km/h;

e.g. you want to set the treadmill at a real speed of 10 km/h:

$$10 = 1.09x + 1.64$$
$$x = 7.5 \text{ km/h}$$

In this example, you would need to set the treadmill display to 7.5 km/h for the treadmill to run at the real speed of 10 km/h.

Data recording

Treadmill Speed Measurements

Date: _____

Tape #1 to #2 = _____ m

Tape #2 to #3 = _____ m

Tape #3 to #1 = _____ m

Total treadmill belt length (sum of the three distances above) = _____ m

	WITH PARTICIPANT WALKING/RUNNING ON TREADMILL	
	5 km/h	**15 km/h**
Treadmill speed	30 revs/____ s	30 revs/____ s
Treadmill speed	____ revs/s	____ revs/s
Revolutions per min	____ revs/min	____ revs/min
Distance covered in 1 min	____ m/min	____ m/min
Treadmill speed	____ km/min	____ km/min
Treadmill speed	____ km/h	____ km/h
% error between displayed and real speed	____ %	____ %

Speed percentage error at 5 km/h acceptable?   YES/NO

Speed percentage error at 15 km/h acceptable?   YES/NO

Create a calibration curve in Figure 1.4 and equation of the line if at least one of the % errors is deemed to be 'unacceptable'.

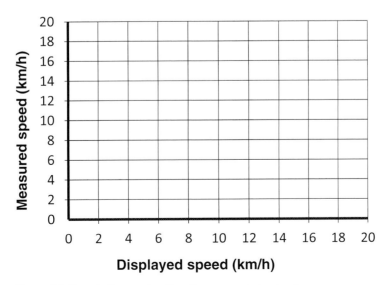

Figure 1.4 Treadmill speed calibration curve data sheet

The equation of the line using $y = mx + c$

where $x1 = $ _____ ; $y1 = $ _____ ; $x2 = $ _____ ; $y2 = $ _____

$$m = (y2 - y1) / (x2 - x1)$$

$$= \text{_____}$$

Then substituting one of the points' coordinates for y (e.g. $y1$) and x (e.g. $x1$) in the equation.

$$y1 = m \times x1 + c$$

$$c = \text{_____}$$

Therefore, the equation of the line is $y = $ _____ $x + $ _____ .

Treadmill Grade Measurements		
	5%	15%
If using an inclinometer		
Treadmill grade	%	%
% error between displayed and real grade	%	%
If using a 1 m long spirit level		
Distance between treadmill and bottom end of the spirit level	cm	cm
Treadmill grade	%	%
% error between displayed and real grade	%	%

Grade percentage error at 5% acceptable?   YES/NO

Grade percentage error at 15% acceptable?   YES/NO

Create a calibration curve in Figure 1.5 and equation of the line if at least one of the percentage errors is deemed to be 'unacceptable'.

The equation of the line using $y = mx + c$

where $x1 = $ _____ ; $y1 = $ _____ ; $x2 = $ _____ ; $y2 = $ _____

$$m = (y2 - y1) / (x2 - x1)$$

$$= \text{\_\_\_\_}$$

Then substituting one of the points' coordinates for y (e.g. $y1$) and x (e.g. $x1$) in the equation:

$$y1 = mx1 + c$$

$$c = \text{\_\_\_}$$

Therefore, the equation of the line is $y = $ _____ $x + $ _____

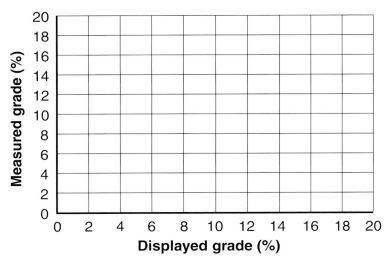

Figure 1.5 Treadmill grade calibration curve data sheet

Activity 1.2 Mechanically braked cycle ergometer verification and calibration

AIM: to calibrate and verify a mechanically braked cycle ergometer.

Background

On a mechanically braked cycle ergometer, the work rate depends on the resistance and the cycling rate or cadence. It is therefore essential that the tension of the belt is accurate. This activity involves dismantling and manipulation of equipment. Given the technical requirements of this skill, please ensure that appropriate permission and technical supervision is obtained prior to attempting this procedure.

The general principles of verification and calibration on a mechanically braked ergometer are as follows:

1 Disconnect the brake belt from the spring. Ensure that the belt does not fall into the flywheel covering by taping it loosely to the outside of the cover.

2 Check that the mark on the pendulum aligns with the '0' mark.

3 Attach a known weight (e.g. 4 kg calibration weight) at the extremity of the belt.

4 If the reading (e.g. 4 kg) is not correct, follow the manufacturer's instructions to adjust the scale and/or the pendulum.

Verification of the following points is also important:

- Check the brake contact surface and make sure it is clean and dry.
- Clean the chain regularly.
- Check the chain for tension.
- Have someone cycle slowly on the ergometer, gradually increasing the cadence. Listen for a clicking noise with every pedal revolution. If the noise increases with the increasing cadence, then this may indicate that the pedals are not tight enough or that the crank is loose. You should then tighten the pedals and/or the crank.

Each cycle ergometer has its own design and calibration processes. Technical documents are usually available on the manufacturer's website. The practical work described below is for the calibration of a well-known cycle ergometer, the Monark 828E (Figure 1.6) and follows the manufacturer's recommendations.

Protocol summary

Verify and calibrate a cycle ergometer by zeroing the scale and adjusting the pendulum to the appropriate reading when the calibration weight is attached to the brake belt.

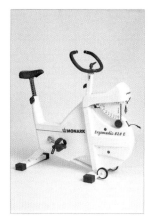

Figure 1.6 Monark 828E mechanically braked cycle ergometer

Used with permission from Monark

Protocol

Scale – zero adjustment

1. Have the cycle ergometer and necessary instrument ready (calibration weight, Allen key, cleaning tissue).

2. Disconnect the brake belt from the spring. Ensure that the belt does not fall into the flywheel covering by taping it loosely to the outside of the cover.

3. Check that the pendulum hangs in a vertical position and that the index on the pendulum (Figure 1.7, #2) weight is aligned with the '0' position on the scale board.

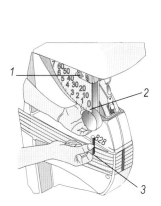

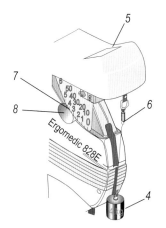

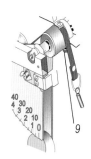

Fig: Scale adjustment
1) Locking nut
2) O-index
3) Adjustment weight, pendulum

Fig: Calibration
4) Calibration weight, 4kg
5) kp-scale
6) Attachment of calibration weight
7) Pendulum at 4kp
8) Screw to adjustment weight

Fig: Adjustment kp-scale window
9) Lock screw for scale indicator

Figure 1.7 Monark 828E mechanically braked cycle ergometer calibration

Source: Monark website https://sport-medical.monarkexercise.se/support-downloads/

4. If adjustment is necessary, first loosen the locking nut (Figure 1.7, #1) and then change the position of the scale board. Tighten the locking nut after the adjustment.

5. Record the results on the calibration report section of the data-recording sheet.

Calibration against the 4 kg calibration weight

1 Disconnect the brake belt from the spring. Ensure that the belt does not fall into the flywheel covering by taping it loosely to the outside of the cover.

2 Attach the calibration weight (4 kg) to the spring (see Figure 1.7, #6). Make sure the weight is hanging independently.

3 Read the number off the scale board where it aligns with the pendulum indicator (Figure 1.8).

4 If the reading is '4', the ergometer is correctly calibrated and there is no need for adjustment.

5 If the reading differs from '4', then you need to adjust the pendulum to the correct weight. To do this, use the adjustment weight that is located inside the pendulum (see Figure 1.7, #3). Adjust the pendulum by moving weight up or down using the relevant methods (e.g. loosen the lock screw on the back of the pendulum weight (Figure 1.9) or the solid bar that runs through the pendulum weight).

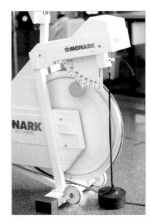

Figure 1.8 Calibration against the 4 kg calibration weight

Used with permission from Monark

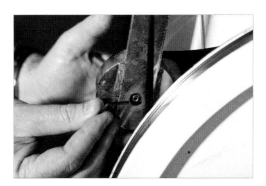

Figure 1.9 Loosening the screw on the pendulum weight

Used with permission from Monark

6 If the index of the pendulum weight is too low, move the adjusting weight upwards in the pendulum. Do the opposite if the pendulum weight is too high.

7 Tighten the lock screw.

8 Complete the calibration report section of the data-recording sheet.

Data recording

Calibration Report — Cycle Ergometer — Zero Adjustment

Date: _____

Index of pendulum align with the zero index of the scale board	Yes ☐ No ☐	Action taken:
Zero adjustment successful	Yes ☐ No ☐	Action taken:

Calibration Report — Cycle Ergometer — 4 kg Calibration Weight

Date: _____

Index of pendulum indicates '4' on the scale board	Yes ☐ No ☐	Action taken:
Calibration successful	Yes ☐ No ☐	Action taken:

Activity 1.3 Metabolic system calibration

AIM: to understand and complete calibration of a metabolic system with respect to gas analysis, flow rates and volumes.

Background

The two main components of metabolic systems are the gas analyser/s and the volume/flow measuring device. Oxygen and carbon dioxide analysers are prone to drift and it is recommended the tester calibrate them immediately before and verify after an exercise test to estimate the drift that occurred during exercise. This value should then be taken into consideration when interpreting the data obtained during the exercise test. All commercially available systems have well-described calibration procedures. Calibration procedures for O_2 and CO_2 gas analysers typically involve two different gas mixtures with low-, mid- or high-range O_2 or CO_2 concentrations. For O_2, the high-concentration gas mixture is usually room air (e.g. $20.93 \pm 0.03\%$, depending on relative humidity). For CO_2 analysers, calibration using both room air (e.g. $0.03 \pm 0.02\%$) and a gas mixture containing physiological concentrations commonly measured during exercise (e.g. 5%–7%) are used. Calibration should be performed with both room air and two tanks containing low- and mid-range O_2 (12%–13% and 16%–17% O_2, respectively) and mid- and high-range CO_2 (3%–4% and 5%–7% CO_2, respectively) reference gases in nitrogen to check the linearity of the analysers. It is important to make sure that the room used for calibration and testing is adequately ventilated.

Flow rate devices can be of different types including pneumotachometers, turbines or pitot tubes. Calibration of flow rate devices extends between a stable baseline of 0 L/min and known calibration syringes (usually 3–4 L). The syringes should be manipulated at different flow rates across the physiological spectrum and appropriate volumes should be detected at each flow rate.

Protocol summary

Using calibration gas tanks and syringes, calibrate the gas analysers, flow rates and volume.

Protocol

Calibration of gas analysers

1 Prior to the start of the test, it will be necessary to switch the metabolic system/analysers/pumps on so they are given adequate time to warm up. The system's manual should be consulted to check the time required, but analysers using zirconia fuel cells should be left on all the time and most pumps need to be on for ∼30 min before testing.

2 If using a drying agent in the inspired air line, this should be changed prior to the calibration whilst the equipment is warming up. Record environmental conditions (room temperature, relative humidity and barometric pressure).

3 Sample the O_2 and CO_2 gases of room air or the first calibration tank.

4 Read the O_2 and CO_2 values returned by the analysers.

5 If the readings do not show ∼$20.93 \pm 0.03\%$ and ∼$0.03 \pm 0.02\%$ for O_2 and CO_2 respectively, for room air or the values of the first calibration tank, then adjust the analysers. Record final values after adjustment.

6 Connect the second calibration tank; read and record the O_2 and CO_2 values returned by the analysers. Adjust as appropriate (± 0.03 for O_2 and ± 0.02 for CO_2). Record final values after adjustment.

7 Let the analyser sample room air and check that the analysers return to appropriate values.

8 The system should be analysed for linearity at regular intervals to confirm the operating status of the analysers.

9 Immediately following testing, verify the O_2 and CO_2 values and compare with initial values to determine whether any analyser drift has occurred during testing.

10 Ensure calibration tanks are completely switched off.

Calibration of flow rates and volumes

1 Use a calibration syringe of appropriate volume to calibrate the volume/flow rates of the system (Figure 1.10).

2 Start by assessing the stability at baseline according to the manufacturer's instructions (it should be ~0 L). Record the result.

3 Connect the syringe to the volume/flow rate device and inject the full volume. Repeat at different flow rates across the physiological spectrum (e.g. from 5 L/min to 300 L/min).

4 Read the volume returned by the device (it should match the volume of the syringe $\pm 2\%$).

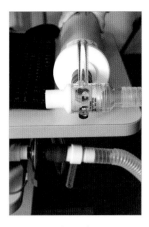

Figure 1.10 Calibration syringe

Used with permission from Vacumed

Data recording

Calibration Report — O_2 and CO_2 Analysers

Calibration mixtures

Room air: 20.93% O_2; 0.03% CO_2 or Tank 1: _____ % O_2 _____ CO_2

Tank 2: _____ % O_2 _____ % CO_2

Date: _____

Room temperature: _____ °C % Humidity: _____ %

Barometric pressure: _____ mmHg

Room air or Tank 1	Readings after adjustment	
	O_2 (%) _____	CO_2 (%) _____
Calibration successful	Yes ☐	Action taken:
	No ☐	
Tank 2	Readings after adjustment	
	O_2 (%) _____	CO_2 (%) _____
Calibration successful	Yes ☐	Action taken:
	No ☐	

Post Exercise Test Readings — Analyser Drift

Room air or tank 1	Readings after adjustment	
	O_2 (%) _____	CO_2 (%) _____
Comparison with pre exercise values	O_2 analyser drift	
	Drift $= [(O_2 \, (\%)_{PRE} - O_2 \, (\%)_{POST})/O_2 \, (\%)_{PRE}]*100$ Drift $=$ _____ $=$ _____ %	

continued overpage

Data recording *(continued)*

Comparison with pre exercise values	CO_2 analyser drift
	Drift $= [(CO_2\ (\%)_{PRE} - CO_2\ (\%)_{POST})/CO_2\ (\%)_{PRE}]*100$ Drift $= \rule{5cm}{0.4pt}$ $= \rule{3cm}{0.4pt} \%$

Calibration Report — Flow/Volume
Date: \rule{4cm}{0.4pt}

Flow/volume rate type: \rule{3cm}{0.4pt}	Volume of syringe (L): \rule{3cm}{0.4pt}
Baseline (~0 L/min)	Reading after adjustment: \rule{3cm}{0.4pt}
Injection of the syringe volume (L)	Reading after adjustment: \rule{3cm}{0.4pt}
Calibration successful	Yes ☐ No ☐ Action taken:

Interpretation

First, consider the four steps of interpretation outlined in Appendix G. Whether the calibration of room air/tank 1, tank 2 and flow/volume are considered successful or unsuccessful depends on the purpose of the test and the intended use of the data. For example, in the Australian state institutes and academies of sport, the following criteria are used to determine whether the results should be accepted.

Room air/tank 1 and tank 2

Accept the test results if the drift from pre-test calibration to post-test verification is less than 0.1% (absolute) in each of the two analysers. For repeat testing sessions on the same participant, the following net changes from the previous testing session calibration report are used to determine successful O_2 and CO_2 calibration:

$<1\%$ = acceptable

$1\%–3\%$ = accept and repeat

$>3\%$ = don't accept and troubleshoot.

Flow/volume

Accept the test results if the variation between the syringe volume and the reading following injection of the syringe is $<1.0\%$ (relative). For repeat testing sessions on the same participant, the following net changes from the previous testing session calibration report are used to determine successful flow/volume calibration:

average difference $\leq 1.0\%$ = acceptable

average difference $>1.0\%$ = don't accept and troubleshoot

range (highest–lowest) $\leq 3.0\%$ = acceptable

range (highest–lowest) $>3.0\%$ = don't accept and troubleshoot.

If there is a large percentage error or drift in the O_2, CO_2 and/or flow/volume calibration, then the accuracy of variables such as $\dot{V}O_2max$, submaximal economy and the respiratory exchange ratio (RER) will be compromised. This will reduce your ability to accurately provide information, including recommended training zones, to the participant, coach and other relevant professionals. Furthermore, asking a participant to return to the laboratory to repeat a test may negatively affect your rapport with the participant and/or coach. Therefore, where any issues with calibration are detected, it is important to check all connections are tightly sealed and the tubing and inspired air line are intact. A comment should be made within the database where the test data are stored to indicate any issues and actions taken. If no issues are clearly visible, report the issue to the lab technician (where available) and/or contact the manufacturer for advice and potential servicing. Before the next test is scheduled, a further set of calibrations should be conducted to determine whether this was a once-off issue or if there is an underlying cause that needs to be addressed.

Reliability

While accuracy is important, it is also important that assessments employ reliable tests and measures. Reliability ensures that the result obtained can be *consistently achieved* and strengthens the accuracy and validity of the test/measure. The consistency (or inconsistency) of the same tester completing two or more of the same measure is termed intra-tester reliability. A skilled, experienced assessor who employs standardised procedures should have a high *intra-tester reliability*. It may be common for the assessments to be conducted by different testers. If this occurs, then the consistency (or inconsistency) of two or more testers completing the same measure is termed *inter-tester reliability*.

Measuring reliability

Calculation of different aspects of measurement error (e.g. inter- and intra-tester reliability) enables greater certainty in the accuracy of the test. Appropriately designed tests should be used to quantify the reliability of an assessment. To design a reliability test, it is important to understand the context of the assessment. For example, is there only one or multiple testers? Will the tests be conducted at various times during the day, and therefore will diurnal reliability need to be established? Is the reliability specifically about the equipment being used? Or will biological reliability, and therefore day-to-day reliability, need to be established? Understanding where the sources of measurement error are likely to come from is necessary to design a reliability study. The most common way to assess measurement error is to calculate the technical error of the measurement (TEM), also known as the typical error (TE) or standard error of the measurement (SEM).[2] Usually this error is determined by measuring a certain number of participants (e.g. 10) on two separate occasions. The following formula is then used to calculate the TEM:

$$TEM = SD_{diff} / \sqrt{2}$$

where SD_{diff} is the difference in the standard deviations

In this manual, reliability will often need to be quantified on a single pair of measures or testers as either inter- or intra-tester reliability. This measure of reliability will be calculated using the following equation:

$$\text{Relative percentage difference} = \left[\frac{\text{largest measure} - \text{smallest measure}}{\text{smallest measure}} \right] \times 100$$

The higher the percentage difference, the lower is the confidence in the reliability of the results and the ability to detect meaningful changes. A typical example of when measuring reliability should be applied in practice is when measures are made before and after an exercise intervention. If the inter- or intra-tester reliability is higher than the observed difference in the measures, then you cannot confidently say that this change is 'real'. In this situation, any difference between the measures made before and after an intervention may just be due to measurement error. For example, your client completes a 12-week diet and exercise intervention and the difference in their waist circumference from before to after the intervention was 1.5%. If your intra-tester reliability for the measurement of waist circumference is $\geq 1.5\%$, then you cannot say that this is a 'real' change in response to the diet and exercise intervention, but rather that it is within the limits of your measurement error. The smaller your inter- and/or intra-tester reliability is, the better you are able to detect small changes in your measures (i.e. greater sensitivity). Training, practice and following a standardised protocol will help to minimise error and maximise inter- or intra-tester reliability.

The International Society for the Advancement of Kinanthropometry (ISAK) provides inter- and intra-tester reliability targets for practitioners to aim for during measurements of physique traits collected on 20 different people on different days. The acceptable range for the intra-tester reliability measurements according to ISAK for a level 1 anthropometrist is 7.5% for skinfolds and 1.5% for girth and breadth measures.[2] To confirm inter-tester reliability, the practitioner's results are compared with a level 3 anthropometrist (expert), with targets set at 10% for skinfold measurement and 2% for girth and breadth measurements.[4] With increased training and experience, the acceptable percentage error is reduced.

Activity 1.4 Inter- and intra-tester reliability

AIM: to calculate inter- and intra-tester reliability.

Background

It is important to determine whether testers are being consistent in their measurements and the amount of error between measurements. Calculation of inter- and intra-tester reliability enables greater confidence in the validity of the test results and the ability to detect meaningful changes.

The waist-to-hip ratio (WHR) has been proven to be one of the most robust measurements of cardiometabolic health, with waist and hip circumferences being reliable predictors of central and peripheral adiposity, respectively.[4] The accuracy of the waist and hip measurements will impact the calculation of the WHR, and consequently its ability to validly determine cardiometabolic health risk with any degree of certainty.[4]

Protocol summary

Measure waist and hip circumferences on multiple occasions to calculate inter- and intra-tester reliability.

Protocol

Testing session 1

1 In a group of three, you (the tester) measure the waist and hip circumferences (trial 1) of another group member (the participant) following the testing procedures outlined in Practical 4 (Activity 4.2). The third group member records the results (the recorder).

2 The tester performs a second measure of waist and hip circumference on the participant (trial 2).

3 Calculate the difference between trials 1 and 2 using the following equation:

$$\text{Relative percentage difference} = \left[\frac{\text{largest measure} - \text{smallest measure}}{\text{smallest measure}} \right] \times 100$$

4 If the difference between trials 1 and 2 in waist and/or hip circumference is $>1.5\%$, the tester performs a third in waist and/or hip circumference.

5 Record the mean of the waist and/or hip circumference measures if two measures are performed. Record the median if three waist and/or hip circumference measures are performed.

6 Group members rotate roles so that each member acts as a tester, participant and recorder until steps #1 to #5 are completed on each group member, by each group member.

Testing session 2

1 After an appropriate amount of time has passed (ideally on a separate day, but separated by as much time as feasibly possible), the tester repeats steps #1 to #5, described above in Testing session 1, on the initial participant.

2 To demonstrate what happens when *incorrect* waist and hip circumference sites are identified, the tester repeats steps #1 to #5 on the initial participant, but places the tape 2 cm below the identified sites.

Data analysis

Record data collected on the same participant by two different testers (tester 1 (you) and tester 2) from testing session 1 to calculate inter-tester reliability. Record data you collected on the same participant from testing sessions 1 and 2 to calculate intra-tester reliability. Record measurements 2 cm below each identified site collected by you from testing session 2.

Data recording

Inter-Tester Reliability: Testing Session 1

Participant's name: _____   Date: _____

Age: _____ years   Sex: _____

Tester 1 (you): _____

MEASURE	TRIAL 1	TRIAL 2	TRIAL 3 (if required)[a]	MEAN OR MEDIAN[b]
Girths				
Waist (cm)				
Gluteal (hip) (cm)				

a. Take a third measure if the difference between trials 1 and 2 differs by >1.5%
b. Record the mean if only two measures are performed. Record the median if three measures are performed

Using the mean/median results, calculate the WHR from tester 1 (you): _____

Tester 2 name: _____

MEASURE	TRIAL 1	TRIAL 2	TRIAL 3 (if required)[a]	MEAN OR MEDIAN[b]
Girths				
Waist (cm)				
Gluteal (hip) (cm)				

a. Take a third measure if the difference between trials 1 and 2 differs by >1.5%
b. Record the mean if only two measures are performed. Record the median if three measures are performed

Using the mean/median results, calculate the WHR from tester 2: _____

Calculate the inter-tester reliability using the following equation and the WHRs from testers 1 and 2:

$$\text{Inter-tester reliability} = \left[\frac{\text{largest WHR measure} - \text{smallest WHR measure}}{\text{smallest WHR measure}} \right] \times 100$$

Inter-tester reliability: ____ %   Acceptable?   Yes / No

continued overpage

Data recording *(continued)*

Intra-Tester Reliability: Testing Session 1

Participant's name: _____   Date: _____

Age: _____ years   Sex: _____

MEASURE	TRIAL 1	TRIAL 2	TRIAL 3 (if required)[a]	MEAN OR MEDIAN[b]
Girths				
Waist (cm)				
Gluteal (hip) (cm)				

a. Take a third measure if the difference between trials 1 and 2 differs by $>1.5\%$
b. Record the mean if only two measures are performed. Record the median if three measures are performed

Using the mean/median results, calculate the participant's WHR for testing

session 1: _____

Intra-Tester Reliability: Testing Session 2

Date: _____

MEASURE	TRIAL 1	TRIAL 2	TRIAL 3 (if required)[a]	MEAN OR MEDIAN[b]
Girths				
Waist (cm)				
Gluteal (hip) (cm)				

a. Take a third measure if the difference between trials 1 and 2 differs by $>1.5\%$
b. Record the mean if only two measures are performed. Record the median if three measures are performed

Using the mean/median results, calculate the participant's WHR for testing

session 2: _____

Calculate the intra-tester reliability using the following equation and the WHRs you measured on the same individual in testing sessions 1 and 2:

$$\text{Intra-tester reliability} = \left[\frac{\text{largest WHR measure} - \text{smallest WHR measure}}{\text{smallest WHR measure}}\right] \times 100$$

Intra-tester reliability: _____ %   Acceptable?   Yes/No

Incorrect Site Assessment: Testing Session 2

MEASURE	TRIAL 1	TRIAL 2	TRIAL 3 (if required)[a]	MEAN OR MEDIAN[b]
Girths				
Waist (cm)				
Gluteal (hip) (cm)				

a. Take a third measure if the difference between trials 1 and 2 differs by $>1.5\%$
b. Record the mean if only two measures are performed. Record the median if three measures are performed

continued

> ## Data recording *(continued)*
>
> Using the mean/median results, calculate the WHR: _____
>
> Calculate the intra-tester reliability using the following equation and (1) the mean WHR from your measures on a participant used to calculate intra-tester reliability above and (2) the mean/median WHR from the incorrect site:
>
> $$\text{Inter-tester reliability} = \left[\frac{\text{largest WHR measure} - \text{smallest WHR measure}}{\text{smallest WHR measure}} \right] \times 100$$
>
> Intra-tester reliability: _____ %   Acceptable?   Yes/No

Interpretation

First, consider the four steps of interpretation outlined in Appendix G.

Treadmill verification and calibration interpretation

Determining the accuracy and reliability of a measurement, and the testers and equipment involved in taking that measure, will clarify whether the results indicate a real change, or are just within the measurement error.

The action(s) to take following the verification and calibration of equipment depends on several factors such as the margin of error calculated, the setting in which the equipment will be used and the feasibility/availability of resources to act upon the verification results. For example, if the equipment is to be used in a research setting and thus the accuracy of equipment is paramount, the acceptable error margin might be set at $<1\%$. However, if the equipment is to be used in a fitness centre environment for general training purposes, then a larger error margin (e.g. $\leq 5\%$) may be deemed acceptable.

Verification and, where possible, calibration of treadmill and cycle ergometers should be performed regularly (i.e. 2–3 times per year, depending on the frequency of their use). If the displayed values on an ergometer that cannot be easily calibrated (e.g. a treadmill) are determined to be inaccurate, then there are several options available for consideration, including creating and using calibration curves, sending the treadmill to the manufacturer for calibration, or using a different treadmill that is more accurate. If the required amount of adjustment on an ergometer that can be calibrated (e.g. a Monark cycle ergometer) is greater than the acceptable error, options for action include creating and using calibration curves to adjust test results conducted between calibration reports, having more-frequent calibration reports moving forwards, sending the cycle ergometer to the manufacturer for servicing, or using another cycle ergometer with less drift in calibration.

Gas analyser, flow rate and volume verification and calibration interpretation

Gas analysers, flow rates and volume should be calibrated before, and verified after, every $\dot{V}O_2max$/peak test. Where the drift in the gas analysers, flow rates and volume from the start to the end of a test is greater than the acceptable error, then options include using calibration curves, repeating the $\dot{V}O_2max$/peak test on a separate day, contacting the manufacturer for servicing, or using another analyser with less drift in calibration.

Inter- and intra-tester reliability interpretation

Intra-tester reliability and, where multiple testers are involved, inter-tester reliability should be calculated before performing a test on a participant. As previously mentioned, ISAK supply recommended targets for inter- and intra-tester reliability. For girth (i.e. waist and hip) measures the recommended inter-tester reliability is $\leq 2\%$ while for intra-tester reliability it is $\leq 1.5\%$. These are calculated from measures collected on 20 different people on different days.[2]

Examine your intra-tester reliability, the inter-tester reliability and the intra-tester reliability for the incorrect sites. Interpretation of the data should involve a comparison with the ISAK values. It is important to recognise whether the reliability of these measurements modifies the interpretation of disease risk for waist circumference or WHR ratio. This will help explain what impact these results and interpretation would have on a client and the actions of a practitioner. In this case, provide examples of how you would deliver the information to your client (e.g. verbal, written), taking into account the reliability of the measure.

Consider how the reliability would impact on detecting true differences from longitudinal measures (e.g. before and after an exercise intervention). Across the different measures of reliability (intra-, inter-, and intra-tester reliability at incorrect/alternative sites), calculate the difference you would need to see to be confident that it is real and explain how you would incorporate these data in feedback to a participant post-intervention.

The higher the inter- or intra-tester reliability measurements, the lower the confidence in the accuracy of the results and the ability to detect meaningful changes. Where inter- and/or intra-tester reliability is below the acceptable limit, then options include undertaking additional training on the skill/s, using calibration curves or having someone with greater accuracy repeat the measure. For example, if the recorded inter- or intra-tester reliability of the waist and/or hip circumference measurements are greater than the ISAK proposed targets, completion of an ISAK anthropometry course and/or additional practice is recommended.

Case studies

Case Study 1

Setting: You are a sports scientist working with the Rowing Australia junior national team. You have been asked to conduct a $\dot{V}O_2$max test on an athlete who has recently joined your squad. The results from this test, and the feedback you will provide to the coach, will influence the type of training program this athlete will receive over the coming few months.

Your task: The calibration report from the rower's $\dot{V}O_2$max test is included below. Follow the four steps of interpretation outlined in Appendix G. Complete the calibration report by indicating whether the calibration of the O_2 and CO_2 analysers and flow/volume rates were successful or unsuccessful. Confirm whether you believe the O_2 and/or CO_2 analyser drift from pre- to post-exercise is acceptable. Clarify what action/s you would take based on the calibration report results.

Data recording

Calibration Report — O_2 and CO_2 Analysers

Calibration mixtures

Room air: 20.93% O_2; 0.03% CO_2 or Tank 1: _____ % O_2 _____ CO_2

Tank 2: _____16.00_____ % O_2 _____5.00_____ % CO_2

Date: _24/10/21_

Room temperature: _____20.2_____ °C %   Humidity: _____36.0_____ %

Barometric pressure: _____754.3_____ mmHg

Room air or Tank 1	Readings after adjustment		
	O_2 (%) _20.94_		CO_2 (%) _0.04_
Calibration successful	Yes ☐	Action taken:	
	No ☐		*continued*

Case studies *(continued)*

Data recording *(continued)*

Tank 2	Readings after adjustment	
	O_2 (%) __16.01__	CO_2 (%) __5.00__
Calibration successful	Yes ☐	Action taken:
	No ☐	

Post Exercise Test Readings — Analyser Drift

Room air or tank 1	Readings after adjustment	
	O_2 (%) __20.93__	CO_2 (%) __0.15__
Acceptable O_2 drift?	Yes ☐	Action taken:
	No ☐	
Acceptable O_2 drift?	Yes ☐	Action taken:
	No ☐	

Calibration Report — Flow/Volume
Date: __24/10/21__

Flow/volume rate type: pneumotachometer _____		Volume of syringe (L): __3.0__
Baseline (~0 L/min)	Reading after adjustment: __0.0__	
Injection of the syringe volume (L)	Reading after adjustment: __3.009__	
Calibration successful	Yes ☐ No ☐	Action taken:

Interpretation

Was the room air or tank 1 calibration successful or unsuccessful?

_____

_____

What action would you take based on the room air or tank 1 calibration?

_____

_____

Was tank 2 calibration successful or unsuccessful?

_____

_____

continued overpage

Case studies (continued)

What action would you take based on the tank 2 calibration?

_____

_____

_____

Was the flow/volume rate calibration successful or unsuccessful?

_____

_____

_____

What action would you take based on the flow/volume rate calibration?

_____

_____

_____

Was the O_2 and/or CO_2 analyser drift from pre- to post-exercise acceptable?

_____

_____

_____

What action would you take based on the O_2 and/or CO_2 analyser drift from pre- to post-exercise?

_____

_____

_____

Case Study 2

Setting: You are completing your Honours on a project exploring the dose–response effect of exercise training on exercise capacity in middle-aged adults. Exercise capacity will be measured via distance walked on a treadmill. You conduct treadmill speed and grade verification on one of the treadmills available for testing and training as part of this study. Given the middle-aged adults participating in the study will vary in their baseline exercise capacities, you choose to initially conduct a two-point verification at 5 and 15 km/h and 5 and 15% speed and grade. You and your supervisor determine the acceptable % error for treadmill speed and grade as <1%.

Your task: Calculate the percentage error for the speed and grade of the treadmill. Create calibration curves and equations of the line if the percentage errors are deemed to be unacceptable. Clarify what action/s you would take based on the verification results.

Data recording

Treadmill Speed Measurements

Tape #1 to #2 = 1.1 m

Tape #2 to #3 = 0.9 m

Tape #3 to #1 = 0.5 m

Total treadmill belt length (= sum of the 3 distances above) _____ m

continued

Case studies *(continued)*

Data recording *(continued)*

	WITH PARTICIPANT WALKING/RUNNING ON TREADMILL	
	5 km/h	**15 km/h**
Treadmill speed	30 revs/46 s	30 revs/16 s
Treadmill speed	revs/s	revs/s
Revolutions per min	revs/min	revs/min
Distance covered in 1 min	m/min	m/min
Treadmill speed	km/min	km/min
Treadmill speed	km/h	km/h
% error between displayed and real speed	%	%

Speed percentage error at 5 km/h acceptable?   *YES/NO*

Speed percentage error at 15 km/h acceptable?   *YES/NO*

Create a calibration curve and equation of the line if at least one of the percentage errors is deemed to be 'unacceptable'.

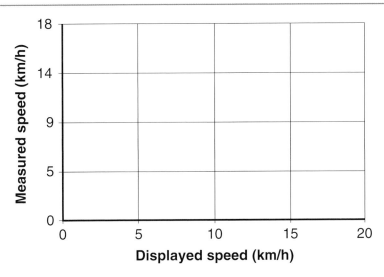

The equation of the line using $y = mx + c$

where $x1 = $ _____; $y1 = $ _____; $x2 = $ _____; $y2 = $ _____:

$$m = (y2 - y1)/(x2 - x1)$$

$$= \underline{\hspace{1.5cm}}$$

Then substituting one of the points' coordinates for y (e.g. $y1$) and x (e.g. $x1$) in the equation:

$$y1 = m \times x1 + c$$

$$c = \underline{\hspace{1.5cm}}$$

Therefore, the equation of the line is $y = $ _____$x + $ _____

continued overpage

Case studies *(continued)*

Treadmill Grade Measurements

	5%	15%
If using a 1 m long spirit level		
Distance between treadmill and bottom end of the spirit level	5.0 cm	14.9 cm
Treadmill grade	%	%
% error between displayed and real grade	%	%

Grade percentage error at 5% acceptable?   YES/NO

Grade percentage error at 15% acceptable?   YES/NO

Create a calibration curve and equation of the line if at least one of the percentage errors is deemed to be 'unacceptable'.

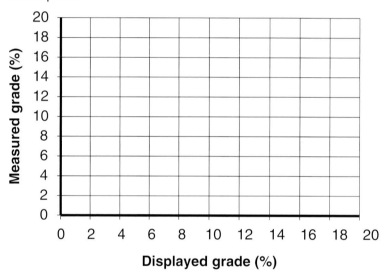

The equation of the line using $y = mx + c$

where $x1 = \underline{\quad}$; $y1 = \underline{\quad}$; $x2 = \underline{\quad}$; $y2 = \underline{\quad}$:

$$m = (y2 - y1)/(x2 - x1)$$

$$= \underline{\quad}$$

Then substituting one of the points' coordinates for y (e.g. $y1$) and x (e.g. $x1$) in the equation:

$$y1 = m \times x1 + c$$

$$c = \underline{\quad}$$

Therefore, the equation of the line is $y = \underline{\quad} x + \underline{\quad}$.

References

[1] Baumgartner RN, Heymsfield SB, Lichtman S, Wang J, Pierson RN, Jr. Body composition in elderly people: effect of criterion estimates on predictive equations. Am J Clin Nutr 1991;53(6):1345–53.

[2] Stewart AD, Marfell-Jones M, Olds T, Hans De Ridder J, Norton K. International standards for anthropometric assessment. Lower Hutt, New Zealand: International Society for the Advancement of Kinanthropometry (ISAK); 2011.

[3] Atkinson G, Nevill AM. Statistical methods for assessing measurement error (reliability) in variables relevant to sports medicine. Sports Med. 1998;26(4):217–38.

[4] Daniel M, Martin AD, Drinkwater DT, Clarys JP, Marfell-Jones MJ. Waist-to-hip ratio and adipose tissue distribution: contribution of subcutaneous adiposity. Am J Hum Biol 2003;15(3):428–32.

PRACTICAL 2
BLOOD ANALYSIS

Jeff Coombes and Cecilia Kitic

LEARNING OBJECTIVES

- Explain the scientific rationale, purposes, reliability, validity, assumptions and limitations of common blood analysis tests
- Identify and explain the common terminology, processes and equipment required to conduct accurate and safe blood analysis tests
- Identify and describe considerations that may require the modification of blood analysis tests, and make appropriate adjustments for relevant populations or participants
- Describe the principles and rationale for the calibration of equipment commonly used for blood analyses
- Conduct appropriate pre-assessment procedures, including explaining the test and obtaining informed consent
- Identify the need for guidance or further information from a relevant health professional
- Select and conduct blood analysis tests
- Record, analyse and interpret information from blood analysis tests and convey the results, including the validity and limitations of the assessments, through verbal and/or written communication to a participant or relevant health professional

Equipment and other requirements

- Information sheet and informed consent form
- Haematocrit centrifuge
- Glucose, cholesterol and haemoglobin analysers
- Consumables for analysers
- Capillary tubes for collection of blood for haematocrit
- Non-latex gloves of various sizes (S, M, L)
- Alcohol swabs and lancets
- Critoseal pad
- Biohazardous waste container
- Sharps containers
- Band-Aids/finger cots
- Sterile cotton wool balls/swabs and tissues

- Bench surface protection paper
- Spray bottle with diluted bleach (bleach:water, 1:10)
- Sink/hand wash area
- Cleaning and disinfecting equipment (see Appendix A)

Personal protective equipment/immunisations

- Laboratory coat
- Protective eyewear (e.g. safety glasses)
- Covered footwear (no thongs, sandals or open toe shoes)
- Hepatitis B and tetanus immunisations (recommended)

INTRODUCTION

The increased availability of small, inexpensive analytical devices has made it easier for exercise professionals to analyse blood and obtain information about a participant's health. Blood analysis and interpretation skills are commonly used in corporate health environments, although, as costs decrease, they are also becoming more popular in health and fitness settings as part of a more comprehensive screening/health assessment process. The Adult Pre-exercise Screening System (APSS) requires information collected from blood measures to more validly risk stratify participants in stage 2 (see Practical 6, Screening). In Practical 3, plasma cholesterol and glucose values will also be used to determine cardiovascular risk scores.

This practical covers the skill of obtaining a blood sample from a finger prick to measure a range of variables. Blood collected from finger prick samples provides values somewhat comparable to using venous blood specimens (i.e. as would be collected in an accredited pathology laboratory).[1–3] However, there may be discrepancies based on the type of sample (e.g. from whole blood vs plasma).

It is important to have some basic biochemistry knowledge of the different compounds being measured and why they are used to assess aspects of health. Of utmost importance is the understanding that the measures *will not* lead to making a diagnosis. Exercise professionals *do not* make diagnoses. Medically trained individuals need to use measures from accredited laboratories in association with additional medical history information to diagnose the presence of a disease (e.g. diabetes, hypercholesterolaemia, anaemia). However, exercise professionals can perform a vital role in identifying potential risk factors for disease and referring the participant to a medical practitioner for follow-up. This may lead to early diagnosis and treatment that could have a significant impact upon the health of an individual.

Quality assurance

When using blood analysis testing devices, appropriate quality assurance protocols should be established to ensure the accuracy of the data being collected. Quality assurance usually consists of both 'internal' and 'external' quality control procedures. Internal quality control covers issues such as the training and skills of the operator, whereas an external quality control process could include comparing measures made with the portable device with those obtained on the same samples from an accredited pathology laboratory. The training of the operator should consist of understanding the basic principles of quality control, troubleshooting skills and the risks of releasing inaccurate data to a participant. It has been recognised that the increased availability of low-cost blood analysis devices has led to many practitioners including blood measures as part of a general health assessment without implementing the appropriate quality assurance processes.[4] This is also usually combined with a typical underestimation of the risk of analytical error and therefore a lack of appreciation of the need for quality assurance.

Resources such as those provided by the International Organization for Standardization (ISO) are recommended to improve accuracy of blood-testing devices.[5] The ISO recommends that users of analytical devices should be trained in the theory and practice of quality assurance. In addition, protocols at the testing site should detail procedures such as storage requirements and preparation of quality control material, frequency of quality control testing, documentation requirements and basic troubleshooting advice.[6] The required knowledge to successfully process and interpret internal quality control should be tested within the competency assessment of users. For an exercise professional these quality assurance protocols may be seen as a burden unless their role in ensuring the accuracy of the blood measures is made clear to the users.

DEFINITIONS

Anaemia: low haemoglobin or decreased oxygen-binding ability to haemoglobin.

Cardiovascular disease (CVD): an umbrella term that refers to any disease that affects the heart or blood vessels. This includes coronary heart disease (CHD), hypertension, peripheral vascular disease and stroke (cerebrovascular accident).

Coronary heart disease (CHD): also known as coronary artery disease (CAD), is a narrowing or blockage of the coronary arteries of the heart, usually caused by atherosclerosis. It can lead to chest pain (angina) or a heart attack (myocardial infarction) and damage to the heart muscle.

Diabetes: a chronic metabolic disease characterised by elevated levels of blood glucose, which leads over time to serious damage to the heart, blood vessels, eyes, kidneys and nerves.

Glucose: a circulating simple sugar. A person with chronically elevated plasma glucose is most likely to have diabetes.

Glycated haemoglobin (HbA$_{1c}$): develops when haemoglobin joins with glucose in the blood, becoming glycated. The higher the level of HbA$_{1c}$, the greater is the risk of developing diabetes-related complications.

Haematocrit: also known as packed cell volume – the percentage of red blood cells relative to total blood fluid. It is an indicator of oxygen-carrying capacity.

Haemoglobin: an iron-containing protein that binds oxygen molecules and is located within the red blood cells. It is an indicator of oxygen-carrying capacity.

High-density lipoprotein cholesterol (HDL cholesterol): also referred to as the 'good cholesterol', this molecule is responsible for removing cholesterol from within the artery wall and transporting it back to the liver for metabolism and excretion.

Low-density lipoprotein cholesterol (LDL cholesterol): also referred to as the 'bad cholesterol', this molecule transports cholesterol to the artery wall. Elevated LDL cholesterol leads to atherosclerosis and increased risk of heart attack and stroke (cerebrovascular accident).

Plasma: the pale yellow liquid component of blood that allows the blood cells to be in suspension. Plasma is obtained by collecting whole blood in a tube that contains an anticoagulant (e.g. heparin) and then centrifuging it such that the blood cells go to the bottom of the tube. Some analytical tests require plasma and therefore the blood needs to be collected using an anticoagulant-containing tube.

Polycythaemia: a condition where the proportion of blood volume that is occupied by red blood cells is increased.

Pre-diabetes: a condition in which blood glucose concentrations are higher than normal, although not high enough to be diagnosed with type 2 diabetes. Also known as **impaired fasting glucose**.

Red flag: used in clinical screening to denote a warning sign, indicating that referral to a relevant health professional is warranted.

Serum: plasma without the clotting factors. It is obtained the same way as plasma except it is collected into a tube without an anticoagulant. Some analytical tests require serum and therefore the blood needs to be collected in tubes that do not contain an anticoagulant.

Total cholesterol: the sum of cholesterol sub-fractions – mainly low-density lipoprotein (LDL), high-density lipoprotein (HDL) and very-low-density lipoprotein (vLDL).

Triglycerides: circulating lipids that are useful for assessing the risk of CHD. Elevated triglycerides are associated with atherosclerosis and an increased risk of heart attack and stroke (cerebrovascular accident).

Very low density lipoprotein cholesterol (vLDL cholesterol): also referred to as a 'bad cholesterol', this molecule mostly comprises of triglycerides and transports cholesterol to the artery wall. Elevated vLDL cholesterol leads to atherosclerosis and increased risk of heart attack and stroke (cerebrovascular accident).

SAFETY[a]

Working with human blood, tissue and body fluids involves a risk of contracting infectious diseases. All blood and body fluid should always be handled as if they are infected.

This practical requires special care to be taken as safety is of utmost importance when sampling and handling blood. It is imperative that all health and safety regulations are followed to minimise the risk of injury or infection. To increase the safety of this practical, the tester will be required to handle and analyse their own blood sample once it has been collected.

The primary methods and equipment chosen to minimise risk are: finger prick rather than venipuncture, use of retractable lancets, wearing of personal protective equipment (see Figure 2.1),

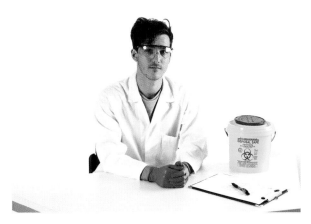

Figure 2.1 Appropriate personal protective equipment is essential for this practical

correct disposal bins, and adherence to procedures (e.g. no eating or drinking in the laboratory).

Lab coats and protective eyewear must be worn at all times in the laboratory. Lab coats should be buttoned up. Avoid lifting safety glasses and resting them on the top of the head. If there is the need to have a break from wearing the glasses, ask to leave the room for a short period.

Gloves must be worn for the entire session (except when having blood drawn out of the respective hand). Gloves should be replaced promptly if torn or damaged. New gloves should be used prior to sample collection and gloves should be replaced if there is blood on them.

All participants must be aware of the first aid involved when dealing with blood and body fluid.[b] Immediately following exposure to blood or body fluids, it is recommended that the exposed person undertakes the following steps as soon as possible:

- If blood gets on the skin, irrespective of whether there are cuts or abrasions, wash well with soap and water.
- Irrigate mucous membranes and eyes (remove contact lenses) with water or normal saline. If the eyes are contaminated, rinse whilst they are open, gently but thoroughly (for at least 30 seconds), with water or normal saline.
- If blood or body fluids get in the mouth, spit them out and then rinse the mouth with water several times.
- If blood gets on clothing, remove the item where possible and launder as appropriate.

Any incidents must be reported to the instructor and medical advice should be sought if first aid has been administered. After reporting the incident, a risk assessment should be performed.

Cleaning and disposal of contaminated items

- Any sharp items (capillary tubes and lancets) must be placed into a biohazard sharps bin immediately after use.
- All other rubbish (e.g. gloves) should be disposed of into a biohazardous waste container. No other bins should be in the room.
- Workstations must be cleaned thoroughly with diluted bleach (bleach:water, 1:10).

Blood spill procedure

- Blood spills need to be decontaminated to prevent the potential transmission of a communicable disease.
- A small amount of blood, if splashed, can cover a large area.
- Spray the blood contaminated surfaces with diluted bleach (bleach:water, 1:10). Be careful not to contaminate the outside of the spray bottle.
- Absorb and remove all traces of the spill with paper towels.
- Respray the cleaned area with the bleach solution and allow to air dry.
- Place all waste materials into a biohazardous waste container.

---

[a] In addition to the safety information provided here, please refer to Appendix A 'Laboratory safety, cleaning and disinfection' section.
[b] See also the 'Laboratory safety, cleaning and disinfection' section at the beginning of this manual.

- Inspect the blood spill area closely, making sure nothing has been missed and that the clean-up process is complete.

All participants in this practical are strongly advised to be immunised against hepatitis B and tetanus.

Activity 2.1 Blood collection and analysis

AIM: to obtain blood from a finger prick and measure haematocrit, haemoglobin, total cholesterol, LDL cholesterol, HDL cholesterol, triglycerides and glucose. Following the measures, interpret the results and provide feedback to a participant.

Background

There are a number of different commercially available analysers that can be used to measure haemoglobin, plasma lipids and glucose concentrations. Haematocrit will be measured using a haematocrit chart.

A commonly used analyser for measuring plasma lipids and glucose combines enzymatic methodology and solid-phase technology on a cassette. Samples used for testing can be whole blood, as the cassette separates the plasma from the blood cells. A portion of the plasma flows to the right and left sides of the cassette where it is transferred to reaction pads. The analyser measures the resultant colour in all the reactions by reflectance photometry (the amount of light reflected from the surface). The amount of light reflected is proportional to the analyte concentration of interest.

A typical haemoglobin analyser also uses photometry and dry chemistry. Once blood is added to the analyser via the micro-cuvette, the red cells are ruptured and haemoglobin is released into a solution. The free haemoglobin binds to a chemical which forms a coloured compound. A photodiode detects the amount of light from the compound after it interacts with light from light-emitting diodes. This is then converted to a haemoglobin concentration.

Protocol summary

Obtain blood from a participant and measure haematocrit, haemoglobin, lipids and glucose.

Protocol

Fasting

If a fasting plasma glucose measure is being obtained then the participant should not have consumed food or beverages (except water) for at least 8 hours, but no more than 16 hours (10–12 hours is optimal).[7] Fasting plasma glucose measures are therefore commonly performed in the morning. It is suggested that the participant brings something to eat after the blood has been collected. In addition, physical activity/exercise should have been limited and alcohol avoided in the previous 24 hours. Fasting is not required for lipid measures,[8] haematocrit and haemoglobin.[9]

Ensure that the correct personal protective equipment is worn (see 'Safety' section above and Appendix A). This should include a requirement to have a clean laboratory coat, protective eyewear (i.e. safety glasses), gloves and covered footwear (no thongs, sandals or open-weave shoes). If cassettes are being used for the analytical device, they should be removed from the refrigerator with sufficient time to reach room temperature for testing.

Workstation set-up

Collect the supplies that will be needed and arrange them in the workstation (Figures 2.2 and 2.3). It may be useful to mentally practise the whole procedure to make sure that everything is in place before the skin is punctured. This will avoid needing to leave the participant so you can retrieve something during the procedure.

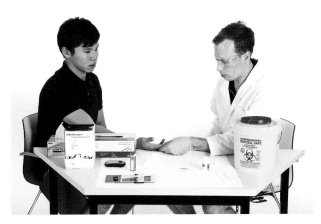

Figure 2.2 Typical workstation set-up

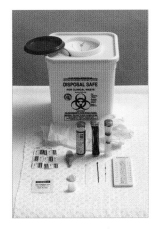

Figure 2.3 Typical arrangement of supplies
Used with permission from Hawksley

Requirements (in order of use) are:

1 bench surface protection paper

2 gloves

3 alcohol swab

4 lancet

5 sharps container

6 blood collection tubes, depending on analysers (for this activity, capillary tubes will be used)

7 Critoseal pad

8 analyser consumables

9 sterile gauze pads

10 sterile cotton wool swabs

11 Band-Aids/finger cots.

Work in groups of two. If there is a group of three, have one person providing blood (participant), one person collecting the blood (tester) and the third person reading the directions and passing the tubes. Once the blood collection is finished, the tester should handle their own sample for the remainder of the practical.

Fainting

Both the participant and tester should be seated during the procedure. The tester should first determine a few important details from the participant, such as how long it has been since the participant has consumed food or a beverage (other than water) and whether the participant has ever had blood collected previously. If they have had blood collected previously, did they have any problems during the procedure (e.g. feel faint)?

The most common time that people faint is when they see their own blood, or someone else's blood entering the collection tube. The likelihood that participants will be fasted increases the probability of fainting. The tester should determine whether the participant has a problem with blood collection and if they have then they should be closely monitored. When people faint during a procedure such as this, there is also an increased likelihood that they will lose control of their bladder and/or bowel. The most common indication that someone is about to faint will be a loss of colour from their face. If this occurs then ask them to lie on the floor, supporting their head and raising their legs (Figure 2.4). If the person faints in the chair, ensure someone strongly supports them to prevent them from falling onto the ground (Figure 2.5). The main goal when someone faints is to avoid any impact with the head. Usually a person will be unconscious for only a few seconds. Having some 'emergency jelly beans' to hand can be useful.

If the participant appears uneasy just prior to the blood draw, use words of encouragement/distraction, which may decrease the participant's stress.

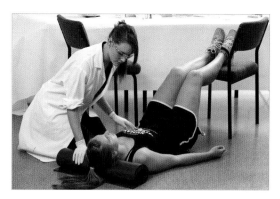

Figure 2.4 When conscious, ask the person to lie on the floor and support their head and raise their feet

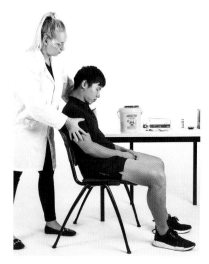

Figure 2.5 If a person faints while seated, ensure that they are well supported

Sample collection

The sample collection method will depend on the analyser. This protocol is for capillary tubes and micro-cuvettes:

1 Follow the pre-exercise test procedures outlined in Appendix B.

2 Many of the contraindications to collecting a blood sample are consistent with those of exercise testing. Therefore, check Appendix C to ensure that there are no contraindications to sample collection.

3 The participant should be sitting quietly for at least 5 minutes prior to the blood collection.

4 Use the participant's second or third finger.

5 Generally, it is harder to get a blood sample from people with cold fingers or when the environment is cold. Ask the participant if they have cold fingers and if they do then ask them to run their hand under warm water, hold something warm and/or clench their fist several times to increase the circulation to the finger where the sample is to be collected.

6 Keep the participant's hand below the level of the heart to improve blood flow.

7 Wipe the finger to be pricked with an alcohol swab (Figure 2.6) and wait a few seconds for the alcohol to evaporate.

8 Place the lancet on the fingertip (perpendicular to fingerprint lines if using a blade lancet). It is suggested to place the lancet away from the midline as there may be a thick fat pad there. Avoid the very side and tip of the finger as there is not as much tissue in these areas and it may be more uncomfortable. Figures 2.7 and 2.8 show an appropriate location.

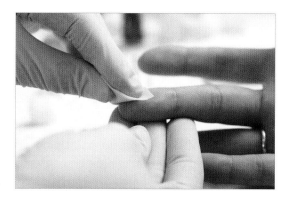

Figure 2.6 Wipe the finger with alcohol wipe

9 Support the back of the finger and hold the lancet firmly on the finger before pushing down on the release mechanism to activate the needle.

> **Note:** common mistakes are:
> - not pushing the lancet down hard enough and/or slightly lifting off when puncturing the skin. As a result, the incision is not deep enough and blood will not flow.
> - squeezing the finger at the same time you depress the lancet.

10 Immediately dispose of the lancet in the sharps container (Figure 2.9). The lancet should not be placed on the table.

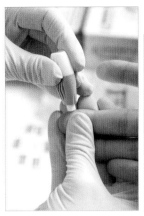
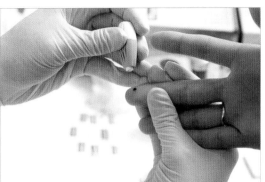
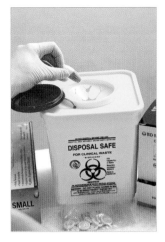

Figures 2.7 and 2.8 Lancet placement

Figure 2.9 Immediately dispose of the lancet

11 Wipe the first drop of blood with a sterile gauze pad as it may contain tissue fluid (Figure 2.10).

12 Determine whether there will be a good amount of blood without additional assistance (gently squeezing or massaging the finger).

13 If the new blood drop is slow to form, gently squeeze the finger. If this does not provide enough blood then gently massage the finger from the base to the tip. As the tester will be wearing gloves, it may be easier to ask the participant to do this – gently. Do not squeeze or massage too hard as this may rupture blood cells, causing invalid test results.

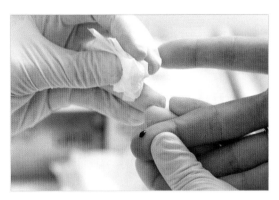

Figure 2.10 Wipe the first drop of blood with a sterile gauze pad

Note: Even with a deep puncture some participants will have more viscous (thicker) blood that will be slow to flow. In contrast, some participants will have lower-viscosity (thinner) blood and cotton wool swabs may be needed to stop the bleeding. If blood stops flowing before the sample has been collected, even after gentle squeezing or massaging of the finger, the tester should ask the participant if another attempt can be made on another finger.

14 Once a good size drop of blood appears, hold the capillary tube at a slight descending angle (Figure 2.11) and *gently touch* it on the blood drop that should have formed. Avoid contact between the skin and capillary tube. It doesn't matter which end of the tube you place against the blood.

15 Capillary action will draw blood along the tube.

16 If the blood stops flowing, wipe the finger firmly with sterile gauze to reopen the puncture and, if needed, gently massage the finger from the base to the tip.

17 Try to fill each tube in less than 10 seconds, avoiding air bubbles. Holding the tube at a very slight downward angle to the horizontal will assist in collection. The number of tubes required to be filled will depend on the analyser used.

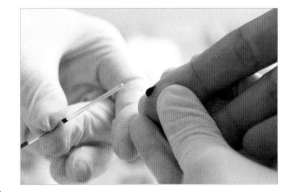

Figure 2.11 Wait until a good-sized drop of blood appears before placing the capillary tube into the blood drop (avoid touching the skin)

18 Seal the end of the capilary tube that was not in contact with the blood to avoid blood being transferred to the Critoseal. Seal the end of the capillary tube by holding it horizontally and the Critoseal vertically and gently pushing the tube into the plasticine (Figure 2.12). To ensure a good seal, push it into the plasticine twice.

19 Place a sterile cotton wool swab on the wound/s and cover with a finger cot (Figures 2.13 and 2.14). If these are not available then a Band-Aid can be used.

Measuring haematocrit using a haematocrit chart

1 Place the capillary tube into the centrifuge. Make sure that the sealed end faces out. Record the numbered position of the tube.

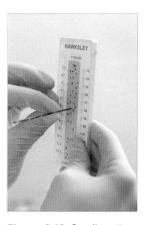

Figure 2.12 Sealing the end of the capillary tube

Used with permission from Hawksley

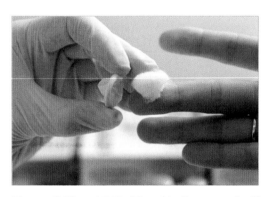 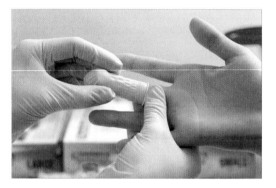

Figures 2.13 and 2.14 Attend to the wound with a sterile cotton swab and a finger cot

2 Ensure that the centrifuge is balanced. If it is not full, make sure tubes are placed directly across from each other. It may be necessary to use an empty tube to balance if there is not an even number of samples to be spun.

3 Check that you have appropriately closed the centrifuge lid/s. Some centrifuges contain a separate screw-top lid in addition to the bucket lid that, if not closed properly, may cause your tubes to shatter while spinning. Most haematocrit centrifuges spin at fixed revolutions per minute (rpm), usually around $15,000 \times g$. Set the centrifuge to 5 minutes to allow sufficient time for the plasma and red cells to separate. While waiting for the centrifuge, it may be more efficient to conduct the measurements for haemoglobin, plasma lipids and glucose using the relevant analyser.

4 Wait until the centrifuge has stopped completely before opening the lid.

5 With the centrifuge open and the capillary tubes still in place, take the opportunity to look at the variability in plasma to red cell ratios among the samples.

6 Carefully remove your tube from the centrifuge and estimate the haematocrit value before measuring it.

7 Using the micro-haematocrit chart (Figure 2.15):

   a place the bottom of the red cells on the 0% line (Figure 2.16A)

   b slide the capillary tube along the chart until the top of the plasma is aligned with the 100% line on the chart (Figure 2.16B)

   c the line on the chart corresponding to the intersection of the red cells and plasma is the haematocrit percentage (Figure 2.16C)

   d if there is not enough blood for A and B to occur, place the bottom of the red cells on the 10% line and slide the capillary tube along the chart until the top of the plasma is aligned with the 90% line; then read the value.

8 Record the haematocrit value on the data sheet.

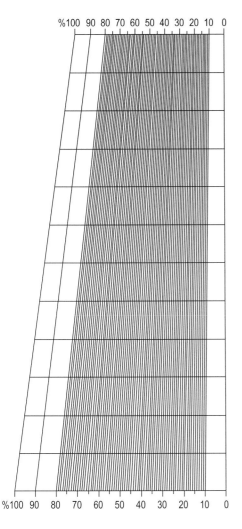

%100 90 80 70 60 50 40 30 20 10 0

%100 90 80 70 60 50 40 30 20 10 0

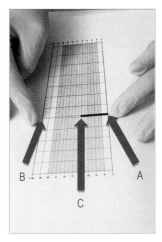

Figure 2.16 Place the bottom of the red cells on the 0% line (A) and slide the capillary tube along the chart until the top of the plasma is aligned with the 100% line on the chart (B). The line on the chart corresponding to the intersection of the red cells and plasma is the haematocrit value (C)

Figure 2.15 Haematocrit chart

Used with permission from The University of Queensland

9 Dispose of the capillary tube in the sharps container.

10 Clean and disinfect the area (see Appendix A).

Measuring haemoglobin, plasma lipids and glucose

There are several different types of analysers available for the measurement of haemoglobin, plasma lipids and glucose. To ensure accurate measurement of these variables, please follow the instructions provided by the manufacturer of the specific analyser you are using.

Data recording

Participant's name: _____   Date: _____

Age: _____ years   Sex: _____

VARIABLE	VALUE	APPROPRIATE VALUE OR RANGE	CLASSIFICATION (e.g. 'LOW')
Haematocrit (%)			
Haemoglobin (g/dL)			
Glucose (mmol/L)			
Total cholesterol (mmol/L)			
HDL cholesterol (mmol/L)			
Triglycerides (mmol/L)			
LDL cholesterol (mmol/L)			

Interpretation

First, consider the four steps of interpretation outlined in Appendix G. To interpret the data, it is essential that there is an understanding of the physiological basis of the measures and the pathophysiology around abnormal results.

Haematocrit and haemoglobin

Table 2.1 provides reference values. A low haematocrit is often accompanied by low haemoglobin and vice versa. This is because haematocrit is the volume of red blood cells and each red blood cell contains haemoglobin. Therefore, the two values should be interpreted together and are used by medical practitioners in the diagnosis of anaemia and polycythaemia.

TABLE 2.1 Reference ranges for haematocrit and haemoglobin in adults		
	MALE	**FEMALE**
Haematocrit (%)	40–54	37–47
Haemoglobin (g/dL)	13.5–17.5	12.0–15.5

Sources: The Royal College of Pathologists of Australasia[7] and Mayo Clinic[9]

 Haematocrit and haemoglobin red flags

- If either of these measures fall outside the reference range.

Plasma glucose

Table 2.2 shows plasma glucose values collected after fasting (8–16 hours following a meal) and when collected between 2 and 8 hours following a meal, sometimes known as a 'random' glucose measure. These values may be useful for participants who have not fasted. If a person has consumed a meal/beverage <2 hours prior to the test and the glucose value is ≥ 7.8 mmol/L then further testing is recommended.[10]

TABLE 2.2 Diagnostic criteria for type 2 diabetes and intermediate hyperglycaemia for adults		
PLASMA GLUCOSE	**FASTING: 8–16 h AFTER A MEAL (mmol/L)**	**RANDOM: 2–8 h AFTER A MEAL (mmol/L)**
Normal	3.0–5.4	3.0–7.7
Higher risk of type 2 diabetes[a]	5.5–6.9	7.8–11.0
Pre-diabetes[a]	6.1–6.9	Not provided
Type 2 diabetes[a]	≥ 7.0	≥ 11.1

[a] See additional diagnostic criteria provided below regarding how a medical practitioner would perform a diagnosis
Sources: The Royal College of Pathologists of Australasia[7] and a Position Statement from the Royal College of Pathologists of Australasia and Australasian Association of Clinical Biochemists[10]

Plasma glucose red flag

- If this measure falls outside the normal ranges.

Throughout this manual there are constant reminders that exercise professionals are not diagnosticians, but it is useful to understand what additional tests and criteria a medical practitioner would use to diagnose diabetes or pre-diabetes, also known as impaired fasting glucose. The best measure of chronic high blood glucose levels is glycated haemoglobin (HbA_{1c}). Glycation refers to glucose attaching to a molecule, in this case haemoglobin, and the resulting molecule is called HbA_{1c}. The degree of haemoglobin glycation reflects the mean plasma glucose over the life of the red blood cell (approximately the previous 3 months). Testing HbA_{1c} is now more commonly used to diagnose diabetes. Although there are point-of-care devices to measure HbA_{1c} using a finger prick blood sample, the cost of these tests makes it too prohibitive to include in this practical.

Another test in the diagnostic process is an oral glucose tolerance test. This is where a person consumes a glucose drink and blood samples are collected afterwards (usually at 1 and 2 hours post-consumption) to determine how quickly the glucose is cleared from the blood.

Additional diagnostic criteria

The following notes are from The Royal College of Pathologists of Australasia (RCPA) manual[7] and should be used with the criteria in Table 2.2 to better understand how a medical practitioner would diagnose diabetes or pre-diabetes.

- In a person with symptoms suggestive of type 2 diabetes, the finding of a fasting plasma glucose level of $\geq$7.0 mmol/L, or a random plasma glucose level of $\geq$11.1 mmol/L at least 2 hours following a meal, is diagnostic of type 2 diabetes. The finding of either of these levels on two occasions even in the absence of symptoms is also diagnostic of type 2 diabetes.

- In patients with fasting plasma glucose levels between 5.5 and 6.9 mmol/L or random plasma glucose levels between 7.8 and 11.0 mmol/L, an oral glucose tolerance test should be performed if the patient is at high risk for diabetes (e.g. morbidly obese).

- Irrespective of any glucose tolerance test results, a fasting plasma glucose level of 6.1–6.9 mmol/L indicates 'impaired fasting glucose'.

- Fasting plasma glucose levels <5.5 mmol/L and/or non-fasting levels <7.8 mmol/L make type 2 diabetes unlikely, and a glucose tolerance test is not indicated.

Plasma lipids (total cholesterol, LDL cholesterol, HDL cholesterol, triglycerides)

Tables 2.3–2.6 provide reference values for plasma lipids.[11]

TABLE 2.3 Classification of total cholesterol for adults	
TOTAL CHOLESTEROL	**(mmol/L)**
High	>6.20
Borderline high	5.17–6.19
Desirable	<5.17

Source: National Cholesterol Education Program Expert Panel on Detection Evaluation and Treatment of High Blood Cholesterol in Adults[11]

TABLE 2.4 Classification of HDL cholesterol for adults	
HDL CHOLESTEROL	**(mmol/L)[a]**
High	$\geq$1.55
Low	<1.03

[a] A value between 1.03 and 1.55 is not categorised in this system
Source: National Cholesterol Education Program Expert Panel on Detection Evaluation and Treatment of High Blood Cholesterol in Adults[11]

TABLE 2.5 Classification of LDL cholesterol for adults	
LDL CHOLESTEROL	**(mmol/L)**
Very high	>4.91
High	4.12–4.91
Borderline high	3.34–4.11
Near optimal	2.58–3.33
Optimal	<2.58

Source: National Cholesterol Education Program Expert Panel on Detection Evaluation and Treatment of High Blood Cholesterol in Adults[11]

PLASMA TOTAL CHOLESTEROL

Elevated total cholesterol is associated with atherosclerosis and increased risk of heart attack and stroke. Although the measurement of total cholesterol is useful for assessing the risk of developing CHD, it does not take into account the important relative proportions of each component (i.e. LDL

TABLE 2.6 Classification of triglycerides for adults	
TRIGLYCERIDES	(mmol/L)
Very high	≥ 5.64
High	2.27–5.64
Borderline high	1.69–2.26
Normal	< 1.69

Source: National Cholesterol Education Program Expert Panel on Detection Evaluation and Treatment of High Blood Cholesterol in Adults[11]

cholesterol, HDL cholesterol and vLDL cholesterol) and is not usually measured alone, except in screening situations. Therefore, interpretation of a total cholesterol value is usually done in conjunction with the HDL and LDL values.

🏴 *Plasma total cholesterol red flag*

- If this measure is above the desirable range.

PLASMA HDL CHOLESTEROL

These lipoproteins are often referred to as the 'good cholesterol'. They act as cholesterol scavengers, picking up excess cholesterol in blood and taking it back to the liver, where it is metabolised. Higher HDL levels are associated with a lower risk of CVD whereas low HDL increases the risk of heart attack and stroke.

🏴 *Plasma HDL cholesterol red flag*

- If this measure is in the low range.

PLASMA LDL CHOLESTEROL

LDL cholesterol contains more lipids than protein and carries most of the circulating cholesterol from the liver to various tissues. Because of this, increased LDL cholesterol constitutes a major risk factor for the development of CHD. Elevated LDL cholesterol leads to atherosclerosis and increased risk of heart attack and stroke.

🏴 *Plasma LDL cholesterol red flag*

- If this measure is above the 'near optimal' range.

PLASMA TRIGLYCERIDES

Triglycerides are fats that are used as an energy source. They are stored as adipose tissue and circulate in the blood. Elevated triglycerides lead to atherosclerosis and increased risk of heart attack and stroke.

🏴 *Plasma triglycerides red flag*

- If this measure is above the normal range.

Feedback and discussion

First, consider the three steps of feedback and discussion outlined in Appendix G. Each measure should be related back to the participant with the value and a qualitative descriptor, for example:

'*Your haematocrit is 45% and your haemoglobin is 12 g/dL. Both of these are in the healthy, normal range.*'

If any value is a red flag, the participant should be referred to a medical practitioner for follow-up. In this situation the priority is to convey the importance of the abnormal measure and the need for medical follow-up. When conveying the pathophysiological importance, the tester needs to do this in a manner that shows concern, but does not cause too much anguish for the participant. Secondly, the participant needs to be aware that this single abnormal measure is not a diagnosis. It has been performed for the purpose of screening and diagnoses are made only by medically trained individuals after receiving results from an accredited pathology laboratory and taking into account additional information such as the participant's medical history.

To convey the importance of the abnormal measure the tester needs to understand the pathological implications. The following statements could be used in association with an abnormal value:

Low haematocrit and/or haemoglobin: *'these are measures that reflect the ability of your blood to carry oxygen. Low values can be associated with constant tiredness and fatigue.'* This can lead to a discussion with the participant regarding whether they have experienced any of these symptoms.

High plasma glucose: *'this can be a sign of diabetes, which is a serious condition that can often go undiagnosed in people for a long period of time. If it is diagnosed early, treatment can be started to decrease the side effects of high blood glucose, which may include kidney and eye problems.'*

Abnormal plasma lipids: *'abnormal blood lipids or fats can place you at a higher risk of heart disease and stroke. Early detection of unusual values can lead to treatments such as lifestyle modification that will significantly decrease your risk of developing heart disease or having a stroke.'* Dietary intake of saturated fats (e.g. deep-fried fast foods) can lead to elevated LDL cholesterol and total cholesterol.[12] If a participant has abnormal plasma lipids then this can lead into a discussion around their eating habits and a potential referral to an Accredited Practising Dietitian.

As discussed in the 'interpretation, feedback and discussion' section in Appendix G, any negative news should be balanced with a positive statement at the end. For example, in the diabetes case, the tester could finish with: *'if you were to be diagnosed with diabetes, then it is important to know that regular exercise and a healthy diet can help manage the condition'*.

Conversely, a participant who has values in the normal healthy ranges can be given positive feedback. For example, a high HDL value is usually associated with good cardiorespiratory fitness and a reduced risk of CVD.[13]

Case studies

Setting: You work for a large company as an Accredited Exercise Scientist and one of your tasks is to offer a range of health screening options for employees. One of these is a fasting blood analysis where you take a finger prick blood sample and measure haematocrit, haemoglobin, lipids and glucose.

Case Study 1

The first employee is a 52-year-old male. Before taking the sample at 8.30 a.m., you confirm that his last food or beverage intake (excluding water) was at around 8.00 p.m. the previous evening.

Your task: The blood results are provided below. Complete the table by indicating what the appropriate value or range is for each variable and the subsequent classification. Follow the four steps of interpretation outlined in Appendix G and clarify how you would interpret the results.

_____

_____

Consider the three steps of feedback and discussion outlined in Appendix G. What questions would you ask the employee and what feedback should be provided?

_____

_____

continued overpage

Case studies (continued)

VARIABLE	VALUE	APPROPRIATE VALUE OR RANGE	CLASSIFICATION (e.g. 'LOW')
Haematocrit (%)	42		
Haemoglobin (g/dL)	13.6		
Glucose (mmol/L)	6.7		
Total cholesterol (mmol/L)	4.52		
HDL cholesterol (mmol/L)	1.34		
Triglycerides (mmol/L)	2.15		
LDL cholesterol (mmol/L)	2.75		

Case Study 2

The second employee is a 29-year-old female. Before taking the sample, you confirm that it has been around 12 hours since she last consumed a meal or beverage (except water).

Your task: The blood results are provided below. Complete the table by indicating what the appropriate value or range is for each variable and the subsequent classification. Follow the four steps of interpretation outlined in Appendix G and clarify how you would interpret the results.

_____

_____

Consider the three steps of feedback and discussion outlined in Appendix G. What questions would you ask the employee and what feedback should be provided?

_____

_____

VARIABLE	VALUE	APPROPRIATE VALUE OR RANGE	CLASSIFICATION (e.g. 'LOW')
Haematocrit (%)	34		
Haemoglobin (g/dL)	11.1		
Glucose (mmol/L)	4.5		
Total cholesterol (mmol/L)	3.56		
HDL cholesterol (mmol/L)	1.62		
Triglycerides (mmol/L)	1.45		
LDL cholesterol (mmol/L)	2.14		

References

[1] Schroeder LF, Giacherio D, Gianchandani R, Engoren M, Shah NH. Postmarket surveillance of point-of-care glucose meters through analysis of electronic medical records. Clin Chem 2016;62:716–24.

[2] Whitehead SJ, Ford C, Gama R. A combined laboratory and field evaluation of the Cholestech LDX and CardioChek PA point-of-care testing lipid and glucose analysers. Ann Clin Biochem 2014;51:54–67.

[3] du Plessis M, Ubbink JB, Vermaak WJ. Analytical quality of near-patient blood cholesterol and glucose determinations. Clin Chem 2000;46:1085–90.

[4] Deemers LM. Regulatory issues and point of care testing. Point of care testing. Washington DC: AACC Press; 1999.

[5] International Organization for Standardization. ISO 22870. Point-of-care testing (POCT) – requirements for quality and competence. Geneva: ISO; 2016. https://www.iso.org/iso/home/store/catalogue_ics/catalogue_detail_ics.htm?csnumber= 71119.

[6] Holt H, Freedman DB. Internal quality control in point-of-care testing: where's the evidence? Ann Clin Biochem 2016;53:233–9.

[7] The Royal College of Pathologists of Australasia. RCPA manual. Surry Hills, NSW: RCPA; 2015. https://www.rcpa.edu. au/Manuals/RCPA-Manual.

[8] Nordestgaard BG, Langsted A, Mora S, Kolovou G, Baum H, Bruckert E, et al.; European Atherosclerosis S, the European Federation of Clinical C, Laboratory Medicine Joint Consensus I. Fasting is not routinely required for determination of a lipid profile: Clinical and laboratory implications including flagging at desirable concentration cutpoints – a joint consensus statement from the European Atherosclerosis Society and European Federation of Clinical Chemistry and Laboratory Medicine. Clin Chem 2016;62:930–46.

[9] Mayo Clinic. Hemoglobin test. 2017. http://www.mayoclinic.org/tests-procedures/hemoglobin-test/basics/results/ prc-20015022.

[10] Royal College of Pathologists of Australasia (RCPA) and Australasian Association of Clinical Biochemists (AACB). Position statement on impaired fasting glucose. Pathology 2008;40:627–8.

[11] National Cholesterol Education Program Expert Panel on Detection Evaluation and Treatment of High Blood Cholesterol in Adults. Third report of the National Cholesterol Education Program (NCEP) expert panel on detection, evaluation, and treatment of high blood cholesterol in adults (Adult Treatment Panel III) final report. Circulation 2002;106:3143–421. https://www.nhlbi.nih.gov/files/docs/resources/heart/atp-3-cholesterol-full-report.pdf.

[12] Sacks FM, Lichtenstein AH, Wu JHY, Appel LJ, Creager MA, Kris-Etherton PM, et al.; American Heart Association. Dietary fats and cardiovascular disease: a presidential advisory from the American Heart Association. Circulation 2017; 136:e1–e23.

[13] Pedersen BK, Saltin B. Exercise as medicine – evidence for prescribing exercise as therapy in 26 different chronic diseases. Scand J Med Sci Sports 2015;25(Suppl 3):1–72.

PRACTICAL 3
CARDIOVASCULAR HEALTH

Jeff Coombes and Andrew Williams

LEARNING OBJECTIVES

- Understand the scientific rationale, purposes, reliability, validity, assumptions and limitations of common cardiovascular health assessments
- Identify and explain the common terminology, processes and equipment required to conduct accurate and safe cardiovascular health assessments
- Conduct appropriate pre-assessment procedures, including explaining the test
- Identify the need for guidance or further information from a relevant health professional
- Conduct appropriate cardiovascular health assessments
- Record, analyse and interpret information from cardiovascular health assessments and convey the results, including the validity and limitations of the assessments, through verbal and/or written communication to a participant or relevant health professional

Equipment and other requirements

- Information sheet and informed consent form
- Stopwatch
- Stethoscope
- Teaching stethoscope
- Chest strap heart rate monitor set (e.g. transmitter, receiver, chest strap)
- Wrist-worn heart rate monitor
- Desk (or similarly portable) sphygmomanometer with various size arm cuffs (with size indicators)
- Sphygmomanometer on stand with various size arm cuffs (with size indicators)
- Semi-automated sphygmomanometer
- Alcohol wipes
- Adult Pre-exercise Screening System (APSS) forms
- Monark cycle ergometer
- Calculator
- Cleaning and disinfecting equipment (see Appendix A)

INTRODUCTION

Coronary heart disease (CHD) is the leading cause of death in Australia.[1] Exercise professionals often have the opportunity to evaluate a person's cardiovascular health in situations such as health screening and during a fitness assessment. In these environments the two main physiological measures of cardiovascular health usually performed are 'resting' heart rate (HR) and blood pressure (BP) and their response to exercise. Practitioners can also use methods that calculate a cardiovascular disease (CVD) risk score based on known risk factors. These are likely to be used in a more general health assessment. In this practical, physiological measures and a risk score calculator will be used to show how exercise professionals can gain information on a person's cardiovascular health.

DEFINITIONS

Absolute disease risk: risk of developing a disease over a period of time.

Acute myocardial infarction (AMI): also known as a heart attack, this refers to an interruption of blood flow to the heart muscle causing cells to die. It is commonly caused by coronary heart disease (CHD).

Ambulatory blood pressure monitoring: measuring blood pressure using a device while a person is carrying out their activities of daily living (ADLs).

Angina: chest pain caused by a decreased blood flow to part of the heart muscle usually caused by coronary heart disease (CHD). Angina may occur at rest or it may only manifest during exercise or other stress when there is a greater demand for coronary blood flow.

Arterial pulse: pressure wave generated by the ejection of blood from the heart.

Auscultation of heart rate: listening to the heartbeat, usually with a stethoscope on the chest.

Blood pressure (BP): the pressure exerted against the artery walls.

Cardiorespiratory fitness: ability of the circulatory and respiratory systems to supply oxygen and support the energy demands during sustained physical activity. Also known as aerobic fitness or aerobic endurance.

Cardiovascular disease (CVD): an umbrella term that refers to any disease that affects the heart or blood vessels. This includes coronary heart disease (CHD), hypertension, peripheral vascular disease and stroke (cerebrovascular accident).

Coronary heart disease (CHD): also known as **coronary artery disease (CAD)**, this is a narrowing or blockage of the coronary arteries of the heart, usually caused by atherosclerosis. It can lead to chest pain (angina) or a heart attack (myocardial infarction) and damage to the heart muscle.

Diastolic blood pressure (DBP): the pressure in the arteries when the heart relaxes between beats.

Inter-tester reliability: also known as between-tester reliability, this is the amount of agreement (reliability) between two different testers measuring the same parameter on the same individual.

Intra-tester reliability: also known as within-tester reliability, this is the amount of agreement (reliability) from the same tester measuring the same parameter on the same individual on different occasions.

Korotkoff sounds: arterial sounds heard through a stethoscope applied to the brachial artery that change with varying cuff pressure and that are used to determine systolic and diastolic blood pressure.

Masked hypertension: when blood pressure measured in a clinic situation is lower than that measured out of the clinic (via home or ambulatory blood pressure measurements).

Mean arterial pressure: the average blood pressure exerted against the arterial walls throughout the cardiac cycle.

MET: or metabolic equivalent is a measure of the energy cost of physical activities relative to the energy cost at rest. At rest it is convention that 1 MET of energy is being expended, which is obtained by consuming and using 3.5 mL/kg/min of oxygen.

Orthostatic hypotension: also known as **postural hypotension**, occurs when a person's blood pressure suddenly falls when changing posture.

Palpation of heart rate: pressing with fingers onto the surface of the body to detect the arterial pulse.

Pulse pressure: difference between the systolic and diastolic blood pressures.

Rate pressure product: also known as **double product**, this is a measure of the work of the heart and depends on the rate at which it is contracting (heart rate) and the force that must be produced to expel blood into the systemic circulation (systolic blood pressure).

Relative disease risk: used to compare the risk of developing a disease in two different groups of people (e.g. smokers and non-smokers).

Resting blood pressure: the blood pressure when a person is awake, in a neutrally temperate environment, and has not had any recent exertion or stimulation.

Resting heart rate: the heart rate when a person is awake, in a neutrally temperate environment, and has not had any recent exertion or stimulation.

Sustained hypertension: when a person is hypertensive in the clinic and out of the clinic (via home or ambulatory blood pressure measurements).

Systolic blood pressure (SBP): the pressure in the arteries when the heart contracts.

True normotension: when a person is normotensive in the clinic and during ambulatory monitoring.

White coat hypertension: raised clinic blood pressure but normal out-of-clinic blood pressure.

HEART RATE

The heart rate is primarily regulated by the inotropic and chronotropic effects of both branches of the autonomic nervous system (ANS) acting on the sinoatrial node and the myocardium. Sympathetic stimulation increases the heart rate and comes from the release of norepinephrine (noradrenaline) from the accelerans nerve. The vagus nerve provides parasympathetic input to slow the heart rate by secreting acetylcholine. A measure of the resting heart rate is best obtained on waking (e.g. before getting out of bed) and this value will usually be lower than that obtained in a clinical situation.[2] A person's resting heart rate typically rises with age, and individuals with higher cardiorespiratory fitness will generally have a lower resting heart rate.[3] This has led to its use in non-exercise fitness tests to predict cardiorespiratory fitness.[4] Importantly, an abnormal resting heart rate can be an indicator of an underlying problem with the cardiovascular system.

The heart rate increases immediately at the start of exercise. Indeed, even thinking of doing the exercise may cause an anticipatory heart rate rise. For this reason, a heart rate measured just before exercise should be referred to as a pre-exercise measure rather than a resting measure. During submaximal exercise there is a linear relationship between exercise intensity and heart rate, and this association is used in many submaximal fitness tests to predict cardiorespiratory fitness (as seen in Practical 11).

Methods to measure the heart rate

This practical will measure the heart rate using palpation, auscultation, a telemetric device using a chest strap sensor and a wrist-worn device using an optical sensor. In recent years there has been a rapid development in the technology used to measure heart rate using different approaches. For example, biosensors are now fitted into clothing to measure the heart rate.

Accuracy and reliability of measuring the heart rate

The heart rate is influenced by a number of factors that impact on the ability to obtain an accurate and reliable measure (see Practical 1, Test accuracy, reliability and validity). For a 'resting' measure the physiological state of the participant (e.g. recent exertion or stimulation) and environment (e.g. temperature) will have large effects on whether it is close to a true resting measure. The protocol to obtain a heart rate that is close to a true resting value includes having the participant lying awake in a thermoneutral, dimly lit room for an extended period (e.g. >20 min)[5] prior to obtaining the measure with a heart rate monitor. The accuracy of chest strap monitors has been compared with ECG monitoring across numerous studies, with most showing good agreement (less than 5 beats per minute (bpm) difference between the two measures).[6] A number of wrist-worn heart rate watches have also been shown to accurately measure the heart rate at rest and during exercise (correlations from 0.67 to 0.95 with ECG-measured heart rate).[7]

With regards to reliability, when the participant is in a well-controlled state (i.e. environment, participant preparation) there is good day-to-day reliability with the resting heart rate (coefficient of variation <1.5%).[8]

Validity of heart rate measures to assess cardiovascular health

The resting heart rate has been established as a valid (prognostic) measure of cardiovascular health.[9] Epidemiological studies involving >100,000 participants and follow-up periods of 5–36 years have demonstrated that a lower resting heart rate is associated with decreased all-cause mortality in the general population and in individuals with cardiovascular conditions.[10] Indeed, a 5 bpm decrease in the resting heart rate was related to an 18% reduction of mortality.[11] This association is independent of background CVD risk.[12] As mentioned, the heart rate response to exercise is used to estimate cardiorespiratory fitness. The strong relationship between cardiorespiratory fitness and physical and mental health further emphasises the importance of being able to accurately measure the heart rate.[13]

Activity 3.1 Palpating the heart rate

AIM: measure your heart rate by palpation at the radial and brachial arteries.

Background

The heart rate may be palpated from a number of arteries; however, the three major sites commonly used are:

1 radial artery: around 2–5 cm from the base of the thumb on the anterolateral side of the wrist (Figure 3.1)

2 brachial artery: on the medial third of the antecubital fossa (inside of the elbow joint) (Figure 3.2) or

3 carotid artery: on the neck lateral to the larynx (not recommended).

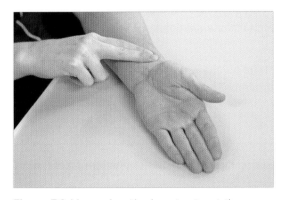

Figure 3.1 Measuring the heart rate at the radial artery

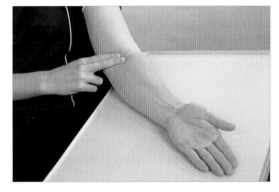

Figure 3.2 Measuring the heart rate at the brachial artery

For safety and proximity purposes you should first try to obtain the heart rate from the radial artery. Pressure should be light; if the artery is pressed too hard, the pulse will disappear. Slightly more pressure is usually needed to locate the brachial artery pulse. You should avoid taking the heart rate at the carotid artery as excessive pressure may block blood flow to the brain. In addition, massaging this area (as you are trying to locate this artery) may stimulate baroreceptors in the artery, resulting in blood pressure fluctuations, which may lead to fainting. To reinforce this, only radial and brachial palpation methods will be covered in this practical.

Protocol summary

Obtain your heart rate at the radial and brachial arteries.

Protocol

Radial heart rate

1　You should be seated with your arm relaxed on a table.

2　Locate your radial artery by palpation.

　　a　Have one of your palms facing upwards (side not important). The location of the radial artery is approximately 2–5 cm proximal to the wrist on the lateral side (thumb side) of the arm (see Figure 3.1).

3　Apply light pressure with the tips of the middle and index fingers[a] from your opposite hand, and try to feel the rhythmical pulsing. If you do not feel it after 5 seconds, move your fingers to a slightly different location and/or apply slightly more pressure, or less pressure if pressing hard.

4　Measuring the heart rate: when you do feel the pulse, count the pulses whilst using a stopwatch to time for 15 seconds and multiply the pulses by four (to determine the heart rate in bpm). It is important to count the first pulse as '0' as you start the stopwatch.

5　Record your value.

Brachial heart rate

1　You should be seated with your arm slightly bent and relaxed on a table.

2　Locate your brachial artery by palpation.

　　a　Have one of your palms facing upwards (side not important). The brachial artery is located in the medial third of the elbow joint (antecubital fossa) (see Figure 3.2).

3　Apply pressure (slightly firmer than for the radial pulse) with the tips of the middle and index fingers from your opposite hand, and try to feel the rhythmical pulsing. If you do not feel it after 5 seconds, move your fingers to a slightly different location and/or apply slightly more pressure. It may be useful to begin again from the centre of the arm (in anatomical stance position) and work your way towards the medial aspect of the elbow joint.

4　Measuring heart rate: when you do feel the pulse, count the pulses while using a stopwatch to time for 15 seconds and multiply the pulses by four (to determine heart rate in bpm). It is important to count the first pulse as '0' as you start the stopwatch.

5　Record your value.

> **Note:** You will also need to locate this artery when measuring blood pressure for positioning of the stethoscope.

Data recording

Your radial HR _____ bpm　　　　Your brachial HR _____ bpm

---

[a] You should not use your thumb to palpate the heart rate as it has an artery near the surface and you may feel your own pulse when trying to measure another person's heart rate.

Activity 3.2 Auscultating heart rate

AIM: measure your heart rate by auscultation with a stethoscope on your chest.

Background

In some individuals it may be difficult to palpate the heart rate. This could be due to an underlying vascular issue. Although one of the objectives of this practical is to measure the heart rate, it is also possible to evaluate the consistency of the beat or the heart rhythm. This can be more easily achieved by auscultation with a stethoscope. A stethoscope consists of removable earpieces, the chestpiece containing the bell and diaphragm, and the tubes (Figure 3.3). For teaching purposes, a dual-user stethoscope (Figure 3.4) is very useful.

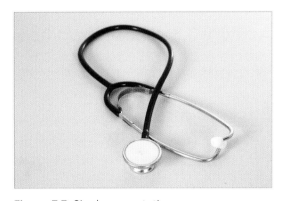

Figure 3.3 Single-user stethoscope

Irregularities in heart rhythm may be an indication of a medical condition with the heart. It is important to recognise that the skill of listening for heart rhythms is gained through much experience and not considered in the standard skill set of an exercise professional. When a heart rhythm irregularity is found, it is important that this is conveyed to the participant's medical practitioner.

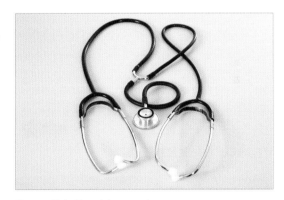

Figure 3.4 Teaching stethoscope

Protocol summary

Obtain your heart rate using a stethoscope on your chest for 15 seconds.

Protocol

1 Clean the earpieces of the stethoscope with alcohol wipes.

2 If the stethoscope has bent earpieces, they should point forward when inserting into the ears so they angle into the ear canal.

3 The chestpiece should be placed on your thorax medial to the left nipple (Figure 3.5).

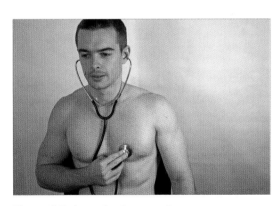

Figure 3.5 Auscultating your heart rate

4 Measuring heart rate: when you hear the heartbeat, count the pulses whilst using a stopwatch to time for 15 seconds and multiply the value by four (to determine heart rate in beats per minute). It is important to count the first pulse as '0' as you start the stopwatch.

5 Record your value.

6 Clean and disinfect all equipment (see Appendix A).

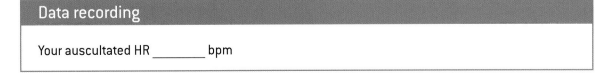

Data recording

Your auscultated HR _____ bpm

If you are required to auscultate the heart rate of another person, first explain where you will be placing the stethoscope and determine whether clothing may need to be removed, or unbuttoned. Avoid breast tissue by starting closer to the midline of the thorax.

Activity 3.3 Chest strap heart rate monitor

AIM: measure your heart rate using a chest strap heart rate monitor.

Background

There are a number of different approaches to monitor heart rate using a device. One method is where the sensor is located on a strap that is worn around the chest. The chest strap heart rate monitor has:

(1) a sensor and transmitter that are either separate to, or integrated into, the chest strap; and (2) a receiver (e.g. wristwatch) (Figure 3.6). The sensor picks up the electrical activity of the heart after the electrical signal has been transmitted to the skin. The signal is detected by electrodes on the surface (sensor). It then sends (transmits) this information to the receiver that displays and/or records the heart rate. Water or a conducting gel is usually needed on the electrodes to improve signal detection.

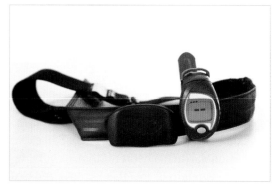

Figure 3.6 Heart rate monitor set consisting of chest strap with integrated transmitter and receiver (watch)

Protocol summary

Obtain your heart rate from the monitor.

Protocol

1 Wet the electrodes on the heart rate electrodes with water or an electrode conducting gel.

2 Secure the sensor/transmitter using the strap around the chest below your pectoral fold. For females this will be just below the bra line.

3 Check that the watch is receiving the signal from the transmitter (allow 30 seconds). There are a variety of techniques to get a signal depending on the make and model. For example, some models may need the watch tapped against the transmitter to trigger signal transference. Others may need the watch to be held within 10 cm from the sensor. Refer to the user's manual for the specific device being used.

4 Record your value.

5 Clean and disinfect all equipment (see Appendix A).

Data recording
Your heart rate using a heart rate monitor _____ bpm

Troubleshooting

- If the watch does not appear to be receiving the signal from the transmitter, check that the sensor/transmitter is firm on the skin and water or an electrode gel has been used on the electrodes.

- It is a common error for the strap to be fitted too loosely owing to difficulties in adjusting the tension.
- If it is still not receiving a signal then move, or ask the participant to move, the sensor/transmitter either slightly up or down on your chest (usually higher, i.e. closer to the pectoral muscles).
- If the heart rate is changing rapidly it may be picking up a signal from another transmitter. Move at least 2 metres away from other transmitters being used.
- For participants with concave chest cavities you may need to move the sensor/transmitter around to the back of the individual.

Activity 3.4 Comparing heart rate methods – concurrent validity

AIM: Compare the heart rate obtained using palpation of the radial artery with that obtained using a chest strap heart rate monitor. Interpret the values and provide feedback to the participant.

Background

Heart rate monitors are very accurate at measuring the heart rate.[6,7] However, given the time it takes to fit the transmitter and the possibility that a signal may be lost during an exercise test, it is important that an exercise professional can accurately measure the heart rate via palpation. This activity will allow you to directly compare your palpation accuracy and provide feedback to a participant regarding baseline heart rate. This is usually provided during a standard health/fitness assessment. Understanding what feedback to provide is also an objective of this activity.

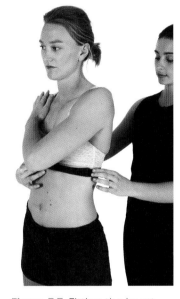

Protocol summary

Fit a heart rate monitor to another individual and compare the value from this device with the heart rate you obtain by palpating.

Protocol

1 Fit the heart rate monitor chest strap and sensor/transmitter to another individual and obtain their heart rate on the receiver (Figure 3.7).

Figure 3.7 Fitting the heart rate transmitter

   a To avoid breast tissue, ask the participant to lift up their own clothing to place the chest strap into position under the pectoral fold. You can secure the ends of the strap either behind or to the side of the participant and then have them move it into position. It is helpful to ask the participant to hold the sensor in position against their chest while it is attached to the strap. Asking the participant to rotate their body will also enable the strap to more easily go around their torso.

   b Check the tension on the strap once it is secured and tighten if necessary.

   c Remind the participant to lower their clothing or put their shirt back on.

2 Ask the participant to be seated until you observe a steady heart rate on the receiver.

3 Measure their radial heart rate via palpation at the radial artery as per Activity 3.1 (Figure 3.8).

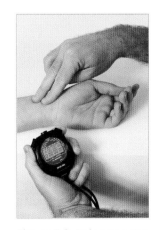

Figure 3.8 Palpating the 'resting' heart rate of another individual

4 Then obtain the value from the heart rate monitor as per Activity 3.3 as soon as possible after you have measured their radial heart rate (as touching the participant will probably increase their heart rate).

5 Enter the values on the data form.

6 Ask the participant to remove the heart rate monitor

7 Clean and disinfect all equipment (see Appendix A).

Data analysis

Determine the concurrent validity by calculating the percentage difference.

> **Note:** The heart rate monitor is accepted to be the more accurate measure in this situation; therefore you are calculating the percentage difference of your palpation measure.
>
> The largest HR measure will be either from the monitor or from palpation. The smallest will be the other HR.

$$\text{Percent difference} = \left[\frac{\text{largest HR measure} - \text{smallest HR measure}}{\text{smallest HR measure}}\right] \times 100$$

As a general rule, the percentage difference should be less than 5% when comparing a technique such as palpating the heart rate against a reference method (heart rate monitor).

Data recording

Radial HR _____ bpm   Heart rate monitor HR _____ bpm

Difference _____ %

Interpretation, feedback and discussion

First, consider the four steps of interpretation and the three steps of feedback and discussion outlined in Appendix G. Box 3.1 can be used to classify an individual's 'resting' heart rate. As previously mentioned, a true 'resting' heart rate' is obtained when the participant is in a neutrally temperate environment and has not been subject to any recent exertion or stimulation, such as stress or surprise. Additional influences on the resting heart rate include caffeine, and certain medications. These factors should be considered when discussing the prognostic validity of your measure with a participant.

Box 3.1 Normal values and terms associated with slow or fast 'resting' heart rates

Classification of 'Resting' Heart Rate
$<$60 bpm = bradycardia (slow rate)
60–100 bpm = normal rate
$>$100 bpm = tachycardia (fast rate)

Resting heart rate red flags

- An unexplained high 'resting' heart rate ($>$100 bpm) may indicate stress, disease, or infection. In athletes, a high 'resting' heart rate may be a sign of overtraining.
- An unexplained low 'resting' heart rate ($<$60 bpm) may be a sign of hypothyroidism or a potassium imbalance. These are unusual. A low resting heart rate is also common in endurance athletes.

If the participant has a high or low 'resting' heart rate you should ask whether they have been made aware of this previously and whether they have been experiencing any dizziness, tiredness, chest pain or any other symptoms that could be indicative of an underlying cardiovascular problem.

If there appears to be no clinical reason explaining the abnormal value then you could suggest they monitor their own heart rate, preferably first thing in the morning or, if possible, come back and see you for a follow-up measure. As always, the participant should be referred to their medical practitioner if there are sufficient concerns.

Blood pressure

Cardiac output, total peripheral resistance and arterial stiffness all impact on blood pressure. It is influenced by a person's emotional state, recent physical activity, cardiorespiratory fitness and health/disease state. In the short-term, blood pressure is regulated by pressure sensitive baroreceptors that influence the nervous and endocrine systems via the brain.

As aerobic exercise intensity increases, so too does systolic blood pressure (SBP). In healthy individuals, the SBP increase varies with age and sex (ranging from around 5 to 8 mmHg per MET of intensity),[14] and will normally continue to increase before plateauing at peak intensity. Diastolic blood pressure (DBP) tends to remain the same, or rise or fall slightly as exercise intensity increases. When the heart is contracting during systole, the increased cardiac output leads to an increase in pressure and vasodilation to accommodate the increased blood flow. When the heart relaxes, the driving pressure due to cardiac outflow is removed; however, the recoil of the elastic arteries ensuring continued flow is balanced by the continued dilation of the peripheral arteries, resulting in minimal change in DBP from rest.

Methods to measure blood pressure

The Royal Australian College of General Practitioners recommend that blood pressure should be measured in all adults from 18 years of age at least every 2 years.[15] Traditionally, blood pressure was measured using a mercury sphygmomanometer owing to its accuracy and reliability.[16] Although these are still used to calibrate other devices, they are no longer routinely used because of concerns about potential mercury toxicity. Thus, non-mercury devices including digital (Figure 3.9) and anaeroid (Figure 3.10) sphygmomanometers and semi-automated approaches are used. Semi-automated devices generally use an oscillometric method to determine the strength of the pressure in the cuff over the artery.

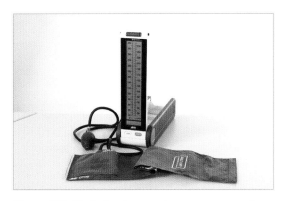

Figure 3.9 Digital column sphygmomanometer
Used with permission from A&D Medical

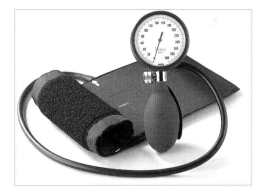

Figure 3.10 Anaeroid sphygmomanometer
Used with permission from Boso

Blood pressure can be readily measured during exercise if following a standardised procedure.[17] Participant movement can introduce artifact (particularly at higher exercise intensities) into measurement accuracy. Generally, oscillometric devices are highly sensitive to movement,[18] and so this is why manual auscultation is the preferred measurement option. However, there are motion-tolerant devices in use in cardiac investigation laboratories.

Accuracy and reliability of measuring blood pressure

Major factors that will impact on the accuracy and reliability of the blood pressure measure include: the skill of the tester, the quality of the sphygmomanometer/device, the calibration state of the sphygmomanometer/device and the physiological state of the participant (see Practical 1, Test accuracy, reliability and validity). Potential sources of error in the measurement of blood pressure are provided in Table 3.1.

TABLE 3.1 Common sources of error when measuring blood pressure

EQUIPMENT	TESTER	PARTICIPANT
Blood pressure cuff • incorrect size – see guideline at 'test preparation' Sphygmomanometer • inaccurate – not calibrated or validated (see Practical 1, Test accuracy, reliability and validity) Stethoscope • not turned on • poor quality	Technique • poor choice of location (e.g. background noise) • poor set-up (e.g. arm at the wrong level) • not enough time allowed for blood pressure to fall to a 'resting' level while in position (e.g. seated) • poor control of valve leading to inflation or deflation being too fast or slow • inaccurate stethoscope placement • too much pressure on the stethoscope • slow reaction time • not palpating radial pulse before auscultatory measurements resulting in failure to detect systolic gap • re-inflating the cuff to repeat measurement before it has fully deflated • rounding off actual reading by more than 2 mmHg • taking a single measurement Hearing • poor auditory acuity	Preparation • has not followed, or been provided with, pre-test instructions During measurement • participant allowed to talk

The Stride blood pressure initiative has developed a comprehensive list of validated blood pressure monitors.[19] Detailed instructions on how to check that a blood pressure monitor is validated for accuracy have also been created.[20,21]

The physiological state of the individual can significantly affect the interpretation of blood pressure readings. For example, some participants experience high 'resting' blood pressures in clinical settings that are not replicated when other forms of blood pressure measurement, such as home or 24-hour ambulatory blood pressure monitoring, are used.[22,23] This condition is known as white coat (false) hypertension. The name is derived from evidence that it is due to anxiety experienced during the procedure. It is important to try and minimise this occurring by creating a positive, friendly environment and trying to make the participant feel as relaxed as possible. In contrast, there are other individuals in whom blood pressure measurements within a clinical setting are normal; however, they experience high blood pressures when measured out of the clinic (via home or ambulatory monitoring). This is referred to as masked hypertension. It has been estimated that more than 50% of normotensive diagnoses based on 'resting' clinic blood pressure may be incorrect (false negative).[24]

Validity of blood pressure measures to assess cardiovascular health

'Resting' blood pressure is measured to detect hypertension, which is a primary risk factor for CVD and is one of the most commonly diagnosed medical conditions. In the 2017–18 National Health Survey, 22.8% (4.3 million people) of Australians aged 18 years and over had a measured high blood pressure reading (systolic/diastolic blood pressure $\geq$140/90 mmHg).[25] It is important to note that many people on blood pressure medication often report having no cardiovascular disease concerns because they are medicated; however, their risk is still elevated compared with a person with normal blood pressure who is not medicated.[26]

A diagnosis of hypertension is made by a medically trained individual and should be based on multiple measures on at least two separate occasions,[27] and involve out-of-clinic monitoring such as home or 24-hour ambulatory measurement. Measuring a participant's blood pressure intermittently over a 24-hour period using a specialised monitor is often used in the diagnosis of hypertension. This is known as ambulatory blood pressure monitoring; measurement frequency is usually set to 20–30 minutes during the day and 30–60 minutes at night with the data recorded automatically. Average values during these two time periods are used to help diagnose hypertension.[22] Since 24-hour ambulatory monitoring is often not available outside of specialist clinics, home BP measurement should be encouraged by the exercise professional to complement in-clinic measurements. Guidance on the correct way to measure and interpret home BP has been created.[28,29]

Hypertension is often called the 'silent killer' because it usually has no warning signs or symptoms, and many people don't know they have the condition. It places extra load on the heart and damages blood vessels making it more likely that cholesterol plaques will form. Hypertension also causes the artery walls to become thicker, stiffer and less able to accommodate changes in blood flow.

Blood pressure should be measured as part of all clinical exercise tests,[30] as abnormal responses may be indicative of elevated cardiovascular disease risk. A low or 'hypotensive' response to exercise (failure for BP to rise with increasing exercise intensity) is a poor prognostic sign and requires immediate specialist follow-up. An excessive rise in blood pressure or 'hypertensive' response is generally defined at maximal exercise intensity as a SBP >210 mmHg (males) and >190 mmHg (females) because it has been associated with cardiovascular events and mortality in some studies. However, a hypertensive response at submaximal exercise intensities, although being associated with increased risk of CVD events and mortality,[31] predicts the future development of hypertension.[32] An exercise SBP $>\sim170$ mmHg at submaximal exercise intensities is likely indicative of poor blood pressure control and should prompt referral to a general practitioner to follow-up care and encouragement of the patient to perform home blood pressure monitoring.[33]

Pulse pressure

The pulse pressure (PP) represents the force that the heart generates each time it contracts. A high pulse pressure at rest indicates increased stiffness in the large arteries and is a risk factor for heart disease.[34] Indeed, a 10 mmHg increase in pulse pressure increased the risk of CVD morbidity and mortality by nearly 20%.[34] PP is calculated using the following formula and the units are mmHg:

$$\text{Pulse Pressure (PP)} = \text{SBP} - \text{DBP}$$

Mean arterial pressure

The mean arterial pressure (MAP) reflects the average pressure in the arteries. It is considered to be the pressure responsible for carrying blood to the organs. A MAP of 65 mmHg or greater is considered to be the pressure needed to decrease risk of ischaemia and subsequent hypoxia to organs.[35] MAP can be loosely approximated using the following formula that assumes the heart spends three times longer in diastole than systole. The clinical relevance and accuracy of these 'form-factor' equations are questionable and should not be used to inform any treatment decisions.[36] The units for MAP are mmHg.

$$\text{Mean Arterial Pressure (MAP)} = \frac{(\text{SBP} - \text{DBP})}{3} + \text{DBP}$$

Rate pressure product

The rate pressure product (RPP), or double product, is an estimate of the workload of the heart muscle.[37] It is primarily used in research to assess the response of the coronary circulation to myocardial metabolic demands. It is calculated using the following formula and is usually expressed without units.

$$\text{Rate Pressure Product (RPP)} = \frac{\text{HR (bpm)} \times \text{SBP (mmHg)}}{100}$$

Activity 3.5 Blood pressure – manual method

AIM: measure blood pressure on a participant using a sphygmomanometer and stethoscope (manual method). Interpret the values and provide feedback to the participant.

Background

The brachial artery at the antecubital fossa (elbow crease) is usually the site for this measurement, owing to its position at approximately heart level. Millimetres of mercury (mmHg) are the standard international units for blood pressure. The equipment used to measure blood pressure includes a sphygmomanometer (commonly called a 'sphygmo') and a stethoscope. The manometer on the sphygmomanometer is usually either a column (see Figure 3.9) or anaeroid (dial) (see Figure 3.10).

After the blood pressure cuff is wrapped around the upper arm, it is inflated so that blood flow to the forearm is occluded. As the cuff is then deflated, pressure within the artery exceeds the occluding pressure of the cuff allowing blood flow to resume. The resumption of blood flow through a partially occluded artery results in turbulent flow, which is the noise that is heard through the stethoscope. The vibrations caused by blood against the arterial wall are known as Korotkoff sounds (Table 3.2).

TABLE 3.2 The phases of Korotkoff sounds	
Phase I (SBP)	Onset of consecutive faint, clear tapping sounds with a gradual increase in intensity
Phase II	Sounds change to swishing or blowing sounds
Phase III	Sound becomes clearer and crisper, creating soft thuds that become louder
Phase IV	Sound becomes suddenly muffled and assumes a soft, blowing character that diminishes
Phase V (DBP)	Sound disappears

SBP = systolic blood pressure; DBP = diastolic blood pressure

The first audible noise (Korotkoff Phase I) indicates the resumption of blood flow through the partially occluded artery and corresponds to SBP. As the cuff continues to deflate, DBP corresponds to the point at which the sounds cease and indicates the lowest (or baseline) pressure within the arterial system. While Korotkoff Phase IV is closer to the actual DBP, it can be difficult to determine and hence Korotkoff Phase V (i.e. the last sound heard) is commonly used and is the reference DBP for normative classification. In some individuals, particularly during exercise, blood flow can be heard until the pressure reads close to zero (e.g. within around 30 mmHg). For these individuals, the onset of the Korotkoff Phase IV (sound becomes softer and muffled) should be used to determine DBP. When the cuff is completely deflated, blood flow is usually laminar and no sound can be heard through the stethoscope.

The following protocol for measuring blood pressure is from the National Heart Foundation of Australia.[27] It is considered best practice to assess blood pressure in both arms. This may lead to diagnosis of a medical condition if a large discrepancy exists (e.g. due to arterial stenosis). It is recommended that when a participant has their blood pressure measured for the first time by a tester it is measured on both arms.

Protocol summary

Measure blood pressure on a participant using a sphygmomanometer and stethoscope.

Protocol

1 Ensure stethoscope earpieces have been swabbed with an alcohol wipe.

2 Many stethoscopes have a head that can rotate to open/close the diaphragm. To check that the stethoscope is open, place the stethoscope earpieces in your ears, rotate the chestpiece and lightly tap the diaphragm. When the sound is loudest the stethoscope is open.

3 The participant should be asked if they have had their blood pressure measured previously, the value and when this was done.

4 Choose an arm to take blood pressure and try to arrange the participant so that they are seated with the chosen arm closest to you on the table.

5 The cuff should be at the level of the heart so having a high table, a low chair and/or a support for the arm is recommended.

6 Ensure that the participant is sleeveless or that a loose-fitting shirt can be rolled up to the shoulder *without* restricting blood flow.

7 Select the appropriate-sized arm cuff (Figure 3.11) using the indicating marks on the cuff – blood pressure will be exaggerated with a cuff that is too small and underestimated with a cuff that is too large. If the cuffs are not marked then the bladder length should be at least 80% and the width at least 40% of the circumference of the mid-upper arm. The bladder is the inflatable bag inside of double layers of cuff material.

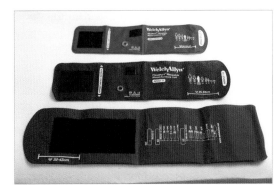

Figure 3.11 Variety of different-sized blood pressure cuffs
Used with permission from Welch Allyn

Measurement

1 A good technique and a calibrated device are critical to an accurate measure of blood pressure. Table 3.1 lists some potential sources of error in blood pressure assessment.

2 The participant should be sitting quietly in a chair with a backrest for at least 5 minutes prior to the measurement of baseline blood pressure.

3 Inform the participant what you are about to do and then locate the brachial artery in the antecubital space (elbow crease) by palpation (Figure 3.12). It may be helpful to mark this position with a pen for future readings (Figure 3.13).

4 Ensure there is no air remaining in the cuff before fitting it to your participant. Wrap the cuff firmly around the person's upper arm. Check that the internal aspect of the cuff is against the participant's skin (i.e. not inside out). The bladder within the cuff should be directly above the artery (indicated by the rubber tubes) and the bottom of the cuff should be 3–4 cm above the antecubital space (Figure 3.14). Avoid twists in the tubes.

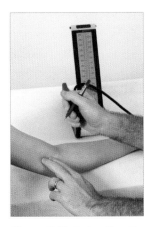

Figure 3.12 Palpating the location of the brachial artery
Used with permission from A&D Medical

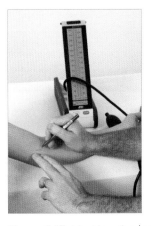

Figure 3.13 Marking the location of the brachial artery
Used with permission from A&D Medical

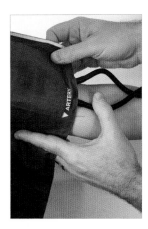

Figure 3.14 Lining up the brachial artery with the arrow on the cuff

5 Turn the sphygmomanometer on and allow it to zero (if digital).

6 Inform the participant about what you intend to do and the sensations to be expected when the cuff is inflated (e.g. pressure on the upper arm, tingling sensation in the fingers) and then palpate the radial artery, as per Activity 3.1. While monitoring this pulse, turn the air-release knob fully clockwise and inflate the cuff at approximately 10 mmHg per second, until the radial pulse can no longer be detected. Mentally note the pressure at this point and then rapidly deflate the cuff by turning the air-release knob counter-clockwise. The point at which the pulse disappears is an estimation of the participant's SBP.

7 Place the diaphragm of the stethoscope gently over the brachial artery, as per Activity 3.1 (Figure 3.15), ensuring that the thumb is not on the stethoscope. It is suggested that this position is marked on the skin with a pen if repeat measurements are going to be performed. Excess pressure will cause turbulent flow past that point independent of cuff pressure so keep only a light pressure on the diaphragm. If the artery cannot be palpated then use the previous troubleshooting advice to identify the brachial artery.

8 Wait at least 30 seconds from the deflation of the cuff from the estimation of the SBP and then inflate the cuff to a pressure 30 mmHg above that detected in step 6.

9 Wait for a few seconds before deflating the cuff to allow for any temporary rise in blood pressure, which may occur in association with the action of the cuff inflation.

10 Carefully deflate the cuff at a rate of 2–3 mmHg per second (Figure 3.16) while watching the bar in the column (or dial on the anaeroid) lower and carefully listening to the brachial artery through the stethoscope.

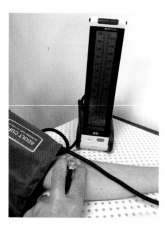

Figure 3.15 Placement of the stethoscope diaphragm over the brachial artery

Used with permission from A&D Medical

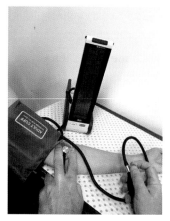

Figure 3.16 Control of deflation is improved with careful handling of the bulb and valve

Used with permission from A&D Medical

11 The highest pressure at which blood flow can be detected is the Korotkoff Phase I sound. You should hear clear rhythmical tapping sounds for three consecutive beats.

> **Note:** The pressure at the first sound is the SBP. It should be recorded to the nearest 2 mmHg and you will need to remember it until the DBP is determined.

12 Continue to deflate the cuff at 2–3 mmHg per second (which will be approximately per pulse beat), noting the changes in Korotkoff sounds, although differentiating between the sounds is not necessary.

13 A 'systolic gap' may occur in some participants when the sounds disappear between the systolic and diastolic pressures. It has no known physiological significance but is one reason why the protocol requires a palpatory estimation of systolic pressure first (in case a silent gap causes the systolic pressure to be missed).

14 Take a reading of the DBP when the repetitive rhythmical sounds disappear. The last sound represents the DBP and should be recorded to the nearest 2 mmHg.

15 Deflate the cuff completely and remove it from the arm.

16 The blood pressure values should be recorded as soon as possible once the cuff is deflated.

17 Wait at least 30 seconds before repeating the measure on the opposite arm. You may need to re-position yourself so that you are close to the other arm.

18 Measure the heart rate (see Activity 3.4) using palpation of the radial artery for determination of rate pressure product.

19 Clean and disinfect all equipment (see Appendix A).

An average of at least two readings should be measured to avoid errors caused by rapid fluctuations in blood pressure. If the two readings differ by more than 10 mmHg systolic or 6 mmHg diastolic, or if initial readings are in the high range, have the participant rest quietly for 5 minutes, then take another reading on the first arm and check that the difference between the measures on the same arm do not vary by greater than these amounts.[27]

Data analysis

Calculate the PP, MAP and RPP and enter these values on the data-recording sheet. For the RPP use the average (of two), or median (of three) SBPs as appropriate.

Data recording

Participant's name: _____   Date: _____

Age: _____ years   Sex: _____

	SBP (mmHg)	DBP (mmHg)	PP (mmHg)	MAP (mmHg)
1st arm				
2nd arm				
3rd measurement on 1st arm (if required)				
Average (of two), or median (of three)[a]				
Rate pressure product: _____				

[a] If the two readings differ by more than 10 mmHg systolic or 6 mmHg diastolic, or if initial readings are in the high range
DBP = diastolic blood pressure; MAP = mean arterial pressure; PP = pulse pressure; SBP = systolic blood pressure

Troubleshooting

- If you hear interference around the points of systole or diastole and you are not confident with the accuracy of the measure you can quickly re-inflate with one or two squeezes and check your measure, or deflate the cuff completely and wait around 30 seconds before trying again.

Interpretation, feedback and discussion

First, consider the four steps of interpretation and the three steps of feedback and discussion outlined in Appendix G. It is important to know that the diagnosis of high blood pressure is made by a medically trained individual and usually based on multiple blood pressure measures on several separate occasions. Taking this into account, Table 3.3 from Australia's National Heart Foundation can be used to categorise (but not diagnose) the blood pressure.

Low blood pressure can be more difficult to interpret and for this reason tables such as Table 3.3 generally do not include this category. It is usually defined as a systolic pressure <90 mmHg and/or a diastolic <60 mmHg. However, if it is not associated with any symptoms, such as lightheadedness or dizziness resulting in a person fainting, it is usually not treated. This usually occurs when a person stands after sitting or lying, and is known as orthostatic or postural hypotension.

🚩 *Blood pressure red flags*

- Blood pressure categorised as high-normal or higher should be discussed in detail with the participant.

TABLE 3.3 Blood pressure classification for adults[a]			
CATEGORY	SBP (mmHg)		DBP (mmHg)
Optimal	<120	and	<80
Normal	120–129	and/or	80–84
High-normal	130–139	and/or	85–89
Grade 1 (mild) hypertension	140–159	and/or	90–99
Grade 2 (moderate) hypertension	160–179	and/or	100–109
Grade 3 (severe) hypertension	≥180	and/or	≥110
Isolated systolic hypertension	>140	and	<90

[a] When a participant's systolic and diastolic pressures fall into different categories, the higher category should be used
Source: National Heart Foundation of Australia[27]

The following feedback assumes you are aware of any medical conditions or medications.

Feedback regarding blood pressure will usually involve telling the participant their blood pressure values and how this is categorised.

If the participant has high-normal or higher you should tell them that their blood pressure is in the respective category (e.g. 'your blood pressure is in the high-normal category').

Then you would ask whether the participant has been made aware of their blood pressure previously. This discussion should include informing them that it is common for people to have elevated blood pressure (white coat hypertension) in a 'clinic' environment. Notwithstanding any caveats, you should strongly suggest that they get their blood pressure measured again, perhaps by you if possible. If they have their blood pressure measured and categorised as grade 1 (mild) hypertension or higher on two separate occasions they should be referred to their medical practitioner.

If the participant has moderate-to-severe hypertension and were unaware of it they should be referred to their medical practitioner straight away.

If the participant has low blood pressure you should ask whether they experience lightheadedness or dizziness. If they do on a semi-regular basis then they should be referred to their medical practitioner.

If they have an abnormal blood pressure you can also suggest that they purchase their own semi-automated blood pressure device for use at home. This suggestion can complement the information regarding white coat hypertension.

Activity 3.6 Inter-tester reliability in blood pressure

AIM: to have your blood pressure measured by two different individuals using the manual method and determine the inter-tester reliability.

Background

This activity is designed to provide extra practice in the manual measurement of blood pressure and show the reliability when different people (inter-tester) measure the same parameter (see Practical 1, Test accuracy, reliability and validity).

Protocol summary

Compare the variability when your blood pressure is measured by two different individuals.

Protocol

1 Using the protocol in Activity 3.5, have two different people measure your blood pressure and record these average/median values in the first two rows of the data-recording sheet.

2 Calculate the pulse pressure (PP) and mean arterial pressures (MAP) from each tester and record these in the first two rows of the data-recording sheet.

3 Calculate the averages of the two testers, measures and record in the third row of the data-recording sheet.

4 Calculate your rate pressure product using the average systolic pressure and the radial heart rate from Activity 3.1.

5 Calculate the inter-tester reliability (percent difference) of the SBP using the following formula:

$$\text{Percent difference} = \left[\frac{\text{largest measure} - \text{smallest measure}}{\text{smallest measure}} \right] \times 100$$

Data recording

Participant's name: _____   Date: _____

Age: _____ years   Sex: _____

	TESTER NAME	SBP (mmHg)	DBP (mmHg)	PP (mmHg)	MAP (mmHg)
1.					
2.					
	Average				

Rate pressure product _____

Inter-tester reliability of SBP _____ %

DBP = diastolic blood pressure; MAP = mean arterial pressure; PP = pulse pressure; SBP = systolic blood pressure

Activity 3.7 Blood pressure – semi-automated device

AIM: measure blood pressure of a participant using a semi-automated device.

Background

Semi-automated blood pressure devices (e.g. Figure 3.17) are useful for obtaining quick blood pressure measures. The quality of these devices differs considerably, affecting the accuracy of the measures. Smaller, more commonly available devices are not accurate when individuals are exercising and therefore exercise professionals need to be skilled in the use of a sphygmomanometer and stethoscope.

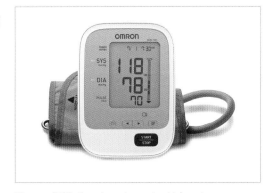

Figure 3.17 Semi-automated blood pressure device

Used with permission from Omron

Protocol summary

Use a semi-automated device to measure blood pressure on a participant.

Protocol

This is dependent on the device but most will require the following steps.

1 Choose the correct size cuff, attach it to the device and then wrap firmly around the participant's upper arm as described in Activity 3.5.

2 Turn the device on and wait for an indication that the measure can be performed.

3 Push the appropriate button to inflate the cuff.

4 The device will inflate and deflate detecting the first and last sounds. Depending upon individual devices, they may also provide the heart rate.

5 Remove the cuff from the arm and record the blood pressure values from the device in the data-recording sheet.

6 Wait at least 30 seconds before repeating the measure on the same arm.

7 Clean and disinfect all equipment (see Appendix A).

An average of at least two readings should be measured to avoid errors caused by rapid fluctuations in blood pressure. If the two readings differ by more than 10 mmHg systolic or 6 mmHg diastolic, or if initial readings are high, have the participant rest quietly for 5 minutes then take additional readings until consecutive readings do not vary by greater than these amounts.

Data analysis

Calculate the pulse pressures and mean arterial pressures (see Activity 3.5).

Data recording

Participant's name: _____   Date: _____

Age: _____ years   Sex: _____

	SBP (mmHg)	DBP (mmHg)	PP (mmHg)	MAP (mmHg)
1st measurement				
2nd measurement				
3rd measurement (if required)				
Average (of two), or median (of three)				
Rate pressure product: _____				

DBP = diastolic blood pressure; MAP = mean arterial pressure; PP = pulse pressure; SBP = systolic blood pressure

Activity 3.8 Exercise blood pressure and accuracy of a wrist-worn heart rate monitor during exercise

AIMS: measure blood pressure of a participant during graded exercise and determine the accuracy of a wrist-worn heart rate monitor during exercise.

Background

A common application of measuring exercise heart rate and blood pressure is during a graded exercise test to provide a safety check on the cardiovascular response to exercise. For example, if the exercise heart rate or blood pressure increases too much during an exercise test then a person may be asked to stop exercising. Blood pressure measurement during sub-maximal exercise intensities may also provide information about high-BP related CVD risk.[33] Exercise stress testing may accompany a measure of cardiorespiratory fitness, but not always. For example, in a cardiac investigation setting the major goal of the test is to see how the ECG pattern and blood pressure change during and after exercise. The ability of exercise professionals to conduct these skills opens career paths working as cardiac technicians in clinical measurement laboratories.

To measure exercise blood pressure it is preferable to use a sphygmomanometer on a stand that can be adjusted so the column is approximately at the level of the heart of the participant (Figure 3.18). Alternatively, a desk sphygmomanometer on an adjustable stand, although not ideal, can also be used.

There are guidelines for the correct measurement of blood pressure during exercise.[38] In general, the methods for measuring exercising blood pressure are similar to that at rest with the following considerations.

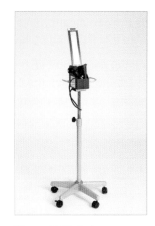

Figure 3.18 Sphygmomanometer on an adjustable stand

Used with permission from A&D Medical

1 The weight of the arm should be supported while blood pressure is being measured to reduce the influence of muscular tension on the brachial artery (Figures 3.19 and 3.20).

2 During exercise it is common to hear the Phase V Korotkoff sounds down to, or close to, 0 mmHg. If this occurs then DBP is measured at the onset of the Korotkoff Phase IV sound (becomes softer and muffled).

In around 2014 the first wrist-worn heart rate monitor was commercially available. These devices have optical sensors that detect the changes in blood volume in vessels close to the skin as a measure of heart rate. The technology is now incorporated into most smart watches and is becoming a popular approach for monitoring the heart rate. Indeed, a number of studies have reported good agreement between heart rates from various different wrist-worn monitors and ECG-derived heart rates at rest and during exercise.[7,39] In this activity we will compare the heart rate values obtained from a wrist-worn device and the chest strap heart rate monitor that have been shown to be accurate.[6]

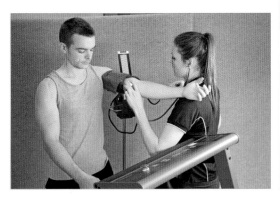
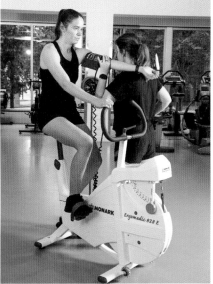

Figures 3.19 and 3.20 Supporting the arm during exercise blood pressure measurement

Protocol summary

The participant cycles for 3 minutes at 300 kilopond metres per minute (kpm/min) and then 3 minutes at 600 kpm/min. The heart rate and blood pressure are measured at rest and during the last minute of each exercise stage.

Protocol

1 Follow the pre-exercise test procedures outlined in Appendix B.

2 Check Appendix C to ensure that there are no contraindications to exercise testing.

3 Fit a chest strap heart rate monitor to the participant (see Activity 3.3).

4 Provide the participant with a wrist-worn heart rate monitor, or allow them to use their own. Start the device so that it is measuring the heart rate.

5 Position the participant on the cycle ergometer and adjust the seat (the knee should be slightly bent at around 5° when the pedal is at the furthest point from the seat in the crank cycle) and handlebars (such that the participant is comfortable).

6 Adjust the sphygmomanometer so that the column/dial is approximately level with the heart of the participant.

7 Place the blood pressure cuff on the participant, support the weight of the arm and measure the pre-exercise blood pressure.

8 Record the pre-exercise heart rate from both watches at the same time (as close as possible).

9 Start the participant exercising at a work rate of 300 kpm/min (to set the Monark, see Table 11.1) and ask them to cycle at this intensity for 3 minutes.

10 Measure the blood pressure during the 3rd minute. You should start inflating the cuff after 2 minutes. This will give you adequate time (1 minute) to take the blood pressure.

11 Record the heart rate at the end of the 3 minutes from both watches at the same time (as close as possible).

12 After the 3rd minute (or after the blood pressure has been obtained) increase the work rate to 600 kpm/min (to set the Monark, see Table 11.1).

13 Measure the blood pressure during the 6th minute.

14 Record the heart rate at the 6th minute from both watches at the same time (as close as possible).

15 Stop the test.

16 Clean and disinfect all equipment (see Appendix A).

Data analysis

Calculate the accuracy (percentage difference) of the wrist-worn heart rate monitor at the three different time points using the following formula:

$$\text{Percent difference} = \left[\frac{\text{largest measure} - \text{smallest measure}}{\text{smallest measure}}\right] \times 100$$

Calculate the average accuracy of the wrist-worn heart rate monitor from the three different time points.

Data recording

Participant's name: _____ Date: _____

Age: _____ years   Sex: _____

TIME	CHEST STRAP HEART RATE MONITOR (BPM)	WRIST-WORN HEART RATE MONITOR (BPM)	SBP (mmHg)	DBP (mmHg)
Pre-exercise				
3rd minute				
6th minute				

continued

Data recording *(continued)*

	CHEST STRAP HEART RATE MONITOR (BPM)	WRIST-WORN HEART RATE MONITOR (BPM)	SBP (mmHg)	DBP (mmHg)
Accuracy of wrist-worn heart rate monitor				
Pre-exercise: _____ %				
3rd minute: _____ %				
6th minute: _____ %				
Average: _____ %				
DBP = diastolic blood pressure; SBP = systolic blood pressure				

Risk scores

There are many tools to assess cardiovascular disease risk using predictive equations.[40] Many of these approaches, including the one to be used in Activity 3.9, are based on the Framingham Risk Equation. This was developed using data from a longitudinal prospective study of over 5000 people, which started in 1948 in Framingham, Massachusetts.[41] This study led to the development of the term 'risk factor'. One of the main findings of the study has been that the probability of an individual developing CVD depends more on the combination and intensity of risk factors than on the presence of any single risk factor. This is because the cumulative effects of multiple factors are synergistic. As a result of this study the Framingham Risk Equation was established. Risk scores are being used in general health and fitness assessments and exercise professionals should be aware of the purposes and limitations of these approaches.

One of the main purposes of using a risk estimator is to raise the awareness of individual CVD risk factors to motivate adherence to recommended lifestyle changes or therapies. In clinical practice, risk prediction algorithms have been used to identify individuals at high risk for developing CVD in the short term and to determine the individuals who need more-intensive preventive interventions. A major limitation of risk scores is that age (an unmodifiable risk factor) is a heavily weighted variable. In addition, as most risk scores are based on the Framingham Study, they have been developed using data from a small, middle-class, predominantly white population from a single town in the USA; therefore prognostic validity is decreased when it is applied to a person from a different ethnicity.[42] The failure to include socioeconomic status and chronic kidney disease, factors known to impact CVD risk, also decreases their validity.[43]

Activity 3.9 Australian Cardiovascular Disease Risk Charts

AIM: use the Australian Cardiovascular Disease Risk Charts to assess the 5-year CVD risk of a participant and provide feedback.

Background

The Australian Cardiovascular Risk Charts are based on guidelines from the National Vascular Disease Prevention Alliance (NVDPA) using the Framingham Risk Equation.[44] They have been developed for people without (Figure 3.21) or with (Figure 3.22) diabetes, aged 45 years or over (and all Aboriginal and Torres Strait Islander adults aged 35–74 years), without known history of CVD and not already known to be at a clinically determined high risk. The charts estimate the risk of developing CVD over the next 5 years. These include coronary heart disease, stroke and other vascular disease including peripheral arterial disease and renovascular disease.

Protocol summary

Assess the 5-year CVD risk of a participant and provide feedback.

Protocol

1 Using either Figure 3.21 (non-diabetes) or Figure 3.22 (diabetes), calculate the 5-year risk of CVD (see Box 3.2) of a participant. Recognise that the charts are not valid (prognostically) in people under 45 years of age. If you are unable to complete this activity on someone of that age then using a younger person will still provide experience in using the charts.

2 Record the value.
   Information required for the Australian Cardiovascular Disease Risk Charts:

   - age
   - sex
   - ethnicity
   - total cholesterol:HDL cholesterol ratio
   - SBP
   - diabetes status
   - smoking status.

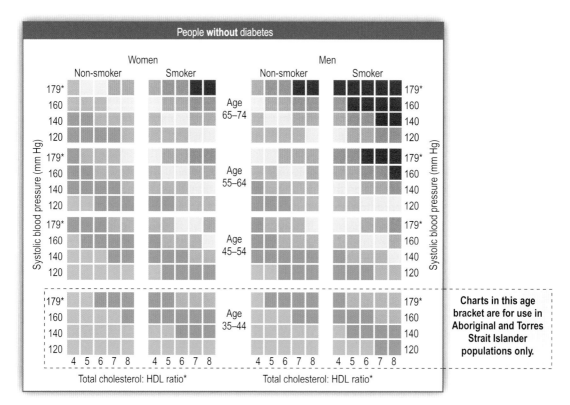

* In accordance with Australian guidelines, patients with systolic blood pressure ≥180 mmHg, or a total cholesterol of >7.5 mmol/L, should be considered at clinically determined high absolute risk of CVD.

Risk level for 5-year cardiovascular (CVD) risk

High risk	Moderate risk	Low risk
≥30%	10–15%	5–9%
25–29%		<5%
20–24%		
16–19%		

Figure 3.21 Australian Cardiovascular Risk Charts for people without diabetes

Source: National Vascular Disease Prevention Alliance[44]

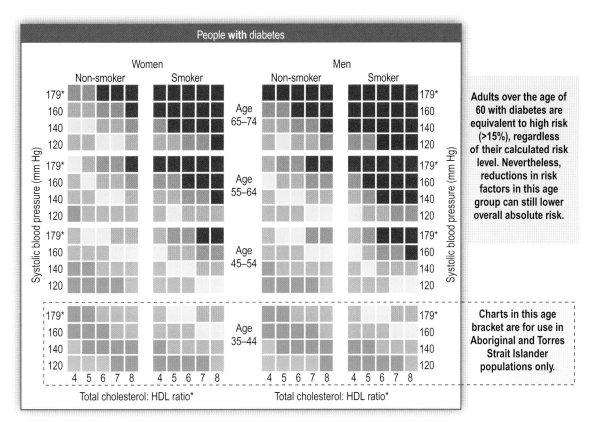

* In accordance with Australian guidelines, patients with systolic blood pressure ≥180 mmHg, or a total cholesterol of >7.5 mmol/L, should be considered at clinically determined high absolute risk of CVD.

Risk level for 5-year cardiovascular (CVD) risk

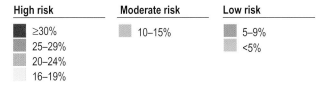

High risk
- ≥30%
- 25–29%
- 20–24%
- 16–19%

Moderate risk
- 10–15%

Low risk
- 5–9%
- <5%

Figure 3.22 Australian Cardiovascular Risk Charts for people with diabetes

Source: National Vascular Disease Prevention Alliance[44]

Box 3.2 How to use the Australian Cardiovascular Disease Risk Charts

Step 1
Identify the chart relating to the person's sex, diabetes status, smoking history and age.

Step 2
Within the chart choose the cell *nearest* to the person's age, SBP and total cholesterol (TC):HDL ratio. If a participant has a value that is exactly between those in the chart (e.g. TC:HDL ratio of 5.5) then the higher value cell should be used.

Step 3
The colour of the cell that the person falls into provides their 5-year absolute cardiovascular risk level (see the legend below each chart for risk category). People who fall exactly on a threshold between cells are placed in the cell indicating higher risk.

Data recording
Participant's 5-year risk of cardiovascular disease _____ %
Risk = _____

Feedback, discussion and implications

First, consider the four steps of interpretation and the three steps of feedback and discussion outlined in Appendix G. The process of calculating the risk score allows for the participant to understand what factors contribute to the level of risk. Feedback should focus on the factors that can be modified and suggestions should be provided to assist the participant to reduce their risk, if necessary. It would be useful to state that these scores are designed to help medical practitioners with decisions regarding initiation, type and intensity of treatment (e.g. cholesterol-lowering treatment and blood pressure management).[45] The risk scores can result in an informed discussion between a medical practitioner and patient regarding lifestyle changes and pharmacological treatment. This may motivate individuals to improve their health-related behaviours, with the ultimate goal to prevent CVD events. They also provide an opportunity to prioritise individuals with the highest CVD risk leading to a targeted allocation of resources.[45]

Risk score red flags

The risk score calculator is colour coded to identify an individual who has a risk factor, or a total risk factor score that should prompt referral to a medical practitioner.

The following are some examples of verbal feedback that could be provided to a participant:

'You have a 5-year risk of cardiovascular disease of less than 5%, which is low risk. This is because you have low cholesterol, normal blood pressure and you do not have diabetes. Your healthy lifestyle has most likely contributed to this low risk. Eating healthy foods and being physically active will keep these values in the healthy range.'

'You have a 5-year risk of cardiovascular disease of between 10% and 15%, which is moderate risk. This is because I have measured your cholesterol and blood pressure and found them to be above normal. These values will need to be checked by a medical practitioner so I would recommend you see your doctor and I would like to send him a letter to explain what I have found. It is important to know that eating healthy foods and being physically active can decrease your cholesterol and blood pressure and I am sure your doctor will discuss this further with you.'

'You have a 5-year risk of cardiovascular disease of more than 30%, which is categorised as high risk. This is because I have measured your cholesterol and blood pressure and found them to be above normal and you smoke. These values will need to be checked by a medical practitioner so I would recommend you see your doctor as soon as possible and I would like to send him a letter to explain what I have found. It is important to know that by stopping smoking, eating healthy foods and being physically active you can decrease your risk of cardiovascular disease and I am sure your doctor will discuss this further with you.'

Case studies

Setting: You work in a health and fitness centre that requires members to undertake a fitness test as part of their membership requirements. When members join they complete the Adult Pre-exercise Screening System (APSS) and are given pre-test instructions for the fitness test. You are responsible for conducting the fitness test, which includes resting heart rate and blood pressure measures. Blood pressure is recorded as the average of two measures separated by at least 30 seconds, with the two readings not differing by more than 10 mmHg systolic or 6 mmHg diastolic. You are expected to provide feedback to the client during the appointment.

Case Study 1

Kelly is a 29-year-old female who has answered 'No' to all questions on the APSS and indicated she has no known medical conditions and is not taking any medications. Before taking the resting measures, you confirm Kelly has followed the pre-test instructions. You obtain the following values and are confident they are accurate:

Heart rate $=$ 74 bpm; average BP $=$ 134/92 mmHg

What questions would you ask Kelly and what feedback would you provide?

Case Study 2

Michael is a 51-year-old male who has answered 'No' to all questions on the APSS and indicated he has no known medical conditions and is not taking any medications. Before taking the resting measures, you confirm he has followed the pre-test instructions. You obtain the following values and are confident they are accurate:

Heart rate $=$ 82 bpm; average BP $=$ 148/106 mmHg

What questions would you ask and what feedback would you provide?

Case Study 3

Emma is a 21-year-old female who has answered 'No' to all questions on the APSS and indicated she has no known medical conditions and is not taking any medications. Before taking the resting measures, you confirm Emma has followed the pre-test instructions. You obtain the following values and are confident they are accurate:

Heart rate $=$ 58 bpm; average BP $=$ 84/64 mmHg

What questions would you ask and what feedback would you provide?

Case Study 4

A participant fills in the attached details on the Australian Cardiovascular Risk Chart:

Sandie – 55-year-old Caucasian female
Total cholesterol:HDL cholesterol ratio $=$ 6.6
SBP $=$ 146/82 mmHg
Diabetes $=$ yes
Smoker $=$ yes

What questions would you ask and what feedback would you provide?

References

[1] Australian Institute of Health and Welfare. Deaths in Australia (2019). PHE 229. 25 June 2021. https://www.aihw.gov.au/reports/life-expectancy-death/deaths-in-australia/contents/leading-causes-of-death.

[2] Lequeux B, Uzan C, Rehman MB. Does resting heart rate measured by the physician reflect the patient's true resting heart rate? White-coat heart rate. Indian Heart J 2018;70:93–8.

[3] Jensen MT, Suadicani P, Hein HO, Gyntelberg F. Elevated resting heart rate, physical fitness and all-cause mortality: a 16-year follow-up in the Copenhagen Male Study. Heart 2013;99:882–7.

[4] Nes BM, Janszky I, Vatten LJ, Nilsen TIL, Aspenes ST, Wisløff U. Estimating $\dot{V}O_2$ peak from a nonexercise prediction model: the HUNT Study, Norway. Med Sci Sports Exerc 2011;43:2024–30.

[5] Vogel CU, Wolpert C, Wehling M. How to measure heart rate? Eur J Clin Pharmacol 2004;60:461–6.

[6] Laukkanen RM, Virtanen PK. Heart rate monitors: state of the art. J Sports Sci 1998;16 Suppl:S3–7.

[7] Wallen MP, Gomersall SR, Keating SE, Wisløff U, Coombes J. Accuracy of heart rate watches: implications for weight management. PLoS One 2016;11:e0154420.

[8] Johansen CD, Olsen RH, Pedersen LR, Kumarathurai P, Mette R, Mouridsen MR, et al. Resting, night-time, and 24 h heart rate as markers of cardiovascular risk in middle-aged and elderly men and women with no apparent heart disease. Eur Heart J 2013;34:1732–9.

[9] Custodis F, Roggenbuck U, Lehmann N, Moebus S, Laufs U, Mahabadi A-A, et al. Resting heart rate is an independent predictor of all-cause mortality in the middle aged general population. Clin Res Cardiol 2016;105:601–12.

[10] Bøhm M, Reil JC, Deedwania P, Kim JB, Borer JS. Resting heart rate: risk indicator and emerging risk factor in cardiovascular disease. Am J Med 2015;128:219–28.

[11] Gillum RF, Makuc DM, Feldman JJ. Pulse rate, coronary heart disease, and death: the NHANES I Epidemiologic Follow-up Study. Am Heart J 1991;121:172–7.

[12] Custodis F, Reil JC, Laufs U, Bøhm M. Heart rate: a global target for cardiovascular disease and therapy along the cardiovascular disease continuum. J Cardiol 2013;62:183–7.

[13] Laukkanen JA, Kurl S, Salonen B, Rauramaa R, Solonen JT. The predictive value of cardiorespiratory fitness for cardiovascular events in men with various risk profiles: a prospective population-based cohort study. Eur Heart J 2004;25:1428–37.

[14] Currie KD, Floras JS, La Gerche A, Goodman JM. Exercise blood pressure guidelines: time to re-evaluate what is normal and exaggerated? Sports Med 2018;48:1763–71.

[15] Royal Australian College of General Practitioners. Guidelines for preventative activities in general practice, 9th ed. The red book, 8.2 Blood pressure. East Melbourne, Vic: RACGP; 2018. https://www.racgp.org.au/your-practice/guidelines/redbook/8-prevention-of-vascular-and-metabolic-disease/82-blood-pressure/.

[16] Parati G, Faini A, Castiglioni P. Accuracy of blood pressure measurement: sphygmomanometer calibration and beyond. J Hypertens 2006;24:1915–18.

[17] Sharman JE, LaGerche A. Exercise blood pressure: clinical relevance and correct measurement. J Hum Hypertens. 2015;29:351–8.

[18] Shinohara T, Tsuchida N, Seki K, Otani T, Yamane T, Ishihara Y, et al. Can blood pressure be measured during exercise with an automated sphygmomanometer based on an oscillometric method? J Phys Ther Sci 2017;29:1006–9.

[19] Stride blood pressure. Validated blood pressure monitors. https://stridebp.org/bp-monitors.

[20] Menzies Institute for Medical Research. How to check that a blood pressure monitor has been properly tested for accuracy. https://www.menzies.utas.edu.au/documents/pdfs/Blood-pressure-devices.pdf

[21] Picone DS, Padwal R, Campbell NRC, Boutouyrie P, Brady TM, Olsen MH, et al. How to check whether a blood pressure monitor has been properly validated for accuracy. J Clin Hypertens 22;12, 2167–74.

[22] Head GA, McGrath BP, Mihailidou AS, Nelson MR, Schlaich MP, Stowasser M, et al. Ambulatory blood pressure monitoring in Australia: 2011 consensus position statement. J Hypertens 2012;30:253–66.

[23] Parati G, Stergiou GS, Bilo G, Kollias A, Pengo M, Ochoa JE, et al. Home blood pressure monitoring: methodology, clinical relevance and practical application: a 2021 position paper by the Working Group on Blood Pressure Monitoring and Cardiovascular Variability of the European Society of Hypertension. J Hypertens 2021;39(9):1742–67.

[24] Selenta C, Hogan BE, Linden W. How often do office blood pressure measurements fail to identify true hypertension? An exploration of white-coat normotension. Arch Fam Med 2000;9:533–40.

[25] Australian Bureau of Statistics. 2017/18. National health survey. https://www.abs.gov.au/ausstats/abs@.nsf/Lookup/by%20Subject/4364.0.55.001~201718~Main%20Features~Hypertension%20and%20measured%20high%20blood%20pressure~60.

[26] Ho CLB, Breslin M, Doust J, Reid CM, Nelson MR. Effectiveness of blood pressure-lowering drug treatment by levels of absolute risk: post hoc analysis of the Australian National Blood Pressure Study. BMJ Open 2018;8:e017723.

[27] National Heart Foundation of Australia. Guideline for the diagnosis and management of hypertension in adults – 2016. Melbourne, Vic: National Heart Foundation of Australia; 2016. https://www.heartfoundation.org.au/getmedia/c83511ab-835a-4fcf-96f5-88d770582ddc/PRO-167_Hypertension-guideline-2016_WEB.pdf.

[28] Sharman JE, Howes FS, Head GA, McGrath BP, Stowasser M, Schlaich M, et al. Home blood pressure monitoring: Australian Expert Consensus Statement. J Hypertens 2015;33:1721–8.

[29] Heart Foundation of Australia. Measuring your blood pressure at home. https://www.hbprca.com.au/wp-content/uploads/2021/08/Home-BP-monitoring-infographic.pdf.

[30] Fletcher GF, Ades PA, Kligfield P, Arena R, Balady GJ, Bittner VA, et al. Exercise standards for testing and training: a scientific statement from the American Heart Association. Circulation 2013;128:873–934.

[31] Schultz MG, Otahal P, Cleland VJ, Blizzard L, Marwick TH, Sharman JE. Exercise-induced hypertension, cardiovascular events, and mortality in patients undergoing exercise stress testing: a systematic review and meta-analysis. Am J Hypertens 2013;26:357–66.

[32] Schultz MG, Otahal P, Picone DS, Sharman JE. Clinical relevance of exaggerated exercise blood pressure. J Am Coll Cardiol. 2015;66:1843–5.

[33] Schultz MG, La Gerche A and Sharman JE. Blood pressure response to exercise and cardiovascular disease. Curr Hypertens Rep 2017;19:89.

[34] Blacher J, Staessen JA, Girerd X, Gasowski J, Thijs L, Liu L, et al. Pulse pressure not mean pressure determines cardiovascular risk in older hypertensive patients. Arch Intern Med 2000;160:1085–9.

[35] Thooft A, Favory R, Salgado DR, Taccone FS, Donadello K, De Backer D, et al. Effects of changes in arterial pressure on organ perfusion during septic shock. Crit Care 2011;15:R222.

[36] Schultz MG, Picone DS, Armstrong MK, Black JA, Dwyer N, Roberts-Thomson P, et al. The influence of SBP amplification on the accuracy of form-factor-derived mean arterial pressure. J Hypertens 2020;38:1033–9.

[37] Gobel FL, Norstrom LA, Nelson RR, Jorgensen CR, Wang Y. The rate-pressure product as an index of myocardial oxygen consumption during exercise in patients with angina pectoris. Circulation 1978;57:549–56.

[38] Sharman JE, LaGerche A. Exercise blood pressure: clinical relevance and correct measurement. J Hum Hypertens 2015;29:351–8.

[39] Wang R, Blackburn G, Desai M, Phelan D, Gillinov L, Houghtaling P, et al. Accuracy of wrist-worn heart rate monitors. JAMA Cardiol 2017;2:104–6.

[40] Lloyd-Jones DM. Cardiovascular risk prediction: basic concepts, current status, and future directions. Circulation 2010;121:1768–77.

[41] Wilson PW, D'Agostino RB, Levy D, Belanger AM, Silbershatz H, Kannel WB. Prediction of coronary heart disease using risk factor categories. Circulation 1998;97:1837–47.

[42] Chia YC, Gray SY, Ching SM, Lim HM, Chinna K. Validation of the Framingham general cardiovascular risk score in a multiethnic Asian population: a retrospective cohort study. BMJ Open 2015;5:e007324.

[43] Backholer K, Hirakawa Y, Tonkin A, Giles G, Magliano DJ, Colagiuri S, et al. Development of an Australian cardiovascular disease mortality risk score using multiple imputation and recalibration from national statistics. BMC Cardiovasc Disord 2017;17:17.

[44] National Vascular Disease Prevention Alliance. Absolute cardiovascular disease risk management, quick reference guide for health professionals. 2012. ©2012 National Stroke Foundation. https://www.cvdcheck.org.au/pdf/Absolute_CVD_Risk-Quick_Reference_Guide.pdf.

[45] Usher-Smith JA, Silarova B, Schuit E, Moons KGM, Griffin SJ. Impact of provision of cardiovascular disease risk estimates to healthcare professionals and patients: a systematic review. BMJ Open 2015;5:e008717.

PRACTICAL 4
PHYSIQUE ASSESSMENT

Tina Skinner, Gary Slater and Kellie Pritchard-Peschek

LEARNING OBJECTIVES

- Explain the scientific rationale, purposes, reliability, validity, assumptions and limitations of common measures of physique traits
- Identify and explain the common terminology, processes and equipment required to conduct accurate and safe measures of physique traits
- Identify and describe considerations that may require modification to measures of physique traits, and make appropriate adjustments for relevant populations or participants
- Describe the principles and rationale for the calibration of equipment commonly used for measures of anthropometry
- Conduct appropriate pre-assessment procedures, including explaining the test
- Identify the need for guidance or further information from a relevant health professional
- Select and conduct appropriate protocols for safe and effective anthropometry, bioelectrical impedance analysis, dual-energy x-ray absorptiometry and air displacement plethysmography measurements
- Record, analyse and interpret information from anthropometric assessments and convey the results, including the validity and limitations of the assessments, through relevant verbal and/or written communication to a participant

Equipment and other requirements

- Information sheet and informed consent form
- Skinfold calipers
- Self-retracting, flexible metal anthropometry tape
- Marker pen
- Alcohol swabs
- Segmometer
- Anthropometry box (dimensions 40 cm $\times$ 50 cm $\times$ 30 cm)
- Stadiometer (wall-mounted or portable)
- Body mass scales
- Bioelectrical impedance analysis (BIA) device
- BOD POD system
- Dual-energy x-ray absorptiometry (DXA) scanner
- Calculator

INTRODUCTION

Assessments of physique traits by exercise professionals are routine measurements, with applications across a broad range of situations, including:

- general health screening in lifestyle-related disease risk assessment
- monitoring the effectiveness of lifestyle (i.e. diet and/or exercise) or other (e.g. pharmacological or surgical) interventions
- assessing long-term change in body composition
- talent identification within the sporting environment.

A strong association exists between lifestyle, disease risk and overweight or obesity. Specifically, the central distribution of body fat significantly increases the risk of a range of diseases, including type 2 diabetes mellitus, hypertension and hyperlipidaemia.[1] In an attempt to assess and monitor changes in the central distribution of body fat, and the risk of cardiometabolic disease of an individual, anthropometric measurements such as the body mass index (BMI) and waist-to-hip ratio (WHR) are commonly used screening tools in many settings, owing to their simplicity and low cost.[2] The use of waist circumference is an alternative measurement to WHR, as it appears to be unaffected by either sex or the degree of overall adiposity of an individual.[2] BMI, WHR and waist circumference, or derivations of this, are the most common assessment measures that are used to screen an individual for metabolic disease risk.

A relationship between competitive success and physique traits has been identified in an array of sports, including football codes,[3] aesthetically judged sports,[4] swimming,[5] track and field events[6] and skiing,[7] as well as lightweight[8] and heavyweight rowing.[9] The specific physique traits associated with competitive success vary with the sport. For athletes participating in aesthetically judged sports, maintenance of low body fat levels is associated with positive outcomes.[10–12] A similar relationship exists in sports where frontal surface area, power-to-weight ratio and/or thermoregulation are important.[13] However, in sports demanding high force production, muscle mass may be more closely associated with performance outcomes.[3,5] Likewise, in sports such as rowing, other physique traits such as a shorter sitting height (relative to height) and longer limb lengths are related to competitive success,[14] with such information used successfully in talent identification.[15] Because of these relationships, it has become common practice to monitor physique traits of athletes in response to growth, training and/or dietary interventions.

Despite the association between physique traits and competitive success, the assessment of body composition among athletes, especially female athletes and dancers, has been questioned owing to the possibility of promoting anxiety and disordered eating.[16] This comes despite recognition that evidence supporting a causal relationship between body composition assessments and disordered eating has yet to be established. Furthermore, when performed in conjunction with a suitably designed education program, current evidence indicates physique assessments can be performed without promoting adverse affective consequences.[17] Given this, concurrent education of athletes on the rationale for assessments makes good sense and should be actively promoted, with consideration given to the sensitivity of such assessments during both data capture and reporting.

An array of techniques is available for the measurement of physique traits, including anthropometric measurements, radiographic (computed tomography (CT), dual-energy x-ray absorptiometry (DXA)) and other medical imaging techniques (magnetic resonance imaging (MRI), ultrasound), metabolic (creatinine, 3-methylhistidine) and nuclear (total body potassium, total body nitrogen) tests and bioelectrical impedance analysis (BIA). When selecting the most appropriate approach, a range of factors should be considered, including technical issues such as the safety, validity, reliability and accuracy of measurement. Practical issues must also be taken into account such as equipment availability, financial implications, portability, invasiveness, time effectiveness and technical expertise necessary to conduct the procedures. Consideration must also be given to the ability of physique trait assessment methodologies to accommodate the unique body composition characteristics of some participants, including particularly tall, broad and muscular individuals or those with extremely high or low body fat levels.

For reasons of timeliness, practicality and cost effectiveness, the routine monitoring of body composition is most often performed using anthropometric measurement of body mass, subcutaneous skinfold thicknesses and girths at specific anatomical landmarks. In addition, surface anthropometry requires relatively inexpensive equipment that is easily portable (Figure 4.1); therefore, this practical reviews the use of surface anthropometry and indices of heaviness (including scale weight as well as BMI), as these are the most commonly used techniques to assess the physique traits of the majority of participants.

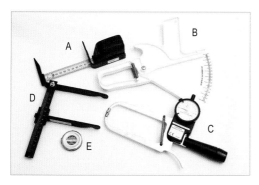

Figure 4.1 Surface anthropometry equipment: A, segmometer; B and C, skinfold calipers; D, small bone calipers; E, anthropometry tape

Used with permission from University of Western Australia, Baty International Limited, Harpenden, Rosscraft and Lufkin

DEFINITIONS

Body mass index (BMI): a population-based measure of obesity-related disease risk calculated as body mass (in kilograms) divided by height (in metres) squared (kg/m^2).

Frankfort plane: position of the head when the orbitale (lower edge of the eye socket) is in the same horizontal plane as the tragion (the notch superior to the tragus of the ear).

Index of central obesity (ICO): also known as waist-to-height ratio, this is a population-based measure of central obesity and obesity-related disease risk calculated as waist circumference (in centimetres) divided by height (in centimetres).

Inter-tester reliability: also known as between-tester reliability, this is the amount of agreement (reliability) between two different testers measuring the same parameter on the same individual.

Intra-tester reliability: also known as within-tester reliability, this is the amount of agreement (reliability) from the same tester measuring the same parameter on different occasions.

Mid-prone position: the participant assumes a relaxed standing position with the arm hanging by the side and the thumb pointing forwards.

Osteopenia: a medical condition in which the protein and mineral content of bone tissue is reduced, but less severely than in osteoporosis.

Osteoporosis: a medical condition in which the bones become brittle and fragile from loss of tissue. It is characterised by decreased bone mineral density (2.5 standard deviations or more below the mean for young adults) and altered micro-architecture, resulting in compromised bone strength and increased risk for fracture.

Reliability: the ability of a measure to provide consistent/repeatable data.

Visceral adipose tissue: also known as intra-abdominal fat or visceral fat, this describes the fat tissue located deep in the abdomen and around the internal organs.

PARTICIPANT PRESENTATION

For all body composition assessments, participants should present in a euhydrated state. Hydration status should be confirmed using at least one of the techniques described in Appendix B. Participants should ideally undergo body composition assessment after an overnight fast with no physical activity for at least 8 hours. The bladder should be emptied and all metal objects removed. The facility for assessment should offer privacy for the participant and be maintained to ensure thermoneutral conditions.

Body mass can be acutely influenced by an array of factors, independent of changes in fat mass or skeletal muscle mass. Adults can exhibit diurnal variation of approximately 1% in height and 2 kg in body mass over the course of the day.[18] Consequently, body mass measurements should be made at the same time of day (preferably upon waking, before breakfast or training but after voiding the bladder and bowel), at least when serial measurements are performed over time, and wearing minimal clothing,[19] so as to minimise the influence of extraneous factors that can impact on body mass. Other considerations to improve the accuracy of body mass measurements include consistency in the scales used,[20] the phase of the menstrual cycle in females[21] and hydration status.

In preparation for a DXA test, the participant should be advised to wear minimal clothing free of metal (e.g. zippers, bras with underwire) and reflective material (e.g. as found on many exercise tights), and not too compressive of the skin. While small amounts of food and fluid do not appear to influence results,[22] larger volumes influence the measurement of lean body mass, and thus measurements should be performed in a fasted state wherever possible.[23]

In preparation for air displacement plethysmography testing, the participant should be advised to wear a tight-fitting swimsuit or single-layer compression garments with a swim cap, and to remove excess facial hair.

SURFACE ANTHROPOMETRY

Among population groups such as athletes or the obese, consideration must be given to the unique physique traits these individuals may possess, including particularly tall, broad and/or muscular individuals as well as those with very low or high body fat levels. Taken together, height, body mass, girths and skinfolds comprise surface anthropometry. Taken separately, the measures comprising surface anthropometry can be used to determine obesity-related disease risk calculations – that is, height and body mass to determine the BMI, waist and hip circumferences to determine the waist:hip ratio, and skinfolds to determine sum of six skinfolds and body fat percentage. Surface anthropometry continues to be utilised for the routine monitoring of body composition, although BIA and DXA are becoming more popular as their accessibility increases.[24]

Precise assessment of anthropometric traits, in particular skinfold thickness, can be difficult; therefore extreme care in site location and measurement is required if meaningful results are to be obtained.[25] Prior to assessment, the tester should develop the appropriate technique, reducing the level of error in repeated measurements, and thus enhancing the ability to detect small but potentially important changes. The standard assessment protocol of the International Society for the Advancement of Kinanthropometry (ISAK)[26] is recommended. Testers wishing to monitor the physique traits of individuals using surface anthropometry are strongly encouraged to undertake professional training through accredited courses.

Activity 4.1 Body mass index (BMI)

AIMS: measure height and body mass to classify obesity-related disease risk within an adult population, interpret the results and provide feedback to a participant.

Background

The BMI measure was developed to classify obesity-related disease risk in large-scale population-based studies. This is where BMI is very useful and gives a good indication of health at a population/sub-population level. However, it is used extensively to interpret the body composition of individuals using population-based category ranges. This is a significant limitation and caution should be taken when interpreting individual results from a test designed for population-based assessment. It is recommended that individual BMI results not be interpreted in isolation; that is, if a participant's BMI is calculated, feedback should be provided only in combination with other measures of physique traits.

When BMI cut-offs are applied at an individual level, a number of assumptions are made that may result in inappropriate classification of disease risk. For example, there is no distinction in the composition of total body mass, thus muscular athletes are often categorised at an increased disease risk owing to their higher body mass relative to their height. As such, BMI is best combined with a measure of body fat distribution such as a waist girth, waist-to-hip (WHR) ratio or an index of central obesity, as this more validly describes disease risk.[27]

Protocol summary

Measure the participant's height and body mass in duplicate (or triplicate as required), dividing the mass in kilograms by the height in metres squared to determine BMI.

Protocol

Height (stretch stature)

1 Follow the pre-test procedures outlined in Appendix B.

2 Two people are required to measure the participant's height: the measurer and a recorder.

3 Ask the participant to remove their shoes.

4 The participant then stands directly under the stadiometer with their feet together and their heels, buttocks, and upper part of their back touching the wall or the stadiometer.

5 The participant's head should be positioned in the Frankfort plane. This plane is achieved by placing the tips of the thumbs on each orbitale, and the index fingers on each tragion, then horizontally aligning the two (Figure 4.2a). You then relocate your thumbs posteriorly towards the participant's ears, and far enough along the line of the jaw to ensure that upward pressure, when applied, is transferred through the mastoid processes (Figure 4.2b).

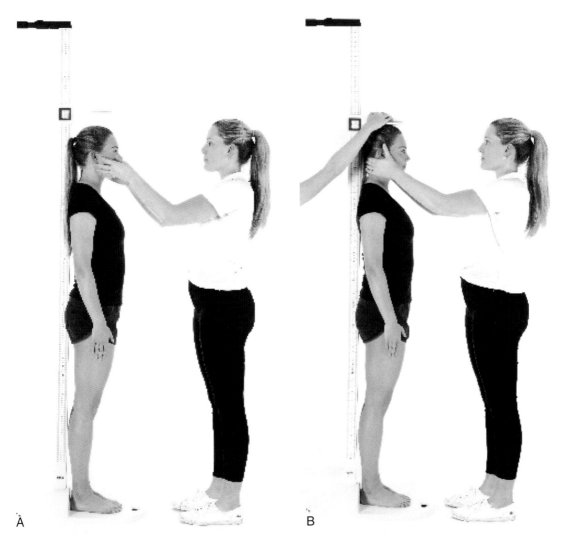

A   B

Figure 4.2 a: The Frankfort plane. b: Application of upward pressure through the mastoid processes for measurement of stretch stature

Used with permission from Seca

6 Instruct the participant to take in and hold a deep breath while keeping the head in the Frankfort plane.

7 Apply a gentle upward lift through the mastoid processes.

8 The recorder brings the stadiometer tape down until it is placed firmly on the vertex, crushing the participant's hair as much as possible. Ensure that the heels do not leave the floor and that the position of the head is maintained in the Frankfort plane.

9 Depending on the stadiometer and the height of the tester, it may be helpful for the tester to stand on an anthropometry box so that the reading is made at eye level.

10 The measurement is recorded at the end of a deep inward breath.

Body mass

1 Follow the pre-test procedures outlined in Appendix B.

2 The bladder should be voided prior to assessment.

3 If using scales with an analogue dial, position the scales where you will be able to read the dial clearly and directly from the front (i.e. reading the dial upside down) (Figure 4.3).

4 Where possible, calibrate the scales to ensure that they are reading zero.

5 The participant should be dressed in minimal clothing with shoes removed and pockets emptied.

6 Ask the participant to stand on the centre of the scales without support and with the body mass evenly distributed on both feet.

7 Ask the participant to hold their head up and look directly ahead.

8 When the body mass measure stabilises, record the result.

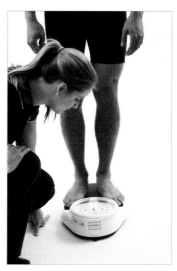

Figure 4.3 Positioning of head directly over the scales to avoid parallax error when measuring body mass

Used with permission from Ecomed Products

Data analysis

Perform measures for two rotations (trial 1 and trial 2) of height and body mass. If there is $\leq 1.5\%$ difference between the two measures (i.e. trial 1 height vs trial 2 height; trial 1 body mass vs trial 2 body mass), record the mean (average) of these measures. If there is $>1.5\%$ difference between the two measures, perform a third measure and record the median. To calculate whether your measures are $\leq 1.5\%$:

$$\text{Percent difference} = \left[\frac{\text{largest measure} - \text{smallest measure}}{\text{smallest measure}} \right] \times 100$$

Data recording

Participant's name: _____ Date: _____

Age: _____ years   Sex: _____

MEASURE	TRIAL 1	TRIAL 2	TRIAL 3 (IF REQUIRED)ᵃ	MEAN OR MEDIANᵇ
Height (cm)				
Body mass (kg)				

ᵃ Take a third measure if the difference between trials 1 and 2 is $>1.5\%$.
ᵇ Record the mean if only two measures are performed. Record the median if three measures are performed.

Calculate BMI for participants using the mean/median of body mass and height in the equation:

BMI = body mass (kg)/height^2 (m)

BMI = _____ kg/m^2

continued overpage

Data recording *(continued)*

Classification (according to Table 4.1 for participants 21 years or older, percentile according to Figures 4.4 or 4.5 for participants <21 years, or Table 4.2 for boys and girls aged 5–19 years, respectively): _____

Risk of obesity-related diseases from BMI and waist circumference (according to Table 4.1):

_____

TABLE 4.1 Combining BMI and waist circumference for lifestyle-related disease risk in adults

BMI		WAIST CIRCUMFERENCE (cm)	
CLASSIFICATION	(kg/m^2)	MALE (94–102 cm) FEMALE (80–88 cm)	MALE (>102 cm) FEMALE (>88 cm)
Underweight	<18.5	—	—
Normal weight	18.5–24.9	—	Increased[a]
Overweight	25.0–29.9	Increased[a]	High[a]
Obese	30.0–34.9	High[a]	Very high[a]

[a] Risk of obesity-related diseases (e.g. diabetes, hypertension and cardiovascular disease)
Note: The waist circumference norms presented above are for adult Caucasians
Source: National Health and Medical Research Council[1]

Interpretation, feedback and discussion

First, consider the four steps of interpretation and the three steps of feedback and discussion outlined in Appendix G. Refer to Table 4.1 to classify obesity-related disease risk within an adult population (i.e. 21 years or older). To classify obesity-related disease risk for children and adolescent populations 5–19 years of age, refer to Table 4.2.[28] As previously stated, individual BMI results should not be interpreted in isolation, but rather in combination with other measures of physique traits such as a waist girth, WHR ratio or index of central obesity, as this more validly describes disease risk.[27] For individuals <21 years of age, BMI-for-age percentile charts should be used (Figures 4.4 and 4.5). Amongst elderly populations, all-cause mortality is not increased until BMI reaches the obese range,[29] with evidence of elevated risk at a BMI below 24.0 kg/m^2.[30] The optimal BMI range for adults >65 years appears to be between 24.0 and 30.9 kg/m^2.[30] Evidence suggests the association between BMI, body fat and fat distribution differ across ethnic groups. As such, population-specific cut-off points for BMI have been proposed,[31] including a lowering of cut-offs to define overweight and obesity for Asian populations.[32] This is due to the higher risk of type 2 diabetes and cardiovascular disease at a BMI <25.0 kg/m^2 in the Asian population. Thus, it has been proposed that for people from Asia to include BMI cut-offs of 23.0, 27.5, 32.5 and 37.5 kg/m^2 along the BMI continuum, in addition to the existing classifications. Furthermore it has been suggested that BMI cut-offs should differ for Polynesian individuals owing to their relatively higher proportion of lean body mass for a given BMI; however, this has been recently refuted.[33] The WHO Consultation, therefore, has recommended that the current WHO BMI cut-offs remain in place as an international classification system.[33]

Factors to consider include:

- How would the participant react to being labelled within one of the BMI categories (i.e. would categorising your participant as 'underweight' or 'obese' be received favourably or unfavourably)?
- Does the participant appear to have a large amount of muscle mass that may have influenced the results (e.g. resistance-trained athletes)?

2 to 20 years: Boys
Body mass index-for-age percentiles

NAME _____

RECORD # _____

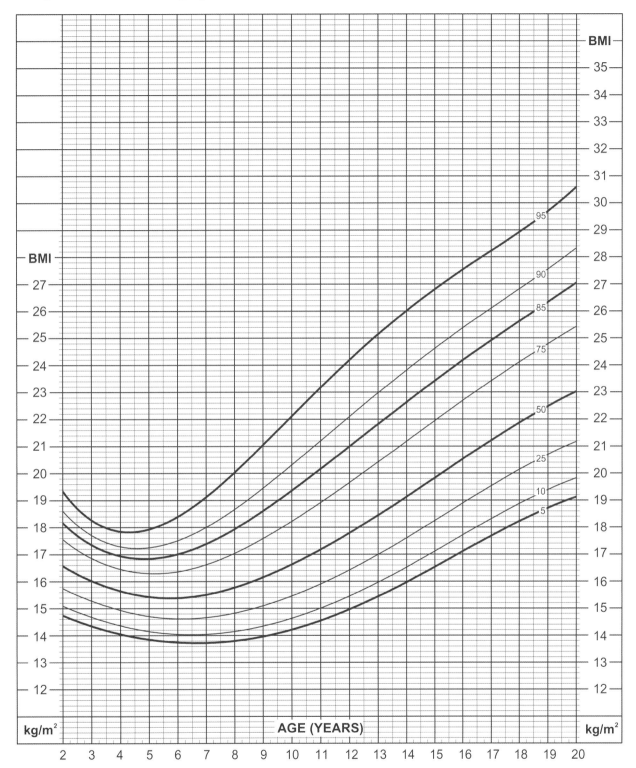

Figure 4.4 Boys: body mass index-for-age percentiles

Source: National Center for Health Statistics in collaboration with the National Center for Chronic Disease Prevention and Health Promotion: http://www.cdc.gov/growthcharts

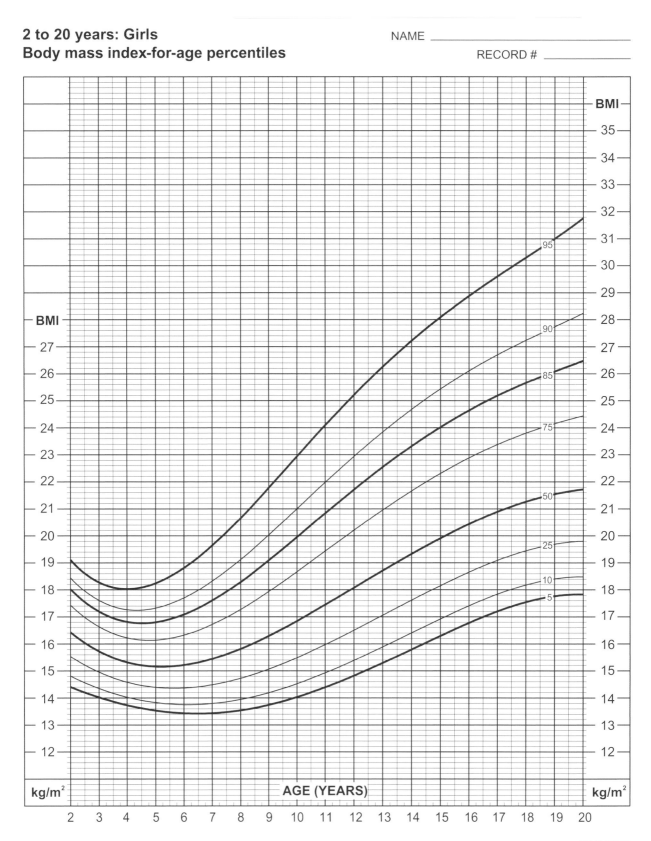

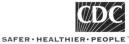

Figure 4.5 Girls: body mass index-for-age percentiles

Source: National Center for Health Statistics in collaboration with the National Center for Chronic Disease Prevention and Health Promotion: http://www.cdc.gov/growthcharts

TABLE 4.2 BMI-for-age cut-points for adolescents (5–19 years)

	BMI FOR AGE (kg/m^2)			
	THIN	NORMAL WEIGHT	OVERWEIGHT	OBESE
Boys				
5 years	<13.0	13.0–16.5	16.6–18.2	≥18.3
6 years	<13.1	13.1–16.8	16.9–18.7	≥18.8
7 years	<13.2	13.2–17.1	17.2–19.2	≥19.3
8 years	<13.4	13.4–17.6	17.7–20.0	≥20.1
9 years	<13.6	13.6–18.1	18.2–20.8	≥20.9
10 years	<13.9	13.9–18.7	18.8–21.8	≥21.9
11 years	<14.3	14.3–19.5	19.6–22.9	≥23.0
12 years	<14.7	14.7–20.3	20.4–24.1	≥24.2
13 years	<15.2	15.2–21.2	20.3–25.2	≥25.3
14 years	<15.8	15.8–22.1	22.2–26.3	≥26.4
15 years	<16.3	16.3–23.0	23.1–27.3	≥27.4
16 years	<16.7	16.7–23.8	23.9–28.2	≥28.3
17 years	<17.1	17.1–24.5	24.6–28.8	≥28.9
18 years	<17.4	17.4–25.1	25.2–29.4	≥29.5
19 years	<17.6	17.6–25.3	25.4–29.6	≥29.7
Girls				
5 years	<12.7	12.7–16.8	16.9–18.9	≥19.0
6 years	<12.7	12.7–17.0	17.1–19.4	≥19.5
7 years	<12.8	12.8–17.4	17.5–20.0	≥20.1
8 years	<13.0	13.0–17.9	18.0–20.9	≥21.0
9 years	<13.3	13.3–18.6	18.7–21.9	≥22.0
10 years	<13.7	13.7–19.3	19.4–23.0	≥23.1
11 years	<14.1	14.1–20.2	20.3–24.2	≥24.3
12 years	<14.7	14.7–21.2	21.3–25.5	≥25.6
13 years	<15.2	15.2–22.2	22.3–26.7	≥26.8
14 years	<15.7	15.7–23.0	23.1–27.7	≥27.8
15 years	<16.0	16.0–23.7	23.8–28.5	≥28.6
16 years	<16.3	16.3–24.2	24.3–29.0	≥29.1

continued overpage

TABLE 4.2 BMI-for-age cut-points for adolescents (5–19 years) *(continued)*				
	BMI FOR AGE (kg/m^2)			
	THIN	NORMAL WEIGHT	OVERWEIGHT	OBESE
17 years	<16.4	16.4–24.5	24.6–29.3	≥ 29.4
18 years	<16.5	16.5–24.8	24.9–29.5	≥ 29.6
19 years	<16.5	16.5–24.9	25.0–29.6	≥ 29.7

Based on data from 11,410 boys and 11,507 girls from the Health Examination Survey (HES) Cycle II (6–11 years) and Cycle III (12–17 years); and the Health and Nutrition Examination Survey (HANES) Cycle I (birth to 74 years), from which only data from the 1–24 years age range were used. Data are median baseline values. Thin <-2 SD from the median; overweight $>+1$ SD from the median; obese $>+2$ SD from the median
Source: World Health Organization[28]

- Is the participant involved in sporting or other activities in which a higher BMI (e.g. Sumo wrestling) or lower BMI (e.g. long-distance running) may be beneficial?

Most participants will generally be aware of their BMI category even before you conduct the test. Most obese individuals will be aware that they are obese, yet hearing that they are obese may be a negative experience. Therefore, delivering the results will require sensitivity and tact to ensure that the feedback and discussion is a positive and productive experience.

For participants who have a large muscle mass for which you believe that the results may not reflect their actual risk of obesity-related diseases, highlighting the limitations of BMI to differentiate between muscle mass and fat mass will be important. For participants whose performance is dependent on higher or lower BMI, the feedback and discussion should focus around this; however, it may still be important to ensure that the participant is aware of their risk of obesity-related diseases.

Activity 4.2 Girths

AIMS: measure waist and hip circumferences to classify obesity-related disease risk within an adult population, interpret the results and provide feedback to a participant.

Background

Waist and hip circumferences can be used as a measure of body fat distribution. Higher values of waist relative to hip circumference indicate greater adiposity in the abdominal region (android or 'apple' shape), whereas lower values indicate greater adiposity in the hip and gluteal region (gynoid or 'pear' shape). Android obesity is an indirect measure of visceral adipose tissue, which is associated with an increased risk of cardiovascular disease (CVD). Indeed, waist circumference has shown greater clinical utility than other measures of obesity, such as those derived from CT, DXA and BMI, for the identification of adults with elevated cardiometabolic risk factors.[34]

Protocol summary

Measure the participant's waist and hip circumferences in duplicate (or triplicate as required), dividing the waist by the hip circumference to determine waist-to-hip ratio.

Protocol

Follow the pre-test procedures outlined in Appendix B and 'general methods for measuring girths' in Box 4.1.

> **Box 4.1 General methods for measuring girths**
>
> 1 It is recommended that two people measure the participant's girth – the measurer and a recorder.
>
> 2 Have the participant assume the necessary position for each girth measurement, making use of an anthropometric box where appropriate to ensure that the tester's eyes are at the level of the site being measured.
>
> 3 Employ the 'cross-hand' technique by holding the case of the tape in your right hand and the stub in the left. Feed the stub of the tape measure in a clockwise direction around the area to be measured. Gauge whether you may have difficulties reaching all the way around the area; if so, ask the participant to hold one end of the tape while you walk the other end around to meet the ends together.
>
> 4 Secure the stub and case with the right hand to allow the left hand to manipulate the tape. When the tape has been positioned correctly, regain control of the stub in your left hand by reaching underneath the right hand.
>
> 5 Where possible, measurements should be performed on the participant's right side, ensuring you remain outside of the participant's personal space.
>
> 6 The tape is to be held at right angles to the long axis of the body segment being measured, with the tape manipulated so the zero marking can be read laterally. The middle fingers can be used to further manipulate the tape.
>
> 7 Once in place, regain control of the stub in your left hand by reaching underneath the right hand. Your right hand is always above the left hand, ensuring the zero marking on the tape can be aligned with the millimetre notches that appear on the bottom of the tape (see Figure 4.6). Allow the tape to self-retract, maintaining constant tension sufficient to minimise gaps between skin and tape but not so much that there is any compression of the underlying skin and subcutaneous tissue.
>
> 8 Ensure there is sufficient space between the fingers and thumb from the zero mark and read the girth with your eyes level to the tape.

Adapted from: Stewart et al[26]

Waist circumference

Definition: the circumference of the abdomen at its narrowest point between the lower costal (10th rib) border and the top of the iliac crest, perpendicular to the long axis of the trunk.[26]

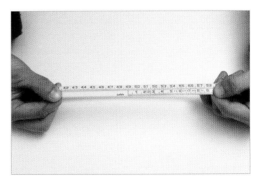

Figure 4.6 Anthropometry tape showing free end of tape aligned with millimetre notches on the bottom

Used with permission from Lufkin

Location: ask the participant to fold their arms across their chest with their hands-on opposite shoulders. Stand in front of the participant and pass the tape around the abdomen. The stub of the tape and the housing are then both held in the right hand while using the left hand to adjust the level of the tape at the back to the adjudged level of the narrowest point. Resume control of the stub with the left hand using the cross-hand technique and position the tape in front at the target level (Figure 4.7). If there is no obvious narrowing, the measurement is performed at the mid-point between the lower costal (10th rib) border and the iliac crest. Once the tester is confident that the tape measure is perpendicular to the long axis of the body, located around the minimum circumference of the waist and flush against the skin with no tension on the tape, the measurement is performed at the end of normal expiration. The tester should not provide breathing instructions to the participant, as even the instruction to 'breathe normally' may inadvertently alter their breathing rate. As the participant breathes in the measure will get slightly larger, as they breathe out the measure will get smaller. Take the measure after watching 2–3 breathing cycles at the end of normal expiration (end tidal).

Gluteal (hip) circumference

Definition: the circumference of the buttocks at the level of the greatest posterior protuberance, perpendicular to the long axis of the trunk.[26]

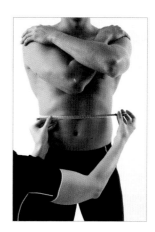

Figure 4.7 Waist circumference
Used with permission from Lufkin

Location: ask the participant to stand with their feet together, the gluteal muscles relaxed and rest their hands on their opposite shoulders. Stand to the right of the participant and pass the tape around the hips from the side. The stub of the tape and the housing are then both held in the right hand while the left hand adjusts the level of the tape at the back to the level of the greatest posterior protuberance of the buttocks. Resume control of the stub with the left hand and using the cross-hand technique position the tape at the side (Figure 4.8). Double-check with the recorder that the tape is in a horizontal plane at the target level, before taking the measurement. If the participant is wearing thick clothing (jeans, etc.), pull the tape measure very slightly to compress any clothing.

Data analysis

Waist and hip measurements should be performed one after the other – that is, waist circumference then hip circumference (trial 1), before a second measurement of each (trial 2). If there is ≤1.5% difference between the two measures (trial 1 waist circumference vs trial 2 waist circumference; trial 1 hip circumference vs trial 2 hip circumference), record the mean (average) of these measures. If there is >1.5% difference, perform a third measure and record the median (middle value) of the three values. To calculate whether your measures vary by ≤1.5%:

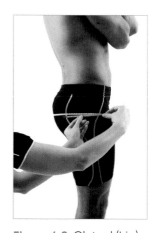

Figure 4.8 Gluteal (hip) circumference
Used with permission from Lufkin

$$\text{Calculating reliability} = \left[\frac{\text{Largest measure} \times 100}{\text{Smallest measure}} \right] - 100$$

Data recording

Participant's name: _____   Date: _____

Age: _____ years   Sex: _____

MEASURE	TRIAL 1	TRIAL 2	TRIAL 3 (IF REQUIRED)[a]	MEAN OR MEDIAN[b]
Girths				
Waist (cm)				
Gluteal (hip) (cm)				

[a] Take a third measure if the difference between trials 1 and 2 is >1.5%.
[b] Record the mean if only two measures are performed. Record the median if three measures are performed.

Waist circumference = _____ cm

continued

Data recording *(continued)*

Risk of obesity-related diseases from the mean/median waist circumference (according to Table 4.3): _____

Calculate waist-to-hip ratio using the mean/median of waist and hip circumferences in the equation:

WHR = waist circumference (cm) / hip circumference (cm)

WHR = _____

Risk of obesity-related diseases from WHR (according to Table 4.4): _____

Calculate waist-to-height ratio, using the mean/median of waist circumference and height in the equation:

Waist-to-height ratio = waist circumference (cm)/height (cm)

Waist-to-height ratio = _____

TABLE 4.3 Risk criteria for waist circumference in adults

RISK CATEGORY[a]	MALES (cm)	FEMALES (cm)
Very low	<80	<70
Low	80–99	70–89
Moderate	100–120	90–109
High	>120	>110

[a] Risk of obesity-related diseases (e.g. diabetes, hypertension and cardiovascular disease)
Source: Bray[35]

TABLE 4.4 Waist-to-hip ratio to define lifestyle-related disease risk in adults

RISK CATEGORY[a]	MALES		FEMALES	
	<60 years	>60 years	<60 years	>60 years
Low	<0.90	<0.95	<0.80	<0.85
Moderate	0.90–0.95	0.95–1.03	0.80–0.86	0.85–0.90
High	>0.95	>1.03	>0.86	>0.90

[a] Risk of obesity-related diseases (e.g. diabetes, hypertension and cardiovascular disease)
Adapted from: Folson et al [36] and Heyward and Stolarczyk[37]

Interpretation, feedback and discussion

First, consider the four steps of interpretation and the three steps of feedback and discussion outlined in Appendix G. Disease risks associated with waist circumferences for both males and females are specified in Table 4.3 [35] while the disease risks when both BMI and waist circumference data are combined are found in Table 4.1. Use Table 4.4 to classify WHR.[36,37]

Waist-to-height ratio has been proposed as a simple anthropometric index to classify disease risk across age ranges (i.e. from childhood to adulthood) and ethnic groups (i.e. it can be used internationally), with the purpose of using one clear message of an individual's disease risk over the lifespan. A waist-to-height ratio, also known as the index of central obesity (ICO), of 0.5 or more indicates increased health risk independent of sex, ethnicity and possibly age.[38] It is also purported to be more sensitive than BMI at detecting early signs of health risks.[38]

When providing feedback to the participant, it is encouraged that multiple assessments of body composition (e.g. BMI, WHR, ICO, waist circumference and skinfolds) are combined to provide a more comprehensive overview of their current disease risk and minimise the limitations of each individual test. For example, providing feedback on WHR in isolation will provide a good indication of the participant's relative body fat distribution; however, it will not provide any absolute measure of fat mass. A participant may be at 'low risk' when classifying their waist relative to their hip circumference; however, their actual waist circumference may classify them at an increased risk of obesity-related diseases. Providing this information independently may confuse the participant.

Activity 4.3 Skinfolds

AIMS: to measure subcutaneous skinfold thicknesses at specific anatomical landmarks, interpret the results and provide feedback to the participant.

Background

The measurement of 'skinfolds' refers to the thickness of a double fold of skin and compressed subcutaneous adipose tissue.[39] To infer fat mass (FM) or percentage of total body fat from skinfold measurement requires a number of assumptions to be made, including:

- constant compressibility of skinfolds across sites on the body
- skin thickness at any one site is negligible or a constant fraction of a skinfold
- fixed adipose tissue patterning across the body.

While it is estimated that subcutaneous fat comprises one-third of total body fat, this can range from 20% to 70% depending on sex, degree of fatness, age and fitness.[40] Despite the obvious flaws in these assumptions, a strong relationship does exist between subcutaneous adiposity and whole-body adiposity, and between direct skinfold thickness measures and whole-body adiposity.[41]

Aside from the convenience for assessing physique traits, skinfolds are very robust and are not readily influenced by factors such as hydration status,[42] although the hyperaemia of subcutaneous tissue associated with exercise may promote a small increase in skinfold measurements.[43] Skilled technicians are required if accurate and reliable data are to be collected (see Practical 1, Test accuracy, reliability and validity).[25] Two people are required to measure the participant's surface anthropometry: the measurer and a recorder.

Protocol summary

Identify and mark specific anatomical landmarks on the participant's body before measuring and recording the subcutaneous skinfold thickness at each site.

Protocol

The following protocol for the use of surface anthropometry has been developed by ISAK. It relates specifically to the measurement of subcutaneous fat thickness via the use of skinfold measures. The reader is directed elsewhere for details on the procedure for other measures such as lengths and breadths.[44]

Follow the pre-test procedures outlined in Appendix B and general methods for landmarks in Box 4.2.

Box 4.2 General methods for landmarking

1. Where possible, all sites should be marked and measured on the right side of the body.

2. Identify the landmark with your thumb or index finger.

3. Release the site to remove skin distortion.

4. Mark with a fine pen directly over the site.

5. All landmarks are marked with a small horizontal line $(-)$.

6. All skinfold sites are marked with a small cross $(+)$.

7. Re-check that the location of the landmark is correct.

8. Mark all sites before measuring.

Adapted from: Stewart et al[26]

Anatomical landmarks

1. ACROMIALE
Definition: the point on the superior aspect of the most lateral part of the acromion border.

Location: stand behind and on the right side of the participant and palpate along the spine of the scapula to the corner of the acromion. This represents the start of the lateral border, which usually runs anteriorly, slightly superiorly and medially. Apply the straight edge of a pen to the lateral and superior aspect of acromion to confirm the location of the most lateral part of the border. Palpate superiorly to the top margin of the acromion border in line with the most lateral aspect and mark this most lateral aspect (Figure 4.9).

> **Note:** The most lateral part of the acromion border is typically slightly posterior to the midline of the shoulder.

2. RADIALE
Definition: the point at the proximal and lateral border of the head of the radius (Figure 4.10).

Location: palpate downwards into the lateral dimple of the right elbow. It should be possible to feel the space between the capitulum of the humerus and the head of the radius. Move the thumb distally onto the most lateral part of the proximal radial head and make a small indentation on the skin at this point with the thumbnail for accurate marking. Correct location can be checked by slight rotation of the forearm, which causes the head of the radius to rotate.

3. ACROMIALE–RADIALE
Definition: the linear distance between the acromiale and radiale sites.

Location: the participant assumes a relaxed standing position with the arms hanging by the sides and the right forearm pronated. Use of a large sliding caliper or segmometer instead of a tape will allow for clearance of the deltoids. One branch of the caliper or segmometer is anchored on the acromiale while the other branch is placed on the radiale. This represents the upper arm length. You need this length to identify the mid-acromiale–radiale landmark (Figure 4.11).

4. MID-ACROMIALE–RADIALE
Definition: the mid-point of the straight line joining the acromiale and the radiale.

Location: measure the linear distance between the acromiale and radiale with the arm relaxed and extended by the side. Measure this distance using a segmometer or large sliding caliper as it is not acceptable to follow the curvature of the arm with a tape measure. Bring the lower edge of the

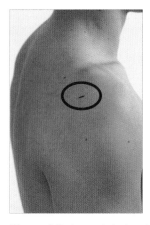

Figure 4.9 Acromiale landmark

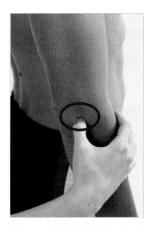

Figure 4.10 Radiale landmark

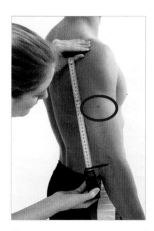

Figure 4.11 Mid-acromiale–radiale landmark

Used with permission from the University of Western Australia

segmometer or large sliding caliper up to the level of the mid-point between these two landmarks and make a small indentation on the skin with the instrument. Place a small horizontal mark at this point.

5. TRICEPS SKINFOLD SITE

Definition: the point on the posterior surface of the arm in the mid-prone position, in the midline, at the level of the marked mid-acromiale–radiale landmark.

Location: using a tape measure, project the mid-acromiale–radiale site perpendicularly to the long axis of the arm around the back of the arm (Figure 4.12). Intersect the projected line with a vertical line in the middle of the arm when viewed from behind (Figure 4.13). It may be necessary to slightly abduct the arm to find the midline of the arm.

6. BICEPS SKINFOLD SITE

Definition: the point on the anterior surface of the arm, in the mid-prone position, at the level of the mid-acromiale–radiale landmark, in the middle of the muscle belly (Figure 4.14).

Location: similar to the triceps skinfold site, using a tape measure, project the mid-acromiale–radiale site perpendicularly to the long axis of the arm around to the front of the arm, and intersect the projected line with a vertical line in the middle of the muscle belly when viewed from the front. It may be necessary to slightly abduct the arm to find the middle of the muscle belly.

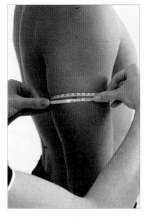

Figure 4.12 Technique to project the mid-acromiale–radiale landmark to the triceps and biceps skinfold site

Used with permission from Lufkin

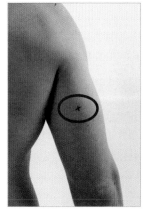

Figure 4.13 Triceps skinfold site

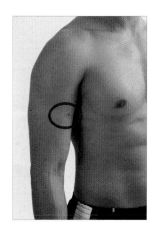

Figure 4.14 Biceps skinfold site

> **Note:** This may be medial from the midline of the anterior surface of the arm.

7. SUBSCAPULARE
Definition: the undermost tip of the inferior angle of the scapula.

Location: ensure that the participant maintains a relaxed standing position as the skin at this site is quite pliable and prone to error with participant movement. Palpate the inferior angle of the scapula with the left thumb, starting medially and running the thumb under the undermost tip of the scapula. If there is extreme difficulty locating the inferior angle of the scapula, the participant should slowly reach behind the back with the right arm. The inferior angle of the scapula should be felt continuously as the hand is again placed by the side of the body. A final check of this landmark should be made ensuring the arm is released completely back to the relaxed position. Always release the site and re-check this mark.

8. SUBSCAPULAR SKINFOLD SITE
Definition: the site 2 cm along a line running laterally and obliquely downwards from the subscapular landmark at a 45° angle.

Location: use a tape measure to locate the point 2 cm from the subscapular in a line 45° laterally downwards (Figure 4.15). You may need to ask female participants to reach behind their back with their left arm to move their bra strap out of the way.

9. ILIOCRISTALE
Definition: the point on the iliac crest where a line drawn from the mid-axilla (middle of the armpit), on the longitudinal axis of the body, meets the ilium.

Location: ask the participant to put their right hand on their left shoulder. Use your left hand to stabilise the body by providing resistance on the left side of the pelvis. Find the general location of the top of the iliac crest with the right hand by rolling the heel of the thumb or using the palms of the fingers. Once the general position has been located, find the specific edge of the crest by horizontal palpation with the tips of the fingers. Once identified, draw a horizontal line at the level of the iliac crest (Figure 4.16). Draw an imaginary line from the mid-axilla down the midline of the body. The landmark is at the intersection of the two lines.

10. ILIAC CREST SKINFOLD SITE
Definition: the site at the centre of the skinfold raised immediately above the marked iliocristale.

Location: ask the participant to put their right hand on their left shoulder. This skinfold is raised superior to the iliocristale. To do this, place your left thumb tip on the marked iliocristale site, and raise the skinfold between the thumb and index finger of the left hand (Figure 4.17). The fold runs slightly

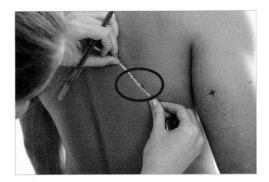

Figure 4.15 Subscapular skinfold site
Used with permission from Lufkin

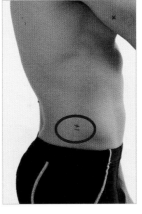

Figure 4.16 Iliocristale and iliac crest skinfold site

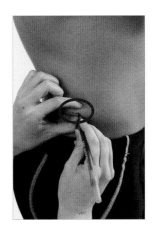

Figure 4.17 Technique to locate iliac crest skinfold site

downwards anteriorly as determined by the natural fold of the skin. Once the skinfold has been raised, mark its centre with a cross (+) (see Figure 4.16).

11. ILIOSPINALE

Definition: the most inferior or undermost part of the tip of the anterior superior iliac spine (Figure 4.18).

Location: as this landmark is usually below the level of the waistband, it may be appropriate to ask the participant to assist with the identification of this site by lowering their pant-line on the right side. Palpate the superior aspect of the ilium and follow anteriorly and inferiorly along the crest until the prominence of the ilium runs posteriorly. The landmark is marked at the lower margin or edge where the bone can just be felt. Difficulty in appraising the landmark can be assisted by the participant lifting the heel of their right foot and rotating the femur outwards. Because the sartorius muscle originates at the site of the iliospinale, this movement of the femur enables palpation of the muscle and tracing to its origin.

> **Note**: On females, the landmark is usually proportionally lower on the trunk, owing to the flatter and broader shape of the female pelvis.

12. SUPRASPINALE SKINFOLD SITE

Definition: the point at the intersection of two lines: (1) the vertical line from the marked iliospinale to the anterior axillary border; and (2) the horizontal line at the level of the marked iliocristale.

Location: using a tape measure, locate the line that runs from the anterior axillary border (i.e. the front of the armpit) to the iliospinale and draw a short line along the side roughly at the level of the iliocristale (see Figure 4.18). It may be useful to ask the participant to hold the tape at the anterior axillary border with their left hand. Then run the tape horizontally around from the marked iliocristale to intersect the vertical line (Figure 4.19).

13. ABDOMINAL SKINFOLD SITE

Definition: the point 5 cm horizontally to the right-hand side of the omphalion (mid-point of the navel) (Figure 4.20).

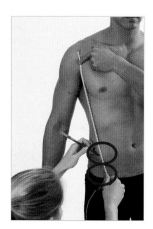

Figure 4.18 Iliospinale part 1: technique used for the location of the supraspinale skinfold site

Used with permission from Lufkin

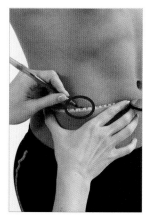

Figure 4.19 Iliospinale part 2: technique used for the horizontal intersection for the supraspinale skinfold site

Used with permission from Lufkin

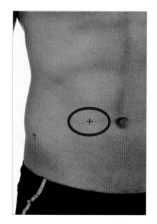

Figure 4.20 Abdominal skinfold site

Location: using a tape measure, this site is measured horizontally across 5 cm to the right from the mid-point of the navel.

> **Note**: The distance of 5 cm assumes an adult height of approximately 170 cm. Where height differs markedly from this, the distance should be scaled for height. For example, if the height is 120 cm, the distance will be $5 \times 120/170 = 3.5$ cm.

14. FRONT THIGH SKINFOLD SITE

Definition: the mid-point of the linear distance between the inguinal point (the point at the intersection of the inguinal fold and the midline of the anterior thigh) and the patellare (the mid-point of the posterior superior border of the patella).

Location: the participant assumes a seated position with the torso erect and the arms hanging by the sides. The knee of the right leg should be bent at a right angle. The measurer stands facing the right side of the seated participant on the lateral side of the thigh. If there is difficulty locating the inguinal fold (the crease at the angle of the trunk and the anterior thigh), the participant should flex the hip to make a fold. Using a segmometer or large sliding caliper, measure from the inguinal fold to the posterior superior border of the patella (Figure 4.21). Mark the point that is equidistant between these two landmarks in the midline of the thigh (Figure 4.22).

15. MEDIAL CALF SKINFOLD SITE

Definition: the point on the most medial aspect of the calf at the level of the maximal girth.

Location: ask the participant to stand on top of an anthropometric box with their feet separated and their body mass evenly distributed. Using a tape measure, find the maximum circumference of the calf. Begin measuring girths proximally and using your middle fingers to manipulate the position of the tape in a series of distal and proximal movements (Figure 4.23). Once the maximal level is located, the point is marked on the medial aspect of the calf with a small cross (+).

Skinfolds

1 Prior to the measurement of skinfolds, verify that the skinfold caliper is accurately measuring the distance between the centre of its contact faces with the use of vernier calipers.

2 The fold is picked up with the near edge of the thumb and finger in line with the marked site, and the back of the hand facing the measurer (Figure 4.24). The fold should be grasped and lifted so that a parallel, double fold of skin (including the underlying subcutaneous adipose tissue) is held between the thumb and index finger of the left hand.

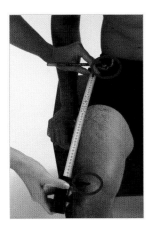

Figure 4.21 Technique to locate front thigh skinfold site

Used with permission from the University of Western Australia

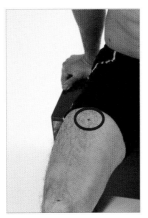

Figure 4.22 Front thigh skinfold site

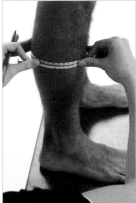

Figure 4.23 Technique to locate medial calf skinfold site

Used with permission from Lufkin

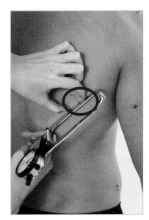

Figure 4.24 Technique to ensure that fingers pinch exactly on the located skinfold site

Used with permission from Harpenden

Note: Avoid grasping large folds creating a 'mushroom' effect or small folds where the caliper may slip off and cause pain and discomfort.

---

3 The nearest edge of the caliper is applied 1 cm away from the edge of the thumb and finger. The centre of the caliper faces should be placed at a depth of approximately mid-fingernail.

4 The caliper is held at 90° to the surface of the skinfold in the three spatial planes at all times. Ensure the fold is held while the caliper is in contact with the skin.

5 Measurement is performed 2 seconds after full pressure of the caliper is applied.

Note: The caliper handles should be released during measurement.

6 Skinfold sites are measured in succession (i.e. one trial of each skinfold measure is performed before returning to each site for the duplicate measure, reducing the effects of skinfold compressibility and technician bias).

7 Skinfold measurements are performed in duplicate. A third measurement should be performed if the difference between the two trials is >7.5%.

1. TRICEPS

Definition: the skinfold measurement taken parallel to the long axis of the arm at the triceps skinfold site.

Location: the right arm of the participant should be relaxed with the shoulder joint slightly externally rotated to the mid-prone position and elbow extended by the side of the body. The skinfold is raised with the left thumb and index finger on the marked posterior mid-acromiale–radiale line. The fold is vertical and parallel to the line of the upper arm. Ask the participant to extend, then relax, and then take the skinfold measurement (Figure 4.25).

2. SUBSCAPULAR

Definition: the skinfold measurement taken with the fold running obliquely downwards at the subscapular skinfold site.

Location: the skinfold is taken at the subscapular skinfold site which is marked 2 cm laterally and obliquely downwards from the subscapular landmark at a 45° angle as determined by the natural fold lines of the skin (Figure 4.26). You may need to ask female participants to reach behind their back with their left arm to move their bra strap out of the way.

3. BICEPS

Definition: the skinfold measurement taken parallel to the long axis of the arm at the biceps skinfold site (Figure 4.27).

Location: the right arm of the participant should be relaxed with the shoulder joint slightly externally rotated to the mid-prone position and the elbow extended by the side of the body. The skinfold is raised with the left thumb and index finger on the marked anterior mid-acromiale–radiale line. The fold is

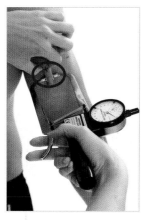

Figure 4.25 Triceps skinfold

Used with permission from Harpenden

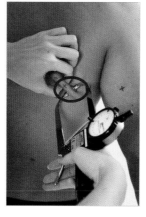

Figure 4.26 Subscapular skinfold

Used with permission from Harpenden

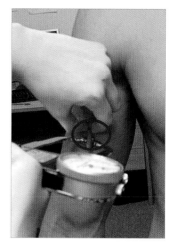

Figure 4.27 Biceps skinfold

Used with permission from Harpenden

vertical and parallel to the line of the upper arm. Take the skinfold while the arm is relaxed. As the biceps skinfold is generally a small skinfold, take care not to pinch too deep causing a triple fold of the skin.

4. ILIAC CREST
Definition: the skinfold measurement taken near horizontal at the iliac crest skinfold site.

Location: the right arm of the participant should be either abducted or placed across the trunk. This skinfold is raised immediately superior to the iliocristale on the mid-axilla line. This fold runs slightly downwards posterior–anterior, as determined by the natural fold lines of the skin (Figure 4.28). This skinfold is equivalent to that described by Durnin and Womersley[45] as the suprailiac skinfold.

5. SUPRASPINALE
Definition: the skinfold measurement taken with the fold running obliquely and medially downwards at the supraspinale skinfold site.

Location: the participant assumes a relaxed standing position with the arms hanging by the sides. The fold runs medially downwards and anteriorly at about a 45° angle as determined by the natural fold lines of the skin (Figure 4.29).

6. ABDOMINAL
Definition: the skinfold measurement taken vertically at the abdominal skinfold site.

Location: the participant assumes a relaxed standing position with the arms hanging by the sides. This is a vertical fold raised 5 cm from the right-hand side of the mid-point of the navel (Figure 4.30). Make sure the initial grasp is firm and broad as often the underlying musculature is poorly developed. This may result in an underestimation of the thickness of the subcutaneous layer of tissue. Do not place the fingers inside the navel. If the skinfold is thick enough for this to occur, move the mark over to the right so the fingers are placed beside the navel. Record the distance from the mid-point of the fold to the mid-point of the navel for re-test measures.

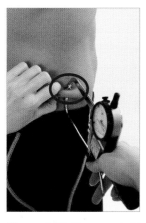

Figure 4.28 Iliac crest skinfold
Used with permission from Harpenden

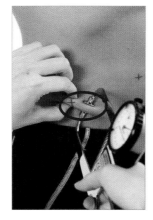

Figure 4.29 Supraspinale skinfold
Used with permission from Harpenden

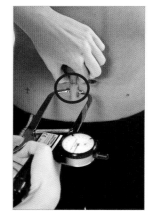

Figure 4.30 Abdominal skinfold
Used with permission from Harpenden

7. FRONT THIGH
Definition: the skinfold measurement taken parallel to the long axis of the thigh at the front thigh skinfold site.

Location: the participant assumes a seated position at the front edge of the anthropometric box with the torso erect, the arms supporting the hamstrings and the leg extended. The measurer stands facing the right side of the participant on the lateral side of the thigh.

> **Note:** The site is marked while the knee is bent; however, the skinfold measurement is taken with the leg extended. The participant can assist by raising the underside of the thigh to relieve the tension of the skin. If the participant has particularly tight skinfolds, the recorder can assist by standing on the left and raising the fold with both hands, at about 6 cm either side of the landmark (Figure 4.31). The measurer then raises the skinfold at the marked site and takes the measurement.

8. MEDIAL CALF

Definition: the skinfold measurement taken vertically at the medial calf skinfold site.

Location: the participant assumes a relaxed standing position with the right foot placed on the box and calf relaxed. The right knee is bent at 90°.

> **Note:** The site is marked with the participant standing on the anthropometric box; however, the skinfold measurement is taken with the right foot placed on the box. The vertical fold is raised on the medial aspect of the calf at a level where it has maximal circumference. The fold is parallel to the long axis of the leg (Figure 4.32).

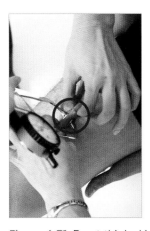

Figure 4.31 Front thigh skinfold
Used with permission from Harpenden

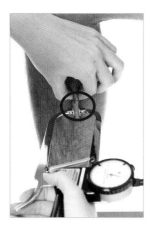

Figure 4.32 Medial calf skinfold
Used with permission from Harpenden

Data analysis

1 After landmarking your participant, measure the specified skinfolds and girths in duplicate or triplicate as required.

2 Estimate body density (required for the subsequent estimation of percentage body fat) using the following three regression equations for males and females below, and record values.

Females

Withers et al[46] – six-site formula

$$\text{Body density} = 1.20953 - [0.08294 \times (\log_{10} X_1)]$$

where X_1 = sum of six skinfolds (in mm): triceps, subscapular, supraspinale, abdominal, front thigh and medial calf.

Participants were female athletes ($n = 182$) aged 11–41 years who were state representatives across 14 sports. Harpenden calipers were used to measure skinfolds according to the technique described by Ross and Marfell-Jones.[47]

Jackson and Pollock[48] – three-site formula

$$\text{Body density} = 1\,099421 - [0.0009929 \times (X_1)] + [0.0000023 \times (X_1)^2] - [0.0001392 \times (\text{age})]$$

where $X_1 =$ sum of three skinfolds (in mm): triceps, iliac crest and front thigh.

Participants were women ($n = 331$) aged 18–55 years who varied considerably in body structure, composition and habitual activity. Lange calipers were used to measure skinfolds according to the technique described by the Committee on Nutritional Anthropometry of the Food and Nutrition Board of the National Research Council.[49]

Jackson et al[49] – four-site formula

$$\text{Body density} = 1.096095 - 0.0006952\,(X_1) + 0.0000011\,(X_1)^2 - 0.0000714\,(\text{age})$$

where $X_1 =$ sum of four skinfolds (in mm): triceps, iliac crest, abdomen and front thigh.

Participants were women ($n = 331$) aged 18–55 years who varied considerably in body structure, composition and habitual activity. Lange calipers were used to measure skinfolds according to the technique described by the Committee on Nutritional Anthropometry of the Food and Nutrition Board of the National Research Council.[50]

Males

Withers et al[46] – seven-site formula

$$\text{Body density} = 1.0988 - [0.0004 \times (X_1)]$$

where $X_1 =$ sum of seven skinfolds (in mm): triceps, subscapular, biceps, supraspinale, abdominal, front thigh and medial calf.

Participants were male athletes ($n = 207$) aged 15–39 years who were state representatives across 18 sports. Harpenden calipers were used to measure skinfolds according to the technique described by Ross and Marfell-Jones.[47]

Durnin and Womersley[45] – four-site formula

$$\text{Body density} = 1.1765 - [0.0744(\log_{10}X_1)]$$

where $X_1 =$ sum of four skinfolds (in mm): triceps, biceps, subscapular and, iliac crest.

Participants were apparently healthy men ($n = 209$) aged 17–72 years deliberately selected to represent a variety of body types. Either Harpenden or Lange calipers were used to measure skinfolds according to the technique described by Weiner and Lourie.[51]

Katch and McArdle[52] – three-site formula

$$\text{Body density} = 1.09665 - [0.00103 \times X_1] - [0.00056 \times X_2] - [0.00054 \times X_3]$$

where $X_1 =$ triceps (in mm), $X_2 =$ subscapular (in mm), $X_3 =$ abdominal (in mm).

Participants were men ($n = 53$) aged 19 ± 2 years enrolled in physical education at college. Lange calipers were used to measure skinfolds according to the technique described by Katch and McArdle.[52]

3 Use the calculated body density to estimate body fat using the following equation and record values.

Siri equation[53]

$$\% \text{ body fat} = [(4.95/\text{body density}) - 4.50] \times 100$$

Data recording

Participant's name: _____　　Date: _____

Age: _____ years　　Sex: _____

Skinfolds

MEASURE (MM)	TRIAL 1	TRIAL 2	TRIAL 3 (IF REQUIRED)[a]	MEAN OR MEDIAN[b]
Triceps				
Subscapular				
Biceps				
Iliac crest				
Supraspinale				
Abdominal				
Front thigh				
Medial calf				
Sum of 7 (no iliac crest)				
Sum of 6 (no iliac crest and front thigh)				
Sum of 6 skinfolds[c] percentile (according to Table 4.5)[54]:				

[a] Take a third measure if the difference between trials 1 and 2 is >7.5%
[b] Record the mean if only two measures are performed. Record the median if three measures are performed
[c] The skinfolds assessed were triceps, subscapular, biceps, supraspinale, abdominal and medial calf

Female body density and body fat percentage

EQUATION	BODY DENSITY	BODY FAT (%)
Withers et al[46]		
Jackson and Pollock[48]		
Jackson et al[49]		

Male body density and body fat percentage

EQUATION	BODY DENSITY	BODY FAT (%)
Withers et al[46]		
Durnin and Womersley[45]		
Katch and McArdle[52]		

Interpretation, feedback and discussion

First, consider the four steps of interpretation and the three steps of feedback and discussion outlined in Appendix G, and refer to Table 4.5. If making repeated measures on the same participant over time, consider whether the changes, if any, in body mass and sum of skinfolds are likely due to changes in muscle mass and/or body fat (Table 4.6).

TABLE 4.5 Sum of six skinfolds reference data[a]

PERCENTILES	AGE (years)					
	18–29	30–39	40–49	50–59	60–69	70–78
Males						
5	30.3	31.7	49.1	42.8	46.5	34.3
25	41.5	64.1	69.1	68.7	66.4	53.5
50	62.8	80.6	88.5	88.5	80.6	73.5
75	89.6	102.9	106.9	106.4	101.9	87.2
95	140.2	146.6	156.1	138.7	144.6	109.0
Mean	71.7	84.4	92.2	89.3	86.4	72.0
Standard deviation	37.8	32.0	32.2	28.8	27.9	20.9
Participants (n)	92	120	137	110	108	32
Females						
5	51.6	49.5	66.1	60.7	67.1	65.8
25	79.1	74.7	91.1	105.9	106.5	98.4
50	103.2	100.3	129.8	141.5	134.7	129.1
75	141.9	140.7	168.2	174.1	160.3	149.2
95	204.2	201.4	222.3	211.0	201.4	193.4
Mean	112.5	110.1	133.3	139.7	134.6	127.8
Standard deviation	45.7	45.7	48.0	43.8	38.6	34.7
Participants (n)	85	130	139	125	87	26

[a] Skinfolds assessed were triceps, subscapular, biceps, supraspinale, abdominal and medial calf measured in mm
Source: Gore and Edwards[54]

TABLE 4.6 Interpretation of changes in physique traits based on skinfold and body mass data

ANTHROPOMETRIC TRAIT		INTERPRETATION – PHYSIQUE TRAIT	
BODY MASS	SKINFOLDS	MUSCLE MASS	BODY FAT
Increase	Stable	Gain	No change
Decrease	Stable	Loss	No change
Stable	Increase	Loss	Gain
Stable	Decrease	Gain	Loss
Increase	Increase	Potential gain	Gain
Increase	Decrease	Gain	Loss
Decrease	Increase	Loss	Gain
Decrease	Decrease	Potential loss	Loss

Source: Gary Slater, University of the Sunshine Coast

Issues to consider include:

- How much did body fat differ depending on the equation used? Consider the possible reasons for these discrepancies in body fat percentage (e.g. differences in equipment, technique, or characteristics of the reference data vs your participant).
- Do the results appear to be a valid representation of body fat, taking into consideration observation, training status, body mass, BMI and WHR?

As demonstrated, estimates of body density, fat mass (FM) and/or fat-free mass (FFM) are derived from skinfold data using one of many available equations. Because these equations are population specific, only equations derived from individuals with similarities in age, sex, body composition and activity levels should be considered for use. Consequently, amongst athletes, skinfold equations derived from athletic populations such as that of Withers et al[46] are likely to offer a more valid estimate of body composition.[55] Furthermore, compatibility in technical aspects of data collection, including anatomical landmarking and high-quality anthropometric equipment, is also essential.

Despite the advancement in physique assessment techniques, and the notable desire of participants wishing to know their 'body fat percentage', practitioners are advised to use raw anthropometric data (e.g. sum of six skinfold $= 54$ mm) rather than attempt to make estimates of whole-body composition from available equations[56] (see Tables 4.5 and 4.6).

Amongst obese populations achieving only modest weight loss, visceral adipose tissue may decrease preferentially over subcutaneous fat mass, although this effect is attenuated with greater weight loss.[26] Given this, consideration should be given to routine measures of visceral fat mass, including field-based options such as girth measures.

BODY COMPOSITION ASSESSMENTS

Activity 4.4 Bioelectrical impedance analysis

AIMS: to assess total body water, fat mass (FM) and fat-free mass (FFM) using a bioelectrical impedance (BIA) device, interpret the results and provide feedback to a participant.

Background

BIA has become increasingly popular as a tool for assessing the physique traits of individuals given its relative ease of use, portability and cost effectiveness. It is a safe and non-invasive method to assess physique traits that is based on the differing electrical conductivity of FM and FFM.[57,58] FFM contains water and electrolytes and is a good electrical conductor, whereas anhydrous fat mass is not. The method involves measuring the resistance (R) to flow of a low level current/s.[59] Resistance is proportional to the length (L) of the conductor (in this case the human body) and inversely proportional to its cross-sectional area. A relationship then exists between the impedance quotient (i.e. L^2/R) and the volume of water (total body water), which contains electrolytes that conduct the electrical current. In practice, height in centimetres is substituted for length. Therefore, a relationship exists between FFM (approximately 73% water) and height (cm)^2/R. FM is obtained from FFM by subtracting the value for FFM from total body mass.[57]

Although the relationship between FFM and impedance is readily accepted, there are several assumptions associated with the use of BIA to measure body composition. First, the human body is assumed to be a cylinder with a uniform length and cross-sectional area. Rather, the human body more closely resembles several cylinders. The body parts with the smallest FFM (the limbs) have the greatest influence on whole-body resistance. The trunk, which is a shorter, thicker segment, contains $\approx 50\%$ of body mass but contributes only a minor amount to the overall resistance. Second, it is assumed the conducting material within the cylinder is homogeneous. Finally, the resistance to current flow per unit length of a specific conductor is assumed to be constant. However, this will vary depending on tissue structure, hydration status and electrolyte concentration of the tissue.[59]

Due to the relevance of body water to conductivity of electrical current, there is substantial evidence that BIA is not valid (concurrent) for assessment of individuals with abnormal hydration such as visible oedema, ascites, kidney, liver and cardiac disease and pregnancy.[58] Exercise-induced hypohydration to a level of 3% body mass has been shown to decrease the estimate of FM via BIA by 1.7%. Conversely, acute rehydration increased estimates of FM by 3.2%, with a further increase in the estimate of FM as a state of hyperhydration was achieved.[60] Even the ingestion of relatively small volumes of fluid (591 mL) has been shown to increase estimates of FM.[61] Consequently, participants should remain fasted and euhydrated for at least 8 hours prior to assessment.[58] Given this, it would be prudent to undertake assessments in the morning prior to breakfast wherever possible, with participants encouraged to present in a euhydrated state. The following protocol is for a BIA device that uses hand and foot electrodes.

A wide range of BIA devices is available. Strategically placed gel electrodes or pressure-contact metal electrodes are used for generating and measuring electrical current, which passes from leg to leg, arm to arm or leg to arm, depending on the device. Irrespective of the device used, pre-test standardisation of body position, previous exercise, dietary intake and skin temperature must be respected. For specific guidance, refer to the user manual of your particular device.

Protocol summary

Have the participant lie in a supine position, locate the anatomical landmarks on the right hand/wrist and foot/ankle before attaching the BIA electrodes to determine total body water, FM and FFM.

Protocol

1 Follow the pre-test procedures outlined in Appendix B, strongly encouraging the participant to arrive in a euhydrated state.

2 Undertake calibration procedures in accordance with manufacturer's guidelines.

3 Given the significant influence of hydration on BIA results,[62] measurement of the hydration status of the participant is recommended (see Appendix B).

4 Weigh the participant on a calibrated scale in minimal clothing (see Activity 4.1).

5 Measure height using a wall-mounted stadiometer (see Activity 4.1).

6 Obtain relevant demographic data from the participant, including ethnicity, age, sex, etc., ensuring the most valid (concurrent) equations can be used in the subsequent analysis.

7 Place the participant in a supine position on a flat, even surface free of any metal. The limbs should be abducted: arms at 30° from the trunk and legs separated at 45°. This position should be maintained for at least 10 minutes prior to assessment to minimise the influence of body water shifts between compartments (Figure 4.33).

8 Follow the set-up instructions of the user manual of the particular device you are using for the correct electrode placement.

9 Initiate data collection and record results as displayed on the monitor.

10 Clean and disinfect all equipment (see Appendix A).

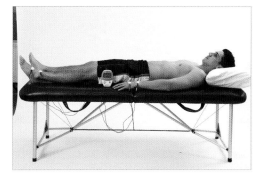

Figure 4.33 Bioelectrical impedance analysis
Used with permission from ImpediMed

Data recording

Participant's name: _____   Date: _____

Age: _____ years   Sex: _____

Record the data presented on the BIA device:

Fat-free mass: _____ kg _____ %

Fat mass: _____ kg _____ %

Total body water: _____ L _____ %

Intracellular water: _____ L _____ %

Extracellular water: _____ L _____ %

Calculate percentage of body fat by dividing fat mass by body mass:

% body fat: _____ %

Fat mass percentile (according to Table 4.7): _____

% body fat percentile (according to Table 4.7): _____

Interpretation

First, consider the four steps of interpretation outlined in Appendix G, and refer to Table 4.7.[63] Given the range of devices available, outputs can vary significantly. However, all BIA devices will provide body composition (fat-free mass, fat mass) and total body water (potentially also including intracellular and extracellular water). Devices targeted at the medical industry may also include a range of other variables, including estimates of visceral adipose tissue and bone mineral content, the validity (concurrent) of which remains to be confirmed. The presentation of raw impedance data provides an opportunity to utilise a regression equation with character traits similar to the participant population under investigation. Selection of such equations probably enhances precision of body composition estimates.

TABLE 4.7 Fat mass and % body fat reference data				
	FAT MASS (kg)		BODY FAT (%)	
PERCENTILES	MALES	FEMALES	MALES	FEMALES
0	1.9	4.4	2.4	8.1
20	17.4	20.1	24.0	34.1
40	21.3	24.4	27.5	38.4
50	23.0	26.5	29.0	40.2
60	24.9	28.8	30.4	41.9
80	29.4	35.0	33.6	45.8
100	79.1	94.2	52.5	63.0

Based on data from 16,969 men and 24,344 women aged 27–75 years enrolled in the Melbourne Collaborative Cohort Study from 1990 to 1994. Data were collected using a single frequency (50 Hz) BIA-101A RJL system analyser (RJL Systems, Detroit, Michigan). Data are median baseline values. Very poor >80th percentile; poor = 80th–61st percentile; average = 60th–41st percentile; good = 40th–20th percentile; excellent <20th percentile
Source: Simpson et al[63]

Issues to consider include:

- How much did body fat differ from the BIA device to the percentage body fat calculated from the skinfold measures? Consider the possible reasons for these discrepancies in body fat percentage.
- Do the BIA results appear to be a valid representation of body fat, taking into consideration observation, training status, body mass, BMI and WHR? Due consideration of the limitations and assumptions of body fat calculations via BIA and the extraneous factors influencing each measure (e.g. hydration status, activity level) are essential.

Activity 4.5 Dual-energy x-ray absorptiometry (DXA)

AIMS: to assess fat mass, fat-free mass and percentage body fat using DXA, interpret the results and provide feedback to a participant.

Background

DXA technology is based on the differential attenuation of transmitted photons at two energy levels by bone, fat and lean tissue.[64] DXA was originally developed for the diagnosis of osteoporosis and remains the gold standard tool for this assessment when combined with peripheral quantitative CT.[65] However, DXA technology is also able to measure soft tissue body composition, which has rapidly gained popularity in recent years as one of the most widely used and accepted laboratory-based methods for body composition analysis.

Whole-body DXA scans are quick ($\approx$5 min), non-invasive and associated with very low radiation doses ($\approx$0.5 µSv or approximately 1/500th of annual natural background radiation), making the technology relatively safe for longitudinal monitoring of body composition. DXA provides a measure of fat mass and fat-free mass, but also regional body composition (i.e. arms, legs, trunk, differences between left and right side), making DXA appealing when assessing the effectiveness of targeted exercise training programs or during periods of rehabilitation from injury in athletic populations.

While there are several manufacturers of DXA technology, all models comprise an x-ray source, scanning table, detector and computer interface with complex algorithm software for the conversion of raw data into estimates of body composition. The systems differ in analysis software and the geometry of scanning (fan, narrow fan or pencil beam technology); therefore, longitudinal monitoring of an individual should be performed on the same DXA machine.[66-68]

Compared with the four-compartment model, the current 'gold standard' body composition tool, DXA demonstrates good agreement in young, apparently healthy males and females,[69] but underestimates body fat[70] in leaner individuals.[71] However, DXA appears to be sufficiently sensitive to detect small changes in body composition with longitudinal monitoring.[72,73]

The precision of measurement for DXA in sedentary populations has been shown to be superior to hydrodensitometry and surface anthropometry,[74] with a coefficient of variation of less than 1.0 kg for fat mass, fat-free mass and total mass.[64,75] Accurate positioning of the participant on the DXA scanner is essential to enhance precision of the measure.[76,77] Where possible, it is recommended that longitudinal monitoring of an individual is conducted by the same technician.[78] Positioning of the arms and legs should be standardised, ensuring clear separation from the torso; foam blocks, not recognised by the scanner, can be particularly helpful. The defined scanning area available for assessment is generally limited (e.g. $\approx$60–65 cm $\times$ 193–198 cm), which makes it difficult to perform whole-body DXA scans on particularly tall or broad individuals. Hence, taller individuals are typically scanned without their head or feet, have their knees bent so as to fit within the scanned area[79] or data is summed from two partial scans – the latter appearing to be the method of choice, with the body divided at the neck resulting in the most valid estimates of bone and soft tissue composition.[80] For very broad individuals, newer DXA scanners contain software that allows an estimate of whole-body composition from a half-body scan,[81] which has been validated (concurrent) in obese individuals.[82]

Protocol summary

Have the participant lie quietly on the DXA bed while body composition is measured (Figure 4.34).

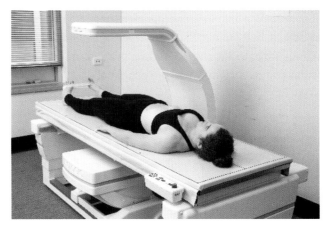

Figure 4.34 Dual-energy x-ray absorptiometry
Used with permission from Hologic

Protocol

1 Follow the pre-test procedures outlined in Appendix B.

2 Weigh the participant on a calibrated scale in minimal clothing (see Activity 4.1).

3 Measure height using a wall-mounted stadiometer (see Activity 4.1).

4 Obtain relevant demographic data from the participant, including age, sex, etc.

Conducting a DXA scan requires appropriate training and certification, such as completion of the bone densitometry short courses conducted by the Australian and New Zealand Bone and Mineral Society. DXA technicians are also required to obtain a radiation user licence prior to using any equipment that uses ionising radiation. Further details regarding how to conduct a DXA scan are subsequently beyond the scope of this practical. However, given the wide availability of DXA scanning services available across Australia and New Zealand, exercise professionals should have the ability to interpret the findings of a DXA scan and apply the findings to optimise outcomes for their participant.

Data recording

Participant's name: _____   Date: _____

Age: _____ years   Sex: _____

Record the following data presented on the DXA report:

Lean mass: _____ kg _____ %

Lean mass + bone mineral content (BMC): _____ kg _____ %

Fat-free mass index (lean mass / height^2): _____ kg/m^2 _____ percentile compared with age-matched control

Fat mass: _____ kg _____ %

Fat mass index (fat mass / height^2): _____ kg/m^2 ____ percentile compared with age-matched control

Total body fat: _____ % _____ percentile compared with age-matched control

Android:gynoid ratio: _____

Risk of obesity-related diseases from android:gynoid ratio (according to Table 4.4): _____

Interpretation

First, consider the four steps of interpretation outlined in Appendix G. There is a selection of reports that can be generated depending on the information required and the DXA scanner used. These include bone density, body composition, and metabolic and visceral fat. Some DXA models afford an opportunity to create reports that populate data from the current assessment with prior scans, creating an excellent medium for interpreting changes in physique traits longitudinally. Most DXA reports provide details on several variables. Understanding their concurrent validity and application will assist in interpreting scan results for participants.

Indices of bone health

Although indices of bone health such as bone mineral content and density are included in whole-body scans, neither is diagnostic, and should not be used to classify someone as having normal bone density, osteopenia or osteoporosis. When an assessment of bone health is desired, or a whole-body scan potentially indicates low bone density, a dual femur and/or anterior–posterior lumbar spine DXA scan should be performed for diagnostic purposes.

Fat mass

Although individuals are often drawn to the measure of body fat percentage, there are several other variables which offer greater insight into disease risk. Given that there are no reference ranges for body fat, percentiles offer a convenient way of providing context to results. Furthermore, it is important to remember that changes in percentage body fat are influenced just as much by changes in lean mass as they are by fat mass. Given this, practitioners are encouraged to focus on absolute fat mass values, especially when monitoring participants longitudinally. The android (located centrally and often described as male fat distribution) and gynoid (located on the lower body and often described as female fat distribution) body fat estimates help describe fat patterning and ultimately disease risk. Higher android body fat (and thus android:gynoid ratio) is associated with higher visceral adipose tissue (VAT), which is an independent risk factor for atherosclerosis in men.[83] VAT diagnostic thresholds for increased risk (>100 cm^2) and high risk (>160 cm^2) have been established for use in general populations.[84]

Lean mass

Practitioners (and participants alike) should be equally interested in lean mass results, which incorporates both metabolically highly active internal organs and skeletal muscle mass. Given there are no reference ranges for lean mass, percentiles also offer a convenient way of providing context to results. Regional lean mass data may be of interest among some populations, including athletes or individuals recovering from injury associated with disuse atrophy. Although a small degree of asymmetry is common between left and right sides as a consequence of laterality, marked differences may need to be addressed. Among older adults, relative lean mass (lean mass/height^2 (m)) can be assessed as part of the diagnostic criteria for sarcopenia,[85,86] with appropriate interventions applied accordingly.

Activity 4.6 Air displacement plethysmography

AIMS: to assess body density, fat mass, fat-free mass and percentage body fat using air displacement plethysmography via a BOD POD, interpret the results and provide feedback to a participant.

Background

The BOD POD (Life Measurement, Inc., Concord, CA) is a quick, relatively comfortable, automated, non-invasive and safe technique to estimate percentage fat from body density. It uses air displacement plethysmography and the inverse relationship between pressure and volume in two enclosed chambers to calculate body density and body composition.

A BOD POD report provides reference information on both body volume and body density, as well as derived body composition data (i.e. fat mass and fat-free mass). When assessments are performed longitudinally, reports can also be generated that consolidate data across time, creating an easily interpreted platform for tracking changes. The BOD POD also provides an estimate of resting energy expenditure, applying body composition data to a previously validated (concurrent) regression equation for estimating energy expenditure.

The two-compartment technique of the BOD POD involves measurement of the volume of air displaced by the body whilst sitting in an enclosed chamber. Lung functional residual capacity is then measured using pulmonary plethysmography. If measurement of lung functional residual capacity is not feasible (e.g. in the elderly, children or those with pulmonary dysfunction), it can be predicted based on age, sex and height. Body density is calculated by dividing the measured body mass by the corrected body volume, with percentage body fat then estimated using either the Siri[53] or Brozek[87] equations.

The BOD POD's ability to validly measure body density is comparable to underwater weighing without requiring the participant to be submerged under water,[88] although it has been shown to slightly underestimate body fat in males ($-1.2 \pm 3.1\%$) and slightly overestimate body fat in females ($1.0 \pm 2.5\%$), independently of age, body mass or height.[89] The BOD POD is able to detect changes in body mass within a 2 kg range.[90] The test–retest reliability of the BOD POD is high,[91] with a between-day coefficient of variation for body fat of 2.0%–5.3%,[92] although large discrepancies (up to 12%) have been reported between trials.[91] Although there is good reliability between different BOD POD systems,[93] it is always recommended that repeat measures be performed using the same system.

The use of measured versus predicted lung volume can deviate estimates of body fat by as much as 3%.[94] Therefore, lung volume should be measured wherever possible and never used interchangeably with predicted thoracic gas volumes. Although measurement of functional residual capacity using pulmonary plethysmography is considered both reliable and valid (concurrent),[95] it can change in response to alterations in body composition.[96]

Protocol summary

Have the participant sit quietly in an enclosed chamber while the volume of air displaced by the body is measured to determine body density and estimate fat mass, fat-free mass and percentage body fat.

Protocol

1 Follow the pre-test procedures outlined in Appendix B.

2 Power on the computer to launch the BOD POD application and log in at least 30 minutes prior to the start of quality control procedures.

3 Undertake quality control procedures on the BOD POD and the scales in accordance with manufacturer's guidelines.

4 Measure height using a wall-mounted stadiometer (see Activity 4.1).

5 Enter participant's name and relevant demographic data into the computer.

6 Follow the manufacturer's instructions and computer screen prompts to conduct volume calibration. If thoracic gas volumes are to be measured as part of the test procedure (recommended), connect the disposable tube to the filter, then attach it filter end first into the nozzle in the BOD POD test chamber.

7 At the end of the first half of the volume calibration, place the calibration volume in the test chamber (Figure 4.35).

8 During the second half of the volume calibration the mass of the participant is measured, typically for between 6 and 20 seconds.

9 Remove the calibration volume from the test chamber.

10 Ask the participant to put on the swim cap, ensuring all of the participant's hair is in the swim cap and any air pockets under the cap are pushed out, and enter the test chamber for the body volume measurements (Figure 4.36).

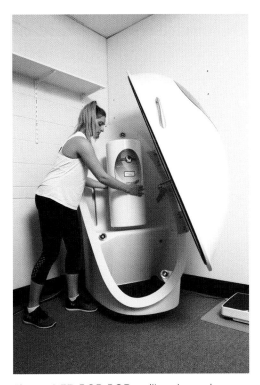

Figure 4.35 BOD POD calibration volume measurement

Used with permission from BOD POD

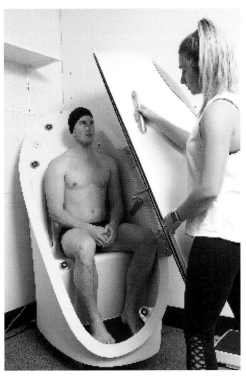

Figure 4.36 BOD POD participant preparation

Used with permission from BOD POD

11 Once seated in the BOD POD test chamber, ask the participant to relax, limit their movement and breathe normally for the next minute while their body volume is measured.

12 Once the first body volume measurement has been completed, open the door, check on the participant and then repeat the body volume instructions and measurement procedures.

13 If the screen prompts indicate that the first two volume measurements were not consistent, an additional volume measurement is performed. In this case, repeat the previous step.

14 If no combination of two body volume measurements out of the three performed is consistent, the software provides the operator with the option to repeat the test (recommended) or to continue with the test sequence.

15 If thoracic gas volume is to be measured, the success of the thoracic gas volume measurement procedure will be improved by completing a practice run as follows:

a Take the tube out of the BOD POD and hold the filter side.

b Have the participant hold the other end of the tube.

c Verbally instruct the participant to put the tube in their mouth, plug their nose (if not using a nose clip) and take two breaths.

d Watch the rise and fall of their chest. In the middle of the second exhalation (chest falling), completely cover up your end of the tube with your hand while simultaneously instructing the participant to huff three times in a row.

    e Ensure that the participant's cheeks do not puff out, there is a tight seal around the tube and that they do not huff too hard.

    f Repeat the practice procedures as many times as required to ensure that the participant is familiar with the process and the repeatability of the measurement is optimised.

    g Put the tube back into the BOD POD and proceed with the thoracic gas volume measurement process.

16 Instruct the participant that '*Using the tube and filter, this portion of the test will measure the amount of air in your lungs and can be divided into three main steps. You will be in the BOD POD for about 50 seconds.*'

17 Step 1: '*After I close the door, please hold the breathing tube in one hand and watch the monitor for the purple and green progress bar telling you when to breathe IN and OUT. Breathe at the same rate as the progress bar.*'

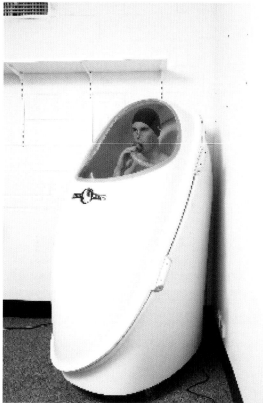

Figure 4.37 BOD POD thoracic gas volume measurement

Used with permission from BOD POD

18 Step 2: '*After about 4 breaths a message will appear on the screen that says "Prepare to put tube in mouth and plug up nose". Simply bring the tube close to your mouth. Immediately after, you will see a message that says, "Put tube in mouth". Please put the tube in your mouth, pinch your nose (if not using a nose clip) and continue breathing according to the progress bar. You will hear some pops and clicks inside of the BOD POD.*' (Figure 4.37).

19 Step 3: '*After a few more breaths you will see a message on the screen that says "Prepare to huff". This will alert you that during the next exhalation the airway connected to the tube will close for 2 seconds. Immediately after, you will see the final message that says "HUFF, HUFF, HUFF". At this point please huff very gently three times in a row as if you were blowing away a feather or fogging up your glasses.*' At the end of the third huff the thoracic gas volume measurement is complete.

20 If the result of the thoracic gas volume test displays a Merit and/or airway pressure of 'High', this usually indicates the participant either closed their glottis during the huffing (i.e. unknowingly performed a Valsalva manoeuvre), huffed too hard, did not maintain a tight seal around the tube during huffing or the participant's measured thoracic gas volume was outside of what was expected. Instruct the participant on these likely contributing factors and repeat the thoracic gas measurement test.

21 The thoracic gas measurement test can be repeated as many times as necessary; however, if time is a constraint, change the option on the thoracic gas volume selection screen to Predicted, Entered or, if available, Previously measured (recommended).

22 Ask the participant to exit the test chamber and then close the test chamber door.

23 Repeat steps 6 to 21 to perform BOD POD measures in duplicate.

24 If there is ≤ 150 mL difference in body volume and $\leq 0.5\%$ difference in percent body fat between the two measures, record the mean (average) of these measures. If there is >150 mL difference in body volume or $>0.5\%$ difference in percent body fat between the two measures, perform a third measure. If body volume is ≤ 150 mL and percent body fat is $\leq 0.5\%$ between any two of the three measures, record the median. If no two measurements meet the acceptance criteria, the entire test procedure (including recalibration) should be repeated.

25 Clean and disinfect all equipment (see Appendix A).

Data recording

Participant's name: _____   Date: _____

Age: _____ years   Sex: _____

Record the following data presented on the BOD POD report:

% Fat: _____ %

% Fat-free mass: _____ %

Fat mass: _____ kg

Fat-free mass: _____ kg

Body fat rating: _____

Interpretation

First, consider the four steps of interpretation outlined in Appendix G, and refer to Table 4.7.

Issues to consider are:

- How much did body fat estimated by the BOD POD differ from the percentage body fat calculated from the skinfold, BIA, DXA or air displacement plethysmography measures? Consider the possible reasons for these discrepancies in body fat percentage.
- Do the BOD POD results appear to be a valid representation of body fat, taking into consideration training status, body mass, BMI and WHR?

Due consideration of the limitations and assumptions of each mode of body fat calculation (i.e. skinfold equations, BIA, DXA and air displacement plethysmography) and the extraneous factors influencing each measure (e.g. hydration status, activity level) are essential when determining which body fat measurement is most valid for your participant according to their current situation.

Feedback and discussion

First, consider the three steps of feedback and discussion outlined in Appendix G. Physique assessments can be a highly personal issue. Given this, ensure that you provide feedback on physique trait results in a private location, and consider whether anyone else should be in the room (e.g. a parent or coach) to support the individual, and ensure gender compatibility between the athlete and staff. Where multiple physique trait tests have been performed, feedback should be combined to be delivered as a collective message, emphasising the results of the more appropriate tests (e.g. if both BMI and DXA results have been calculated for a participant, feedback should not focus on the BMI results). Ensure that you keep the results confidential and release them only as necessary (i.e. to their coach, parent and/or other relevant professionals) and after seeking approval of the individual. It is not appropriate for other athletes to be privy to the physique trait results of their teammates.

Before providing feedback on physique traits to an individual, you should first consider the purpose of the test and the language you will use to ensure that the mental and physical health of the participant is optimised. You should deliver feedback in a manner that is highly sensitive to the personal nature of physique assessment using positive, supportive language.

Given that physique assessments are usually performed concurrently with other measures of fitness/ performance, it is wise to provide combined feedback across all assessments. The focus of feedback on physique trait results should, more often than not, be on the potential for exercise and/or nutrition to improve these measures, and the subsequent effect this would have on the participant's health and/or sporting performance as appropriate. If providing feedback on repeated routine measures of physique traits, ensure that the participant is aware of the likely range and time frame to detect significant differences, to reduce their feelings of disappointment or failure. Where results warrant referral for specialist practitioner follow-up, you should discuss this with the participant during the consult.

Case studies

Case Study 1

Setting: You are an accredited sports scientist providing scientific services for the national rowing squad, as part of a multidisciplinary practitioner team. As you are in regular contact with the squad, it is part of your role to measure the body composition of the rowers throughout the season. The assessments are made in the morning before training, in a controlled environment at the sport science laboratory, and include height, body mass and sum of seven skinfolds.

Task: Matthew is a 21-year-old heavyweight rower who was selected to join the national squad. The coach asked you to assess Matthew's body composition when he joined the team, and then again after 3 months of training.

DATE	BODY MASS	HEIGHT	SUM OF SEVEN SKINFOLDS
10 March	98.5 kg	199 cm	78 mm
14 June	97.1 kg	199.1 cm	66 mm

How would you interpret Matthew's change in body composition after 3 months training?

The coach wants to increase Matthew's power-to-weight ratio over the next training phase. What recommendations would you make regarding the changes to be made to Matthew's body composition? Would you involve other members of the multidisciplinary team to achieve this goal, and why or why not?

Case Study 2

Setting: You are an Accredited Exercise Physiologist working in an exercise physiology clinic. When new members join your clinic, they have the opportunity to complete a physique assessment to stratify their risk of cardiometabolic and lifestyle-related diseases. You are responsible for conducting these assessments on your clients, and designing the exercise program appropriate for each client's condition.

Task: Marcus is a 45-year-old male who has been prescribed exercise by his doctor in order to improve his cardiometabolic health and reduce his risk of lifestyle-related diseases. At your initial consultation, you make the following measurements:

BMI: 30.4 kg/m^2

WHR: 0.98

Waist circumference: 102 cm

What feedback would you provide to Marcus about his current disease risk? What considerations would you need to make when designing his program based on this result?

Case Study 3

Setting: You work as an Accredited Exercise Scientist working in a health and fitness gymnasium. When new members join your centre, you are responsible for conducting initial consultations on clients.

continued

Case studies *(continued)*

Task: Jerry is a 43-year-old male who is training to compete in a body building competition in 6 months. At your initial consultation, Jerry provides you with copies of DXA and BOD POD scans (Figures 4.38 and 4.39) he had completed on the same morning a week ago. He asks for your help interpreting the fat mass, fat-free mass and percentage fat results, how they compared with other guys his age, and whether they are 'accurate'. He asks you for advice as to what he should do regarding measuring his fat and fat-free mass in the lead-up to his competition.

What feedback would you provide to Jerry about his DXA and BOD POD scans? What considerations would you need to make when providing Jerry with his results?

Name:	Sex: Male	Height: 183.0 cm
Patient	Ethnicity: White	Weight: 99.0 kg
DOB: 11 May 1971		Age: 43

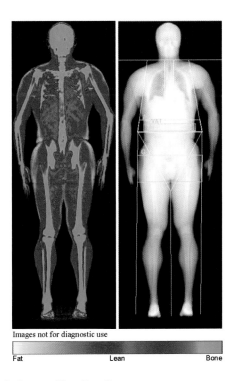

Images not for diagnostic use

Fat Lean Bone

Total Body % Fat

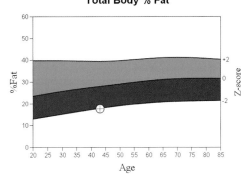

Source: 2008 NHANES White Male

World Health Organization Body Mass Index Classification
BMI = 29.6 WHO Classification Overweight

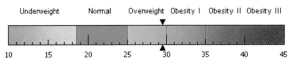

BMI has some limitations and an actual diagnosis of overweight or obesity should be made by a health professional. Obesity is associated with heart disease, certain types of cancer, type 2 diabetes, and other health risks. The higher a person's BMI is above 25, the greater their weight-related risks.

Body Composition Results

Region	Fat Mass (g)	Lean + BMC (g)	Total Mass (g)	% Fat	% Fat Percentile YN	% Fat Percentile AM
L Arm	1097	5262	6359	17.2	20	7
R Arm	1198	5417	6616	18.1	23	8
Trunk	7287	38752	46039	15.8	10	2
L Leg	3120	13351	16472	18.9	12	6
R Leg	3425	14140	17565	19.5	13	7
Subtotal	16127	76923	93050	17.3	11	3
Head	1407	4766	6173	22.8		
Total	**17535**	**81689**	**99223**	**17.7**	**12**	**2**
Android (A)	1086	5199	6284	17.3		
Gynoid (G)	3024	11499	14523	20.8		

Scan Date:
Scan Type: a Whole Body
Analysis:
　　Auto Whole Body Fan Beam
Operator:
Model: Discovery A (S/N 80714)
Comment:

Adipose Indices

Measure	Result	Percentile YN	Percentile AM
Total Body % Fat	**17.7**	**12**	**2**
Fat Mass/Height^2 (kg/m^2)	5.24	32	14
Android/Gynoid Ratio	0.83		
% Fat Trunk/% Fat Legs	0.82	23	6
Trunk/Limb Fat Mass Ratio	0.82	15	4
Est. VAT Mass (g)	339		
Est. VAT Volume (cm^3)	367		
Est. VAT Area (cm^2)	70.4		

Lean Indices

Measure	Result	Percentile YN	Percentile AM
Lean/Height^2 (kg/m^2)	23.2	93	91
Appen. Lean/Height^2 (kg/m^2)	10.8	93	93

Est. VAT = Estimated Visceral Adipose Tissue
YN = Young Normal
AM = Age Matched

Figure 4.38 Dual-energy x-ray absorptiometry (DXA) scan results

Used with permission from Hologic

SUBJECT INFORMATION

NAME	
AGE	
GENDER	Male
HEIGHT	184.1 cm
ID_1	
ID_2	
ETHNICITY	General Population
OPERATOR	
TEST DATE	
TEST NUMBER	

BODY COMPOSITION RESULT

% FAT	17.5	%
% FAT FREE MASS	82.5	%
FAT MASS	17.207	kg
FAT FREE MASS	80.840	kg
BODY MASS	98.046	kg
BODY VOLUME	92.609	L
BODY DENSITY	1.0587	kg/L
THORACIC GAS VOLUME	4.385	L

OPERATOR COMMENTS

TEST PROFILE

DENSITY MODEL	Siri
THORACIC GAS VOLUME MODEL	Predicted

Body Fat: A certain amount of fat is absolutely necessary for good health. Fat plays an important role in protecting internal organs, providing energy, and regulating hormones. The minimal amount of "essential fat" is approximately 3-5% for men, and 12-15% for women. If too much fat accumulates over time, health may be compromised (see table below).

Fat Free Mass: Fat free mass is everything except fat. It includes muscle, water, bone, and internal organs. Muscle is the "metabolic engine" of the body that burns calories (fat) and plays an important role in maintaining strength and energy. Healthy levels of fat-free mass contribute to physical fitness and may prevent conditions such as osteoporosis.

BOD POD Body Fat Rating Table*

*Applies to adults ages 18 and older. Based on information from the American College of Sports Medicine, the American Council on Exercise, Exercise Physiology (4th Ed.) by McArdle, Katch, and Katch, and various scientific and epidemiological studies.

	BODY FAT RATING	MALE	EXPLANATION
	Risky (high body fat)	> 30%	Ask your health care professional about how to safely modify your body composition.
	Excess Fat	20 - 30%	Indicates an excess accumulation of fat over time.
X	Moderately Lean	12 - 20%	Fat level is generally acceptable for good health.
	Lean	8 - 12%	Lower body fat levels than many people. This range is generally excellent for health and longevity.
	Ultra Lean	5 - 8%	Fat levels often found in elite athletes.
	Risky (low body fat)	< 5%	Ask your health care professional about how to safely modify your body composition.

ENERGY EXPENDITURE RESULTS

Est. Resting Metabolic Rate (RMR) kcal/day	*Est. Total Energy Expenditure (TEE) kcal/day	Daily Activity Level
	2758	Sedentary
	3254	Low Active
2155	3750	Active
	4482	Very Active
(See RMR Info Sheet for additional info)	*Est. TEE = Est. RMR x Daily Activity Level	

Applies to adults ages 18 and older. Based on information from the Institute of Medicine (2002), Dietary Reference Intakes For Energy, Carbohydrate, Fiber, Fat, Fatty Acids, Cholesterol, Protein, And Amino Acids, Part I, pp93-206. Washington, D.C., National Academy of Sciences.

Figure 4.39 BOD POD scan results

Used with permission from BOD POD

References

[1] National Health and Medical Research Council. Clinical practice guidelines for the management of overweight and obesity in adults, adolescents and children in Australia. Canberra, ACT: NHMRC; 2013. https://www.nhmrc.gov.au/about-us/publications/clinical-practice-guidelines-management-overweight-and-obesity#block-views-block-file-attachments-content-block-1.

[2] Taylor RW, Keil D, Gold EJ, Williams SM, Goulding A. Body mass index, waist girth, and waist-to-hip ratio as indexes of total and regional adiposity in women: valuation using receiver operating characteristic curves. Am J Clin Nutr 1998;67:44–9.

[3] Olds T. The evolution of physique in male rugby union players in the twentieth century. J Sports Sci 2001;19:253–62.

[4] Claessens AL, Lefevre J, Beunen G, Malina RM. The contribution of anthropometric characteristics to performance scores in elite female gymnasts. J Sports Med Phys Fitness 1999;39:355–60.

[5] Siders WA, Lukaski HC, Bolonchuk WW. Relationships among swimming performance, body composition and somatotype in competitive collegiate swimmers. J Sports Med Phys Fitness 1993;33:166–71.

[6] Claessens AL, Hlatky S, Lefevre J, Holdhaus H. The role of anthropometric characteristics in modern pentathlon performance in female athletes. J Sports Sci 1994;12:391–401.

[7] White AT, Johnson SC. Physiological comparison of international, national and regional alpine skiers. Int J Sports Med 1991;12:374–8.

[8] Rodriguez FA. Physical structure of international lightweight rowers. In: Reilly T, Watkins J, Borms J, eds. Kinanthropometry III. London: E & FN Spon; 1986, p. 255–61.

[9] Shephard RJ. Science and medicine of rowing: a review. J Sports Sci 1998;16:603–20.

[10] Claessens AL, Lefevre J, Beunen G, Malina RM. The contribution of anthropometric characteristics to performance scores in elite female gymnasts. J Sports Med Phys Fitness 1999;39:355–60.

[11] Fry AC, Ryan AJ, Schwab RJ, Powell DR, Kraemer WJ. Anthropometric characteristics as discriminators of body-building success. J Sports Sci 1991;9:23–32.

[12] Faria IE, Faria EW. Relationship of the anthropometric and physical characteristics of male junior gymnasts to performance. J Sports Med Phys Fitness 1989;29:369–78.

[13] Norton K, Olds T, Olive S, Craig N. Anthropometry and sports performance. In: Norton K, Olds T, eds. Anthropometrica. Sydney: University of New South Wales Press; 1996, p. 287–364.

[14] DeRose EH, Crawford SM, Kerr DA, Ward R, Ross WD. Physique characteristics of Pan American Games lightweight rowers. Int J Sports Med 1989;10:292–7.

[15] Hahn A. Identification and selection of talent in Australian rowing. Excel 1990;6:5–11.

[16] Carson JD, Bridges E; Canadian Academy of Sport M. Abandoning routine body composition assessment: A strategy to reduce disordered eating among female athletes and dancers. Clin J Sport Med 2001;11:280.

[17] Whitehead JR, Eklund RC, Williams AC. Using skinfold calipers while teaching body fatness-related concepts: cognitive and affective outcomes. J Sci Med Sport 2003;6:461–76.

[18] Reilly T, Tyrrell A, Troup JD. Circadian variation in human stature. Chronobiol Int 1984;1:121–6.

[19] Maughan R, Shirreffs S. Exercise in the heat: challenges and opportunities. J Sports Sci 2004;22:917–27.

[20] Stein RJ, Haddock CK, Poston WS, Catanese D, Spertus JA. Precision in weighing: a comparison of scales found in physician offices, fitness centers, and weight loss centers. Public Health Rep 2005;120:266–70.

[21] Bunt JC, Lohman TG, Boileau RA. Impact of total body water fluctuations on estimation of body fat from body density. Med Sci Sports Exerc 1989;21:96–100.

[22] Vilaca KH, Ferrioli E, Lima NK, Paula FJ, Moriguti JC. Effect of fluid and food intake on the body composition evaluation of elderly persons. J Nutr Health Aging 2009;13:183–6.

[23] Horber FF, Thomi F, Casez JP, Fonteille J, Jaeger P. Impact of hydration status on body composition as measured by dual energy x-ray absorptiometry in normal volunteers and patients on haemodialysis. Br J Radiol 1992;65:895–900.

[24] Meyer NL, Sundgot-Borgen J, Lohman TG, Ackland TR, Stewart AD, Maughan RJ, et al. Body composition for health and performance: a survey of body composition assessment practice carried out by the ad hoc research working group on body composition, health and performance under the auspices of the IOC medical commission. Br J Sports Med 2013;47:1044–53.

[25] Hume P, Marfell-Jones M. The importance of accurate site location for skinfold measurement. J Sports Sci 2008;26:1333–40.

[26] Stewart AD, Marfell-Jones M, Olds T, Hans De Ridder J. International standards for anthropometric assessment. Lower Hutt, New Zealand: International Society for the Advancement of Kinanthropometry (ISAK); 2011.

[27] Reis JP, Macera CA, Araneta MR, Lindsay SP, Marshall SJ, Wingard DL. Comparison of overall obesity and body fat distribution in predicting risk of mortality. Obesity (Silver Spring) 2009;17:1232–9.

[28] de Onis M, Onyango AW, Borghi E, Siyam A, Nishida C, Siekmann J. Development of a WHO growth reference for school-aged children and adolescents. Bull World Health Organ 2007;85:660–7.

[29] Janssen I, Mark AE. Elevated body mass index and mortality risk in the elderly. Obes Rev 2007;8:41–59.

[30] Winter JE, MacInnis RJ, Wattanapenpaiboon N, Nowson CA. BMI and all-cause mortality in older adults: a meta-analysis. Am J Clin Nutr 2014;99:875–90.

[31] Rush EC, Freitas I, Plank LD. Body size, body composition and fat distribution: comparative analysis of European, Maori, Pacific Island and Asian Indian adults. Br J Nutr 2009;102:632–41.

[32] Stevens J, Nowicki EM. Body mass index and mortality in Asian populations: implications for obesity cut-points. Nutr Rev 2003;61:104–7.

[33] World Health Organisation Expert Consultation. Appropriate body-mass index for Asian populations and its implications for policy and intervention strategies. Lancet 2004;363:157–63.

[34] Katzmarzyk PT, Heymsfield SB, Bouchard C. Clinical utility of visceral adipose tissue for the identification of cardiometabolic risk in white and African American adults. Am J Clin Nutr. 2013;97:480–6.

[35] Bray GA. Don't throw the baby out with the bath water. Am J Clin Nutr 2004;79:347–9.

[36] Folsom AR, Kaye SA, Sellers TA, Hong CP, Cerhan JR, Potter JD, et al. Body fat distribution and 5-year risk of death in older women. JAMA 1993;269:483–7.

[37] Heyward VH, Stolarczyk LM. Applied body composition assessment. Champaign, IL: Human Kinetics; 1996.

[38] Ashwell M, Hsieh SD. Six reasons why the waist-to-height ratio is a rapid and effective global indicator for health risks of obesity and how its use could simplify the international public health message on obesity. Int J Food Sci Nutr 2005;56:303–7.

[39] Martin AD, Ross WD, Drinkwater DT, Clarys JP. Prediction of body fat by skinfold caliper: assumptions and cadaver evidence. Int J Obes 1985;9(Suppl 1):31–9.

[40] Lohman TG. Skinfolds and body density and their relation to body fatness: a review. Hum Biol 1981;53:181–225.

[41] Clarys JP, Provyn S, Marfell-Jones MJ. Cadaver studies and their impact on the understanding of human adiposity. Ergonomics 2005;48:1445–61.

[42] Norton K, Hayward S, Charles S, Rees M. The effects of hypohydration and hyperhydration on skinfold measurements. In: Norton K, Olds, T, Dollman J, eds. Sixth scientific conference of the International Society for the Advancement of Kinanthropometry. Sydney, NSW: University of New South Wales Press; 1998, p. 253–66.

[43] Araujo D, Teixeira VH, Carvalho P, Amaral TF. Exercise induced dehydration status and skinfold compressibility in athletes: an intervention study. Asia Pac J Clin Nutr 2018;27:189–94.

[44] Norton K, Whittingham N, Carter L, Kerr D, Gore CJ, Marfell-Jones M. Anthropometrica. Sydney, NSW: University of New South Wales Press; 1996.

[45] Durnin JV, Womersley J. Body fat assessed from total body density and its estimation from skinfold thickness: measurements on 481 men and women aged from 16 to 72 years. Br J Nutr 1974;32:77–97.

[46] Withers RT, Craig NP, Bourdon PC, Norton KI. Relative body fat and anthropometric prediction of body density of male athletes. Eur J Appl Physiol Occup Physiol 1987;56:191–200.

[47] Ross WD, Marfell-Jones MJ. Physiological testing of the elite athlete. Ottawa: Mutual Press; 1982.

[48] Jackson AS, Pollock ML. Practical assessment of body composition. Phys Sportsmed 1985;13:76–90.

[49] Jackson AS, Pollock ML, Ward A. Generalized equations for predicting body density of women. Med Sci Sports Exerc 1980;12:175–81.

[50] Keys A. Recommendations concerning body measurements for the characterization of nutritional status. Human Biol 1956;28:111–23.

[51] Weiner JS, Lourie JA. International biological programme handbook no. 9. Oxford, UK: Blackwell Scientific; 1969.

[52] Katch FI, McArdle WD. Prediction of body density from simple anthropometric measurements in college-age men and women. Hum Biol 1973;45:445–55.

[53] Siri WE. Body composition from fluid spaces and density: analysis of methods. In: Brozek J, Henschel A, eds. Techniques for measuring body composition. Washington, DC: National Academy of Sciences; 1961, p. 223–44.

[54] Gore CJ, Edwards DA. Australian fitness norms: a manual for fitness assessors. North Adelaide, SA: Health Development Foundation; 1992.

[55] Reilly T, George K, Marfell-Jones M, Scott M, Sutton L, Wallace JA. How well do skinfold equations predict percent body fat in elite soccer players? Int J Sports Med 2009;30:607–13.

[56] Johnston FE. Relationships between body composition and anthropometry. Hum Biol 1982;54:221–45.

[57] National Institute of Health. NIH consensus statement. Bioelectrical impedance analysis in body composition measurement. National Institutes of Health technology assessment conference statement. December 12–14, 1994. Nutrition 1996;12:749–62.

[58] Kyle UG, Bosaeus I, De Lorenzo AD, Deurenberg P, Elia M, Gomez JM, et al. Composition of the EWG. Bioelectrical impedance analysis – part I: review of principles and methods. Clin Nutr 2004;23:1226–43.

[59] Kushner RF. Bioelectrical impedance analysis: a review of principles and applications. J Am Coll Nutr 1992;11:199–209.

[60] Saunders MJ, Blevins JE, Broeder CE. Effects of hydration changes on bioelectrical impedance in endurance trained individuals. Med Sci Sports Exerc 1998;30:885–92.

[61] Dixon CB, Ramos L, Fitzgerald E, Reppert D, Andreacci JL. The effect of acute fluid consumption on measures of impedance and percent body fat estimated using segmental bioelectrical impedance analysis. Eur J Clin Nutr 2009;63:1115–22.

[62] Kerr A, Slater GJ, Byrne N. Impact of food and fluid intake on technical and biological measurement error in body composition assessment methods in athletes. Br J Nutr 2017;117:591–601.

[63] Simpson JA, MacInnis RJ, Peeters A, Hopper JL, Giles GG, English DR. A comparison of adiposity measures as predictors of all-cause mortality: the Melbourne Collaborative Cohort Study. Obesity (Silver Spring) 2007;15:994–1003.

[64] Mazess RB, Barden HS, Bisek JP, Hanson J. Dual-energy x-ray absorptiometry for total-body and regional bone-mineral and soft-tissue composition. Am J Clin Nutr 1990;51:1106–12.

[65] Lewiecki EM. Clinical applications of bone density testing for osteoporosis. Minerva Med 2005;96:317–30.

[66] Tothill P, Avenell A, Love J, Reid DM. Comparisons between Hologic, Lunar and Norland dual-energy x-ray absorptiometers and other techniques used for whole-body soft tissue measurements. Eur J Clin Nutr 1994;48:781–94.

[67] Hull H, He Q, Thornton J, Javed F, Allen L, Wang J, et al. IDXA, Prodigy, and DPXL dual-energy x-ray absorptiometry whole-body scans: a cross-calibration study. J Clin Densitom 2009;12:95–102.

[68] Soriano JM, Ioannidou E, Wang J, Thornton JC, Horlick MN, Gallagher D, et al. Pencil-beam vs fan-beam dual-energy x-ray absorptiometry comparisons across four systems: body composition and bone mineral. J Clin Densitom 2004;7:281–9.

[69] Prior BM, Cureton KJ, Modlesky CM, Evans EM, Sloniger MA, Saunders M, et al. In vivo validation of whole body composition estimates from dual-energy x-ray absorptiometry. J Appl Physiol (1985) 1997;83:623–30.

[70] Deurenberg-Yap M, Schmidt G, van Staveren WA, Hautvast JG, Deurenberg P. Body fat measurement among Singaporean Chinese, Malays and Indians: a comparative study using a four-compartment model and different two-compartment models. Br J Nutr 2001;85:491–8.

[71] Van Der Ploeg GE, Withers RT, Laforgia J. Percent body fat via DEXA: comparison with a four-compartment model. J Appl Physiol (1985) 2003;94:499–506.

[72] Weyers AM, Mazzetti SA, Love DM, Gomez AL, Kraemer WJ, Volek JS. Comparison of methods for assessing body composition changes during weight loss. Med Sci Sports Exerc 2002;34:497–502.

[73] Houtkooper LB, Going SB, Sproul J, Blew RM, Lohman TG. Comparison of methods for assessing body-composition changes over 1 y in postmenopausal women. Am J Clin Nutr 2000;72:401–6.

[74] Pritchard JE, Nowson CA, Strauss BJ, Carlson JS, Kaymakci B, Wark JD. Evaluation of dual energy x-ray absorptiometry as a method of measurement of body fat. Eur J Clin Nutr 1993;47:216–28.

[75] Tothill P, Hannan WJ, Wilkinson S. Comparisons between a pencil beam and two fan beam dual energy x-ray absorptiometers used for measuring total body bone and soft tissue. Br J Radiol 2001;74:166–76.

[76] Lohman M, Tallroth K, Kettunen JA, Marttinen MT. Reproducibility of dual-energy x-ray absorptiometry total and regional body composition measurements using different scanning positions and definitions of regions. Metabolism 2009;58:1663–8.

[77] Lambrinoudaki I, Georgiou E, Douskas G, Tsekes G, Kyriakidis M, Proukakis C. Body composition assessment by dual-energy x-ray absorptiometry: comparison of prone and supine measurements. Metabolism 1998;47:1379–82.

[78] Burkhart TA, Arthurs KL, Andrews DM. Manual segmentation of DXA scan images results in reliable upper and lower extremity soft and rigid tissue mass estimates. J Biomech 2009;42:1138–42.

[79] Silva AM, Minderico CS, Rodrigues AR, Pietrobelli A, Sardinha LB. Calibration models to estimate body composition measurements in taller subjects using DXA. Int J Body Compos Res 2004;2:165–73.

[80] Evans EM, Prior BM, Modlesky CM. A mathematical method to estimate body composition in tall individuals using DXA. Med Sci Sports Exerc 2005;37:1211–15.

[81] Rothney MP, Brychta RJ, Schaefer EV, Chen KY, Skarulis MC. Body composition measured by dual-energy x-ray absorptiometry half-body scans in obese adults. Obesity (Silver Spring) 2009;17:1281–6.

[82] Tataranni PA, Ravussin E. Use of dual-energy x-ray absorptiometry in obese individuals. Am J Clin Nutr 1995;62:730–4.

[83] Lear SA, Humphries KH, Kohli S, Frohlich JJ, Birmingham CL, Mancini GB. Visceral adipose tissue, a potential risk factor for carotid atherosclerosis: Results of the multicultural community health assessment trial (M-CHAT). Stroke 2007;38:2422–9.

[84] Pickhardt PJ, Jee Y, O'Connor SD, del Rio AM. Visceral adiposity and hepatic steatosis at abdominal CT: association with the metabolic syndrome. Am J Roentgenol 2012;198:1100–7.

[85] Reijnierse EM, Trappenburg MC, Leter MJ, Blauw GJ, de van der Schueren MA, Meskers CG, et al. The association between parameters of malnutrition and diagnostic measures of sarcopenia in geriatric outpatients. PloS One 2015;10:e0135933.

[86] Meng NH, Li CI, Liu CS, Lin WY, Lin CH, Chang CK, et al. Sarcopenia defined by combining height- and weight-adjusted skeletal muscle indices is closely associated with poor physical performance. J Aging Phys Act 2015;23:597–606.

[87] Brozek J, Grande F, Anderson JT, Keys A. Densitometric analysis of body composition: Revision of some quantitative assumptions. Ann N Y Acad Sci 1963;110:113–40.

[88] Fields DA, Hunter GR, Goran MI. Validation of the BOD POD with hydrostatic weighing: influence of body clothing. Int J Obes Relat Metab Disord 2000;24:200–5.

[89] Biaggi RR, Vollman MW, Nies MA, Brener CE, Flakoll PJ, Levenhagen DK, et al. Comparison of air-displacement plethysmography with hydrostatic weighing and bioelectrical impedance analysis for the assessment of body composition in healthy adults. Am J Clin Nutr 1999;69:898–903.

[90] Secchiutti A, Fagour C, Perlemoine C, Gin H, Durrieu J, Rigalleau V. Air displacement plethysmography can detect moderate changes in body composition. Eur J Clin Nutr 2007;61:25–9.

[91] Noreen EE, Lemon PW. Reliability of air displacement plethysmography in a large, heterogeneous sample. Med Sci Sports Exerc 2006;38:1505–9.

[92] Anderson DE. Reliability of air displacement plethysmography. J Strength Cond Res 2007;21:169–72.

[93] Ball SD. Interdevice variability in percent fat estimates using the BOD POD. Eur J Clin Nutr 2005;59:996–1001.

[94] Collins AL, McCarthy HD. Evaluation of factors determining the precision of body composition measurements by air displacement plethysmography. Eur J Clin Nutr 2003;57:770–6.

[95] Davis JA, Dorado S, Keays KA, Reigel KA, Valencia KS, Pham PH. Reliability and validity of the lung volume measurement made by the BOD POD body composition system. Clin Physiol Funct Imaging 2007;27:42–6.

[96] Minderico CS, Silva AM, Fields DA, Branco TL, Martins SS, Teixeira PJ, et al. Changes in thoracic gas volume with air-displacement plethysmography after a weight loss program in overweight and obese women. Eur J Clin Nutr 2008;62:444–50.

PRACTICAL 5
PHYSICAL ACTIVITY

Jeff Coombes, Stewart Trost and Sjaan Gomersall

LEARNING OBJECTIVES

- Explain the scientific rationale, purposes, reliability, validity, assumptions and limitations of common measures of physical activity

- Identify and explain the common terminology, processes and equipment required to conduct accurate measures of physical activity

- Describe the principles and rationale for the calibration of equipment commonly used to measure physical activity

- Select and conduct appropriate protocols for effective measures of physical activity, including instructing clients on the correct use of equipment

- Record, analyse and interpret information from measures of physical activity and convey the results, including the validity and limitations of the measures, through relevant verbal and/or written communication to a participant

Equipment and other requirements

- International Physical Activity Questionnaire[1]
- Smartphone
- Step counter (e.g. app in smartphone)
- 10-metre measuring tape/wheel
- Accelerometer and associated software
- Calculator
- Internet access

INTRODUCTION

It is well established that people must maintain adequate levels of physical activity to enjoy healthy and productive lives. People who meet physical activity guidelines have a decreased risk of developing chronic diseases such as cardiovascular disease, diabetes, cancer or osteoporosis.[2] Physical activity can prevent unhealthy weight gain and assist with weight loss[3] and physically active people have better mental health with lower rates of depression and anxiety.[4]

Exercise professionals can assist individuals to become more active. Valid measures of physical activity may be useful in this process and are important to understand the success of interventions/programs. Knowledge of a person's physical activity level along with when and how they are being physically active will allow for the development of strategies to increase activity. However, physical activity is a complex behaviour with multiple dimensions (e.g. mode, frequency, intensity, duration) and domains (e.g. leisure time, occupational, transportation and household). Trying to assess physical activity is not easy. Unlike other health behaviours such as tobacco use, physical activity does not come in easy-to-measure packages (e.g. packets of cigarettes/day).

Physical activity assessment can be broadly divided into subjective and device-based or objective methods (Table 5.1). Device-based methods may be separated into research or consumer devices. The most basic

TABLE 5.1 Methods for assessing physical activity

SUBJECTIVE	DEVICE-BASED OR OBJECTIVE
• Physical activity records/diaries • Physical activity logs • Recall surveys • Global assessment tools	• Direct observation • Doubly labelled water • Heart rate monitoring • Pedometers • Accelerometers • Consumer-based activity trackers

monitoring device is a pedometer that counts steps only; however, these are now rarely used. Most current devices (e.g. smartphone, wearable device) offer a measure of steps using a triaxial accelerometer as their primary sensor, but often include other sensors (e.g. altimeter, gyroscope, global positioning system (GPS), photoplethysmograph). A generally accepted and widely promoted health criterion is for individuals to obtain 10,000 steps per day. Assessing step counts has become a common method to measure physical activity. There is good evidence that asking people to count their steps is associated with significant increases in steps and significant decreases in body mass index and blood pressure.[5]

Wearable devices are now usually worn on the wrist, although some are contained within armbands, clothing or shoes. They are commonly referred to as an 'activity tracker' and are capable of being synchronised (synced) to an app. The app becomes a central component of the activity monitoring approach and it might contain, or be able to access via the internet, algorithms to combine inputs from the different sensors to attempt a more valid and detailed measure of physical activity. Furthermore, advances in heart rate monitoring have allowed heart rate data to be more easily collected and combined with the other motion data. Indeed, most smart watches will contain multiple sensors that also allow them to monitor activity more precisely.

In this practical we will use one subjective (International Physical Activity Questionnaire, IPAQ) and a number of device-based (smartphone and app, wearable device and app, and research-based accelerometer) approaches. Desirable attributes of a physical activity assessment method include: reliability, validity (concurrent), non-reactivity, ability to assess usual/habitual physical activity, being economical, and not being a burden for participants and testers. It is impossible for one method to have all of these attributes. Therefore, the selection of a tool to measure physical activity is typically determined by the resources at your disposal and the intended use of the measure.

DEFINITIONS

Accelerometers: measure accelerations produced by body movement.

Concurrent validity: the degree to which an assessment (e.g. test or measure) accurately measures what it is intended to measure. May refer to the validity of a test (e.g. physical activity is not a valid measure of cardiorespiratory fitness) or the validity of a measure (e.g. a step counter accurately measures the number of steps).

Direct observation: involves observing an individual in a defined behaviour setting (home, school, office, factory) for extended time periods and systematically recording a rating of activity type, intensity level and other relevant contextual information.

Doubly labelled water: assesses total energy expenditure by estimating carbon dioxide production using an isotope dilution method.

Exercise: planned, structured and repetitive movements carried out to sustain or improve fitness and health.

Global assessment tool: contains general questions regarding the type, amount and intensity of physical activity performed over a specified period of time.

Heart rate (HR) monitoring: relies on the linear relationship between heart rate and oxygen consumption to assess physical activity. However, this relationship is not strong at the low end of the physical activity spectrum.

MET: or **m**etabolic **e**quivalent, is a measure of the energy cost of physical activities relative to the energy cost at rest. At rest it is convention that 1 MET of energy is expended, which is obtained by consuming 3.5 mL/kg/min of oxygen.

MET-minute: a measure of energy expenditure. Calculated by multiplying the MET score of an activity by the minutes performed. MET-minute scores are equivalent to kilocalories for a 60 kg person.

Non-reactivity: a measure is made without the participant's awareness.

Pedometers: simple electronic devices used to estimate distance walked or the number of steps taken.

Physical activity: any bodily movement produced by skeletal muscle that results in energy expenditure.

Physical activity log: provides a predefined list of activities for the participant to select. There may also be additional items (e.g. intensity) related to that activity.

Physical activity record/diary: a blank sheet or blank form with defined times. The participant records the details of their physical activity (e.g. mode, intensity and duration) as it occurs.

Recall surveys: participant recalls their physical activity over a specified period of time.

Reliability: the ability of a measure to provide consistent/repeatable data.

Activity 5.1 International Physical Activity Questionnaire (IPAQ)

AIMS: administer the IPAQ, interpret the responses and provide feedback to a participant.

Background

The IPAQ was developed to measure the physical activity levels in large population studies across different countries.[6] The instrument can also be used on individuals to classify whether they are meeting physical activity guidelines. The IPAQ has become the most widely used physical activity questionnaire,[7] with two versions available: the 31-item long form (IPAQ-LF) and the 9-item Short Form (IPAQ-SF). It is publicly available and no permissions are required to use it. This practical will use the IPAQ-SF telephone version that asks about three specific types of activity (walking, moderate-intensity and vigorous-intensity activities) performed in four domains (leisure time, domestic/gardening, work-related and transport-related). Computation of the total score for the Short Form requires summation of the duration (in minutes) and frequency (in days) of walking, moderate-intensity and vigorous-intensity activities. Domain-specific estimates (e.g. work-related vs leisure time-related physical activity) cannot be obtained with the Short Form, which is a limitation as there is strong evidence that the domain in which physical activity occurs influences the relationship between physical activity and health.[4,8] The frequency of physical activity is also an important concept, which is reflected by its inclusion in current public health guidelines.[9] Therefore, both the total volume and the number of days and sessions are included in the IPAQ analysis algorithms.

Validity and reliability

The validity (concurrent) of the IPAQ has been assessed in numerous studies. A systematic review summarised 23 studies and found that a large majority of these found the correlation between the IPAQ

Short Form and device-based measures to be lower than the acceptable standard (0.50), typically overestimating physical activity levels by an average of 84%.[10] Indeed, overreporting of physical activity using a questionnaire approach is well recognised.[11] Therefore, although the IPAQ is easily administered and freely available, poor concurrent validity is a major limitation (see Practical 1, Test accuracy, reliability and validity). However, given the widespread use of physical activity assessment questionnaires, the authors of this practical deemed it important that an activity using a questionnaire was included and that the limitations of this approach are presented. With regards to reliability, the IPAQ has been shown to demonstrate excellent test–retest reliability (intra-class coefficient $= 0.76$).[12] Although validity is low, due to high repeatability if using it in a repeated-measures way, you should be able to see/assess change in that one individual.

Protocol summary

Administer the IPAQ to a participant, interpret the responses and provide feedback.

Protocol

1 Administer the 'Short Last 7 Days Telephone IPAQ' to a participant by reading the script on the questionnaire to the participant along with the 'interviewer clarification'.

2 If the participant is unable to answer the questions asking for specific days per week and time per day (questions 1–6) then use the 'interviewer probe' question.

3 Use the directions in 'data analysis' to obtain a continuous score and a categorical assessment – record these values.

IPAQ short form

READ: I am going to ask you about the time you spent being physically active in the last 7 days. Please answer each question even if you do not consider yourself to be an active person. Think about the activities you do at work, as part of your house and yard work, to get from place to place, and in your spare time for recreation, exercise or sport.

READ: now think about all the vigorous activities which take *hard physical effort* that you did in the last 7 days. Vigorous activities make you breathe much harder than normal and may include heavy lifting, digging, aerobics or fast bicycling. Think only about those physical activities that you did for at least 10 minutes at a time.

Q1 During the **last 7 days**, on how many days did you do **vigorous** physical activities?

_____ days per week

or (circle if appropriate)

Don't know/Not sure

Refused

[**Interviewer clarification**: think only about those physical activities that you do for at least 10 minutes at a time.]

[**Interviewer note**: if respondent answers zero, refuses or does not know, skip to question 3.]

Q2 How much time did you usually spend doing **vigorous** physical activities on one of those days?

_____ hours per day

_____ minutes per day

or (circle if appropriate)

Don't know/Not sure

Refused

[**Interviewer clarification**: think only about those physical activities that you do for at least 10 minutes at a time.]

[**Interviewer probe**: an average time for one of the days on which the respondent does vigorous activity is being sought. If the respondent can't answer because the pattern of time spent varies widely from day to day, ask: '*How much time in total would you spend over the last 7 days doing vigorous physical activities?*']

      _____ hours per week

      _____ minutes per week

or (circle if appropriate)

Don't know/Not sure

Refused

READ: now think about activities which take *moderate physical effort* that you did in the last 7 days. Moderate physical activities make you breathe somewhat harder than normal and may include carrying light loads, bicycling at a regular pace, or doubles tennis. Do not include walking. Again, think about only those physical activities that you did for at least 10 minutes at a time.

Q3 During the **last 7 days**, on how many days did you do **moderate** physical activities?

      _____ days per week

or (circle if appropriate)

Don't know/Not sure

Refused

[**Interviewer clarification**: think only about those physical activities that you do for at least 10 minutes at a time.]

[**Interviewer note**: if respondent answers zero, refuses or does not know, skip to question 5.]

Q4 How much time did you usually spend doing **moderate** physical activities on one of those days?

      _____ hours per day

      _____ minutes per day

or (circle if appropriate)

Don't Know/Not Sure

Refused

[**Interviewer clarification**: think only about those physical activities that you do for at least 10 minutes at a time.]

[**Interviewer probe**: an average time for one of the days on which the respondent does moderate activity is being sought. If the respondent can't answer because the pattern of time spent varies widely from day to day, or includes time spent in multiple jobs, ask: '*What is the total amount of time you spent over the* last 7 days doing moderate physical activities?*']

      _____ hours per week

      _____ minutes per week

or (circle if appropriate)

Don't know/Not sure

Refused

READ: now think about the time you spent *walking* in the last 7 days. This includes at work and at home, walking to travel from place to place, and any other walking that you might do solely for recreation, sport, exercise or leisure.

Q5 During the **last 7 days**, on how many days did you **walk** for at least 10 minutes at a time?

_____ days per week

or (circle if appropriate)

Don't know/Not sure

Refused

[**Interviewer clarification**: think only about the walking that you do for at least 10 minutes at a time.]

[**Interviewer note**: if respondent answers zero, refuses or does not know, skip to question 7.]

Q6 How much time did you usually spend **walking** on one of those days?

_____ hours per day

_____ minutes per day

or (circle if appropriate)

Don't know/Not sure

Refused

[**Interviewer probe**: an average time for one of the days on which the respondent walks is being sought. If the respondent can't answer because the pattern of time spent varies widely from day to day, ask: '*What is the total amount of time you spent walking over the last 7 days?*']

_____ hours per week

_____ minutes per week

or (circle if appropriate)

Don't know/Not sure

Refused

READ: now think about the time you spent *sitting* on weekdays during the last 7 days. Include time spent at work, at home, while doing course work and during leisure time. This may include time spent sitting at a desk, visiting friends, reading or sitting or lying down to watch television.

Q7 During the last 7 days, how much time did you usually spend **sitting** on a **weekday**?

_____ hours per weekday

_____ minutes per weekday

or (circle if appropriate)

Don't know/Not sure

Refused

[**Interviewer clarification**: include time spent lying down (awake) as well as sitting.]

[**Interviewer probe**: an average time per day spent sitting is being sought. If the respondent can't answer because the pattern of time spent varies widely from day to day, ask: '*What is the total amount of time you spent sitting last Wednesday?*']

_____ hours on Wednesday

_____ minutes on Wednesday

or (circle if appropriate)

Don't know/Not sure

Refused

Data analysis

The IPAQ suggests obtaining a categorical assessment and a continuous score.

Continuous score

National physical activity guidelines recommend between 500 and 1000 MET-minutes per week.[13] Therefore, the MET-minutes per week score should be first calculated and then compared with this recommendation.

Calculate the MET-minutes per week by first obtaining the MET-minutes per week for the three domains (vigorous, moderate and walking) using either:

a   responses to the questions with specific days per week and time per day

or

b   response to the 'interviewer probe' questions.

The necessary multiplication factors for each domain are on the data-recording sheet.

Data recording

Participant's name: _____   Date: _____

Age: _____ years   Sex: _____

Continuous Score

Vigorous: _____ days per week (Q1) × _____ time (Q2) = _____ (min/week) × 8 = _____ MET-minutes/week

or from interviewer probe question = _____ (min/week) × 8 = _____ MET-minutes/week

Moderate: _____ days per week (Q3) × _____ time (Q4) = _____ (min/week) × 4.4 = _____ MET-minutes/week

or from interviewer probe question = _____ (min/week) × 4.4 = _____ MET-minutes per week

Walking: _____ days per week (Q5) × _____ time (Q6) = _____ (min/week) × 3 = _____ MET-minutes per week

or from interviewer probe question = _____ (min/week) × 3 = _____ MET- minutes per week

Total MET-minutes/week = vigorous + moderate + walking = _____ MET-minutes/week

Participant meeting the 500 MET-minutes per week guideline (circle)   YES / NO

Categorical assessment

Place the participant into one of the following three categories based on their responses.

CATEGORY 3: HIGH

The participant has met any one of the following two criteria:

- vigorous-intensity activity on at least 3 days and accumulating at least 1500 MET-minutes/week

OR

- 7 or more[a] days of any combination of walking, moderate-intensity or vigorous-intensity activities accumulating at least 3000 MET-minutes/week.

---

[a] Participant could complete physical activity twice in one day and therefore have more than 7 days of activity.

CATEGORY 2: MODERATE

The participant has met any one of the following three criteria:

- 3 or more days of vigorous activity of at least 20 minutes/day

OR

- 5 or more days of moderate-intensity activity and/or walking of at least 30 minutes/day

OR

- 5 or more days of any combination of walking, moderate-intensity or vigorous-intensity activities achieving a minimum of at least 500 MET-minutes/week.

CATEGORY 1: LOW

This is the lowest level of physical activity. Those individuals who did not meet criteria for categories 2 or 3 are considered low physical activity/inactive.

Data recording

Categorical assessment (circle): High / Moderate / Low

Sitting time

Too much sitting is associated with poor health outcomes, including cardiometabolic risk biomarkers, type 2 diabetes and premature mortality.[14] Sitting time is also known as sedentary behaviour and involves activities that have a very low energy expenditure, such as television viewing and deskbound work. It is recommended that most individuals need to reduce the total amount of time they sit during the day. Currently, there is no specific threshold/recommendation for sitting time and interpreting the data (question 7) should be done in conjunction with the continuous score and categorical assessment. For example, if a participant is in the 'high' physical activity category but sits for 8 hours per day, this would be less of a concern than someone who is sitting for the same time but in the 'low' physical activity category.[15]

Interpretation, feedback and discussion

First, consider the four steps of interpretation and the three steps of feedback and discussion outlined in Appendix G. When providing feedback on physical activity levels calculated using the IPAQ, you need to consider the poor concurrent validity of this approach. It is recommended you use the word *'estimated'* when providing feedback to assist in conveying this knowledge.

The relationship between physical activity and health is curvilinear.[16] Figure 5.1 shows the associations between daily physical activity duration and intensity (moderate or vigorous). Across both intensities the curves have a steeper initial slope, meaning at the lower end of the activity scale there is a greater rate of all-cause mortality reduction with increases. This implies that adults who do no moderate or vigorous activity will have significant health benefits if they are able to start exercising. Importantly, there is no obvious lower threshold, indicating that any moderate or vigorous activity is better than none. There is also no consensus on an optimal amount. It is known that substantial health benefits are gained from an overall volume of 500–1000 MET-minutes/week.[13] This can be achieved by doing 150–300 minutes of moderate-intensity activity or 75–150 minutes of vigorous activity each week, or various combinations of moderate and vigorous activity. There is no obvious upper threshold, but there may be risks (e.g. from overuse, injury or infection) when physical activity reaches >5000 MET-minutes/week.[13]

Although physical activity levels expressed using MET-minutes are not easily understood, conveying the overall continuous score using this unit and a comparison with the recommended

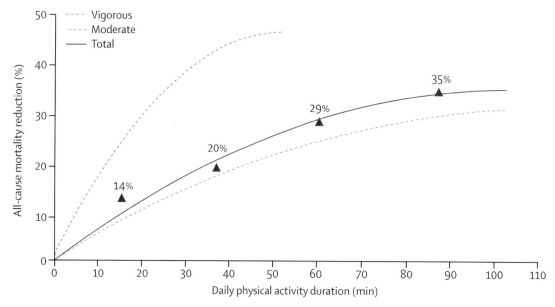

Figure 5.1 Curvilinear relationship between physical activity and all-cause mortality varies with intensity
Used with permission from The Lancet[16]

range of 500–1000 MET-minutes per week is a good starting point when providing feedback. From there, it is important to convey the dose–response relationship that exists between physical activity and health benefits, both within the 500–1000 MET-minutes per week range and above and below this range.[13] The use of the categorical assessment should be able to complement this feedback, for example:

> 'Based on your responses, it is estimated that you completed 750 MET-minutes per week of physical activity. This is in the recommended range of 500–1000 MET-minutes per week to achieve health benefits and places you in the moderately active category.'

Depending on the situation, it may be better to state the minutes of moderate- and vigorous-intensity activity for feedback. This may be easier for the participant to understand. When using this approach, physical activity guidelines suggest that 150–300 minutes of moderate-intensity activity per week could be regarded as approximately equivalent to 500–1000 MET-minutes per week. Indeed, 3.3 METs intensity for 150 minutes per week is equal to 500 MET-minutes per week. Therefore, if adults complete at least 150–300 minutes of moderate-intensity activity per week, they will achieve 500–1000 MET-minutes per week if the intensity is 3.3 METs or greater.

For vigorous-intensity activity, 500 MET-minutes per week can be achieved if a person completes 62.5 minutes per week at an intensity of 8 METs.

Discussion regarding a participant's physical activity level will depend on the context and the aims of the assessment. Improvement of physical activity levels generally requires the identification of a wide range of activities that should meet the individual's interests, needs, schedule and environment. You should take into consideration family, work and social commitments, with options for inclement weather and travel.[17] Specific advice may include the Australian Physical Activity and Sedentary Behaviour Guidelines (Box 5.1). Materials for the education and counselling of participants are available from numerous sources including the Heart Foundation[18] and Exercise and Sports Science Australia.[19] Suggestions for reducing sitting time are found in Table 5.2.[20] A major contributor to increased sitting time is recreational screen time use (e.g. TVs, computers, tablets). The Australian 24-Hour Movement Guidelines for Children and Young People (5–17 years) include recommendations to limit sedentary recreational screen time to no more than 2 hours per day.[21] Furthermore, when using screen-based electronic media, positive social interactions and experiences are encouraged. It is expected that similar guidelines will soon be developed for adults to limit sedentary behaviour.

Box 5.1 Australian Physical Activity and Sedentary Behaviour Guidelines

1 Doing any physical activity is better than doing none. If you currently do no physical activity, start by doing some and gradually build up to the recommended amount.

2 Be active on most, preferably all, days every week.

3 Accumulate 150–300 minutes (2½–5 hours) of moderate-intensity physical activity or 75–150 minutes (1¼–2½ hours) of vigorous-intensity physical activity, or an equivalent combination of both moderate and vigorous activities, each week.

4 Do muscle-strengthening activities on at least 2 days each week.

5 Minimise the amount of time spent in prolonged sitting.

6 Break up long periods of sitting as often as possible.

Source: Department of Health[9]

TABLE 5.2 Suggestions for reducing sitting time

AT HOME	AT WORK	WHILE TRAVELLING
• Get off the couch and walk around the home during commercial breaks. • Do household chores, such as folding clothes, washing dishes or ironing, while watching television. • Stand to read the morning newspaper. • Wash your car by hand rather than using a drive-through car wash. • Move around the house while checking text messages and/or email on your mobile phone.	• Stand and take a break from your computer every 30 minutes. • Take breaks in sitting time in long meetings. • Stand to greet a visitor to your workspace. • Use the stairs. • Stand during phone calls. • Walk to your colleagues' desk rather than phoning or emailing. • Drink more water – going to the water cooler and toilet will break up sitting time. • Move your bin away from your desk so you have to get up to put something in it. • Use a height-adjustable desk so you can work standing or sitting. • Have standing or walking meetings. • Use headsets or the speaker phone during teleconferences so you can stand. • Eat your lunch away from your desk. • Stand at the back of the room during presentations.	• Leave your car at home and take public transport so you walk to and from stops/stations. • Walk or cycle at least part way to your destination. • Park your car further away from your destination and walk the rest of the way. • Plan regular breaks during long car trips. • On public transport, stand and offer your seat to a person who really needs it. • Get on/off public transport one stop/station earlier and walk the rest of the way.

Source: Heart Foundation[20]

Activity 5.2 Consumer-based physical activity monitoring approaches

AIM: understand different approaches used in consumer-based physical activity monitoring.

Background

The popularity of physical activity monitoring means that exercise professionals should understand what is available (e.g. smartphones, wearable devices and apps) and how they can be used by participants. To develop these skills the following activity will ask you to document approaches being used to monitor physical activity using smartphones, wearable devices and apps. Box 5.2 provides four

> **Box 5.2 Common approaches used to monitor physical activity-related measures with smartphone/wearable device/app**
>
> 1 Smartphone with a native app. Motion data from sensor/s in the smartphone are used by an app on the phone that calculates and displays physical activity-related data.
>
> 2 Wearable device with a native app on a smartphone/tablet/computer. Motion data from the device are synced to an app on a smartphone/tablet or an application/program on a computer where the physical activity-related data is calculated and displayed.
>
> 3 App (not native to a smartphone or device) that uses data from a smartphone or wearable device/s.
>
> 4 Wearable device alone (e.g. waist-worn accelerometer, wrist-worn multi-sensor). Physical activity related data are calculated and displayed on the device alone.

common approaches. Smartphone and wearable device manufacturers will generally have developed an app (or apps) that accesses motion data from the device; this will be referred to as the 'native' app for that device. For example, Apple smartphones have the Health app and Samsung smartphones have the Samsung (S) Health app to record steps from the inbuilt accelerometer, the Apple Watch is associated with the Apple Activity app and Fitbit devices have the associated Fitbit app.

A device (smartphone or wearable) is usually constantly measuring physical activity. When people start to do specific exercises (e.g. go for a run, ride a bike), many devices and their associated apps allow the user to start recording data on the activity separate to the ongoing monitoring, which then provides more detailed information about that activity (e.g. distance of a run or bike ride and energy expenditure of that discrete activity).

Validity and reliability

The validity (concurrent) of the approach will depend on the variable of interest (e.g. steps, distance, energy expenditure), the quality of the measuring device (e.g. the triaxial accelerometer in the smartphone), the algorithm used to determine steps/distance/energy expended, an ability to manually calibrate or have the device self-calibrate and the way the smartphone or wearable device (e.g. correct wear position as intended by the manufacturer) is used (see Practical 1, Test accuracy, reliability and validity).

Studies that have assessed the concurrent validity of these approaches have found that the step-counting and distance values are measured with a high degree of accuracy; however, estimates of energy expenditure are poor and would have implications for people using these devices for monitoring physical activity intensity and energy balance.[22,23] For example, the percentage estimate of energy expenditure from four commonly used heart rate wristwatches were 9%–43% below the measured values.[22]

Reliability has been assessed by having participants wear two of the same devices at the same time (inter-device reliability). A systematic review reported high inter-device reliability for steps, distance and energy expenditure.[24] For example, Fitbit trials indicated consistently high inter-device reliability for steps (Pearson and ICC 0.76–1.00), distance (ICC 0.90–0.99) and energy expenditure (Pearson ICC 0.71–0.97).

Limitations

Strengths and weaknesses of consumer-based physical activity monitors are summarised in Table 5.3.[25] The primary limitation of step-based approaches to monitoring physical activity is that they do not consider the intensity of the movement. Hence, movement above a given threshold is counted as a step regardless of whether it occurs during walking, running or jumping.

TABLE 5.3 Strengths and weaknesses of consumer-based physical activity monitors[25]

DEVICE	STRENGTHS	WEAKNESSES
Pedometer	<ul><li>Low cost.</li><li>Low burden.</li><li>Easy data processing.</li><li>Applicable to large numbers of individuals.</li><li>Can be used to motivate people.</li></ul>	<ul><li>Doesn't measure intensity/duration.</li><li>Doesn't measure mode/type.</li><li>Not valid (concurrent) for energy expenditure.</li><li>False steps can be recorded.</li></ul>
Accelerometer	<ul><li>Concurrent measure of movement.</li><li>Provides detailed intensity, frequency and duration data.</li><li>Can store data for weeks at a time.</li><li>Low burden.</li><li>Relatively inexpensive.</li></ul>	<ul><li>Cannot account for all activities, such as cycling, stair use, or activities that require lifting a load.</li><li>Upper-body activities neglected with hip or lower-back wear.</li><li>Black box estimates – data-processing procedures and algorithms to predict PA outcomes are proprietary and unknown to end user.</li></ul>
Multisensing units	<ul><li>Accuracy improved compared with single-sensing assessments.</li></ul>	<ul><li>Higher cost.</li><li>Increased burden of wear for some devices.</li></ul>

Device-based predictions of physical activity intensity and/or energy expenditure are also subject to limitations. Depending on the algorithm and the use and sensitivity of an altimeter, they may also not detect the increased energy cost associated with walking up stairs or an incline. Certain physical activities such as lifting or carrying objects are also not validly quantified. Using the smartphone and app approach requires the user to have the smartphone with them at all times. Furthermore, the location of the smartphone/device can impact accuracy. For example, when the device is located in a different place (e.g. pants pocket, chest, wrist), accuracy is decreased.[26] A device that stays in the one location (e.g. on the wrist) will not have similar issues.

Protocol summary

Complete the data-recording sheet documenting how smartphones, wearable devices and apps work together to provide physical activity-related measures.

Protocol

A. Smartphones and native apps

1 Using your own smartphone (or work with a partner if you don't have one), document on the data-recording sheet the native app that allows physical activity monitoring with the smartphone.

2 Answer the questions that follow.

3 From the internet, choose a different brand of smartphone and, using web pages from the manufacturer, document on the data-recording sheet the associated native app that allows physical activity monitoring.

4 Answer the questions that follow.

B. Wearable devices and native apps

1 Using your own wearable device (or a partner, or use the internet to find one), document on the data-recording sheet the native app associated with the device that allows physical activity monitoring.

2 Answer the questions that follow.

3 From the internet, choose a different wearable device and, using web pages from the manufacturer, document on the data-recording sheet the associated native app that allows physical activity monitoring.

4 Answer the questions that follow.

C. Physical activity apps

1 Use the internet or an app store to find two apps that can be used to monitor physical activity-related measures during an activity. On the data-recording sheet, document the approaches that they use.

2 Answer the questions that follow.

Data recording

A. Smartphones and Native Apps

Your smartphone and native app: _____

Physical activity-related measures: _____

_____

_____

Does the native app allow you to monitor a discrete 'workout' (circle)?   Yes / No

What (if any) physical activity-related measures are provided at the end of a 'workout'?

_____

_____

Second smartphone and native app: _____

Physical activity-related measures: _____

_____

_____

Does the native app allow you to monitor a discrete 'workout' (circle)?   Yes / No

What (if any) physical activity-related measures are provided at the end of a 'workout'?

_____

_____

With regards to physical activity monitoring, what are the similarities and differences between the approaches used by the two smartphones and their native apps?

Similarities: _____

_____

_____

_____

_____

Differences: _____

_____

_____

_____

_____

continued

Data recording *(continued)*

B. Wearable Devices and Native Apps

First wearable device and native app: _____

Physical activity-related measures: _____

_____

_____

Does the native app allow you to monitor a discrete 'workout' (circle)?   Yes / No

What (if any) physical activity-related measures are provided at the end of a 'workout'?

_____

_____

Second wearable device and native app: _____

Physical activity-related measures: _____

_____

_____

Does the native app allow you to monitor a discrete 'workout' (circle)?   Yes / No

What (if any) physical activity-related measures are provided at the end of a 'workout'?

_____

_____

With regards to physical activity monitoring, what are the similarities and differences between the approaches used by the two wearable devices and their native apps?

Similarities:

_____

_____

_____

_____

Differences:

_____

_____

_____

_____

C. Physical Activity Apps

First physical activity app: _____

Physical activity-related measures:

_____

_____

Does the app allow you to monitor a discrete 'workout' (circle)?   Yes / No

continued overpage

Data recording *(continued)*

What (if any) physical activity-related measures are provided at the end of a 'workout'?

Second physical activity app: _____

Physical activity-related measures:

Does the app allow you to monitor a discrete 'workout' (circle)?   Yes / No

What (if any) physical activity related measures are provided at the end of a 'workout'?

With regards to physical activity monitoring, what are the similarities and differences between the approaches used by the physical activity apps?

Similarities:

Differences:

Activity 5.3 Using consumer-based physical activity monitors

AIMS: use consumer-based physical activity monitoring approaches to:

- measure steps, distance walked and energy expended
- determine the accuracy of the step counter
- determine the agreement between two approaches
- determine the effects of changing the location of a smartphone on measured steps.

Background

From the previous activity you identified a number of devices and approaches to measure physical activity. In this activity, you will use two of these approaches: (1) smartphone and app and (2) a wearable device with an app. The accuracy of the step count and the agreement between the two approaches will be determined. We will also try to influence the accuracy of the smartphone by changing the position of the arm of the person wearing the device or the location of the smartphone.

Protocol summary

Complete a walking task twice (out and back) using: (1) a smartphone and app (native or otherwise) and (2) a wearable device with an app (native or otherwise) to monitor physical activity. On completion of each walk, the steps, distance covered and energy expended will be documented from each approach. In addition, participants will count the steps they take during each walk.

Protocol

Choice of devices

For this activity each student will need a (1) smartphone and app (native or otherwise) and a (2) wearable device with an app (native or otherwise). Both combinations will need to measure steps taken, distance moved and energy expended. Some combinations may allow for a discrete workout to be started (zeroing the measures) whereas for others you may have to subtract the starting values.

Walking tasks

1 Select a destination that will take around 10 minutes to walk to. Select a route that is as flat as possible.

2 Go to the start location.

3 The participant starts a new discrete workout on their own (1) smartphone and app combination, and (2) wearable device and app combination. If starting a new workout is not an option then record the starting values.

4 All participants walk to the destination at a brisk walking speed. Each participant manually counts the number of steps they take.

5 At the destination, from both combinations, record the step count, distance walked and energy expended (you may need to subtract starting values, sometimes referred to as 'active energy'). Document the number of steps you manually counted on the data-recording sheet. Energy expenditure may be provided in 'Calories', which is often used as an abbreviation for kilocalories (or kCal). To convert this to kJ, multiply by 4.2 (i.e. 1 kCal = 4.2 kJ). A 10-minute walk should expend approximately 200 kJ.

6 Start or reset both combinations.

7 All participants walk back along the same route at the same speed to the original start position. Try to influence the accuracy of the smartphone (e.g. by folding your arms, by mimicking pushing a pram/ trolley or using an assistive device like a walker, or by moving the smartphone to a different location (e.g. in a bag, backpack, pocket in a different piece of clothing, or held in hand)). Each participant manually counts the steps they take.

8 Back at the start position, on both combinations, record the step count, steps counted distance walked and energy expended. Document the number of steps you manually counted on the data-recording sheet.

Data recording

1 Smartphone and App Combination

Smartphone brand: _____ app name: _____

Smartphone location (on/near body) for walk to destination: _____

2 Wearable Device and App Combination

Wearable device brand: _____ app name: _____

Wearable device location (on body): _____

Influencing accuracy during return walk. Document your attempt (e.g. hold smartphone in hand while walking, move smartphone to a different pocket, etc.):

_____

continued overpage

Data recording *(continued)*

	STEPS (n)			DISTANCE (m)		ENERGY EXPENDITURE (kJ)	
	SMARTPHONE AND APP	WEARABLE DEVICE AND APP	STEPS COUNTED MANUALLY	SMARTPHONE AND APP	WEARABLE DEVICE AND APP	SMARTPHONE AND APP	WEARABLE DEVICE AND APP
Starting location to destination							
Destination to starting location							

Data analysis

A. Accuracy

To determine accuracy as a percentage error of the different approaches, we will use the steps counted manually as the reference value.

1 Calculate the accuracy of the step counts for (a) to (d) below using the following equation:

$$\text{Percentage error} = 100 - \left[\frac{\text{measured steps} \times 100\%}{\text{manually counted steps}} \right]$$

   a Smartphone and app from starting location to destination:

$$\text{Percentage error} = 100 - \left[\frac{\text{measured steps} \times 100\%}{\text{manually counted steps}} \right]$$
$$= \underline{\hspace{2cm}} \%$$

   b Wearable device and app from starting location to destination:

$$\text{Percentage error} = 100 - \left[\frac{\text{measured steps} \times 100\%}{\text{manually counted steps}} \right]$$
$$= \underline{\hspace{2cm}} \%$$

   c Smartphone and app from destination to starting location:

$$\text{Percentage error} = 100 - \left[\frac{\text{measured steps} \times 100\%}{\text{manually counted steps}} \right]$$
$$= \underline{\hspace{2cm}} \%$$

   d Wearable device and app from destination to starting location:

$$\text{Percentage error} = 100 - \left[\frac{\text{measured steps} \times 100\%}{\text{manually counted steps}} \right]$$
$$= \underline{\hspace{2cm}} \%$$

INTERPRETATION OF ACCURACY

It is important to know the accuracy of a measure as this allows the user to take this into account when analysing and interpreting data. In the context of step counting it would be expected that the approach should be accurate to less than 5%. As 10,000 steps/day is often used as a goal, if the approach had 5% error and the approach said the person did 10,000 steps/day then the real value may be 500 steps fewer or more than this. This level of accuracy for this measure would be acceptable for most individuals. In a research setting it would be preferable for the inaccuracy to be below 1%.

Comment on the accuracy of the different approaches to count steps:

_____

_____

_____

_____

B. Agreement

2 Determine the agreement between the smartphone and app for (a) to (f) below with the wearable device and app using the following equation:

$$\text{Percentage difference} = \left[\frac{\text{largest measure} - \text{smallest measure}}{\text{smallest measure}} \right] \times 100$$

a Steps: from starting location to destination:

$$\text{Percentage difference} = \left| \underline{\hspace{3cm}} \right| \times 100$$
$$= \underline{\hspace{1.5cm}} \%$$

b Steps: from destination to starting location:

$$\text{Percentage difference} = \left| \underline{\hspace{3cm}} \right| \times 100$$
$$= \underline{\hspace{1.5cm}} \%$$

c Distance: from starting location to destination:

$$\text{Percentage difference} = \left| \underline{\hspace{3cm}} \right| \times 100$$
$$= \underline{\hspace{1.5cm}} \%$$

d Distance: from destination to starting location:

$$\text{Percentage difference} = \left| \underline{\hspace{3cm}} \right| \times 100$$
$$= \underline{\hspace{1.5cm}} \%$$

e Energy expenditure: from starting location to destination:

$$\text{Percentage difference} = \left| \underline{\hspace{3cm}} \right| \times 100$$
$$= \underline{\hspace{1.5cm}} \%$$

f Energy expenditure: from destination to starting location:

$$\text{Percentage difference} = \left| \underline{\hspace{3cm}} \right| \times 100$$
$$= \underline{\hspace{1.5cm}} \%$$

INTERPRETATION OF AGREEMENT

When different approaches are used to make the same measure, it is important to know their agreement. In the context of step counting, distance and energy expenditure it would be expected that the disagreement between two approaches to measure these should be less than 5%. In a research setting, if two approaches are being used it would be preferable for the disagreement between them to be below 1%.

Comment on the agreement between the two approaches across the different measures:

_____

_____

_____

_____

_____

_____

_____

_____

_____

_____

Activity 5.4 Behaviour change techniques in consumer-based physical activity monitors

AIMS: identify the behaviour change techniques used in a physical activity-monitoring approach.

Background

In addition to monitoring physical activity, apps also have features and functionality that are available for a participant who may be seeking to increase physical activity levels. Although evidence for the long-term success of these apps to increase physical activity levels is lacking, goal setting and self-monitoring have been shown to be an effective way to promote physical activity.[27] The effectiveness of apps to change behaviour will probably depend on the features or functionality, based on accepted behaviour change techniques. The Behaviour Change Wheel is a model developed by Michie and colleagues to characterise and design behaviour change interventions.[28] Items from the associated Behaviour Change Technique Taxonomy V1 will be used in this activity.[29]

Protocol summary

Identify which Behaviour Change Taxonomy techniques from the list below are used in your physical activity monitoring app.

Protocol

1 Students may use either the physical activity monitoring app that comes with their own smartphone or wearable device, or another that they may have or choose to download.

2 Using the list of behaviour change techniques, identify which ones are being used on the app by circling YES/NO on the data-recording sheet. This may require use of the internet to get a better understanding of the different features and functionality of the app via the company's website.

Data recording

1 **Provides information on consequences of behaviour in general**   YES/NO
   Likely consequences in the general case, usually based on epidemiological data, and not personalised for the individual.
   e.g. The app provides information to the user about why physical activity is good for health.

   continued

Data recording *(continued)*

2 **Provides normative information about others' behaviour**   YES/NO

Involves providing information about what other people are doing, i.e. indicates that a particular behaviour or sequence of behaviours is common or uncommon.

e.g. Does the app allow or provide comparison of users' data to average data by all people wearing that device?

3 **Goal setting (behaviour)**   YES/NO

The person is encouraged to make a behavioural resolution (e.g. engage in more exercise next week).

e.g. Does the app set, or encourage the user to set, a daily step goal or other activity-related goals?

4 **Goal setting (outcome)**   YES/NO

The person is encouraged to set a general goal that can be achieved by behavioural means but is not defined in terms of behaviour (e.g. to reduce blood pressure or lose/maintain weight), as opposed to a goal based on changing behaviour.

e.g. Does the app encourage users to set any other health goals (e.g. blood pressure, body weight) that can be achieved at least in part by physical activity?

5 **Prompts review of behavioural goals**   YES/NO

Involves a review or analysis of the extent to which previously set behavioural goals (e.g. engage in more exercise next week) were achieved.

e.g. Does the app provide a daily or weekly review of goal achievement and encourage users to act on this information?

6 **Provides rewards contingent on successful behaviour**   YES/NO

Reinforcing successful performance of the specific target behaviour can include praise and encouragement as well as material rewards, but the reward/incentive must be explicitly linked to the achievement of the specific target behaviour (i.e. the person receives the reward if they perform the specified behaviour but not if they do not perform the behaviour).

e.g. Does the app provide rewards (like medals, or some kind of credit) when behavioural goals are achieved?

7 **Prompts self-monitoring of behaviour**   YES/NO

The person is asked to keep a record of specified behaviour(s) as a method for changing behaviour.

e.g. Does the app store activity data to allow the user to self-monitor their behaviour?

8 **Prompts self-monitoring of behavioural outcome**   YES/NO

The person is asked to keep a record of specified measures expected to be influenced by the behaviour change (e.g. blood pressure, blood glucose, weight loss, physical fitness).

e.g. Does the app allow the user to record other health outcome data such as body weight or blood pressure?

9 **Plans social support/social change**   YES/NO

Involves prompting the person to plan how to elicit social support from other people to help them achieve their target behaviour/outcome.

e.g. Does the app allow opportunities to share goals, data and experiences with others or interact with other users? This may be through links to social media accounts, for example.

continued overpage

Data recording *(continued)*

10   **Relapse prevention/coping planning**   YES/NO
This relates to planning how to maintain behaviour that has been changed.

e.g. Does the app encourage the user to think about or plan strategies to continue meeting their physical activity goals?

Activity 5.5 Research-based physical activity monitoring

AIMS: use a research-based physical activity monitor to assess physical activity levels over one day. Interpret the results and provide feedback to a participant.

Background

Compared with the consumer-based devices, research-based monitors tend to not display data (participants are unaware of the data that are being recorded); data are downloaded and analysed offline by a researcher and/or relevant health professional. This is because most research projects that use these devices do not want participants to change their behaviour during data collection. As mentioned previously, devices that provide feedback to a participant are more likely to result in behaviour change (reactivity). Research-based monitors use the same sensors as consumer tracking devices, but the formulas or algorithms used to convert the accelerometer data to steps, physical activity intensity or energy expenditure are based on published research and fully transparent to end users.

Accelerometers are an established method for assessing physical activity in research settings. They record date- and time-stamped information about the acceleration of the trunk or other body segments during normal human movement performed in free-living or 'real-life' situations. To estimate daily or weekly time spent in sedentary, light, moderate and vigorous activities from accelerometer output (counts or gravitational units), prediction equations or algorithms have been developed to estimate energy expenditure (METs) or physical activity intensity category. A typical approach has been to develop a regression equation that defines the linear relationship between counts and energy expenditure. Once the equation has been developed, the activity counts obtained by an individual performing an unknown activity can be used to estimate energy expenditure.[30] Activity count thresholds or cut-points denoting the dividing line between sedentary-and-light (1.5 METs), light-and-moderate (3 METs) and moderate-and-vigorous physical activity (6 METs) are typically identified. Advantages in using accelerometers include: small size and low participant burden, real-time data storage capacity over many days, measurement of physical activity intensity and ability to detect incidental activity accumulated throughout the day.

Validity and reliability

Numerous studies have investigated the validity (concurrent) of accelerometers under both laboratory and field conditions. The most common criterion measure for these studies has been energy expenditure measured by indirect calorimetry.[31] In addition, energy expenditure measured by doubly labelled water and activity intensity measured by direct observation have also been used. The majority of studies report a strong positive correlation between accelerometer output and energy expenditure and/or exercise intensity.[30–32] However, when accelerometer output (counts or gravitational units (Gs)) is used to estimate physical activity intensity or energy expenditure via prediction equations or 'cut-points', the concurrent validity is dependent on:

- the make and model of the accelerometer
- the types of activities included in the calibration sample

- the characteristics of the sample used in the calibration study
- the statistical methodology used to develop the prediction equations.[32,33]

Validation studies involving independent samples indicate that regression-based cut-point approaches underestimate the true intensity of physical activity 35%–45% of the time.[34,35] However, despite these limitations, the application of cut-points continues to be standard research practice. The measurement errors associated with regression-based energy expenditure prediction equations typically exceed 2 METs per minute, resulting in gross under- and overestimations of physical activity energy expenditure over an entire day.[36] A recent study evaluated the validity of the most commonly used accelerometer for research purposes (the ActiGraph – to be used in the Activity in this practical) for predicting physical activity energy expenditure and found the correlation to be around $r = 0.4$, which they described as reasonable.[37] An emerging approach to accelerometer data reduction that promises to significantly improve accelerometer-based measurement of physical activity is pattern recognition or machine learning. In this approach, recurring patterns or distinguishing time- and frequency-domain features in the raw tri-axial accelerometer data are 'extracted' and entered into sophisticated statistical-learning models. These are then used to predict the physical activity type and/or energy expenditure.[30,35]

The intra-device reliability of various accelerometers has been determined by attaching two devices to one person. The ActiGraph has been shown to be reliable with the limits of agreement of ± 51 min for sedentary time, ± 18.2 min for light physical activity, ± 6.3 min for moderate physical activity, ± 3.5 min for vigorous physical activity and ± 6.7 min for moderate-to-vigorous physical activity.[38]

Limitations

Limitations of accelerometers include:

- cost (usually at least $250 per device)
- failure to account for the increased energy cost associated with walking up stairs or an incline
- less sensitive to some forms of movement such as cycling, lifting or carrying objects
- uncertainty or measurement error related to energy expenditure prediction equations or cut-points
- inability to measure relative exercise intensity
- require additional software and data management skills as data are not automatically processed as is the case for consumer tracking devices.

Protocol summary

Fit an accelerometer on a participant and ask them to wear it for 1 day. During this time you will also ask them to complete a physical activity diary.

Protocol

Accelerometer set-up

1 Open the ActiLife software (Figure 5.2).

2 Attach the accelerometer using the USB cable (Figure 5.3).

3 Wait for the ActiLife to recognise the ActiGraph (Figure 5.4).

4 Initialising the ActiGraph: initialising means preparing the ActiGraph to collect data. Data collection parameters such as start and stop time, date, sampling frequency and other options should be specified (Figure 5.5). A sampling rate of 30 Hz is sufficient for monitoring physical activity. To initialise, click on 'Initialize' in the top left-hand corner. Set start and stop times and other options if applicable. Click on 'Enter Subject Information' and enter the relevant information (Figure 5.6).

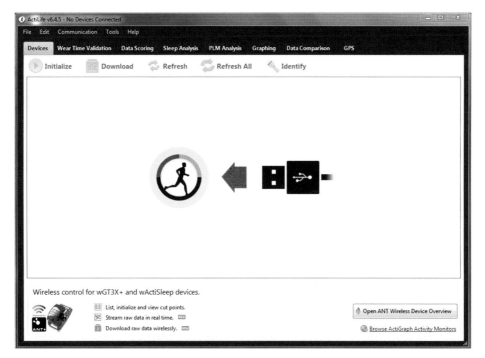

Figure 5.2 ActiLife software

Used with permission from ActiGraph

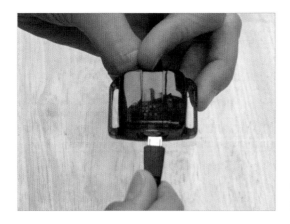

Figure 5.3 Attaching the USB cable to the ActiGraph

Used with permission from ActiGraph and Stewart Trost

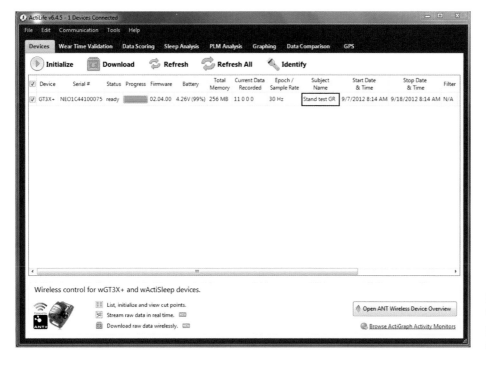

Figure 5.4 ActiLife recognising the ActiGraph

Used with permission from ActiGraph

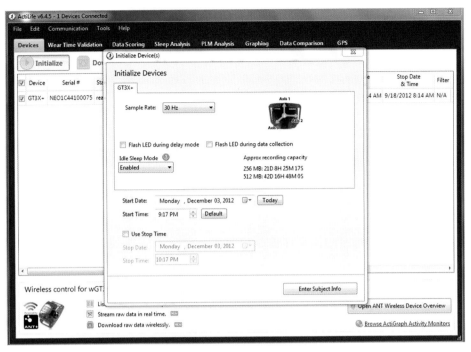

Figure 5.5 Initialising the ActiGraph
Used with permission from ActiGraph

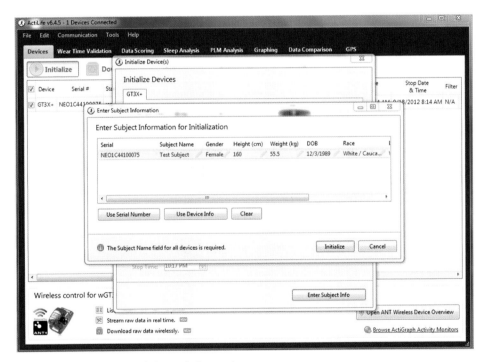

Figure 5.6 Entering participant information
Used with permission from ActiGraph

5   When completed, click 'Initialize'. Wait for the program to complete the initialisation. When the status
column indicates the device has 'finished initializing' (Figure 5.7), you are now able to disconnect
the ActiGraph from the USB cable.

Fitting the accelerometer

1   The accelerometer should be attached according to the manufacturer's instructions. If using an
ActiGraph, it is attached to an adjustable belt worn around the waist. The belt should be snug but not

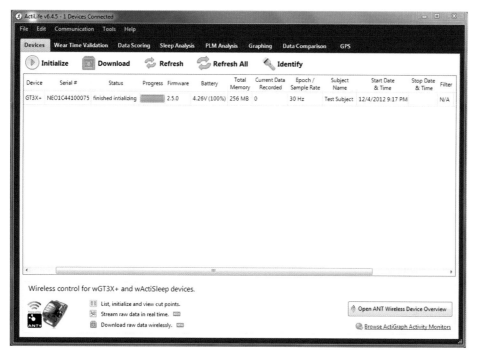

Figure 5.7 Disconnecting the ActiGraph from the USB cable when the status column displays 'finished initializing'

Used with permission from ActiGraph

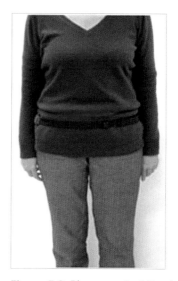

overly tight. It does not need to make contact with the skin (i.e. can be worn over or under clothing). The only requirement is that it is held against the body so it does not move around.

2 The ActiGraph is positioned at the level of the iliac crest on the right hip (Figure 5.8).

3 The monitor should be removed when in water (e.g. swimming, bathing).

Physical activity

1 Provide the participant with a physical activity diary (Table 5.4) and explain that the purpose of the diary is to aid in the interpretation of the accelerometer output. In addition, provide the following advice regarding the diary:

- if there were periods of time longer than 10 minutes that you did not wear the accelerometer, tick the 'not worn box' and record the times

Figure 5.8 Placement of the ActiGraph.
Used with permission from ActiGraph

- also record the times in which you did some physical activity that was longer than 10 minutes in duration

- record the activities that you completed during these times

- record the time you went to bed and the time you woke up.

2 Ask the participant to return the accelerometer and diary to you at around the same time the next day to enable 24 hours of data collection.

3 Clean and disinfect all equipment (see Appendix A).

TABLE 5.4 Physical activity diary

TIME	INFORMATION	DESCRIPTION
to	☐ NOT WORN ☐ PHYSICAL ACTIVITY	
to	☐ NOT WORN ☐ PHYSICAL ACTIVITY	
to	☐ NOT WORN ☐ PHYSICAL ACTIVITY	
to	☐ NOT WORN ☐ PHYSICAL ACTIVITY	
to	☐ NOT WORN ☐ PHYSICAL ACTIVITY	
to	☐ NOT WORN ☐ PHYSICAL ACTIVITY	
to	☐ NOT WORN ☐ PHYSICAL ACTIVITY	
to	☐ NOT WORN ☐ PHYSICAL ACTIVITY	

Start time wearing monitor _____

Finish time wearing monitor _____

What time did you go to bed last night? _____

What time did you get up this morning? _____

Did you wear the accelerometer to bed?   ☐ Yes   ☐ No

Downloading data

1 To download the data, connect the accelerometer to the computer containing the ActiLife software using the USB cable. A dialogue box will appear (Figure 5.9).

2 For 'Download Naming Convention' choose 'Subject Name'.

3 Tick the box for 'Create AGD File'.

4 Set 'Epoch' to 60 seconds, and '# of Axis' to 3.

5 Check the box for 'Steps'.

6 Calculation of daily energy expenditure and time spent in sedentary, light, moderate and vigorous physical activity is a two-step process that involves wear time validation and data scoring. To start, click on the 'Wear Time Validation' tab (Figure 5.10).

7 Click on 'Add Dataset(s)' and select your AGD file.

8 Under 'Define Non-Wear Period' set minimum length to 60 minutes, and spike tolerance to 2 minutes. Leave the other options unselected.

9 Then click on 'Calculate'. The program looks for strings of zero counts lasting 60 minutes or longer, which is indicative of non-wear. The program will calculate the minutes of wear time and non-wear time over the monitoring period. You can click on 'Details' to obtain detailed wear time information for each day and individual segments of the day.

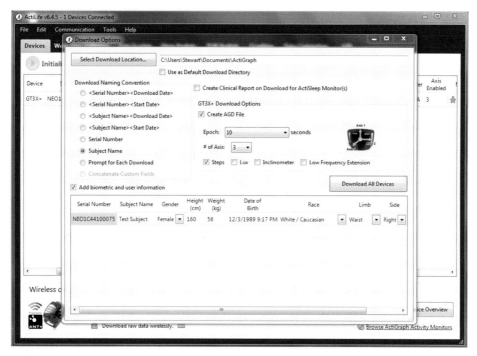

Figure 5.9 Dialogue box for entering information to download the data

Used with permission from ActiGraph

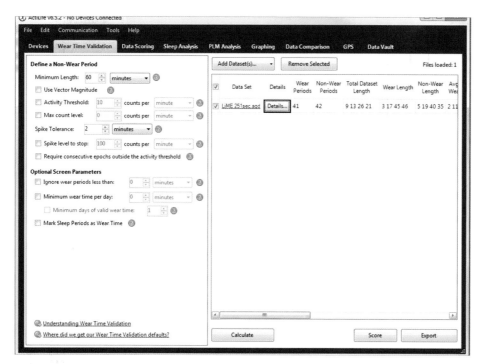

Figure 5.10 Wear time validation dialogue box

Used with permission from ActiGraph

10 After calculating wear time and flagging intervals of non-wear, you are now ready to calculate physical activity summary variables. To do this, click on the 'Data Scoring' tab. The dialogue box in Figure 5.11 will appear.

11 Choose which algorithm/cut points you wish to use (suggest Freedson and colleagues[39]) and other options. You can also 'filter' the data and select certain dates and segments of the day. Ensure that the 'Exclude Non-Wear Times from Analysis' box is checked. Then press 'Calculate'. The physical activity estimates will then populate the table as shown in Figure 5.12.

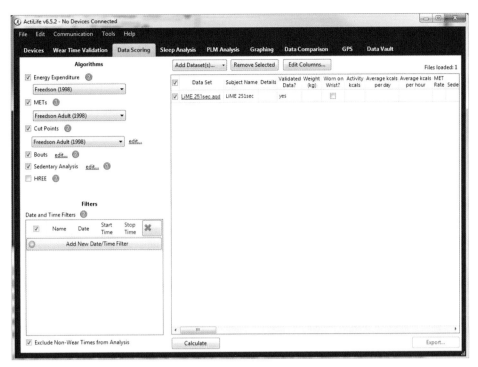

Figure 5.11 Data-scoring dialogue box
Used with permission from ActiGraph

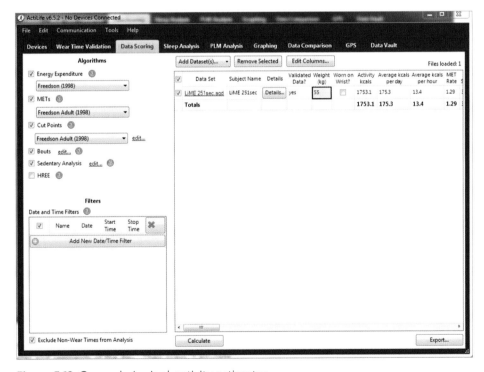

Figure 5.12 General physical activity estimates
Used with permission from ActiGraph

12 Click 'Details' to get daily (Figure 5.13) or hourly estimates.

13 Click 'Export' to export the data into Excel or other applications. Select the information you wish to include (Figure 5.14). Figure 5.15 shows an example of the exported data.

14 To view a graph of the data over the week-long monitoring period, click on the 'Graphing' tab and select your AGD file (Figure 5.16).

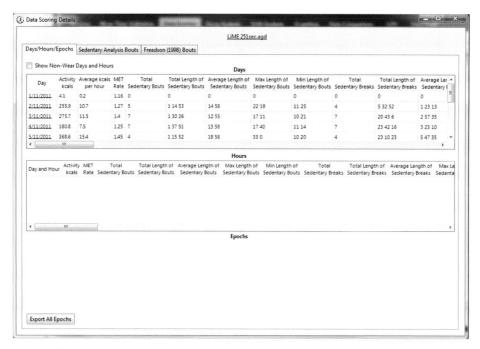

Figure 5.13 Daily physical activity estimates
Used with permission from ActiGraph

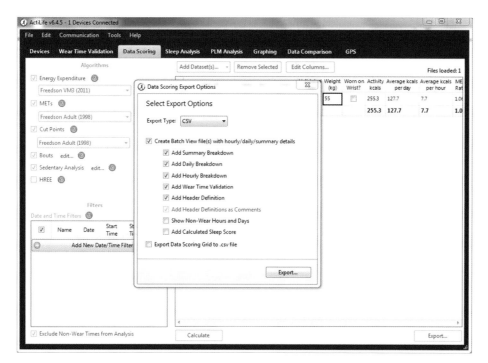

Figure 5.14 Exporting the data
Used with permission from ActiGraph

15 Figure 5.17 has an example of accelerometry data from 2 days. The y axes contain the counts and the x axes the times of day. The counts have ranges categorised as vigorous, moderate, or light intensity. For example, on Thursday the participant was completing some vigorous activity around 4.30 p.m.

Data analysis

1 Data analysis starts by comparing the accelerometer data against the physical activity diary entries. This should allow for an identification of the time the device was worn and will help to identify any

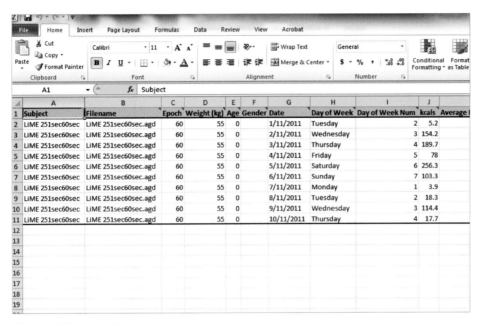

Figure 5.15 Example of the exported data
Used with permission from ActiGraph

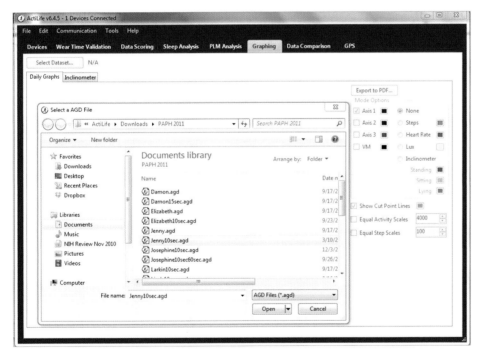

Figure 5.16 Selecting a file to view a graph of the data
Used with permission from ActiGraph

spurious data. It will also assist the tester to understand what general activities were performed over the period.

2 After this comparison, complete the data-recording sheet by obtaining the data from the software (e.g. Figure 5.13) or from the exported CSV or Excel file (see Figure 5.15).

3 Record the values.

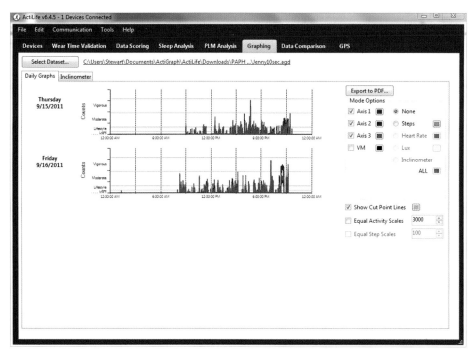

Figure 5.17 Example of a physical activity graph
Used with permission from ActiGraph

Data recording

Participant's name: _____   Date: _____

Age: _____ years   Sex: _____

Sedentary time (min)	
Light physical activity (min)	
Moderate physical activity (min)	
Vigorous physical activity (min)	
Counts	
Steps	
Estimated energy expenditure (kJ)	

Interpretation, feedback and discussion of accelerometry data

First, consider the four steps of interpretation and the three steps of feedback and discussion outlined in Appendix G. Interpretation of accelerometer data can be a complex procedure. For this practical a very simplified approach will be suggested where the collated data (including energy expenditure) from Activity 5.5 will be compared against physical activity guidelines.

1   Time spent in various intensity-level activities: the current physical activity guideline is to complete a minimum of 150 minutes per week of moderate-intensity or 75 minutes per week of vigorous-intensity activity.[9] Compare the 1-day accelerometry data from Activity 5.5 with these guidelines. You will need to multiply the 1-day data by seven to get a weekly estimate.

2 Estimated energy expenditure: the minimum physical activity guidelines (150 minutes of moderate-intensity activity per week) equates to a physical activity energy expenditure of 600 kJ/day.[9]

For feedback, the participant should be first provided with their one-day accelerometry data from Activity 5.5. Then, after explaining the assumption that you have multiplied this by seven to get an estimated weekly physical activity level, this can be compared with the physical activity guidelines (including energy expenditure). Where additional feedback and discussion is needed to address low physical activity levels, refer to the feedback section after the IPAQ activity (Activity 5.1 in this practical). Feedback should include a mention of the limitations of measuring physical activity with accelerometers.

Case studies

Case Study 1

Setting: You work as an Accredited Exercise Scientist in a community health centre in a remote mining community. Your tasks include conducting health assessments and one of your goals is to improve the physical activity levels of the residents.

Mohammed is a 38-year-old male teacher who completes a health check with you. One of the components you have introduced into the health check is an assessment of physical activity levels using the IPAQ. He completes the form and his responses are below.

Task: Analyse and interpret the IPAQ data and provide feedback for Mohammed.

IPAQ SHORT FORM — SUMMARY SHEET

1 During the **last 7 days**, on how many days did you do **vigorous** physical activities?

   _4_ days per week

2 How much time did you usually spend doing **vigorous** physical activities on one of those days?

   _1_ hours per day

   _____ minutes per day

   [**Interviewer probe**: if the respondent can't answer because the pattern of time spent varies widely from day to day, or includes time spent in multiple jobs, ask: *'What is the total amount of time you spent over the last 7 days doing* vigorous *physical activities?'*]

   _____ hours per week

   _____ minutes per week

3 During the **last 7 days**, on how many days did you do **moderate** physical activities?

   _3_ days per week

4 How much time did you usually spend doing **moderate** physical activities on one of those days?

   _____ hours per day

   _30_ minutes per day

   [**Interviewer probe**: if the respondent can't answer because the pattern of time spent varies widely from day to day, or includes time spent in multiple jobs, ask: *'What is the total amount of time you spent over the last 7 days doing* moderate *physical activities?'*]

   _____ hours per week

   _____ minutes per week

5 During the **last 7 days**, on how many days did you **walk** for at least 10 minutes at a time?

   _3_ days per week

continued overpage

Case studies *(continued)*

6 How much time did you usually spend **walking** on one of those days?

_____ hours per day

_20_ minutes per day

[**Interviewer probe**: if the respondent can't answer because the pattern of time spent varies widely from day to day, ask: '*What is the total amount of time you spent* walking *over the last 7 days?*']

_____ hours per week

_____ minutes per week

7 During the last 7 days, how much time did you usually spend *sitting* on a **week day**?

_8_ hours per weekday

_____ minutes per day

[**Interviewer probe**: an average time per day spent sitting is being sought. If the respondent can't answer because the pattern of time spent varies widely from day to day, ask: '*What is the total amount of time you spent* sitting *last Wednesday?*']

_____ hours on Wednesday

_____ minutes on Wednesday

Case Study 2

Setting: You have been employed as a research assistant on a project that is using two consumer-based physical activity monitoring approaches: (1) smartphone and app and (2) a wearable device with an app. You have been asked to determine the accuracy of these approaches to count steps, and the agreement between the two approaches to count steps, distance moved and energy expended. You conduct an experiment using the protocol (steps 1–5) from Activity 5.3 and the data collected are provided below.

Task: Calculate the accuracy (steps) and agreement (steps, distance and energy expended) and interpret the results.

	STEPS (n)			DISTANCE (m)		ENERGY EXPENDITURE (kJ)	
	SMARTPHONE AND APP	WEARABLE DEVICE AND APP	STEPS COUNTED MANUALLY	SMARTPHONE AND APP	WEARABLE DEVICE AND APP	SMARTPHONE AND APP	WEARABLE DEVICE AND APP
Starting location to destination	1178	1162	1150	840	830	206	282

References

[1] International Physical Activity Questionnaire Group. 2013. International Physical Activity Questionnaire (IPAQ). https://sites.google.com/site/theipaq/.

[2] Booth FW, Roberts CK, Laye MJ. Lack of exercise is a major cause of chronic diseases. Compr Physiol 2012;2:1143–211.

[3] Lee IM, Djousse L, Sesso HD, Wang L, Buring JE. Physical activity and weight gain prevention. JAMA 2010;303:1173–9.

[4] White RL, Babic MJ, Parker PD, Lubans DR, Astell-Burt T, Lonsdale C. Domain-specific physical activity and mental health: a meta-analysis. Am J Prev Med 2017;52:653–66.

[5] Bravata DM, Smith-Spangler C, Sundaram V, Gienger AL, Lin N, Lewis R, et al. Using pedometers to increase physical activity and improve health: a systematic review. JAMA 2007;298:2296–304.

[6] Craig CL, Marshall AL, Sjostrom M, Bauman AE, Booth ML, Ainsworth BE, et al. International physical activity questionnaire: 12-country reliability and validity. Med Sci Sports Exerc 2003;35:1381–95.

[7] van Poppel MN, Chinapaw MJ, Mokkink LB, van Mechelen W, Terwee CB. Physical activity questionnaires for adults: a systematic review of measurement properties. Sports Med 2010;40:565–600.

[8] Mahmood S, MacInnis RJ, English DR. Domain-specific physical activity and sedentary behaviour in relation to colon and rectal cancer risk: a systematic review and meta-analysis. Int J Epidemiol 2017;46:1797–813.

[9] Australian Government Department of Health. 2014. Australia's physical activity AND sedentary behaviour guidelines for adults (18–64 years). https://www1.health.gov.au/internet/main/publishing.nsf/Content/health-pubhlth-strateg-phys-act-guidelines#npa1864.

[10] Lee PH, Macfarlane DJ, Lam TH, Stewart SM. Validity of the International Physical Activity Questionnaire Short Form (IPAQ-SF): a systematic review. Int J Behav Nutr Phys Act 2011;8:115.

[11] Sallis JF, Saelens BE. Assessment of physical activity by self-report: status, limitations, and future directions. Res Q Exerc Sport 2000;71:S1–14.

[12] Silsbury Z, Goldsmith R, Rushton A. Systematic review of the measurement properties of self-report physical activity questionnaires in healthy adult populations. BMJ Open 2015;5:e008430.

[13] Brown WJ, Bauman AE, Bull FC, Burton NW. Development of evidence-based physical activity recommendations for adults (18–64 years). Report prepared for the Australian Government Department of Health, August 2012. http://www.health.gov.au/internet/main/publishing.nsf/content/3768EA4DC0BF11D0CA257BF0001ED77E/$File/DEBPA Adults.PDF.

[14] Dunstan DW, Howard B, Healy GN, Owen N. Too much sitting – a health hazard. Diabetes Res Clin Pract 2012;97:368–76.

[15] Nauman J, Stensvold D, Coombes JS, Wisløff U. Cardiorespiratory fitness, sedentary time, and cardiovascular risk factor clustering. Med Sci Sports Exerc 2016;48:625–32.

[16] Wen CP, Wai JP, Tsai MK, Yang YC, Cheng TYD, Lee M-C, et al. Minimum amount of physical activity for reduced mortality and extended life expectancy: a prospective cohort study. Lancet 2011;378:1244–53.

[17] Haskell WL, Lee IM, Pate RR, Powell KE, Blair SN, Franklin BA, et al. Physical activity and public health: updated recommendation for adults from the American College of Sports Medicine and the American Heart Association. Circulation 2007;116:1081–93.

[18] Heart Foundation. 2013. Healthy living – be active every day. https://www.heartfoundation.org.au/images/uploads/main/Active_living/Be-active-everyday.pdf.

[19] Exercise and Sport Science Australia. 2018. Exercise right. http://exerciseright.com.au/.

[20] Heart Foundation. 2012. Sitting less for adults. https://www.heartfoundation.org.au/images/uploads/main/Active_living/Sitting_less_adults.pdf.

[21] Australian Government Department of Health. 2014. Australian 24-hour movement guidelines for children and young people (5–17 years) – an integration of physical activity, sedentary behaviour and sleep. https://www1.health.gov.au/internet/main/publishing.nsf/Content/health-24-hours-phys-act-guidelines.

[22] Wallen MP, Gomersall SR, Keating SE, Wisløff U, Coombes J. Accuracy of heart rate watches: implications for weight management. PLoS One 2016;11:e0154420.

[23] Xie J, Wen D, Liang L, Jia Y, Gao L, Lei J. Evaluating the validity of current mainstream wearable devices in fitness tracking under various physical activities: comparative study. JMIR Mhealth Uhealth 2018;6:e94.

[24] Evenson KR, Goto MM, Furberg RD. Systematic review of the validity and reliability of consumer-wearable activity trackers. Int J Behav Nutr Phys Act 2015;12:159.

[25] Strath SJ, Kaminsky LA, Ainsworth BE, Ekelund U, Freedson PS, Gary RA, et al. Guide to the assessment of physical activity: clinical and research applications: a scientific statement from the American Heart Association. Circulation 2013;128:2259–79.

[26] Alinia P, Cain C, Fallahzadeh R, Shahrokni A, Cook D, Ghasemzadeh H. How accurate is your activity tracker? A comparative study of step counts in low-intensity physical activities. JMIR Mhealth Uhealth 2017;5:e106.

[27] Schoeppe S, Alley S, Van Lippevelde W, Bray NA, Williams SL, Duncan MJ, et al. Efficacy of interventions that use apps to improve diet, physical activity and sedentary behaviour: a systematic review. Int J Behav Nutr Phys Act 2016;13:127.

[28] Michie S, van Stralen MM, West R. The behaviour change wheel: a new method for characterising and designing behaviour change interventions. Implement Sci 2011;6:42.

[29] Michie S, Richardson M, Johnston M, Abraham C, Francis J, Hardeman W, et al. The behavior change technique taxonomy (v1) of 93 hierarchically clustered techniques: building an international consensus for the reporting of behavior change interventions. Ann Behav Med 2013;46:81–95.

[30] Trost SG, O'Neil M. Clinical use of objective measures of physical activity. Br J Sports Med 2014;48:178–81.

[31] Trost SG. Measurement of physical activity in children and adolescents. Am J Lifestyle Med 2007;1:299–314.

[32] Trost SG, McIver KL, Pate RR. Conducting accelerometer-based activity assessments in field-based research. Med Sci Sports Exerc 2005;37:S531–43.

[33] Bassett DR, Jr, Rowlands A, Trost SG. Calibration and validation of wearable monitors. Med Sci Sports Exerc 2012;44: S32–8.

[34] Lyden K, Kozey SL, Staudenmeyer JW, Freedson P. A comprehensive evaluation of commonly used accelerometer energy expenditure and MET prediction equations. Eur J Appl Physiol 2011;111:187–201.

[35] Trost SG, Wong WK, Pfeiffer KA, Zheng Y. Artificial neural networks to predict activity type and energy expenditure in youth. Med Sci Sports Exerc 2012;44:1801–9.

[36] Hills AP, Mokhtar N, Byrne NM. Assessment of physical activity and energy expenditure: an overview of objective measures. Front Nutr 2014;1:5.

[37] Chomistek AK, Yuan C, Matthews CE, Troiano RP, Bowles HR, Rood J, et al. Physical activity assessment with the ActiGraph GT3X and doubly labeled water. Med Sci Sports Exerc 2017;49:1935–44.

[38] Aadland E, Ylvisaker E. Reliability of the Actigraph GT3X+ accelerometer in adults under free-living conditions. PLoS One 2015;10:e0134606.

[39] Freedson PS, Melanson E, Sirard J. Calibration of the Computer Science and Applications, Inc. accelerometer. Med Sci Sports Exerc 1998;30:777–81.

PRACTICAL 6
PRE-EXERCISE HEALTH SCREENING

Jeff Coombes and Kevin Norton

LEARNING OBJECTIVES

- Demonstrate an understanding of the rationale, purpose, terminology, application, assumptions and prognostic validity of pre-exercise health screening
- Identify and explain common processes used to conduct pre-exercise health screenings including the stages of the screening system
- Perform pre-exercise health screening using the Adult Pre-exercise Screening System (APSS)
- Analyse and interpret information from a pre-exercise health screening, and convey the results, including the validity and limitations, through relevant verbal and/or written communication with the participant or relevant health professional
- Identify and describe the limitations of pre-exercise health screenings
- Identify when there is a need for guidance or further information from a relevant health professional

Equipment and other requirements

- Adult Pre-exercise Screening System (APSS) form (version 2, 2019).[1]

INTRODUCTION

Pre-exercise screening is part of exercise professionals' duty of care. It should be completed whenever any one or more of the following conditions are met:

- **Beginning an exercise program from a sedentary or low baseline physical activity.** Examples may include a participant who has been relatively inactive for an extended period of time and decides to start walking as part of a walking-for-fitness group.
- **Significantly upgrading an exercise program, especially when the intensity is elevated substantially.** Examples may include progressing from a walking-based program to a running or high-intensity interval training (HIIT)-based program.
- **When personal health status changes significantly.** Examples may include a recent diagnosis of a chronic disease or a significant injury.

If an exercise professional has access to their participant's original/recent screening assessment that was conducted by a different trainer, another assessment is required regardless of whether there has been any change in health status or program intensity. The main reason is to ensure that the person delivering the exercise service has collected the necessary screening information. An exercise professional may operate in various environments (i.e. multiple gyms, beach or parklands); however, this shouldn't require their participant to complete additional screening assessments for these situations.

Pre-exercise screening results should be kept as confidential files. They may be shared, with the client's consent, if there are other exercise professionals involved with the client's exercise program and general wellbeing.

The purpose of screening is to identify individuals: (1) with medical contraindications to exercise, (2) who demonstrate signs or symptoms of clinical disease, (3) who may have risk factors that need to be considered when prescribing exercise, and (4) with special needs.[2] There are many different screening processes and it is useful to see these lying on a continuum. At one end may be a simple verbal question: '*Do you have any medical or physical condition that may require special consideration for you to exercise?*'

At the other end of the spectrum may be a full medical examination with an exercise stress test, exercise echocardiography, cardiac magnetic resonance imaging (MRI) and blood analysis. In practice, it is always a balance between what is possible with the time, expertise and resources available for the screening and the relative risk of not identifying someone who will have an adverse event due to exercise.

DEFINITIONS

Acute myocardial infarction (AMI): also known as a heart attack, this refers to an interruption of blood flow to part of the heart muscle causing cells to die. It is commonly caused by coronary artery disease.

Adverse event: refers to something unexpected resulting in ill health, physical harm or death to an individual.

Angina: chest pain caused by a decreased blood flow to part of the heart muscle, usually caused by CAD. Angina may occur at rest or it may manifest only during exercise or other stress when there is a greater demand for coronary blood flow.

Angioplasty: technique of mechanically widening narrowed or obstructed arteries.

Atherosclerosis: thickening of an arterial wall due to an accumulation of fatty deposits/plaques.

Cardiac arrhythmias: abnormal heart rhythms that may compromise cardiac output.

Cardiovascular disease (CVD): an umbrella term that refers to any disease that affects the heart or blood vessels. This includes coronary artery disease, hypertension, peripheral vascular disease and stroke (cerebrovascular accident).

Cerebrovascular accident: also known as a stroke. It is a rapid loss of brain functions due to a lack of blood flow to the brain. It may indicate systemic vascular disease.

Coronary artery bypass graft (CABG): a surgical technique where a healthy artery or vein from the body is connected to a blocked coronary artery to improve blood flow.

Coronary artery disease (CAD): also known as coronary heart disease (CHD) or ischaemic heart disease (IHD), this refers to a narrowing or blockage of the coronary arteries of the heart, usually caused by atherosclerosis. It can lead to chest pain (angina) or a heart attack (myocardial infarction) and damage to the heart muscle.

Exercise: planned, structured and repetitive movements carried out to sustain or improve fitness and health.

Exercise professional: a qualified and registered/accredited person who supplies exercise services to the public.

Fitness professional: in Australia, this refers to individuals with either a Certificate or Diploma of Fitness studies.

Heart attack: also known as a myocardial infarction, this refers to an interruption of blood flow to part of the heart muscle causing cells to die. It is commonly caused by CAD.

Heart failure: occurs when the heart muscle doesn't pump blood as well as it should. Certain conditions, such as CAD or high blood pressure, often lead to heart failure.

Heart murmurs: an extra or unusual sound heard during a heartbeat. Most are harmless but some may be a result of a medical condition (e.g. heart valve disease).

Hyperglycaemia: when blood glucose (sugar) levels remain high.[a]

Hypoglycaemia: when blood glucose (sugar) levels remain low.

Medical practitioner: a professional with a medical degree who practises medicine. In Australia this includes physicians (specialists) such as general practitioners (GPs).

Myocardial infarction: also known as a heart attack, this refers to an interruption of blood flow to part of the heart muscle causing cells to die. It is commonly caused by CAD.

Orthostatic hypotension: sudden fall in blood pressure that occurs when a person changes posture (e.g. stands up).

Peripheral arterial disease: a common circulatory problem in which narrowed arteries reduce blood flow to the limbs, usually the legs.

Physical activity: any bodily movement produced by skeletal muscle that requires energy expenditure.

Sensitivity: correctly identifying participants with relevant health conditions.

Silent angina: decreased blood flow to the heart muscle without pain.

Sinus rhythm: normal beating rhythm of the heart.

Specificity: correctly identifying participants without relevant health conditions.

Stenting: placing a tube in a blood vessel to improve blood flow.

Stroke: also known as a cerebrovascular accident. It is a rapid loss of brain functions due to a lack of blood flow to the brain. It may indicate systemic vascular disease.

Vascular claudication: discomfort, tiredness or pain in the legs from a vascular cause that impairs walking and is relieved by rest. It is usually associated with peripheral vascular disease.

Adult pre-exercise screening system (APSS)

In this Practical we will use a screening process, the Adult Pre-exercise Screening System (APSS) version 2, that is recommended for use in most settings where people are beginning or upgrading their exercise patterns.

The APSS was developed in Australia from a collaboration between the major exercise, sport and fitness associations: Exercise and Sports Science Australia (ESSA), Sports Medicine Australia (SMA) and Fitness Australia (FA). The first version of the APSS was published in 2011, with version 2 (Figure 6.1) available in 2019.

The APSS consists of two parts: (1) the questions in stage 1 and stage 2, and (2) the algorithms that provide guidance on how to use the information collected. One algorithm is contained within the tool (Figure 6.1) and one in the user manual (Figure 6.2).[1] The APSS is also available via the Exercise Science Toolkit (http://www.exercisesciencetoolkit.com). This free resource allows students to check risk factors and investigate the absolute risk of an untoward event due to exercise of a virtual participant.

Version 2 of the APSS was developed to:

- simplify interpretation of the screening process, specifically to encourage people to remain active if they are already active, or to begin light–moderate exercise if they are free from chronic conditions or signs or symptoms of serious disease

---

[a] See Practical 2, Table 2.2 for diagnostic criteria.

ADULT PRE-EXERCISE SCREENING SYSTEM (APSS)

This screening tool is part of the Adult Pre-Exercise Screening System (APSS) that also includes guidelines (see User Guide) on how to use the information collected and to address the aims of each stage. No warranty of safety should result from its use. The screening system in no way guarantees against injury or death. No responsibility or liability whatsoever can be accepted by Exercise & Sport Science Australia, Fitness Australia, Sports Medicine Australia or Exercise is Medicine for any loss, damage, or injury that may arise from any person acting on any statement or information contained in this system.

Full Name: _____

Date of Birth: _____ Male: ☐   Female: ☐   Other: ☐

STAGE 1 (COMPULSORY)

AIM: To identify individuals with known disease, and/or signs or symptoms of disease, who may be at a higher risk of an adverse event due to exercise. An adverse event refers to an unexpected event that occurs as a consequence of an exercise session, resulting in ill health, physical harm or death to an individual.

This stage may be self-administered and self-evaluated by the client. Please complete the questions below and refer to the figures on page 2. Should you have any questions about the screening form please contact your exercise professional for clarification.

Please tick your response

	YES	NO
1. Has your medical practitioner ever told you that you have a heart condition or have you ever suffered a stroke?		
2. Do you ever experience unexplained pains or discomfort in your chest at rest or during physical activity/exercise?		
3. Do you ever feel faint, dizzy or lose balance during physical activity/exercise?		
4. Have you had an asthma attack requiring immediate medical attention at any time over the last 12 months?		
5. If you have diabetes (type 1 or 2) have you had trouble controlling your blood sugar (glucose) in the last 3 months?		
6. Do you have any other conditions that may require special consideration for you to exercise?		

IF YOU ANSWERED 'YES' to any of the 6 questions, please seek guidance from an appropriate allied health professional or medical practitioner prior to undertaking exercise.

IF YOU ANSWERED 'NO' to all of the 6 questions, please proceed to question 7 and calculate your typical weighted physical activity/exercise per week.

7. Describe your current physical activity/exercise levels in a typical week by stating the frequency and duration at the different intensities. For intensity guidelines consult figure 2.

Intensity	Light	Moderate	Vigorous/High
Frequency (number of sessions per week)	_____	_____	_____
Duration (total minutes per week)	_____	_____	_____

Weighted physical activity/exercise per week

Total minutes = (minutes of light + moderate) + (2 x minutes of vigorous/high)

TOTAL = _____ minutes per week

- If your total is less than 150 minutes per week then light to moderate intensity exercise is recommended. Increase your volume and intensity slowly.
- If your total is more than or equal to 150 minutes per week then continue with your current physical activity/exercise intensity levels.

- It is advised that you discuss any progression (volume, intensity, duration, modality) with an exercise professional to optimise your results.

I believe that to the best of my knowledge, all of the information I have supplied within this screening tool is correct.

Client signature: _____ Date: _____

ADULT PRE-EXERCISE SCREENING SYSTEM (APSS) V2 (2018)

ExeℝXcise is Medicine® Australia   Fitness Australia   SPORTS MEDICINE AUSTRALIA   ESSA· EXERCISE & SPORTS SCIENCE AUSTRALIA

Figure 6.1 Adult Pre-exercise Screening System tool (version 2)

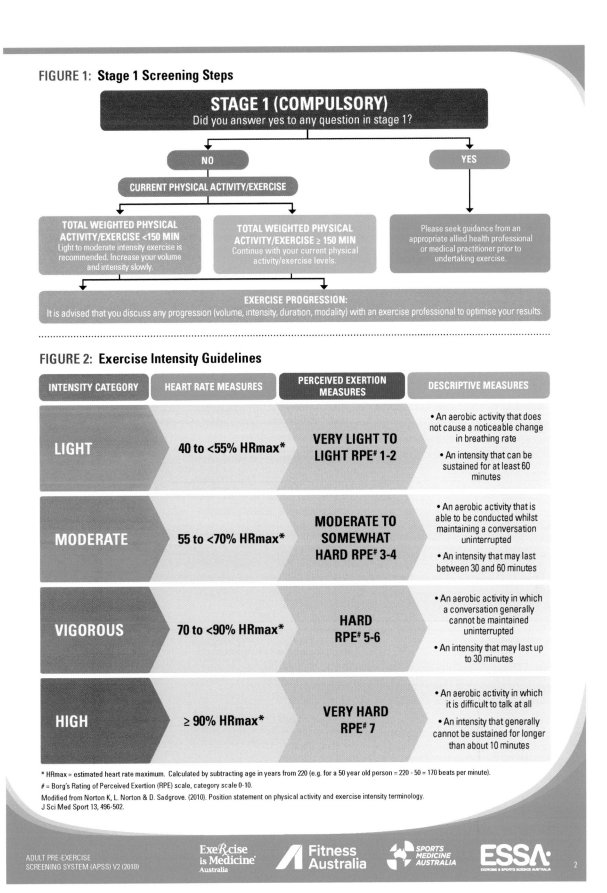

FIGURE 1: Stage 1 Screening Steps

STAGE 1 (COMPULSORY)
Did you answer yes to any question in stage 1?

NO

YES

CURRENT PHYSICAL ACTIVITY/EXERCISE

TOTAL WEIGHTED PHYSICAL ACTIVITY/EXERCISE <150 MIN
Light to moderate intensity exercise is recommended. Increase your volume and intensity slowly.

TOTAL WEIGHTED PHYSICAL ACTIVITY/EXERCISE ≥ 150 MIN
Continue with your current physical activity/exercise levels.

Please seek guidance from an appropriate allied health professional or medical practitioner prior to undertaking exercise.

EXERCISE PROGRESSION:
It is advised that you discuss any progression (volume, intensity, duration, modality) with an exercise professional to optimise your results.

FIGURE 2: Exercise Intensity Guidelines

INTENSITY CATEGORY	HEART RATE MEASURES	PERCEIVED EXERTION MEASURES	DESCRIPTIVE MEASURES
LIGHT	40 to <55% HRmax*	**VERY LIGHT TO LIGHT RPE# 1-2**	• An aerobic activity that does not cause a noticeable change in breathing rate • An intensity that can be sustained for at least 60 minutes
MODERATE	55 to <70% HRmax*	**MODERATE TO SOMEWHAT HARD RPE# 3-4**	• An aerobic activity that is able to be conducted whilst maintaining a conversation uninterrupted • An intensity that may last between 30 and 60 minutes
VIGOROUS	70 to <90% HRmax*	**HARD RPE# 5-6**	• An aerobic activity in which a conversation generally cannot be maintained uninterrupted • An intensity that may last up to 30 minutes
HIGH	≥ 90% HRmax*	**VERY HARD RPE# 7**	• An aerobic activity in which it is difficult to talk at all • An intensity that generally cannot be sustained for longer than about 10 minutes

* HRmax = estimated heart rate maximum. Calculated by subtracting age in years from 220 (e.g. for a 50 year old person = 220 - 50 = 170 beats per minute).
\# = Borg's Rating of Perceived Exertion (RPE) scale, category scale 0-10.
Modified from Norton K, L. Norton & D. Sadgrove. (2010). Position statement on physical activity and exercise intensity terminology. J Sci Med Sport 13, 496-502.

ADULT PRE-EXERCISE SCREENING SYSTEM (APSS) V2 (2018)

ExeRcise is Medicine® Australia

Fitness Australia

SPORTS MEDICINE AUSTRALIA

ESSA·
EXERCISE & SPORTS SCIENCE AUSTRALIA

2

Figure 6.1, cont'd

STAGE 2 (RECOMMENDED)

AIM: This stage is to be completed with an exercise professional to determine appropriate exercise prescription based on established risk factors.

CLIENT DETAILS	GUIDELINES FOR ASSESSING RISK
8. Demographics Age: _____ Male ☐ Female ☐ Other ☐	Risk of an adverse event increases with age, particularly males ≥ 45 yr and females ≥ 55 yr.
9. Family history of heart disease (e.g. stroke, heart attack)? Relationship (e.g. father) Age at heart disease event _____ _____ _____ _____ _____ _____	A family history of heart disease refers to an event that occurs in relatives including parents, grandparents, uncles and/or aunts before the age of 55 years.
10. Do you smoke cigarettes on a daily or weekly basis or have you quit smoking in the last 6 months? Yes ☐ No ☐ If currently smoking, how many per day or week? _____	Smoking, even on a weekly basis, substantially increases risk for premature death and disability. The negative effects are still present up to at least 6 months post quitting.
11. Body composition Weight (kg) _____ Height (cm) _____ Body Mass Index (kg/m²) _____ Waist circumference (cm) _____	Any of the below increases the risk of chronic diseases: $BMI \geq 30$ kg/m^2 Waist > 94 cm male or > 80 cm female
12. Have you been told that you have high blood pressure? Yes ☐ No ☐ If known, systolic/diastolic (mmHg) _____ Are you taking any medication for this condition? Yes ☐ No ☐ If yes, provide details _____	Either of the below increases the risk of heart disease: Systolic blood pressure ≥ 140 mmHg Diastolic blood pressure ≥ 90 mmHg
13. Have you been told that you have high cholesterol/blood lipids? Yes ☐ No ☐ If known: Total cholesterol (mmol/L) _____ HDL (mmol/L) _____ LDL (mmol/L) _____ Triglycerides (mmol/L) _____ Are you taking any medication for this condition? Yes ☐ No ☐ If yes, provide details _____	Any of the below increases the risk of heart disease: Total cholesterol ≥ 5.2 mmol/L HDL < 1.0 mmol/L LDL ≥ 3.4 mmol/L Triglycerides ≥ 1.7 mmol/L

 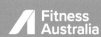

Figure 6.1, cont'd

CLIENT DETAILS	GUIDELINES FOR ASSESSING RISK
14. Have you been told that you have high blood sugar (glucose)? Yes No If known: Fasting blood glucose (mmol/L) _____ Are you taking any medication for this condition? Yes No If yes, provide details _____	Fasting blood sugar (glucose) ≥ 5.5 mmol/L increases the risk of diabetes.
15. Are you currently taking prescribed medication(s) for any condition(s)? These are additional to those already provided. Yes No If yes, what are the medical conditions?	Taking medication indicates a medically diagnosed problem. Judgment is required when taking medication information into account for determining appropriate exercise prescription because it is common for clients to list 'medications' that include contraceptive pills, vitamin supplements and other non-pharmaceutical tablets. Exercise professionals are not expected to have an exhaustive understanding of medications. Therefore, it may be important to use common language to describe what medical conditions the drugs are prescribed for.
16. Have you spent time in hospital (including day admission) for any condition/illness/injury during the last 12 months? Yes No If yes, provide details _____	There are positive relationships between illness rates and death versus the number and length of hospital admissions in the previous 12 months. This includes admissions for heart disease, lung disease (e.g., Chronic Obstructive Pulmonary Disease (COPD) and asthma), dementia, hip fractures, infectious episodes and inflammatory bowel disease. Admissions are also correlated to 'poor health' status and negative health behaviours such as smoking, alcohol consumption and poor diet patterns.
17. Are you pregnant or have you given birth within the last 12 months? Yes No If yes, provide details _____ _____	During pregnancy and after recent childbirth are times to be more cautious with exercise. Appropriate exercise prescription results in improved health to mother and baby. However, joints gradually loosen to prepare for birth and may lead to an increased risk of injury especially in the pelvic joints. Activities involving jumping, frequent changes of direction and excessive stretching should be avoided, as should jerky ballistic movements. Guidelines/fact sheets can be found here: 1) www.exerciseismedicine.com.au 2) www.fitness.org.au/Pre-and-Post-Natal-Exercise-Guidelines
18. Do you have any diagnosed muscle, bone, tendon, ligament or joint problems that you have been told could be made worse by participating in exercise? Yes No If yes, provide details _____ _____	Almost everyone has experienced some level of soreness following unaccustomed exercise or activity but this is not really what this question is designed to identify. Soreness due to unaccustomed activity is not the same as pain in the joint, muscle or bone. Pain is more extreme and may represent an injury, serious inflammatory episode or infection. If it is an acute injury then it is possible that further medical guidance may be required.

ADULT PRE-EXERCISE SCREENING SYSTEM (APSS) V2 (2018)

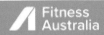   ESSA·

Figure 6.1, cont'd

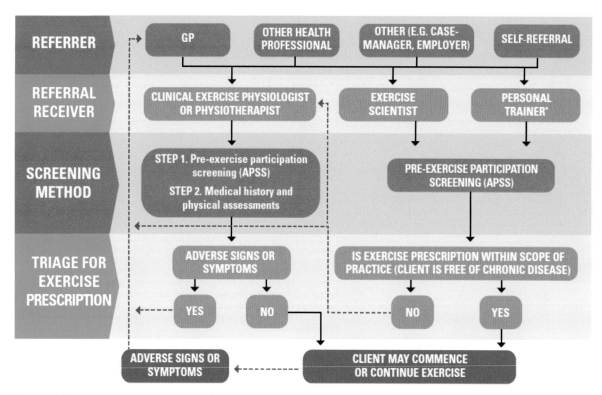

Figure 6.2 Exercise screening, referral and assessment pathways for exercise professionals[1]

- help client management by providing guidance about referral pathways linked to screening outcomes
- remove the process of counting risk factors
- continue to reduce and optimise medical referral pathways to minimise potential barriers to exercise participation.
  The APSS takes into account:
- the considerable evidence that exercise is safe for most people and has many associated health and fitness benefits
- exercise-related cardiovascular events are often preceded by warning signs/symptoms
- that cardiovascular risks associated with exercise lessen as individuals become more physically active/fit.
  Therefore, the main changes between version 1 and 2 of the APSS are:
- version 2 no longer uses the cardiovascular disease risk factors to stratify individuals into high, moderate or low risk
- stage 3 has been incorporated into the recommended stage 2
- an individual's current level of physical activity and desired exercise intensity are considered when applying information obtained with the APSS Tool.

Stage 1 of the APSS screens individuals based on three factors: (1) the presence of signs or symptoms of, and/or known, cardiovascular or metabolic disease, (2) the individual's current level of physical activity and (3) intended exercise intensity. These variables have been identified as the most important risk modulators of exercise-related cardiovascular events.[3]

Stage 2 of the APSS collects information on cardiovascular disease risk factors for more appropriate exercise prescription, but not for risk factor profiling.

Figure 1 in the APSS (see Figure 6.1) contains an algorithm to assist with clinical decision making. It is similar to the recent American College of Sports Medicine (ACSM) screening guidelines algorithm[3] and provides guidance for client management after completing stage 1 of the screening process.

Figure 6.2 is the second algorithm used in the APSS (contained in the user guide)[4] and provides additional guidance on the referral, assessment and prescription of exercise relative to different exercise professionals and referral pathways.[5]

The APSS addresses concerns that excessive referrals to doctors may have been creating a barrier to exercise participation[6] and GPs in Australia questioning the medico-legal issues if they provide clearance to exercise and there is an adverse event.[7] The word 'clearance' is not used within the APSS, instead the individual is asked to 'seek guidance' from relevant health professionals or a medical practitioner. This allows a suitably qualified exercise professional to be a gate keeper for clinical decision making, which may mean that a person does still seek further clinical guidance from their GP.

This also allows suitably qualified exercise professionals to use their knowledge, skills and expertise to assess and manage any risks related to the prescription and delivery of appropriate exercise programs. It is anticipated that removing unjustified barriers to exercise participation will improve the uptake of exercise by the unacceptably high proportion of the population who do not undertake sufficient physical activity for health benefit.

The two algorithms used in the APSS (one in the tool and one in the user guide) (see Figure 6.1) are not a replacement for sound clinical judgment, and decisions about referral to a healthcare provider for guidance before the initiation of an exercise program should continue to be made on an individual basis.

It is expected that the consistent recognition and use of the APSS by fitness professionals,[b] Accredited Exercise Scientists, Accredited Sports Scientists, Accredited Exercise Physiologists, physiotherapists and other allied health practitioners will greatly enhance screening practices.

Validity

Version 2 of the APSS is now similar to the ACSM's updated pre-participation guidelines.[3] To investigate the prognostic validity of the new ACSM approach, a study compared referrals for medical clearance in the new guidelines with other screening approaches (e.g. previous ACSM questionnaire) in around 3500 participants.[8] It found that the new ACSM guidelines resulted in around 40% fewer referrals. Given the similarity in the approaches between version 2 of the APSS and the most recent ACSM guidelines, it would be expected that the APSS would have a similar rate of referrals. The study recognised that additional validation is needed to determine whether the algorithm correctly identifies those at risk for cardiovascular complications. It would also be useful to know if the algorithm positively influences individuals' exercise participation.

Limitations

The major limitation of the APSS, which is similar to other pre-exercise screening systems, is that it relies on the participant to have the necessary knowledge about their health and/or answer questions truthfully. Failure to provide accurate responses would limit the sensitivity and specificity of the system. The system also moves towards more clinical decision making from the exercise professional rather than a medical practitioner. The accuracy of this decision making will depend on the exercise professional's communication skills to retrieve the necessary information, their knowledge of anatomy, physiology, pathophysiology, pharmacology, exercise prescription and experience using the system.

Activity 6.1 Self-screening

AIM: screen yourself using the APSS.

Background

The form contains two stages:

- **Stage 1** has been designed to be self-administered and self-evaluated. It aims to identify individuals with known disease, and/or signs or symptoms of disease, who may be at a higher risk of an adverse event due to physical activity/exercise. It also asks the individual to describe their current physical activity levels to assist with determining whether an individual is ready to begin or continue exercise, or whether they should seek guidance from a health professional prior to commencing such activity.

- **Stage 2** should be administered by an appropriately qualified exercise professional (e.g. fitness professionals,[b] Accredited Exercise Scientists, Accredited Sports Scientists, Accredited Exercise Physiologists, Physiotherapists). This stage identifies CVD risk factors that should be considered when prescribing or modifying a physical activity/exercise program.

---

[b] In Australia, this refers to individuals with either a Certificate or Diploma of Fitness.

Protocol

Using your data from Practicals 2–5, complete the two stages of the APSS form in Figure 6.1 and determine what intensity you may begin/continue exercising. Box 6.1 provides some explanatory notes to assist with questions in stage 1.

Box 6.1   Explanatory notes for stage 1 of the APSS

The following notes provide further information regarding the stage 1 questions:

Question 1. Has your medical practitioner ever told you that you have a heart condition or have you ever suffered a stroke?

Heart conditions include, but are not limited to: post myocardial infarction (heart attack), angina, coronary artery bypass, coronary angioplasty, heart failure, cardiomyopathy, heart transplant, pacemaker insertion, congenital heart disease, heart valve disease and peripheral arterial disease.

Question 2. Do you ever experience unexplained pains or discomfort in your chest at rest or during physical activity/exercise?

Any unexplained chest pains, characterised by: constriction, burning, knifelike pains, and/or dull ache.

Question 3. Do you ever feel faint, dizzy or lose balance during physical activity/exercise?

There are many causes of feeling faint or dizzy. Examples of dizziness may include, but are not limited to: lightheadedness or the feeling of nearly fainting, loss of balance or other sensations such as floating or swimming. This question is attempting to identify individuals with conditions such as blood pressure regulation problems (e.g. orthostatic hypotension) or cardiac arrhythmias. Although dizziness after exercise should not always be ignored, this may occur even in healthy individuals. Dizziness after exercise may not always indicate a serious medical issue.

Question 4. Have you had an asthma attack requiring immediate medical attention at any time over the last 12 months?

Medical attention refers to a medical practitioner or hospital visit following an asthma attack. It does not include the self-administration of medications prescribed for asthma.

Question 5. If you have diabetes (type 1 or 2), have you had trouble controlling your blood sugar (glucose) in the last 3 months?

Trouble controlling blood sugar refers to suffering from hyperglycaemia (high) or hypoglycaemia (low). Abnormal blood sugar levels may impede the individual's ability to exercise. In addition, participants with diabetes have an increased risk for coronary artery disease and can have a reduced ability to feel chest pain (silent angina). It is important to consider blood sugar levels and risk for coronary artery disease in patients with diabetes.

Question 6. Do you have any other conditions that may require special consideration for you to participate in exercise?

Examples include: acute injury, pregnancy, epilepsy, transplants and cancer.

Question 7. Describe your current physical activity/exercise levels in a typical week by stating the frequency and duration at the different intensities. For intensity guidelines, consult Figure 2 in the screening tool.

From the information collected, calculate the total number of minutes of exercise per week.

If weighted physical activity level <150 min/week, the client has a higher risk of chronic disease.

Activity 6.2 Screen a participant

AIM: screen a participant (a classmate) using the APSS.

Background

Screening another individual may require the tester to answer specific questions from the participant. For this activity, the classmate completing the APSS should role-play as the participant and pose some questions to the tester regarding the APSS form and processes. When one person has completed the process, swap roles. Box 6.1 provides additional information regarding the questions in stage 1. A thorough understanding of pathophysiology/pharmacology and their relationships with the exercise/physical activity intentions of the participant will assist in answering questions appropriately across the stages.

Protocol summary

Screen a classmate using the APSS (see Figure 6.1)

Protocol

- Administer stages 1 and 2 of the APSS (see Figure 6.1) to a participant.
- Using the participant's data from Practicals 2–5, complete all stages of the APSS and determine what intensity the participant may begin exercising.

Interpretation, feedback and discussion

First, consider the four steps of interpretation and the three steps of feedback and discussion outlined in Appendix G. Figure 1 on page 2 of the APSS (see Figure 6.1) provides an algorithm to direct action. The outcome will be that participants will:

1 be requested to seek medical guidance before starting or continuing to exercise

2 be able to start exercising at a low-to-moderate-intensity

3 be able to continue to exercise at their current intensity, or

4 be able to start or continue to exercise at a higher intensity (e.g. vigorous).

Figure 2 in the APSS Form is the exercise intensity guidelines table (see Figure 6.1) from Norton and colleagues.[9] This will assist in understanding what is meant by light, moderate, vigorous and high exercise intensities. Note that the thresholds used to define some of the intensities in this table vary from other similar definitions (e.g. ACSM).[2] For example, the ACSM uses 64%–76% maximal heart rate (HR_{max}) for moderate-intensity, whereas Norton and colleagues [9] use 55%–<70% HR_{max}.

As discussed in Practicals 2 and 3, certain abnormal values are 'red flags' (e.g. blood pressure, plasma lipids, plasma glucose) and the participant will need to be referred to their doctor for follow-up. Because of the wide variety of health questions asked across the APSS, it is likely that some aspects will prompt further discussion. Clearly the knowledge and experience of the tester will be the main factor in determining how a participant's questions are answered and discussions led, to accurately obtain information. It is important to give responses that are as evidence based as possible and it is always appropriate for a tester to admit they are not sure of the answer to a question. In this situation, the tester may offer to find out the answer and get back to the participant.

Professional judgment should be used when deciding whether to provide specific feedback to a participant regarding their risk factors. It should depend on the purpose of the screening; in most cases a tester will not give feedback on a participant's specific risk factors identified using the APSS.

Seeking guidance from a general practitioner (GP) or appropriate allied health professional

If you are requesting the participant seeks guidance from their GP/allied health professional, it is vital that this is appropriately conveyed to all involved. Key points to convey when requesting your participant seeks medical guidance are outlined below.

- Minimise the possibility that the participant may feel like they have failed the first part of what may be a big step (e.g. attempting to start an exercise program with professional help).
- The additional information requested from the GP/allied health professional should help in the design of the exercise program.
- The approach to the GP/allied health professional needs to be professional and individualised. Instead of a pro forma letter, it is recommended that your correspondence provides:
  - the specific information from the participant's health history that has led to the request
  - the exact request; avoid the term 'requesting clearance to exercise' and use the APSS term 'seeking guidance'
  - details of the exercise program that you are likely to suggest to the participant
  - an offer to be involved further in the ongoing management of the participant's health (e.g. by offering ongoing updates on the participant's exercise adherence and test results).

Case studies

Case Study 1

Setting: You work in a health and fitness centre.

Participant: Rosa comes into your centre wishing to participate in a group fitness class. The centre's policy is that all clients must complete stage 1 of the APSS before they are able to use the facilities. You provide Rosa with the questionnaire and she completes it in your presence (Figure 6.3).

What questions would you ask Rosa based on her response?

After further questioning you find out that in the last few weeks she has been getting pains in her chest when she walks quickly or goes up stairs.

What action would you take?

_____

_____

_____

_____

Case Study 2

Setting: You own a mobile personal training business.

Participant: Jedda is a new client who has been training under the supervision of another trainer at another business. He has been doing a combination of moderate- and high-intensity exercise. He completes stages 1 and 2 of the APSS (Figure 6.4).

Calculate his weighted physical activity:

_____

_____

continued on page 165

Case studies *(continued)*

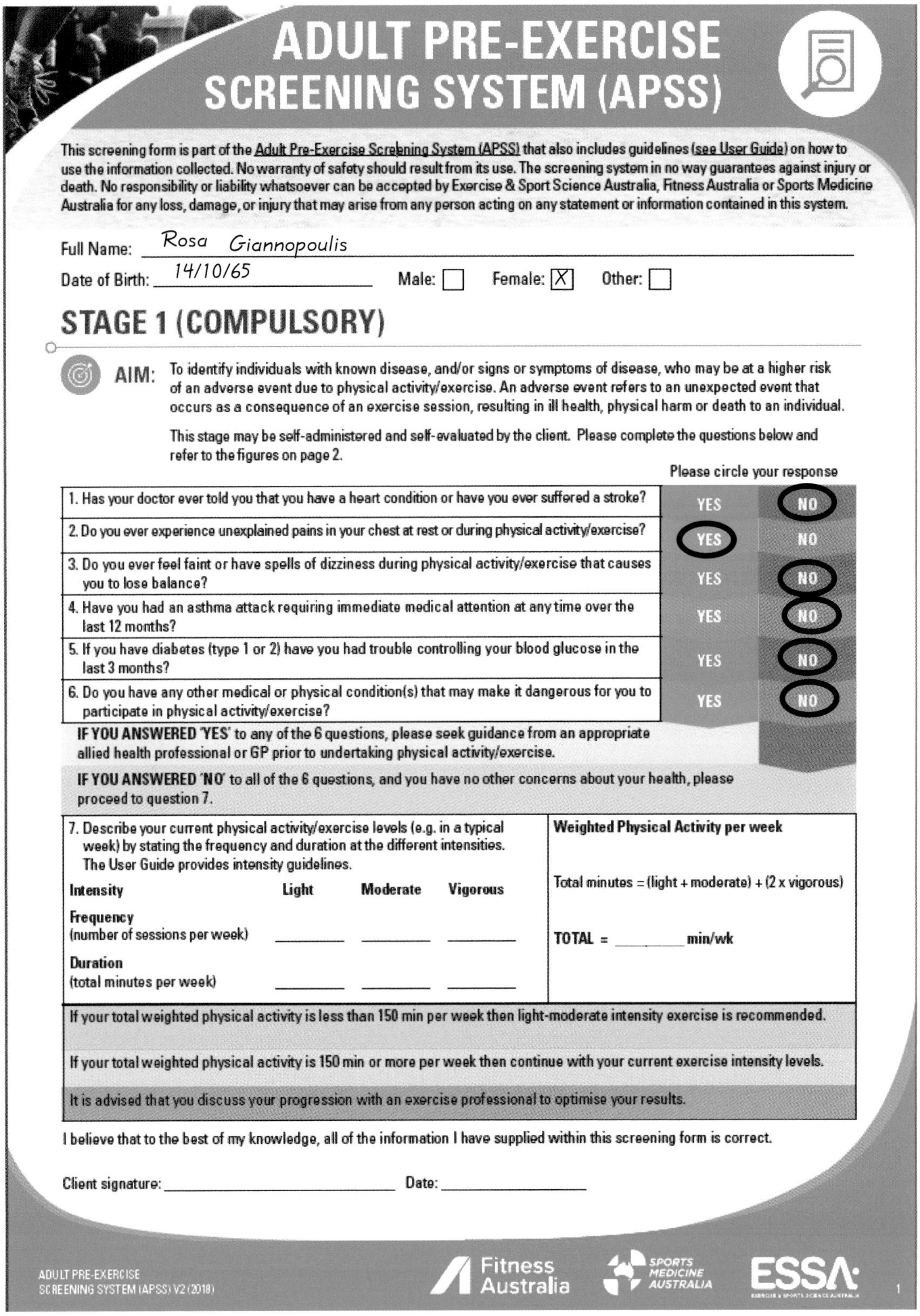

ADULT PRE-EXERCISE SCREENING SYSTEM (APSS)

This screening form is part of the Adult Pre-Exercise Screening System (APSS) that also includes guidelines (see User Guide) on how to use the information collected. No warranty of safety should result from its use. The screening system in no way guarantees against injury or death. No responsibility or liability whatsoever can be accepted by Exercise & Sport Science Australia, Fitness Australia or Sports Medicine Australia for any loss, damage, or injury that may arise from any person acting on any statement or information contained in this system.

Full Name: ___Rosa Giannopoulis___

Date of Birth: ___14/10/65___   Male: ☐   Female: ☒   Other: ☐

STAGE 1 (COMPULSORY)

AIM: To identify individuals with known disease, and/or signs or symptoms of disease, who may be at a higher risk of an adverse event due to physical activity/exercise. An adverse event refers to an unexpected event that occurs as a consequence of an exercise session, resulting in ill health, physical harm or death to an individual.

This stage may be self-administered and self-evaluated by the client. Please complete the questions below and refer to the figures on page 2.

Please circle your response

1. Has your doctor ever told you that you have a heart condition or have you ever suffered a stroke?	YES	**(NO)**
2. Do you ever experience unexplained pains in your chest at rest or during physical activity/exercise?	**(YES)**	NO
3. Do you ever feel faint or have spells of dizziness during physical activity/exercise that causes you to lose balance?	YES	**(NO)**
4. Have you had an asthma attack requiring immediate medical attention at any time over the last 12 months?	YES	**(NO)**
5. If you have diabetes (type 1 or 2) have you had trouble controlling your blood glucose in the last 3 months?	YES	**(NO)**
6. Do you have any other medical or physical condition(s) that may make it dangerous for you to participate in physical activity/exercise?	YES	**(NO)**

IF YOU ANSWERED 'YES' to any of the 6 questions, please seek guidance from an appropriate allied health professional or GP prior to undertaking physical activity/exercise.

IF YOU ANSWERED 'NO' to all of the 6 questions, and you have no other concerns about your health, please proceed to question 7.

7. Describe your current physical activity/exercise levels (e.g. in a typical week) by stating the frequency and duration at the different intensities. The User Guide provides intensity guidelines.

Weighted Physical Activity per week

Total minutes = (light + moderate) + (2 x vigorous)

Intensity	Light	Moderate	Vigorous
Frequency (number of sessions per week)	_____	_____	_____
Duration (total minutes per week)	_____	_____	_____

TOTAL = _____ min/wk

If your total weighted physical activity is less than 150 min per week then light-moderate intensity exercise is recommended.

If your total weighted physical activity is 150 min or more per week then continue with your current exercise intensity levels.

It is advised that you discuss your progression with an exercise professional to optimise your results.

I believe that to the best of my knowledge, all of the information I have supplied within this screening form is correct.

Client signature: _____   Date: _____

ADULT PRE-EXERCISE SCREENING SYSTEM (APSS) V2 (2018)

Fitness Australia   **SPORTS MEDICINE AUSTRALIA**   **ESSA·**   1

Figure 6.3 Case study 1: APSS

continued overpage

Case studies (continued)

ADULT PRE-EXERCISE SCREENING SYSTEM (APSS)

This screening form is part of the Adult Pre-Exercise Screening System (APSS) that also includes guidelines (see User Guide) on how to use the information collected. No warranty of safety should result from its use. The screening system in no way guarantees against injury or death. No responsibility or liability whatsoever can be accepted by Exercise & Sport Science Australia, Fitness Australia or Sports Medicine Australia for any loss, damage, or injury that may arise from any person acting on any statement or information contained in this system.

Full Name: _Jedda Murphy_

Date of Birth: _12/11/88_   Male: [X]   Female: [ ]   Other: [ ]

STAGE 1 (COMPULSORY)

AIM: To identify individuals with known disease, and/or signs or symptoms of disease, who may be at a higher risk of an adverse event due to physical activity/exercise. An adverse event refers to an unexpected event that occurs as a consequence of an exercise session, resulting in ill health, physical harm or death to an individual.

This stage may be self-administered and self-evaluated by the client. Please complete the questions below and refer to the figures on page 2.

Please circle your response

1. Has your doctor ever told you that you have a heart condition or have you ever suffered a stroke?	YES	**NO**
2. Do you ever experience unexplained pains in your chest at rest or during physical activity/exercise?	YES	**NO**
3. Do you ever feel faint or have spells of dizziness during physical activity/exercise that causes you to lose balance?	YES	**NO**
4. Have you had an asthma attack requiring immediate medical attention at any time over the last 12 months?	YES	**NO**
5. If you have diabetes (type 1 or 2) have you had trouble controlling your blood glucose in the last 3 months?	YES	**NO**
6. Do you have any other medical or physical condition(s) that may make it dangerous for you to participate in physical activity/exercise?	YES	**NO**

IF YOU ANSWERED 'YES' to any of the 6 questions, please seek guidance from an appropriate allied health professional or GP prior to undertaking physical activity/exercise.

IF YOU ANSWERED 'NO' to all of the 6 questions, and you have no other concerns about your health, please proceed to question 7.

7. Describe your current physical activity/exercise levels (e.g. in a typical week) by stating the frequency and duration at the different intensities. The User Guide provides intensity guidelines.

Intensity	Light	Moderate	Vigorous
Frequency (number of sessions per week)		3	2
Duration (total minutes per week)		90	30

Weighted Physical Activity per week

Total minutes = (light + moderate) + (2 x vigorous)

TOTAL = _____ min/wk

If your total weighted physical activity is less than 150 min per week then light-moderate intensity exercise is recommended.

If your total weighted physical activity is 150 min or more per week then continue with your current exercise intensity levels.

It is advised that you discuss your progression with an exercise professional to optimise your results.

I believe that to the best of my knowledge, all of the information I have supplied within this screening form is correct.

Client signature: _____   Date: _____

ADULT PRE-EXERCISE
SCREENING SYSTEM (APSS) V2 (2018)

Fitness Australia   SPORTS MEDICINE AUSTRALIA   ESSA·   1

Figure 6.4 Case study 2: APSS

continued

Case studies *(continued)*

STAGE 2 (RECOMMENDED)

 AIM: To identify those individuals with risk factors or other conditions that may result in them being at a higher risk of an adverse event. This stage aims to assist the exercise professional to determine appropriate exercise prescription.

CLIENT DETAILS	GUIDELINES FOR ASSESSING RISK
8. Demographics Age: _____*30*_____ Male [X] Female [ ] Other [ ]	Risk of an adverse event increases with age, particularly males ≥ 45 yr and females ≥ 55 yr.
9. Family history of heart disease (e.g. stroke, heart attack) Age Age Father _*72*_ Mother _____ Brother _____ Sister _____ Son _____ Daughter _____	Risk of heart disease is greater if a first degree relative has suffered a heart attack, stroke or undergone heart surgery and was < 55 yr (males) or < 65 yr (females) when it happened.
10. Do you smoke cigarettes on a daily or weekly basis or have you quit smoking in the last 6 months? Yes [ ] No [X] If currently smoking, how many per day or week? _____	Smoking, even on a weekly basis, substantially increases risk for premature death and disability. The residual negative effects are still present up to at least 6 months post quitting.
11. Body composition Height (cm) _____*175*_____ Weight (kg) _____*92*_____ Waist circumference (cm) _____*102*_____	BMI ≥ 30 kg/m² Waist > 94 cm male or > 80 cm female increases the risk of chronic diseases.
12. Have you been told that you have high blood pressure? Yes [ ] No [X] (If known) Systolic/Diastolic (mmHg) _____	Systolic blood pressure ≥ 140 mmHg or diastolic blood pressure ≥ 90 mmHg increases the risk of cardiovascular disease.

ADULT PRE-EXERCISE SCREENING SYSTEM (APSS) V2 (2018)

3

Figure 6.4, cont'd

continued overpage

Case studies (continued)

CLIENT DETAILS	GUIDELINES FOR ASSESSING RISK
13. Have you been told that you have high cholesterol? Yes ☐ No ☒ (If known) Total cholesterol (mmol/L) _____ HDL (mmol/L) _____ LDL (mmol/L) _____ Triglycerides (mmol/L) _____	Any of the below, increases the risk of heart conditions: Total cholesterol ≥ 5.2 mmol/L HDL < 1.0 mmol/L LDL ≥ 3.4 mmol/L Triglycerides ≥ 1.7 mmol/L
14. Have you been told that you have high blood sugar? Yes ☐ No ☒ (If known) Glucose (mmol/L) _____	Fasting blood glucose ≥ 5.5 mmol/L increases the risk of diabetes.
15. Have you spent time in hospital (including day admission) for any medical condition/illness/injury during the last 12 months? Yes ☐ No ☒ If yes provide details _____	There are positive relationships between illness rates and death versus the number and length of hospital admissions in the previous 12 months. This includes heart disease, lung disease (e.g., COPD and asthma), dementia, hip fractures, infectious episodes and inflammatory bowel disease. Admissions are also correlated to 'poor health' status and negative health behaviours such as smoking, alcohol consumption and nutritional patterns.
16. Are you currently taking prescribed medication(s) for any medical condition(s)? Yes ☐ No ☒ If yes, what is the medical condition? _____	Taking medication indicates a medically diagnosed problem. Judgment is required because it is common for clients to list 'medications' that include contraceptive pills, vitamin supplements and other non-pharmaceutical tablets. Fitness professionals are not expected to have an exhaustive understanding of medications. However, it may be important to use common language to describe what medical conditions the drugs are prescribed for.
17. Are you pregnant or have you given birth within the last 12 months? Yes ☐ No ☐ If yes provide details _____	During pregnancy and after recent childbirth are times to be more cautious with exercise. Appropriate exercise prescription results in improved health to mother and baby. However, joints gradually loosen to prepare for birth and may lead to an increased risk of injury especially in the pelvic joints. Activities involving jumping, frequent changes of direction and excessive stretching should be avoided, as should jerky ballistic movements.
18. Do you have any diagnosed muscle, bone or joint problems that you have been told could be made worse by participating in physical activity/exercise? Yes ☐ No ☒ If yes provide details _____	Almost everyone has experienced some level of soreness following unaccustomed exercise or activity but this is not really what this question is designed to identify. Soreness due to unaccustomed activity is not the same as pain in the joint, muscle or bone. Pain is more extreme and may represent an injury, serious inflammatory episode or infection. If the response is an acute problem then it is possible further medical guidance may be required.

ADULT PRE-EXERCISE SCREENING SYSTEM (APSS) V2 (2019)

Fitness Australia   SPORTS MEDICINE AUSTRALIA   ESSA

4

Figure 6.4, cont'd

continued

Case studies *(continued)*

What questions would you ask Jedda?

Does he have any cardiovascular disease risk factors?

Based on his responses in stages 1 and 2, what would be your action?

Case Study 3

Setting: You work with a corporate fitness company. Your company has a contract with a factory to provide health screening, CVD risk appraisal and exercise prescription.

Participant: Maria completes stages 1 and 2 of the APSS (Figure 6.5) and then has a meeting with you.

Calculate her weighted physical activity:

What questions would you ask Maria?

Does she have any cardiovascular disease risk factors?

Based on her responses in stages 1 and 2, what would be your action?

continued overpage

Case studies *(continued)*

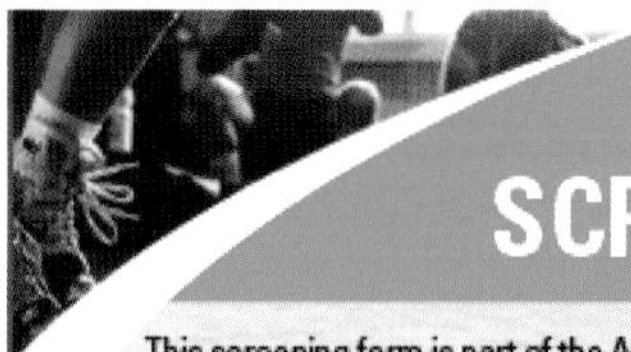

ADULT PRE-EXERCISE SCREENING SYSTEM (APSS)

This screening form is part of the Adult Pre-Exercise Screening System (APSS) that also includes guidelines (see User Guide) on how to use the information collected. No warranty of safety should result from its use. The screening system in no way guarantees against injury or death. No responsibility or liability whatsoever can be accepted by Exercise & Sport Science Australia, Fitness Australia or Sports Medicine Australia for any loss, damage, or injury that may arise from any person acting on any statement or information contained in this system.

Full Name: _Maria Gajanand_

Date of Birth: _21/1/82_   Male: ☐   Female: ☒   Other: ☐

STAGE 1 (COMPULSORY)

AIM: To identify individuals with known disease, and/or signs or symptoms of disease, who may be at a higher risk of an adverse event due to physical activity/exercise. An adverse event refers to an unexpected event that occurs as a consequence of an exercise session, resulting in ill health, physical harm or death to an individual.

This stage may be self-administered and self-evaluated by the client. Please complete the questions below and refer to the figures on page 2.

Please circle your response

1. Has your doctor ever told you that you have a heart condition or have you ever suffered a stroke?	YES	(NO)
2. Do you ever experience unexplained pains in your chest at rest or during physical activity/exercise?	YES	(NO)
3. Do you ever feel faint or have spells of dizziness during physical activity/exercise that causes you to lose balance?	YES	(NO)
4. Have you had an asthma attack requiring immediate medical attention at any time over the last 12 months?	YES	(NO)
5. If you have diabetes (type 1 or 2) have you had trouble controlling your blood glucose in the last 3 months?	YES	(NO)
6. Do you have any other medical or physical condition(s) that may make it dangerous for you to participate in physical activity/exercise?	YES	(NO)

IF YOU ANSWERED 'YES' to any of the 6 questions, please seek guidance from an appropriate allied health professional or GP prior to undertaking physical activity/exercise.

IF YOU ANSWERED 'NO' to all of the 6 questions, and you have no other concerns about your health, please proceed to question 7.

7. Describe your current physical activity/exercise levels (e.g. in a typical week) by stating the frequency and duration at the different intensities. The User Guide provides intensity guidelines.

Intensity	Light	Moderate	Vigorous
Frequency (number of sessions per week)	2		
Duration (total minutes per week)	60		

Weighted Physical Activity per week

Total minutes = (light + moderate) + (2 x vigorous)

TOTAL = _____ min/wk

If your total weighted physical activity is less than 150 min per week then light-moderate intensity exercise is recommended.

If your total weighted physical activity is 150 min or more per week then continue with your current exercise intensity levels.

It is advised that you discuss your progression with an exercise professional to optimise your results.

I believe that to the best of my knowledge, all of the information I have supplied within this screening form is correct.

Client signature: _____   Date: _____

ADULT PRE-EXERCISE
SCREENING SYSTEM (APSS) V2 (2018)

Fitness Australia   SPORTS MEDICINE AUSTRALIA   ESSA

1

Figure 6.5 Case study 3: APSS

continued

Case studies *(continued)*

STAGE 2 (RECOMMENDED)

AIM: To identify those individuals with risk factors or other conditions that may result in them being at a higher risk of an adverse event. This stage aims to assist the exercise professional to determine appropriate exercise prescription.

CLIENT DETAILS	GUIDELINES FOR ASSESSING RISK
8. Demographics Age: _36_ Male ☐ Female ☒ Other ☐	Risk of an adverse event increases with age, particularly males ≥ 45 yr and females ≥ 55 yr.
9. Family history of heart disease (e.g. stroke, heart attack) Father _52_ (Age) Mother ____ (Age) Brother ____ Sister ____ Son ____ Daughter ____	Risk of heart disease is greater if a first degree relative has suffered a heart attack, stroke or undergone heart surgery and was < 55 yr (males) or < 65 yr (females) when it happened.
10. Do you smoke cigarettes on a daily or weekly basis or have you quit smoking in the last 6 months? Yes ☐ No ☒ If currently smoking, how many per day or week? ____	Smoking, even on a weekly basis, substantially increases risk for premature death and disability. The residual negative effects are still present up to at least 6 months post quitting.
11. Body composition Height (cm) _156_ Weight (kg) _78_ Waist circumference (cm) _92_	BMI ≥ 30 kg/m² Waist > 94 cm male or > 80 cm female increases the risk of chronic diseases.
12. Have you been told that you have high blood pressure? Yes ☒ No ☐ (If known) Systolic/Diastolic (mmHg) _140/90_	Systolic blood pressure ≥ 140 mmHg or diastolic blood pressure ≥ 90 mmHg increases the risk of cardiovascular disease.

ADULT PRE-EXERCISE
SCREENING SYSTEM (APSS) V2 (2018)

3

Figure 6.5, cont'd

continued overpage

Case studies *(continued)*

CLIENT DETAILS	GUIDELINES FOR ASSESSING RISK
13. Have you been told that you have high cholesterol? Yes ☐ No ☒ (If known) Total cholesterol (mmol/L) ____ HDL (mmol/L) ____ LDL (mmol/L) ____ Triglycerides (mmol/L) ____	Any of the below, increases the risk of heart conditions: Total cholesterol ≥ 5.2 mmol/L HDL < 1.0 mmol/L LDL ≥ 3.4 mmol/L Triglycerides ≥ 1.7 mmol/L
14. Have you been told that you have high blood sugar? Yes ☐ No ☒ (If known) Glucose (mmol/L) _____	Fasting blood glucose ≥ 5.5 mmol/L increases the risk of diabetes.
15. Have you spent time in hospital (including day admission) for any medical condition/illness/injury during the last 12 months? Yes ☐ No ☒ If yes provide details _____	There are positive relationships between illness rates and death versus the number and length of hospital admissions in the previous 12 months. This includes heart disease, lung disease (e.g., COPD and asthma), dementia, hip fractures, infectious episodes and inflammatory bowel disease. Admissions are also correlated to 'poor health' status and negative health behaviours such as smoking, alcohol consumption and nutritional patterns.
16. Are you currently taking prescribed medication(s) for any medical condition(s)? Yes ☒ No ☐ If yes, what is the medical condition? _*High blood*_____	Taking medication indicates a medically diagnosed problem. Judgment is required because it is common for clients to list 'medications' that include contraceptive pills, vitamin supplements and other non-pharmaceutical tablets. Fitness professionals are not expected to have an exhaustive understanding of medications. However, it may be important to use common language to describe what medical conditions the drugs are prescribed for.
17. Are you pregnant or have you given birth within the last 12 months? Yes ☐ No ☒ If yes provide details	During pregnancy and after recent childbirth are times to be more cautious with exercise. Appropriate exercise prescription results in improved health to mother and baby. However, joints gradually loosen to prepare for birth and may lead to an increased risk of injury especially in the pelvic joints. Activities involving jumping, frequent changes of direction and excessive stretching should be avoided, as should jerky ballistic movements.
18. Do you have any diagnosed muscle, bone or joint problems that you have been told could be made worse by participating in physical activity/exercise? Yes ☐ No ☒ If yes provide details _____	Almost everyone has experienced some level of soreness following unaccustomed exercise or activity but this is not really what this question is designed to identify. Soreness due to unaccustomed activity is not the same as pain in the joint, muscle or bone. Pain is more extreme and may represent an injury, serious inflammatory episode or infection. If the response is an acute problem then it is possible further medical guidance may be required.

ADULT PRE-EXERCISE
SCREENING SYSTEM (APSS) V2 (2019)

4

Figure 6.5, cont'd

References

[1] Exercise and Sport Science Australia. Adult Pre-exercise Screening System (APSS). Ascot, Qld: ESSA; 2019. https://www.essa.org.au/Public/ABOUT_ESSA/Adult_Pre-Screening_Tool.aspx.

[2] American College of Sports Medicine. ACSM's guidelines for exercise testing and prescription, 10th ed. Baltimore, MD: Lippincott, Williams and Wilkins; 2018.

[3] Riebe D, Franklin BA, Thompson PD, Garber CE, Whitfield GP, Magal M, et al. Updating ACSM's recommendations for exercise preparticipation health screening. Med Sci Sports Exerc 2015;47:2473–9.

[4] Exercise and Sport Science Australia. Adult Pre-exercise Screening System (APSS) user guide. Ascot, Qld: ESSA; 2019. https://www.essa.org.au/Public/ABOUT_ESSA/Adult_Pre-Screening_Tool.aspx.

[5] Maiorana AJ, Williams AD, Askew CD, Levinger I, Coombes J, Vicenzino B, et al. Exercise professionals with advanced clinical training should be afforded greater responsibility in pre-participation exercise screening: a new collaborative model between exercise professionals and physicians. Sports Med 2018;48:1293–1302.

[6] Whitfield GP, Pettee Gabriel KK, Rahbar MH, Kohl HW 3rd. Application of the American Heart Association/American College of Sports Medicine Adult Preparticipation Screening Checklist to a nationally representative sample of US adults aged ≥40 years from the National Health and Nutrition Examination Survey 2001 to 2004. Circulation 2014;129:1113–20.

[7] Bradley A. Fresh warnings over 'fit to exercise'. Australian Doctor 2012;23rd April.

[8] Whitfield GP, Riebe D, Magal M, Liguori G. Applying the ACSM preparticipation screening Algorithm to U.S. adults: National Health and Nutrition Examination Survey 2001–2004. Med Sci Sports Exerc 2017;49:2056–63.

[9] Norton K, Norton L, Sadgrove D. Position statement on physical activity and exercise intensity terminology. J Sci Med Sport 2010;13:496–502.

PRACTICAL 7
NEUROMUSCULAR STRENGTH, POWER AND STRENGTH ENDURANCE

Tina Skinner, Robert U Newton and G Greogory Haff

LEARNING OBJECTIVES

- Identify and explain the common terminology, processes and equipment required to conduct accurate and safe measures of neuromuscular strength, power and strength endurance
- Identify and describe the limitations, contraindications or considerations that may require the modification of neuromuscular strength, power and strength endurance assessments, and make appropriate adjustments for relevant populations or participants
- Explain the scientific rationale, purposes, reliability, validity, assumptions and limitations of common neuromuscular strength, power and strength endurance assessments
- Recognise and adjust incorrectly calibrated equipment used in neuromuscular strength, power and strength endurance assessment
- Conduct appropriate pre-assessment procedures, including explaining the test and obtaining informed consent and a focused medical history, and performing a pre-exercise risk assessment
- Identify the need for guidance or further information from an appropriate health professional, and recognise when to cease a test
- Select and conduct appropriate protocols for safe and effective neuromuscular strength, power and strength endurance assessments, including instructing clients on the correct use of equipment
- Record, analyse and interpret information from neuromuscular strength, power and strength endurance assessments and convey the results, including the validity and limitations of the assessments, through relevant verbal and/or written communication with the participant or involved professional

Equipment and other requirements

- Information sheet and informed consent form
- Adult Pre-exercise Screening System (APSS) form
- Rating of perceived exertion (RPE) chart (see Appendix E)
- Grip dynamometer (spring-resistance or hydraulic)
- Uniaxial or triaxial force plate (or similar force measurement system)
- Segmometer (or anthropometric tape)
- Power rack
- Smith machine

170

- Isokinetic dynamometer
- Bench press bench and rack
- Seated row machine
- Leg press machine
- Olympic barbell and weight plates
- Thin floor mat
- Linear potentiometer
- Vertec or yardstick
- Body mass scales
- Long jump mat
- Jump mat
- Masking tape
- Chalk
- 5 cm tall marking cone
- Metronome
- Stopwatch
- Calculator
- Cleaning and disinfecting equipment (see Appendix A)

INTRODUCTION

The relative importance of neuromuscular strength, power and strength endurance in health, sport and exercise varies widely. From a health perspective, neuromuscular strength, power and strength endurance measurements may be useful as part of an evaluation of older adults or various clinical populations to determine risk of accelerated decline in function, loss of independence, reduced ability to perform tasks of daily living and cognitive decline.[1] In addition, such measures are useful for assessing the impact of disease, side effects of treatment and monitoring progress of rehabilitation.

Maximal strength and the ability to increase force output rapidly, and maintain force during rapid movements, are the main determinants of performance in activities requiring one movement sequence with the goal of producing a high velocity at release or impact. Neuromuscular actions, which maximise force magnitude and rate of production, are required in throwing, jumping, sprinting and striking activities. In addition, sudden bursts of power are required when rapidly changing direction or accelerating during various sports or athletic events (e.g. football, basketball, rugby, baseball and gymnastics). For events lasting more than a few seconds the ability to maintain force output becomes more important and this is termed 'strength endurance'. However, maximal strength remains a major component underlying endurance and so assessment of strength, power and strength endurance from single rapid movements to multiple repetitions over time is important to assess the performance spectrum.[2]

As the majority of sporting movements such as sprinting, change of direction, acceleration and jumping require the rapid application of force over a short period of time, force measurements other than maximal strength are required to assess the participant's neuromuscular abilities.

Rate of force development

Maximal rate of force development is calculated as the steepest slope of the force–time curve and can be determined over various time periods, 20 milliseconds (ms) being commonly used. The average rate of force development is calculated from the initiation of the effort to the peak in force. The units of measurement are newtons per second (N/s). This parameter has been demonstrated to correlate well with vertical jump and sprinting performance.[3,4]

Impulse

Impulse is the product of force by time and is the area under the force–time curve over a given time period. Impulse determines the change in velocity or acceleration and so is mechanically the most significant single parameter determining very rapid movements such as sprinting or jumping. Impulse can be measured over various time periods, depending on which athletic movement is to be characterised by the test. For example, foot contact during sprinting is approximately 80 ms, while the time from initiation of a vertical jump to ground take-off is approximately 200 ms. The units of measurement are newtons $\times$ seconds (N·s). Impulse, particularly in the horizontal direction, is associated with sprint acceleration performance in team sport athletes.[5,6]

Similar methods can be used for most major movements specific to sport and tasks of daily living. For example, isolating a bench on the force plate and pressing up against an immovable bar provides a test of isometric bench press. The squat movement can also be performed on a force plate with an immovable bar positioned across the shoulders.

DEFINITIONS

Impulse: product of force by time and the determinant of change in velocity.

Maximum rate of force development (see below): maximum rate of force development during a single effort.

Neuromuscular power: the product of force and velocity of movement, or the rate of doing work.

Neuromuscular strength: the ability of a neuromuscular system to exert force.

Rate of force development (RFD): the ability of a neuromuscular system to rapidly increase force from an initial low level of activation.

Reactive strength index: the ratio of flight time to ground contact time. Typically assessed during drop jumps movements.

Repetition maximum (RM): the maximal weight that can be lifted for a prescribed number of repetitions. For example, a 1RM would be the heaviest weight that can be lifted one time, while a 10RM would be the heaviest weight that can be lifted 10 times.

Strength endurance: the ability of a neuromuscular system to repeatedly exert force against resistance. Strength endurance is typically assessed by tests requiring more than 12 repetitions, or the maximum number of repetitions one can execute without rest over an extended duration or until volitional fatigue.

TYPES OF STRENGTH TESTS

The four types of tests described in this practical are isometric, isokinetic, isoinertial and ballistic.

1 **Isometric tests:** isometric strength is generally measured using dynamometers or force transducers. Dynamometers that are commonly used include those for grip, chest, upper back, lower back and legs. Force plates are particularly useful for measuring isometric strength, can be applied in a wide range of body positions and are readily available in university exercise and sports science departments, institutes and academies of sport. Power cannot be measured using isometric dynamometers as displacement and, therefore, velocity is close to zero. However, many important measures of the ability to rapidly generate force such as maximum rate of force development and impulse over short time periods can be measured accurately during isometric tests. Cable tensiometers can also be used to assess isometric strength for most muscle groups, or grip strength can be combined with other isometric strength tests (e.g. chest, back or leg) to give a total strength score. Muscular endurance can also be measured during isometric tests as the ability to maintain force over a given period of time. The results of isometric tests are specific to the joint angle at which they are conducted, which limits the applicability of these measures to other joints or joint angles.

2 **Isokinetic tests:** measurement of isokinetic strength requires expensive equipment which is generally found in exercise and sports science laboratories or well-equipped rehabilitation practices. In addition to determining the force and power output of a muscle group, isokinetic testing may provide insight into muscle asymmetry (right vs left), or ipsilateral imbalance between agonist (e.g. quadriceps) and antagonist (e.g. hamstrings) strength. Isokinetic strength is measured at a constant velocity and can be concentric (shortening) or eccentric (lengthening), depending on the testing machine being used. Power (watts) can be measured by multiplying peak torque (N·m) (strength) by velocity in radians per second (rad/s). Strength endurance can be measured using a fatigue protocol consisting of multiple repetitions.

3 **Isoinertial tests:** isoinertial testing was formerly known as isotonic testing, implying that the tonicity/tension in the muscle remained constant. However, as an anatomical advantage exists during certain positions within the range of motion, the resistance and therefore the tonicity/tension changes. Isoinertial is a more accurate term as neuromuscular strength is exerted against the resistance of a known inertia (mass) which is being acted upon by the earth's gravity. The most common methods of measuring neuromuscular strength, power and strength endurance are isoinertial tests because the equipment is readily available and the resistance is highly specific as we all have to perform in an environment of the earth's gravity. Strength is usually measured as the maximum weight that can be lifted between 1 and 10 times – that is, 1–10 repetition maximum (1–10RM) tests completed with fixed resistance (e.g. dumbbells or barbells) or variable resistance (e.g. weightlifting) devices. The 1RM test is the most indicative of maximal strength, with reductions in the predictive ability of the test with increases in repetitions (e.g. 3RM or 6RM). There is a perception among clinicians, coaches and scientists that multiple repetition strength testing is less risky than 1RM testing, however, this has not been adequately investigated. Measures of the ability to rapidly exert force such as impulse, maximum rate of force development (RFD), velocity and power can also be measured during isoinertial tests if instrumentation is available to measure force and displacement during the movement. Isoinertial tests can measure neuromuscular strength endurance using various fatigue protocols involving multiple repetitions.

4 **Ballistic tests:** isoinertial tests are not entirely valid for measuring the ability to exert high force rapidly because the load must be decelerated to stop at the end of the ROM. Ballistic movements are preferred for the assessment of these neuromuscular qualities because jumping, throwing or kicking allows the movement to be accelerated up to the point of release or take-off. Examples of ballistic movements include vertical and horizontal (broad) jumping, bench throws, medicine ball throws and ballistic knee extension. Instrumentation is now readily available for the measurement of force output and velocity of movement during ballistic movements providing a plethora of outcome variables, which validly characterise the participant's ability to generate high force rapidly.

NEUROMUSCULAR STRENGTH

Activity 7.1 Grip strength

AIMS: measure the strength of the forearm and finger flexors, interpret the results and provide feedback to a participant.

Background

There are numerous daily activities in which some degree of hand-grip strength is necessary for a successful outcome. Grip strength can be used when a quick and easy estimate of overall body strength is desired. Grip strength has excellent test–retest reliability, with an intra-class correlation of 0.92 for the dominant hand and 0.97 for the non-dominant hand (see Practical 1, Test accuracy, reliability and validity).[7] Grip strength has been shown to correlate with overall body strength,[8] and predict accelerated dependency in activities of daily living (ADLs), cognitive decline in older adults[1] and survival in advanced cancer patients.[9] However, measurement of grip strength lacks specificity to many sporting activities or ADLs as it is an isometric test of the small muscle group of the forearm and finger flexors. In addition, grip strength is typically measured at one specific joint angle so extrapolation to other angles is limited owing to the joint angle/length–tension relationship (Figure 7.1). In saying that, the grip strength test is an extremely useful measure in clinical practice for the assessment of disease and/or rehabilitation progression and, at a national population level, is even able to predict Summer Olympic Games medal success.[10]

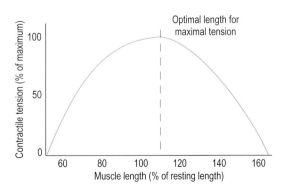

Figure 7.1 Length–tension relationship

Source: Robert Newton, Edith Cowan University, Health and Wellness Institute

Protocol summary

With the upper arm by the side of the body and elbow flexed at 90°, the participant grips the dynamometer and squeezes the handle as hard as possible.

Protocol

1 Follow the pre-exercise test procedures outlined in Appendix B and general methods for neuromuscular strength, power and strength endurance tests described in Table 7.1.[11]

2 Check Appendix C to ensure that there are no contraindications to exercise testing.

3 Demonstrate the test to ensure correct form.

4 For this test you may use either the spring-resistance or the hydraulic dynamometer.

5 Adjust the grip size on the dynamometer (by turning the handle on the spring-resistance device or adjusting the notches on the hydraulic device) so that the hand is comfortable (not too cramped or too stretched) when in the starting position (Figure 7.2).

6 Ask the participant to assume a standing position with the testing upper arm by the side of the body and the elbow flexed at 90°.

7 Check the dial starts on 0 kg, and that the participant is holding the dynamometer with the dial facing outwards.

8 Instruct the participant to squeeze the handle as hard as possible (Figure 7.3).

9 Testers should closely observe to ensure the participant does not use accessory movements to perform the maximal

TABLE 7.1 Recommendations for standardised conditions for neuromuscular strength and strength endurance tests	
GUIDELINE	**RATIONALE**
1 Maintain proper technique	Ensures that the exercise is performed correctly and in a safe fashion.
2 Consistent repetition duration or movement speed	Allows for easier interpretation of the results.
3 Full ROM	Allows for the results of the test to be more easily interpreted and maximises the safety of the exercise.
4 Use of spotters	Used to maximise safety, especially for exercises such as the bench press or back squat.
5 Equipment familiarisation	Maximises the reliability of the assessment.
6 Proper warm-up	Maximises the performance capacity while minimising the potential risks that may be inherent in the testing process.

Adapted from: Whaley et al[11]

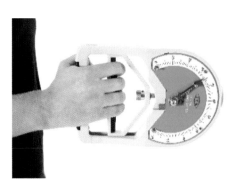

Figure 7.2 Comfortable grip distance on spring-resistance dynamometer

Used with permission from TTM

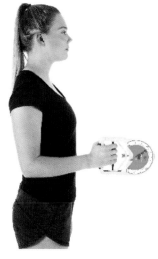

Figure 7.3 Grip strength

Used with permission from TTM

contractions. The hand should stay in a neutral position and should not deviate into supination or pronation. The elbow should remain at 90° and should not leave the side of the body. If the hand rotates, or the elbow deviates from 90° or leaves contact with the body, the test will not be valid and needs to be repeated.

10 Provide encouragement to ensure a maximal result.

11 The participant performs three maximal contractions with each hand, having ≥ 10 seconds rest between trials.

12 Record results and obtain ratings from Tables 7.2 and 7.3 as appropriate. As these tables do not provide a dominant/non-dominant distinction, obtain the rating for the dominant hand from the right-hand data and the non-dominant from the left.

13 Clean and disinfect all equipment (see Appendix A).

Data recording

Participant's name: _____   Date: _____

Age: _____ years   Sex: _____   Dominant hand (circle): Right / Left

DOMINANT HAND:		NON-DOMINANT HAND:	
1.	kg	1.	kg
2.	kg	2.	kg
3.	kg	3.	kg
Best:	kg	Best:	kg
Rating:		Rating:	

Interpretation

First, consider the four steps of interpretation outlined in Appendix G, and refer to Table 7.2 (female) or Table 7.3 (male) as appropriate.[12]

Activity 7.2 Isometric mid-thigh pull

AIMS: measure the strength of the leg and back extensors, interpret the results and provide feedback to a participant.

Background

One of the greatest advantages of the isometric mid-thigh pull test is that it requires little familiarisation and can be implemented across a wide range of populations from children to older adults and across various sports and patient populations. It is used when a quick and easy estimate of overall body strength is desired; however, it requires access to a force plate or other force transducer. A force plate is a relatively common device in biomechanics laboratories and increasingly in performance laboratories and strength facilities throughout the world. Triaxial force plates are designed to measure forces in the three spatial planes and can be used for isometric strength testing; however, uniaxial (single-plane force measurement) force plates are becoming common as they are less expensive and designed

TABLE 7.2 Female isometric grip strength reference data

FEMALES	AGE (YEARS)					
	20–29	30–39	40–49	50–59	60–69	70+
Right hand (kg)						
Very poor	<23.9	<25.5	<24.3	<22.8	<19.5	<15.1
Poor	23.9–28.1	25.5–29.8	24.3–27.9	22.8–26.2	19.5–22.8	15.1–18.6
Average	28.2–31.6	29.9–32.6	28.0–30.7	26.3–29.5	22.9–25.4	18.7–21.3
Good	31.7–35.9	32.7–36.5	30.8–34.0	29.6–33.3	25.5–28.4	21.4–24.9
Excellent	>35.9	>36.5	>34.0	>33.3	>28.4	>24.9
Left hand (kg)						
Very poor	<22.9	<24.0	<23.0	<20.7	<18.7	<14.3
Poor	22.9–26.5	24.0–27.5	23.0–26.7	20.7–24.1	18.7–21.7	14.3–17.7
Average	26.6–29.6	27.6–30.5	26.8–29.3	24.2–27.1	21.8–24.3	17.8–20.4
Good	29.7–33.8	30.6–33.7	29.4–33.2	27.2–30.9	24.4–27.3	20.5–23.4
Excellent	>33.8	>33.7	>33.2	>30.9	>27.3	>23.4

Based on data from 1312 Australian women. Very poor ≤20th percentile; poor = 21st–40th percentile; average = 41st–60th percentile; good = 61st–80th percentile; excellent ≥81st percentile
Adapted from: Massy-Westropp et al[12]

TABLE 7.3 Male isometric grip strength reference data

MALES	AGE (YEARS)					
	20–29	30–39	40–49	50–59	60–69	70+
Right hand (kg)						
Very poor	<38.6	<39.1	<38.4	<38.4	<32.9	<25.9
Poor	38.6–44.3	39.1–44.7	38.4–44.1	38.4–42.9	32.9–37.7	25.9–30.6
Average	44.4–49.1	44.8–49.7	44.2–49.2	43.0–47.0	37.8–42.0	30.7–34.9
Good	49.2–54.7	49.8–55.4	49.3–54.7	47.1–51.9	42.1–47.5	35.0–39.5
Excellent	>54.7	>55.4	>54.7	>51.9	>47.5	>39.5
Left hand (kg)						
Very poor	<37.8	<38.3	<36.9	<36.1	<31.3	<25.7
Poor	37.8–42.7	38.3–44.1	36.9–42.2	36.1–40.8	31.3–36.1	25.7–30.1
Average	42.8–46.9	44.2–49.2	42.3–47.0	40.9–44.9	36.2–39.8	30.2–33.9
Good	47.0–52.2	49.3–54.9	47.1–52.1	45.0–49.3	39.9–45.0	34.0–38.1
Excellent	>52.2	>54.9	>52.1	>49.3	>45.0	>38.1

Based on data from 1366 Australian men. Very poor ≤20th percentile; poor = 20th –40th percentile; average = 41st–60th percentile; good = 61st–80th percentile; excellent ≥81st percentile
Adapted from: Massy-Westropp et al[12]

specifically for measurement of strength and power performance. Alternatively, a force measurement system can be constructed using 'off the shelf' load cells which can be attached to fix a barbell in place and provide a measure of force applied. However, it should be noted that this provides an assessment of force exerted on the barbell rather than at the feet as measured by a force plate.

During the test, force is measured and recorded continuously resulting in a rich data set characterising the participant's ability to generate force. The peak or highest force output obtained is the most commonly recorded parameter and is indicative of maximal strength. This is strongly correlated with overall body strength and with other dynamic strength tests such as the back squat and the power clean.[13]

The following procedures are described for the Fitness Technology 400S force plate and Ballistic Measurement System (BMS) software (Figure 7.4). The protocol is very similar when using other force-measuring systems.

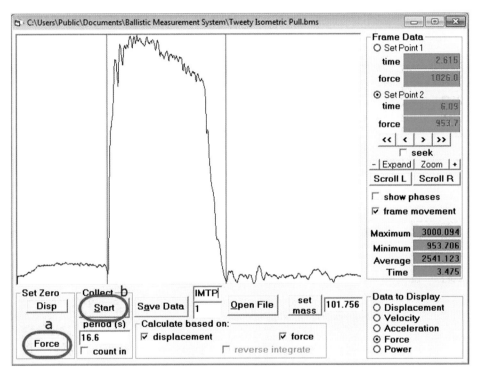

Figure 7.4 Data collection window for Ballistic Measurement System (BMS) software. Buttons to (a) zero the force and (b) start data collection are indicated

Used with permission from BMS

Protocol summary

With the power rack or Smith machine positioned over the force plate, the participant's feet centred on the plate and the participant holding the bar in the mid-thigh pull position, the participant pulls upwards on the bar as hard and fast as possible and tries to exert maximum force until the peak is reached and force starts to decline as fatigue develops.

Protocol

1 Follow the pre-test requirements described in Appendix B and general methods for neuromuscular strength, power and strength endurance tests described in Table 7.1.

2 Measure and record the participant's body mass (as described in Practical 4, Physique assessment).

3 The participant completes a 5-minute general warm-up which may include light jogging, cycling, jumping, rope, etc.

4 For this test, you may use either a uniaxial or a triaxial force plate. If a force plate is not available, load cells placed in series with straps securing the barbell to the floor can be used as an alternative.

5 The power rack or Smith machine should be positioned over the force plate such that the participant's feet will be centred on the plate when they are holding the bar in the mid-thigh pull position.

6 Measure the mid-point of the linear distance between the inguinal point (the point at the intersection of the crease at the angle of the trunk and the anterior thigh and the midline of the anterior thigh) and the patellare (the mid-point of the posterior superior border of the patella) with a segmometer (or anthropometric tape measure). Mark a line (e.g. with tape if wearing pants) across the anterior thigh at the halfway point with a pen.

7 Ensure that neither the participant nor any other object is in contact with the force plate and click the 'Set Zero – Force' button (see Figure 7.4) to set the zero offset.

8 Place the participant in the mid-thigh pull position and adjust the bar height so that it is at this halfway position (Figure 7.5).

9 Demonstrate the test to ensure correct form.

10 Instruct the participant to step onto the plate and assume the mid-thigh pull position. Check that they have the correct body position, with feet shoulder distance apart, knees 5°–10° flexion, back straight, hands in top grip, shoulders set and looking straight ahead.

11 Instruct the participant that '*I will say 3, 2, 1, GO, then pull upwards on the bar as hard and fast as possible and hold the maximum force until instructed to relax. Are you ready?*' If the participant acknowledges they are ready, begin data collection by clicking the 'Collection – Start' button (see Figure 7.4) before instructing the participant to begin by calling out clearly '*3, 2, 1, GO*'.

12 Provide encouragement to ensure a maximal result.

13 Once the force output has passed the peak and begins to decline (Figure 7.6), instruct the participant to relax.

14 The participant performs three maximal contractions providing ≥60 seconds rest between trials.

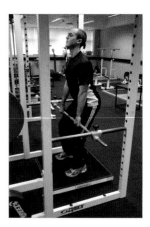

Figure 7.5 Equipment set-up and body position for isometric mid-thigh pull

Source: Robert Newton, Edith Cowan University, Health and Wellness Institute

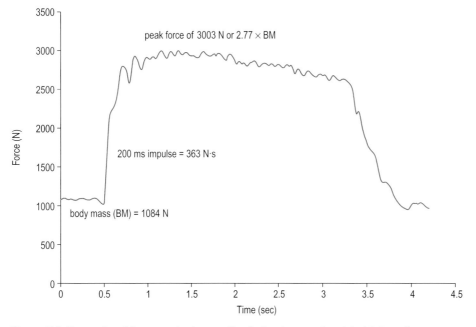

Figure 7.6 Example of force–velocity profile during isometric mid-thigh pull

Source: Robert Newton, Edith Cowan University, Health and Wellness Institute

15 Record results for: peak force including relative to body mass, time to peak, average rate of force development and 200 ms impulse. Compare peak force and rate of force development results with Table 7.4.[13-17]

16 Clean and disinfect all equipment (see Appendix A).

Data recording

Participant's name: _____ Date: _____

Age: _____ years   Sex: _____   Body mass: _____ kg

PEAK FORCE			TIME TO PEAK FORCE		AVERAGE RATE OF FORCE DEVELOPMENT		200 MS IMPULSE	
1	N	N/kg BM	1	s	1	N/s	1	N/s
2	N	N/kg BM	2	s	2	N/s	2	N/s
3	N	N/kg BM	3	s	3	N/s	3	N/s
Best:	N	N/kg BM	Best:	s	Best:	N/s	Best:	N/s

Interpretation

First, consider the four steps of interpretation outlined in Appendix G, and refer to Table 7.4.

TABLE 7.4 Isometric mid-thigh pull strength reference data				
REFERENCE	PARTICIPANTS	BODY MASS (kg)	PEAK FORCE (N)	RATE OF FORCE DEVELOPMENT (N/s)
McGuigan et al[13]	Male recreational athletes ($n = 26$)	90 ± 10	1217 ± 183	5729 ± 2383
Stone et al[14]	Male and female weightlifters ($n = 7$)	98 ± 31	5102 ± 1536	$16,999 \pm 5878$
McGuigan et al[15]	Male American footballers ($n = 22$)	108 ± 23	2159 ± 218	$13,489 \pm 4041$
Nuzzo et al[16]	Males from various sports ($n = 12$)	90 ± 15	3144 ± 792	3555 ± 1026^a

[a] Average rate of force development from time of initiation to peak force
Adapted from: Wrigley and Strauss[17]

Activity 7.3 Isokinetic testing

AIMS: measure isokinetic strength of the knee flexor and extensor muscle groups, interpret the results and provide feedback to a participant.

Background

Isokinetic devices can be used to provide highly accurate measures of specific muscle group strength and identify potential muscle asymmetry. Some dynamometers can be arranged to test various joints and muscle groups (e.g. the knee and shoulder) as well as multi-joint movements such as the chest press or leg press.

Strength capacity is generally measured as the torque (twisting force) at the joint axis produced by the muscles which act about that joint. Although measurement of torque production around the joint is very accurate, isokinetic strength measures are sometimes considered to lack applicability and generalisability to movements replicating activities on the sporting field which are considered to be multiarticular and multidirectional in nature. Isokinetic strength is measured at a constant velocity, which also lacks applicability in sporting contexts where joints move at varying speeds. In addition, the limited range of motion and determination of strength in one plane of movement makes isokinetic strength testing and training more commonly used in injury rehabilitation or risk identification than in sport-specific settings.

There is moderate evidence that muscle asymmetry may place an individual at increased risk of injuries of the muscles acting across the joint (e.g. hamstring strains),[18,19] although further research is required to definitively confirm this. Some studies have demonstrated isokinetic strength measurements can predict musculoskeletal health and athletic performance. For example, deficits in isokinetic shoulder muscle performance were greater in rotator cuff muscles with larger tears and greater degrees of degeneration, and were related to postoperative risk of cuff detachment.[20] Furthermore, knee extension average power was found to positively and significantly affect ball placement in young, competitive tennis players.[21]

Protocol summary

Once the dynamometer is specifically set up for body size and shape, the participant is safely secured on the dynamometer before flexing and extending their lower leg as hard and as fast as possible.

Protocol

Isokinetic strength, power and strength endurance test (knee extension/flexion)

1 Follow the pre-exercise test procedures outlined in Appendix B and general methods for neuromuscular strength, power and strength endurance tests described in Table 7.1.

2 Check Appendix C to ensure there are no contraindications to exercise testing.

3 Measure and record the participant's body mass (see Practical 4, Physique assessment).

4 The participant completes a 5-minute general warm-up which may include light jogging, cycling, jumping rope, etc.

5 While the participant is warming up, turn the isokinetic dynamometer on and follow the onscreen instructions (specific to the dynamometer model) to enter the application and set up the dynamometer.

6 Confirm the participant's details and enter these into the dynamometer application. Ensure that body mass is also correctly entered.

7 Select the appropriate testing protocol, depending on whether muscular strength, strength endurance or both are to be tested.

8 Once the participant has completed the warm-up, position them on the isokinetic dynamometer in an upright position with their hips flexed at 90° and lower legs hanging freely.

9 Follow the onscreen prompts to set up the dynamometer specifically for the participant's body size and shape and finalise the dynamometer positioning ready for the test to begin.

10 Instruct the participant to complete the three practice trial repetitions by flexing and extending their leg. The participant's arms should be positioned across their chest so that it is an 'uninvolved' test.

11 Prior to the performance trial, instruct the participant to flex and extend their lower leg as hard and as fast as possible. Instruct the participant on how many repetitions to perform (i.e. 5 repetitions for muscular strength testing, or 30 repetitions for strength endurance testing). Emphasise that this should be a maximal effort. '*I will say 3, 2, 1, GO, then kick your leg up and pull back as hard and as fast as possible 3 times. Are you ready?*' If the participant acknowledges they are ready call out clearly '*3, 2, 1, GO*' and the test will begin.

12 Provide encouragement during the trial, giving feedback on how many repetitions remain.

13 If performing multiple trials, provide the participant with $\geq$60 seconds rest between trials.

14 For this activity, repeat the tests at both 60° per second and 180° per second to enable evaluation of isokinetic strength at two velocities of movement.

15 Repeat the test on the opposite leg for contralateral comparisons.

16 At the end of the test, warn the participant that their legs may feel weak or wobbly when they get off the seat. Unstrap the participant, ensuring that you are positioned appropriately to support the participant in case of a fall. Direct them to a cycle ergometer to perform an adequate cool-down, followed by appropriate stretches.

17 Follow onscreen prompts to save test data and, if possible, print the report.

18 Record the test results below.

19 Shut down the isokinetic dynamometer.

20 Clean and disinfect all equipment (see Appendix A).

Data recording

Participant's name: _____   Date: _____

Age: _____ years   Sex: _____   Body mass: _____ kg

Dominant leg (circle): R / L

Dominant leg

Peak knee extension torque at 60°/s _____ N·m _____ per kg BM

    Angle at peak torque _____ °

Peak knee flexion torque at 60°/s _____ N·m _____ per kg BM

    Angle at peak torque _____ °

Peak knee extension torque at 180°/s _____ N·m _____ per kg BM

    Angle at peak torque _____ °

Peak knee flexion torque at 180°/s _____ N·m _____ per kg BM

    Angle at peak torque _____ °

Work done (best work repetition) during extension at 180°/s _____ J

Work done (best work repetition) during flexion at 180°/s _____ J

Flexion: extension ratio at 60°/s _____

Average ROM at 60°/s _____

Average ROM at 180°/s _____ °

Dominant leg maximum power at 60°

Power (watts) = torque (N·m) $\times$ angular velocity (rad/s)

Angular velocity at 60° = 1.047 rad/s

Maximum extension power = maximum extension torque at 60° $\times$ 1.047 = _____ W

Maximum flexion power = maximum flexion torque at 60° $\times$ 1.047 = _____ W

Maximum extension power = maximum extension torque at 180° $\times$ 1.047 = _____ W

Maximum flexion power = maximum flexion torque at 180° $\times$ 1.047 = _____ W

continued overpage

Data recording *(continued)*

Non-dominant leg

Peak knee extension torque at $60°/s$ _____ $N \cdot m$ _____ per kg BM

Angle at peak torque _____ $°$

Peak knee flexion torque at $60°/s$ _____ $N \cdot m$ _____ per kg BM

Angle at peak torque _____ $°$

Peak knee extension torque at $180°/s$ _____ $N \cdot m$ _____ per kg BM

Angle at peak torque _____ $°$

Peak knee flexion torque at $180°/s$ _____ $N \cdot m$ _____ per kg BM

Angle at peak torque _____ $°$

Work done (best work repetition) during extension at $180°/s$ _____ J

Work done (best work repetition) during flexion at $180°/s$ _____ J

Flexion: extension ratio at $60°/s$ _____

Average ROM at $60°/s$ _____ $°$

Average ROM at $180°/s$ _____ $°$

Non-dominant leg maximum power at $60°$

Power (watts) = torque $(N \cdot m) \times$ angular velocity (rad/s)

Angular velocity at $60° = 1.047$ rad/s

Maximum extension power = maximum extension torque at $60° \times 1.047 =$ _____ W

Maximum flexion power = maximum flexion torque at $60° \times 1.047 =$ _____ W

Maximum extension power = maximum extension torque at $180° \times 1.047 =$ _____ W

Maximum flexion power = maximum flexion torque at $180° \times 1.047 =$ _____ W

Contralateral comparison

Express the score for the weaker limb (i.e. non-dominant leg) as a percentage of the score for the stronger muscle group (i.e. dominant leg).

Deficit = (stronger limb score – weaker limb score / stronger limb score) $\times$ 100(%)

= _____ significant inter-limb deficit? (circle) Y / N

Ipsilateral comparison

Express the score as a ratio of flexor strength:extensor strength measured at $60°/s$ (e.g. hamstring strength:quadriceps strength)

H:Q ratio = maximum flexion strength / maximum extension strength

Right leg = _____

Left leg = _____

Interpretation

First, consider the four steps of interpretation outlined in Appendix G. There are several components of isokinetic dynamometry testing that should be considered when interpreting the results.

1 Contralateral comparison

A contralateral (right versus left) imbalance requires both limbs to be tested. When comparing between limbs, a significant contralateral deficit is defined as $\geq 10\%$.[15,22]

2 Ipsilateral comparison

a Agonist vs antagonist

Identification of an ipsilateral imbalance involves comparison between agonist and antagonist muscle groups around a joint (e.g. the hamstring:quadriceps (H:Q) ratio). Assuming they exist, confirmation of an 'optimal' functional H:Q ratio still awaits further evidence from controlled studies of injury incidence in people having undergone isokinetic testing prior to injury. There appears to be little consensus of a reference value for the H:Q ratio; however, a conventional value of 0.6 (0.5–0.8 depending on the velocity of the protocol) appears to have gained general acceptance.[23] Table 7.5[24–28] provides comparative isokinetic values for knee flexion and extension (H:Q ratio) at 180°/s.[29]

TABLE 7.5 Comparative isokinetic values for knee flexion and extension (hamstrings:quadriceps ratio) at 180°/s

REFERENCE	PARTICIPANTS	HAMSTRING:QUADRICEPS RATIO
Beam et al[24]	Athletic college men and women	0.70[a]
Gilliam et al[25]	High school footballers	0.79
Housh et al[26]	Track/field athletes	0.80
Housh et al[27]	College footballers	0.78
Wyatt and Edwards[28]	Non-athletic men	0.78
	Non-athletic women	0.79

[a] Hamstring:quadriceps ratio was not different between sexes
Adapted from: Adams[29]

b Peak torque angle

The angle at which peak torque is produced during isokinetic knee flexion may be related to risk of hamstring injury. In comparing uninjured versus previously injured, with regards to the optimal angle for knee flexion torque, Brockett et al[30] reported 30° and 40° respectively. The shorter optimum angle for peak torque of previously injured muscles makes them more prone than uninjured muscles to damage from eccentric exercise; this may account for a higher re-injury rate.

Activity 7.4 Repetition maximum (RM) testing

AIMS: assess neuromuscular strength by determining the maximum weight that can be lifted through: (a) a one repetition maximum (1RM) test for the bench press, and (b) a three repetition maximum (3RM) test for the leg press. Interpret the results and provide feedback to a participant.

Background

RM testing is used to identify the maximum weight that can be lifted for a particular exercise at a given number of repetitions with satisfactory technique. A 1RM is the maximum weight that can be lifted once. A 3RM test measures the maximum weight that can be lifted for three complete repetitions.

RM testing data can be used to monitor improvements in strength, to identify weaknesses in muscle groups or imbalances between muscle groups (e.g. bench press vs bench pull), for talent identification or to evaluate the effectiveness of a period of training. Known RM values for various exercises can be used to prescribe strength-training intensities and direct exercise prescription. Importantly, RM testing has been shown to be positively and significantly correlated with athletic performance. For example, a 1RM bench press was significantly correlated with throwing velocity in male handball players,[31,32] and in American collegiate football players it was able to predict speed and agility,[33] and discriminate between divisions of play and playing ability.[34] Even multiple RM testing has shown to be associated with performance, with a 3RM bench press found to be positively and significantly correlated with 200 m kayak sprint performance,[35] with the smallest important change achieved with a 1.4% ($\pm0.5\%$) change in bench press strength.

Several prediction equations are available to estimate 1RM from multiple RM testing (and vice versa); however, differences in training status[36] and neuromuscular and metabolic demands between low (i.e. 1–6RM) and high (i.e. $\geq$10RM) repetitions[37] may provide erroneous results.

RM testing can be performed using free weights (e.g. barbell), a Smith machine (increased stability) or plate-loaded weight machines in either a flat or an inclined position. Valid (concurrent) comparisons to reference data will depend on the type and leverage system of the equipment used. If specific to the purpose of testing, a tempo could also be set (e.g. with a metronome).

However, there are several limitations of RM testing, including:

- multiple repetition testing provides only an estimate of actual maximal strength
- often subjective methods are used to control the rate of movement and ROM
- it requires educated estimates of the weights to be lifted; this can be difficult with inexperienced testers.

Protocol summary

1RM bench press – the participant lowers the barbell once to lightly touch the chest and presses back to full extension. 3RM leg press – the participant lowers the plate, flexing to 90° of knee flexion before pressing back to full extension three times.

Protocol

1RM bench press protocol

1 Follow the pre-exercise test procedures outlined in Appendix B and general methods for neuromuscular strength, power and strength endurance tests described in Table 7.1.

2 Check Appendix C to ensure there are no contraindications to exercise testing.

3 Measure and record the participant's body mass (see Practical 4, Physique assessment).

4 The participant completes a 5-minute general warm-up which may include light jogging, cycling, jumping rope, etc.

5 Demonstrate the test to ensure correct form, including posture, technique and ideal ROM.

6 Ensure safety procedures are in place. Depending on the type and leverage system of the equipment being used, this may also require setting safety stops and applying collars.

7 Instruct the participant to lie supine with feet in a comfortable position on the bench (Figure 7.7a), so that the back maintains the neutral lumbar arch. Shoulders should be directly under the elbows.

8 Explain to the participant that the starting position is with arms at full extension, then lower them to touch the chest (Figure 7.7b) and press back to full extension. The repetition is successful only if the barbell is pressed back to full extension without assistance.

9 Assume a spotting technique that will enable you to assist the participant to safely return the bar to the rack (Figure 7.7a and b). Stand immediately behind the barbell, with knees and hips slightly

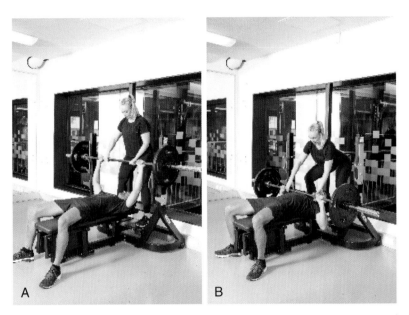

Figure 7.7 a: 1RM bench press initial positioning. b: 1RM bench press technique
Used with permission from Technogym

bent and back straight, so that your shoulders can be directly above the barbell when it is at the bottom of the movement. Assuming a wide split stance for stability, place your hands just inside (towards the middle of the bar) the participant's hands in a reverse grip (one overhand and one underhand). Follow the movement of the barbell by flexing/extending your knees (not changing your elbow angle). Avoid touching the participant or the barbell unless the participant is unable to complete the lift independently.

10 Have the participant warm up by completing 5–10 repetitions at 40%–60% of the estimated 1RM bench press.

11 Allow the participant to rest for 1 minute while you increase the load to 60%–80% of the estimated 1RM bench press.

12 Have the participant complete 3–5 repetitions at 60%–80% of the estimated 1RM bench press.

13 Increase the weight to a heavy but conservative estimate of the participant's 1RM bench press and allow a 1-minute rest before commencing the test.

14 Have the participant attempt one repetition of the selected weight. If the lift is successful, increase the weight conservatively for the next attempt. Observe facial expression and technique, and seek participant feedback to ascertain the next weight increase.

15 The participant should rest for 3 minutes before attempting the next weight increment.

16 Follow this procedure until the participant fails to complete the lift. The 1RM is the maximum weight lifted in the last successful trial.

17 The test is invalid if the barbell is bounced off the chest or fails to touch the chest, or if excessive leg/trunk movement is observed.

18 The 1RM should be achieved within 3–5 trials (not including the warm-ups), with the fewer the better to minimise the effect of fatigue.

19 Avoid, where possible, overestimating the 1RM and reducing the weight after a failed attempt.

20 Record results and compare with Table 7.6.

21 Clean and disinfect all equipment (see Appendix A).

3RM leg press protocol

1 Follow the pre-exercise test procedures outlined in Appendix B and general methods for neuromuscular strength, power and strength endurance tests described in Table 7.1.

TABLE 7.6 1RM bench press and relative strength ratio reference data

	FEMALES		MALES	
	1RM BENCH PRESS (kg)	RELATIVE STRENGTH RATIO	1RM BENCH PRESS (kg)	RELATIVE STRENGTH RATIO
Very poor	<30	<0.48	<70	<0.96
Poor	30–35	0.48–0.55	70–80	0.96–1.05
Average	36–38	0.56–0.62	81–95	1.06–1.17
Good	39–45	0.63–0.71	96–105	1.18–1.31
Excellent	>45	>0.71	>105	>1.31
Mean	37	0.60	88	1.12
Standard deviation	12	0.18	21	0.20
Minimum	10	0.20	45	0.59
Maximum	135	1.9	145	1.73

Based on data from 319 Australian exercise science students (females, $n = 149$) aged 18–30. Very poor ≤20th percentile; poor = 21st–40th percentile; average = 41st–60th percentile; good = 61st–80th percentile; excellent ≥81st percentile

2 Check Appendix C to ensure that there are no contraindications to exercise testing.

3 Measure and record the participant's body mass (see Practical 4, Physique assessment).

4 The participant completes a 5-minute general warm-up which may include light jogging, cycling, jumping rope, etc.

5 Demonstrate the test to ensure correct form, including posture, technique and ROM (90° knee flexion).

6 Ensure safety procedures are in place. Depending on the type and leverage system of the equipment being used, this may include setting safety stops and/or spotting the client.

7 Instruct the participant to sit in the leg press with feet positioned on the middle of the plate, shoulder-width apart. For repeatability, foot position should be marked with masking tape or chalk and/or recorded.

8 Without weight, instruct the participant to lower the plate, flexing to 90° of knee flexion and hold. Mark this plate position on the frame with masking tape or chalk so it is visible to the participant. Explain that this mark indicates how low they must lower the plate on each repetition for the test to have concurrent validity.

9 Have the participant warm up by completing 8–10 repetitions at 40%–60% of the estimated 3RM leg press (Figure 7.8).

10 Allow the participant to rest while you increase the load to 60%–80% of the estimated 3RM leg press.

11 Have the participant complete five repetitions at 60%–80% of the estimated 3RM leg press.

12 Increase the weight to a heavy but conservative estimate of the participant's 3RM leg press and allow a 1-minute rest before commencing the test.

13 Explain to the participant that a valid repetition starts with their legs at full extension, lowering them to the mark on the frame (indicating 90° knee flexion) and pressing back to full extension without assistance.

14 Have the participant attempt three repetitions of the selected weight. If all three repetitions are valid, increase the weight conservatively for the next attempt. The participant should rest for 3 minutes before attempting the next weight increment.

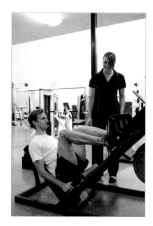

Figure 7.8 3RM leg press technique

15 Follow this procedure until the participant fails to complete three valid repetitions. The 3RM is the maximum weight lifted in the last successful trial.

16 The test is invalid if the mark is not reached or fails to be pressed back to full extension.

17 The 3RM should be achieved within 3–5 trials (the fewer the better) to minimise the effect of fatigue.

18 Avoid, where possible, overestimating the 3RM and reducing the weight after a failed attempt.

19 Record results and compare with Table 7.7.

TABLE 7.7 3RM leg press and relative strength ratio reference data

	FEMALES		MALES	
	3RM LEG PRESS (kg)	RELATIVE STRENGTH RATIO	3RM LEG PRESS (kg)	RELATIVE STRENGTH RATIO
Very poor	<80	<1.30	<185	<2.32
Poor	80–100	1.30–1.63	185–210	2.32–2.82
Average	101–120	1.64–1.86	211–250	2.83–3.16
Good	121–150	1.87–2.24	251–290	3.17–3.64
Excellent	>150	>2.24	>290	>3.64
Mean	114	1.82	236	3.03
Standard deviation	43	0.64	69	0.78
Minimum	40	0.54	80	1.22
Maximum	250	3.78	540	5.19

Based on data from 274 Australian exercise science students (females, $n = 135$) aged 18–30. Very poor ≤20th percentile; poor = 21st–40th percentile; average = 41st–60th percentile; good = 61st–80th percentile; excellent ≥81st percentile

Data recording

Participant's name: _____   Date: _____

Age: _____ years   Sex: _____   Body mass: _____ kg

1RM bench press: _____ kg

Rating: _____

Relative strength ratio (1RM bench press/body mass): _____

Rating: _____

3RM leg press: _____ kg

Rating: _____

Relative strength ratio (3RM leg press/body mass): _____

Rating: _____

Interpretation

First, consider the four steps of interpretation outlined in Appendix G, and refer to Tables 7.6 and 7.7.

Activity 7.5 Multi-stage sit-up test

AIMS: measure abdominal and hip flexor strength, interpret the results and provide feedback to a participant.

Background

The multi-stage sit-up test, otherwise known as the seven-stage sit-up test, is a graded test for assessing abdominal and hip flexor strength. This test is often included in physical testing batteries to discriminate performance among participants. For example, the multi-stage sit-up test was one of the three most effective predictors of success on the Australian Commando Selection and Training Course.[38] The multi-stage sit-up test did not exclude any candidates who passed the Commando Selection and Training Course (zero false negatives) and correctly identified two-thirds of candidates who failed (true negatives). Multi-stage sit-up test performance (i.e. $\geq$level 5) was also a significant contributing predictor of a pass or fail outcome on the 20 km march assessment and 3.2 km battle run performance time.[38]

Protocol summary

The participant lies supine with knees at $90°$ and attempts to complete one repetition at each of the seven progressively challenging sit-up stages until they can no longer successfully complete one of the variations.

Protocol

1 Follow the pre-exercise test procedures outlined in Appendix B and general methods for neuromuscular strength, power and strength endurance tests described in Table 7.1.

2 Check Appendix C to ensure that there are no contraindications to exercise testing.

3 Demonstrate the test to ensure correct form.

4 The participant should remove their shoes before this exercise begins.

5 Instruct the participant to lie down on a mat (e.g. yoga) and perform a warm-up of approximately five abdominal crunches.

6 Position the participant's knees at $90°$ flexion. You may need to check throughout the test to ensure the knee angle doesn't change.

7 Check that the heels of both feet remain on the floor at all times by lightly touching the heels (Figure 7.9). If the heels lift or shift in any way, the test is invalid and should be repeated.

8 Do not anchor the feet down as this has been shown to increase the activation of the hip flexors and hyperextend the lumbar spine during the sit-up.[39]

9 Instruct the participant through attempts at variations 1–7 (detailed below in order) until they can no longer successfully complete one of the variations (Figures 7.10a–7.16b).

10 The sit-up movement should be performed in a controlled manner without swinging or jerking movements. Technique must be maintained to ensure reliable testing of abdominal strength (see Practical 1, Test accuracy, reliability and validity).

11 At least 10 s rest should be allocated between stages.

12 The participant is allowed up to three attempts to pass each stage.

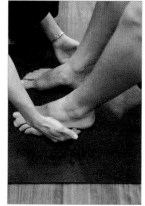

Figure 7.9 Application of very light touch to the heels (not holding) to check for heel movement during the test

Stage 1
Start position: the arms are straight, hands resting on the front of the thighs (Figure 7.10a).
Finish position: the arms are straight, finger tips touching the patella (Figure 7.10b).

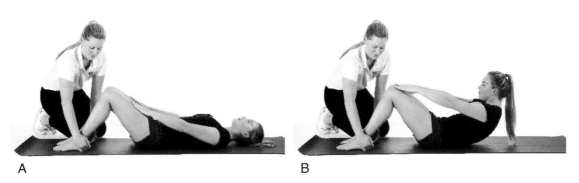

A

B

Figure 7.10 a: Stage 1 start position.   b: Stage 1 finish position

Stage 2
Start position: the arms are straight, hands resting on the front of the thighs (Figure 7.11a).
Finish position: the arms are straight, elbows touching the patella (Figure 7.11b).

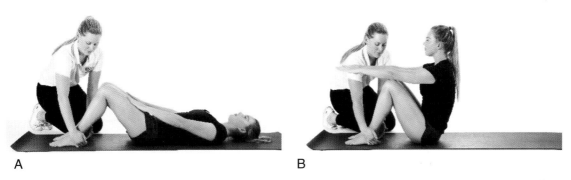

A

B

Figure 7.11 a: Stage 2 start position.   b: Stage 2 finish position

Stage 3
Start position: the hands grip the opposite elbows, forearms in contact with the abdomen (Figure 7.12a).
Finish position: the hands grip the opposite elbows, forearms in contact with the abdomen and thighs.

Note: The arms should remain in contact with the abdomen for the duration of the sit-up (Figure 7.12b).

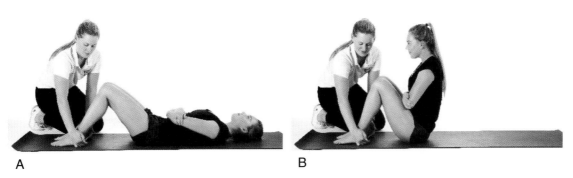

A

B

Figure 7.12 a: Stage 3 start position.   b: Stage 3 finish position

Stage 4

Start position: the hands grip the opposite shoulders, forearms in contact with the chest (Figure 7.13a).
Finish position: the hands grip the opposite shoulders, forearms in contact with the chest and thighs.

> **Note:** The arms should remain in contact with the chest for the duration of the sit-up (Figure 7.13b).

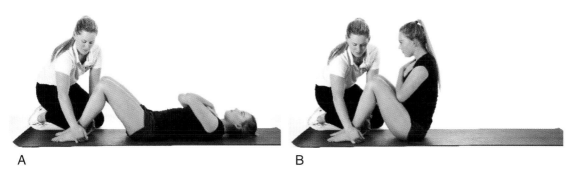

A   B

Figure 7.13 a: Stage 4 start position.   b: Stage 4 finish position

Stage 5

Start position: the arms are flexed behind the head, hands gripping the opposite shoulders (Figure 7.14a).
Finish position: the arms are flexed behind the head, hands gripping the opposite shoulders, chest touching the thighs (Figure 7.14b).

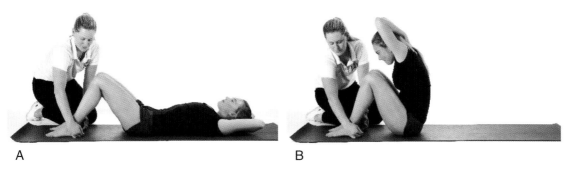

A   B

Figure 7.14 a: Stage 5 start position.   b: Stage 5 finish position

Stage 6

Start position: the arms are flexed behind the head, hands gripping the opposite sides of a 2.5 kg weight (Figure 7.15a).
Finish position: the arms are flexed behind the head, hands gripping the opposite sides of a 2.5 kg weight, chest touching the thighs (Figure 7.15b).

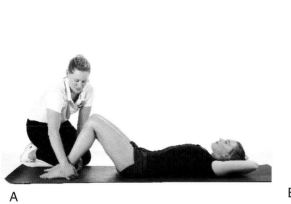
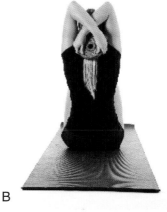

A   B

Figure 7.15 a: Stage 6 start position.   b: Stage 6 finish position

Stage 7
Start position: the arms are flexed behind the head, hands gripping the opposite sides of a 5 kg weight (Figure 7.16a).
Finish position: the arms are flexed behind the head, hands gripping the opposite sides of a 5 kg weight, chest touching the thighs (Figure 7.16b).

13 Clean and disinfect all equipment (see Appendix A).

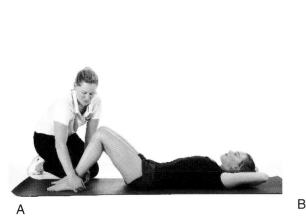
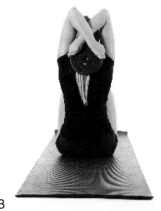

A   B

Figure 7.16 a: Stage 7 start position.   b: Stage 7 finish position

Data recording
Participant's name: _____   Date: _____
Age: _____ years   Sex: _____
Highest stage successfully completed: _____   Rating: _____

Interpretation

First, consider the four steps of interpretation outlined in Appendix G, and refer to Table 7.8. Note that the reference data is the same across sexes owing to female participants having a greater biomechanical advantage (i.e. relatively lower upper body mass) while performing this skill.

TABLE 7.8 Multistage sit-up test ratings	
Stage 1	Very poor
Stage 2	Poor
Stage 3	Fair
Stage 4	Good
Stage 5	Very good
Stage 6	Excellent
Stage 7	Outstanding

MAXIMAL NEUROMUSCULAR POWER

Neuromuscular power is an important component of many sporting and athletic competitions, in addition to the performance of many ADLs. It is a measure of a muscle or muscle group's rate of

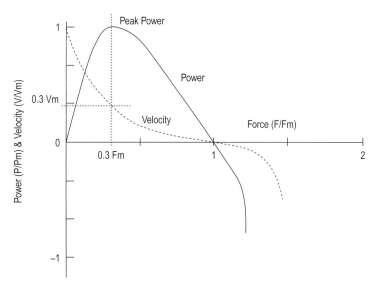

Figure 7.17 Relationships among force, velocity and power for skeletal muscle. Vm = maximum movement velocity; Pm = maximal power output; Fm = maximum isometric force output

Source: Robert Newton, Edith Cowan University, Health and Wellness Institute

work production (work/unit of time) or the product of force by velocity. While power output can be assessed across a wide spectrum of human movement from long-distance cycling through to the highly ballistic single vertical jump or a clean in weightlifting, this section will be focusing on the maximal power capacity during a single movement of duration less than 2 seconds. The classic movement examined and one which provides excellent assessment of leg extensor capabilities is the vertical jump. Qualitatively movements with very-high-power output can be viewed as the combination of neuromuscular strength and speed. In biomechanical terms, such movements involve the application of very high force, the ability to switch the muscles from a relatively low level of activation to maximal very quickly (i.e. maximum RFD) combined with the capacity to continue to produce high force output during rapid joint velocities. The force–velocity relationship of muscle (concentric actions) tells us that the heavier the load (i.e. greater force), the more the speed of movement slows (i.e. lower velocity) (Figure 7.17). Thus, to produce the highest possible power output, both force and velocity of movement need to be optimised. Tests of maximal neuromuscular power are arguably better predictors of athletic performance than are measures of neuromuscular strength or strength endurance.

Various equipment exists (e.g. the dual-force plate system) that can identify differences in RFD and peak force between the dominant and non-dominant limbs. It is typical for there to be a 0.5%–2.2% difference between the peak force and RFD achieved between the right and the left leg during these tests.[40] Furthermore, it is well documented that large inter-limb deficiencies in the RFD and peak force may be related to knee injury risk.[40,41]

Activity 7.6 Bench throw

AIMS: assess upper body strength and power throwing a barbell in a vertical plane of movement, interpret the results and provide feedback to a participant.

Background

Upper body muscle power is often assessed using maximal effort bench throws. The bench throw has been found to discriminate between elite first-division and second-division Australian rugby league athletes,[42] and between professional, semi-professional, academy level and high school level Australian rugby union athletes.[43] Performance on the bench throw test has also demonstrated a positive association with performance of different sport-specific tasks.[44-47] Therefore, the bench throw and other neuromuscular power profiling tests can be used to monitor changes in power, evaluate a training program or intervention, direct exercise prescription and/or identify an optimal training load for power development.

Valid measures of bench throw performance (force, velocity and power of movement) can be obtained using free weights or a Smith machine. Power measures derived from displacement and time data are subject to errors owing to the process of differentiation to obtain velocity and acceleration time data. When possible, it is preferable to measure force output directly, which can be achieved by placing the bench on a force plate.

A bench press movement can be used rather than the bench throw if there are concerns about spotting the barbell. However, true measures of power cannot be measured during traditional, non-ballistic movements owing to the requirement to decelerate to a stop at the end of the movement. Timing lights can be used if a linear position transducer is not available. The Smith machine can be used rather than a free weight barbell to increase safety and reduce the number of spotters required. For the purpose of this practical the protocol will be described using the BMS from Fitness Technology to control the load and further increase safety.

Protocol summary

The participant performs a single repetition rapidly lowering the barbell to the chest without contact and then extends upwards attempting to throw the barbell as high as possible.

Protocol

1 Follow the pre-exercise test procedures outlined in Appendix B and general methods for neuromuscular strength, power and strength endurance tests described in Table 7.1.

2 Check Appendix C to ensure that there are no contraindications to exercise testing.

3 Measure and record the participant's body mass (see Practical 4, Physique assessment).

4 The participant completes a 5-minute general warm-up which may include light jogging, cycling, jumping rope, etc.

5 Demonstrate the test to ensure correct form (i.e. that the participant should rapidly lower the barbell to the chest without contact and then extend upwards attempting to throw the barbell for maximum height).

6 Place a linear position transducer beside the bench directly under where the barbell will track when the participant performs the bench throw. Attach the cord to the barbell (Figure 7.18).

7 Have the participant warm up by completing 8–10 repetitions at 40%–60% of the participant's estimated 1RM. Check the linear position transducer is directly under the barbell as the participant is performing their repetitions.

8 Allow the participant to rest for 1 minute.

9 Instruct the participant that they are to perform a single repetition '*as fast as possible*', reminding them to move through full ROM and aim to throw the bar as high as possible.

10 Begin with an unloaded barbell (generally 20 kg but may gauge the starting weight relative to the strength of the participant).

11 On the computer enter the weight to be lifted.

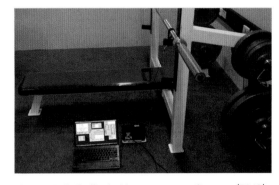

Figure 7.18 Ballistic Measurement System (BMS) with linear position transducer placement for bench press and throw testing

Source: Robert Newton, Edith Cowan University, Health and Wellness Institute. Used with permission from Fitness Technology

12 Assume the correct spotting position. When testing with a free weight load (i.e. not in a Smith Machine) it is essential to have spotters of similar height at either end of the barbell to catch the load. Ensure the spotters closely watch the movement of the bar. They should absorb the weight of the barbell after it has been thrown by flexing their knees.

13 Have the participant move into the starting position (shoulders and elbows extended).

14 Use the computer program to zero the displacement (position) with the participant holding the barbell in the fully extended position by clicking the 'Zero – Disp' button (see Figure 7.4).

15 Initiate data collection by clicking the 'Collection – Start' (see Figure 7.4) and instruct the participant to begin the test. Allow 1–2 seconds before and after completion of the movement to ensure the complete sequence is captured.

16 Repeat the procedure, increasing the weight by 5–10 kg each time until the participant is no longer able to project the weight. Provide ≥60 seconds rest between trials.

17 Record the velocity (m/s) and absolute (W) and relative peak power (W/kg).

18 Clean and disinfect all equipment (see Appendix A).

Data recording

Participant's name: _____   Date: _____

Age: _____ years   Sex: _____   Body mass: _____ kg

Starting weight: _____ kg

Bench press peak power recording sheet

SET	WEIGHT (kg)	VELOCITY (m/s)	PEAK POWER (W)	RELATIVE PEAK POWER (W/kg)
1				
2				
3				
4				
5				
6				
7				
8				
9				

Peak power output: _____ W

Optimal weight for power production: _____ kg

Interpretation

First, consider the four steps of interpretation outlined in Appendix G. Determine and record the highest peak power output and the corresponding weight lifted. This weight is the participant's optimal weight for power production. Compare the participant's results with the reference data in Table 7.9.[43]

TABLE 7.9 Bench throw reference data				
MALE RUGBY UNION PLAYERS	**PROFESSIONAL** $(n = 43)$	**SEMI-PROFESSIONAL** $(n = 19)$	**ACADEMY** $(n = 32)$	**HIGH SCHOOL** $(n = 19)$
Bench throw (W)	1140 ± 220	880 ± 90	800 ± 110	560 ± 140

Adapted from: Argus et al[43]

Activity 7.7 Reactive strength

AIMS: assess the reactive strength of the leg extensors, interpret the results and provide feedback to a participant.

Background

Reactive strength is a very important quality of the neuromuscular power profile. This is the ability to land from a drop height and then perform a rapid stretch shortening cycle to turn the eccentric phase into concentric and produce a good jump height. Reactive strength is needed in ground-based sports or activities requiring very rapid landing and take-off or change of direction. For example, volleyball players and triple jumpers generally have very high reactive strength. Assessment of reactive strength has been shown to be a concurrently valid measure of lower body explosiveness in collegiate female volleyball players[48] and can differentiate among playing positions in basketball players.[49]

Reactive strength is measured during a drop jump where the participant drops down from a height, lands and then immediately jumps, aiming for maximum height while minimising the time on the ground. Ground contact time and flight time can be measured using contact mats or force plates, with the ratio of flight to contact time termed the *reactive strength index*. This test is repeated for increasing heights, the one producing the highest flight time (jump height) being the optimal drop height. With training aimed at increasing reactive strength, you should observe an increase in flight time and reactive strength index at all heights as well as a shift in the optimal drop height to the right (Figure 7.19).

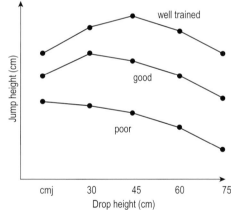

Figure 7.19 Schematic plot of flight time or jump height against drop height. The best score corresponds to the optimal drop height. cmj = countermovement jump

Highly useful measurements of vertical jump can be determined using simple and inexpensive contact mat systems. By measuring the contact and flight times to within an accuracy of ≤ 10 ms, countermovement, static (squat) drop and other jump types can be characterised. In fact, contact timing systems have been found to produce greater accuracy in determining vertical jump (calculated from flight time) than jump and reach devices such as the Vertec.[50,51] They also offer the advantage of measuring the time taken to develop the jump–contact time. For the purpose of this test the Kinematic Measurement System (KMS) developed by Fitness Technology and the SMARTSPEED jump mat developed by Fusion Sport have been described; however, a contact mat system with electronic timing or a force plate can be used.

Protocol summary

The participant steps onto the mat of the contact mat system with both feet, places hands on their hips, dips down to a self-selected depth then jumps as high as possible without tucking their knees up. The test is repeated dropping down from increasing heights.

Protocol

1 Follow the pre-exercise test procedures outlined in Appendix B and general methods for neuromuscular strength, power and strength endurance tests described in Table 7.1.

2 Check Appendix C to ensure that there are no contraindications to exercise testing.

3 Measure and record the participant's body mass (see Practical 4, Physique assessment).

4 The participant completes a 5-minute general warm-up which may include light jogging, cycling, jumping rope, etc.

5 While the participant is warming up, connect and test the contact mat system.

6 On the SMARTSPEED 'Select PROTOCOL' page, select 'jumping'. With the KMS select 'Tests – Jumping – Single'.

7 Demonstrate the test to ensure the correct form.

8 Have the participant stand to the side of the jump mat with feet shoulder-width apart. When ready, they can commence the jump in their own time.

9 The first jump is from a drop height of zero. Instruct the participant to step onto the mat with both feet, crouch down to a self-selected depth (Figure 7.20a) then jump as high as possible without tucking up their knees (Figure 7.20b), landing back on the mat. Hands are to remain on hips for all jumps. The participant should minimise ground contact time then jump as high as possible without tucking up their knees.

10 The data will appear in spreadsheet format recording the flight and contact time.

11 Repeat this sequence but with the participant dropping down from increasing heights. A good scheme is 15, 30, 45, 60, 75 and 90 cm, but this depends on box availability and whether the participant is comfortable dropping from the higher boxes.

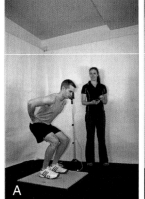
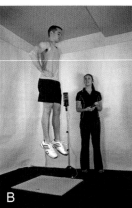

Figure 7.20 a: Flight time crouch to self-selected depth. b: Flight time maximum jump height

Used with permission from Fitness Technology and Fusion Sport

12 It is important to ensure that the participant steps out and drops from the height of the box and does not lower themselves or jump upwards from the box.

13 At least three attempts should be performed at each height, with a minimum of 30 seconds rest allocated between attempts.

14 Record all attempts on the data-recording sheet.

15 Clean and disinfect all equipment (see Appendix A).

Data analysis

Flight time can be used to calculate the jump height in cm with the following equation:

Estimated jump height (cm) $= 9.8 \times FT^2/8$

where: $FT = $ flight time in seconds – if the measure is in milliseconds then divide by 1000.

The jump height can be converted to a power score according to the formula:

$P = 4.9^{0.5} \times BM \times H^{0.5} \times 9.81$

where $P = $ average power (watts), $BM = $ body mass in kg and $H = $ jump height in metres.

Convert the power output into watts per kg by dividing by body mass.

Data recording

Participant's name: _____   Date: _____

Age: _____ years   Sex: _____   Body mass: _____ kg

HEIGHT (cm)	FLIGHT TIME (ms)	CONTACT TIME (ms)	FLIGHT/ CONTACT TIME RATIO	ESTIMATED JUMP HEIGHT (cm)	LEG POWER (W)	RELATIVE POWER (W/kg)
0						
15						
30						
45						
60						
75						
90						
Rating:						

Interpretation

First, consider the four steps of interpretation outlined in Appendix G, and refer to Tables 7.10 and 7.11. Where reactive strength is determined to be limited, plyometric training is often prescribed to optimise performance.

TABLE 7.10 Flight time reference data		
	FEMALES (ms)	MALES (ms)
Very poor	<456	<556
Poor	456–486	556–605
Average	487–505	606–633
Good	506–519	634–668
Excellent	>519	>668
Mean	487	607
Standard deviation	50	43
Minimum	310	426
Maximum	555	840

Based on data from a drop height of zero from 55 Australian exercise science students (females, $n = 25$) aged 18–25 years. Very poor $\leq$20th percentile; poor = 21st–40th percentile; average = 41st–61st percentile; good = 61st–81st percentile; excellent >80th percentile

TABLE 7.11 Leg power reference data

	FEMALES (kgm/s)	MALES (kgm/s)
Very poor	<67.4	<104.7
Poor	67.4–73.9	104.7–113.9
Average	74.0–78.4	114.0–130.7
Good	78.5–100.2	130.8–142
Excellent	>100.2	>142
Mean	83.4	125.3
Standard deviation	23.7	26.6
Minimum	59.0	75.0
Maximum	178.2	189.6

kgm/s = kilogram-metres per second; 1 kgm/s is equal to 9.1 W
Based on data from a drop height of zero from 69 Australian exercise science students (females, $n = 33$) aged 18–25 years. Very poor ≤20th percentile; poor = 21st–40th percentile; average = 41st–60th percentile; good = 61st–80th percentile; excellent ≥81st percentile

Activity 7.8 Countermovement vertical jump test

AIMS: assess leg extensor strength and speed qualities projecting the body in a vertical plane of movement, interpret the results and provide feedback to a participant.

Background

The vertical jump tests are designed to assess maximal leg power by having the participant jump as high as possible using different protocols. The different protocols are representative of various vertical jump techniques typically performed across various sports (e.g. volleyball, netball, Australian Football League (AFL) and basketball).

Vertical jumps can be performed with body weight as well as with the addition of load – either an absolute load (e.g. 40 kg) or a relative load (%BM or %1RM). Additional load can be provided by jumping with a barbell in the back squat position, holding dumbbells in the hands, or using weighted vests or belts. The countermovement vertical jump (CMJ) test has been demonstrated to have acceptable reliability (coefficient of variation < 5%) and good sensitivity (coefficient of variation < smallest worthwhile change).[52] CMJ performance has been shown to be sufficiently sensitive to match load in A-league football, Australian football[53] and rugby union.[54] Although jump height was reduced immediately post-match, flight-to-contraction ratio provided a more sensitive measure of recovery (see Practical 1, Test accuracy, reliability and validity). Thus, the flight-to-contraction ratio may provide an indication of readiness to train or compete,[52] as well as possible overtraining or residual fatigue.[53,54]

Although uniaxial performance force plates are readily available in exercise and sports science laboratories and relatively inexpensive, access for many sports clubs and exercise clinics may not be convenient. It is highly preferable to measure force directly as described below, but linear position transducers, timing systems, contact mats and other devices can also be used to derive measures of jump performance.

For the purpose of this practical, the protocol will be described using the BMS and 400S Performance Force Plate from Fitness Technology.

Protocol summary

On a force plate, the participant squats down to a self-selected depth and then immediately jumps as high as possible.

Protocol

1 Follow the pre-exercise test procedures outlined in Appendix B and general methods for neuromuscular strength, power and strength endurance tests described in Table 7.1.

2 Check Appendix C to ensure that there are no contraindications to exercise testing.

3 Measure and record the participant's body mass (see Practical 4, Physique assessment).

4 The participant completes a 5-minute general warm-up which may include light jogging, cycling, jumping rope, etc.

5 While the participant is warming up, click the 'Set Zero – Force' button (see Figure 7.4) to set the zero offset.

6 Demonstrate the test to ensure correct form.

7 Instruct the participant in the correct jump technique. They begin standing upright with hands on hips. On command, they are to squat down to a self-selected depth and then immediately jump vertically with the intention to maximise height.

8 During the jump, visually inspect the movement to ensure the participant does not dip excessively deep or shallow and maintains an upright body position. Knee angle at the bottom of the dip should be around $90°-110°$.

9 Instruct the participant that '*I will say 3, 2, 1, GO, then squat down and immediately jump upwards as fast as possible, attempting to maximise height. Land back on the force plate and stand upright until I say relax. Are you ready?*' If the participant acknowledges they are ready, say '*3, 2, 1, GO!*' and the test will begin.

10 Commence data collection by clicking the 'Collection – Start' (see Figure 7.4) at least 2 seconds prior to saying '*GO*'. Continue the data collection for 1–2 seconds after the participant has completed the jump. This is to provide a stable force at body mass before and after the jump.

11 Allow three trials, with ≥60 seconds rest between trials. Check the peak velocity of each jump and, if the trial is faster, repeat until the maximal effort is obtained.

12 After each trial, save the data.

13 Repeat with an appropriate load added to the body (e.g. a 20 kg weighted vest or a 10 kg dumbbell in each hand)

14 Record all data from the force plate on the data-recording sheet.

15 Clean and disinfect all equipment (see Appendix A).

Data analysis

The BMS will analyse the jump and use integration of the force–time data (impulse momentum relation) to calculate velocity and displacement time data. Velocity is calculated using the mechanical law that change in velocity or acceleration is a result of the force applied over a period of time. As displacement is simply the product of velocity and time, this too can be calculated by the software. Note that, although this process provides highly accurate force, impulse, power and velocity data, displacement data and thus jump height may be invalid owing to magnification of errors by the integration process.

Data recording

Participant's name: _____   Date: _____

Age: _____ years   Sex: _____   Body mass: _____ kg

Additional load: _____ kg   Stature: _____ cm

	BW ONLY	BW + ADDITIONAL LOAD
Peak force (N)		
Peak force ÷ BW (N/kg)		
Peak power (W)		
Peak power ÷ BW (W/kg)		
Peak velocity (m/s)		
ª Flight time:contraction ratio		

ª Flight time is the time in the air and contraction time is the sum of eccentric and concentric phases

Interpretation and feedback

First, consider the four steps of interpretation and the three steps of feedback and discussion outlined in Appendix G.

Note: There are currently no reference data available for the countermovement vertical jump test; however, this test could be used effectively for pre–post training purposes.

Activity 7.9 Vertical jump and reach tests

AIMS: assess leg power in projecting the body in a vertical plane of movement, interpret the results and provide feedback to a participant.

Background

Similar to the countermovement vertical jump test, the vertical jump and reach tests are designed to assess explosive leg power by having the participant jump as high as possible using different protocols. Three variations of the vertical jump test have been detailed below. Protocol 7.9.1 includes an arm swing, Protocol 7.9.2 excludes an arm swing and Protocol 7.9.3 includes a single step. The arm swing (Protocol 7.9.1) has been shown to contribute a greater extent to jump height in males than in females, probably due to differences in upper body strength.[55]

Each protocol can be performed using a yardstick (measuring rod), Vertec, chalk board or wall. Although highly accessible and easy to perform, using a yardstick, Vertec, chalk board or wall to calculate vertical jump can result in questionable validity of the results relative to the use of force plates (as described in Activity 7.8) owing to the reliance on precise timing and coordination of the arm swing to make contact at peak jump height and sufficient shoulder range of motion.[51] The vertical jump and reach test has good concurrent validity in situations when reaching height during the flight phase is critical for performance (e.g. AFL, basketball and volleyball), but only limited validity for the assessment of vertical impulse production with different jump techniques and conditions.[56] Rugby league players selected to play in the first professional National Rugby League game of the season had superior vertical jump performances to those of non-selected players.[57] Police recruits with the lowest recorded vertical jump heights were more than three times as likely to suffer injury and/or illness as those with highest vertical jump heights.[58]

Protocol summary

After measuring standing reach height, the participant (i) crouches and performs an arm swing prior to take-off from two feet (Protocol 7.9.1), (ii) crouches with no arm swing prior to take-off from two feet (Protocol 7.9.2), or (iii) takes a single preliminary step with an arm swing prior to take-off from one foot (Protocol 7.9.3).

Protocol

For the purpose of this practical, the vertical jump and reach test protocol will be described using the Vertec.

1 Follow the pre-exercise test procedures outlined in Appendix B and general methods for neuromuscular strength, power and strength endurance tests described in Table 7.1.

2 Check Appendix C to ensure that there are no contraindications to exercise testing.

3 Measure and record the participant's body mass (see Practical 4, Physique assessment).

4 The participant completes a 5-minute general warm-up which may include light jogging, cycling, jumping rope, etc.

5 Demonstrate the test to ensure correct form.

6 The participant stands with the preferred side of the body to the apparatus and raises their arm while 'pointing the fingers to the sky'. While remaining flat footed, the participant reaches as high as possible and moves as many vanes as possible (Figure 7.21). Record the number of vanes displaced.

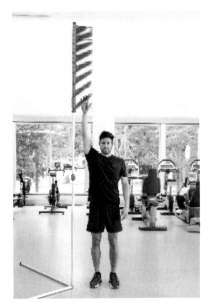

Figure 7.21 Standing reach
Used with permission from Swift Performance

Note: If using a wall, chalk board or yardstick, simply mark a horizontal line at this point.

---

7 The participant is allowed three practice attempts with at least 60 seconds rest before their measured attempts.
   Protocol 7.9.1: with no preliminary steps or shuffling, the participant crouches and performs an arm swing prior to take-off from two feet (Figure 7.22).
   Protocol 7.9.2: with no preliminary steps or shuffling, the participant crouches with no arm swing prior to take-off from two feet (Figure 7.23).
   Protocol 7.9.3: the participant takes a single preliminary step with an arm swing prior to take-off from one foot (Figure 7.24).

8 Ask the participant to jump as high as possible. At the peak of the jump, the participant displaces as many vanes as they can (Figure 7.25). If using a wall, chalk board or a yardstick, mark the peak height with a horizontal line.

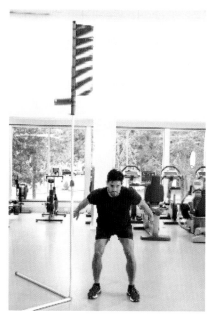

Figure 7.22 Protocol 7.9.1: preparatory crouch with arm swing

Used with permission from Swift Performance

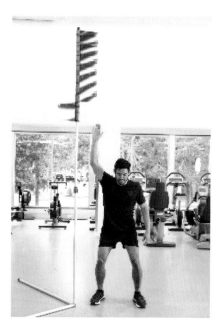

Figure 7.23 Protocol 7.9.2: preparatory crouch without arm swing

Used with permission from Swift Performance

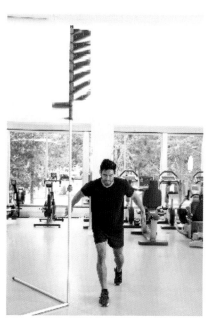

Figure 7.24 Protocol 7.9.3: preparatory step with arm swing

Used with permission from Swift Performance

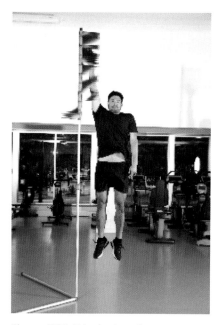

Figure 7.25 Displacing the vanes at peak jump height

Used with permission from Swift Performance

9 At least three attempts are made, with a minimum of 30 seconds rest allocated between attempts.

10 After each jump, record the number of vanes displaced and compare this with Table 7.12.

Data analysis

The effective height jumped is the difference between the number of vanes displaced while standing (standing height mark if using a wall, chalk board or yardstick) and the number of vanes displaced while jumping (peak jump height mark if using a wall, chalkboard or yardstick).

TABLE 7.12 Vertical jump reference data

	FEMALES (cm)			MALES (cm)		
	ARM SWING	NO ARM SWING	SINGLE STEP	ARM SWING	NO ARM SWING	SINGLE STEP
Very poor	<35	<30	<34	<54	<45	<53
Poor	35–39	30–35	34–37	54–59	45–52	53–60
Average	40–43	36–37	38–42	60–65	53–56	61–67
Good	44–49	38–43	43–47	66–74	57–62	68–76
Excellent	>49	>43	>47	>74	>62	>76
Mean	42	37	41	63	54	64
Standard deviation	9	9	9	12	11	15
Minimum	19	12	15	32	22	34
Maximum	71	67	69	92	86	162

Based on data from 356 Australian exercise science students (females, $n = 169$) aged 18–30. Very poor $\leq$20th percentile; poor = 21st–40th percentile; average = 41st–60th percentile; good = 61st–80th percentile; excellent $\geq$81st percentile

Data recording

Participant's name: _____ Date: _____

Age: _____ years   Sex: _____   Body mass: _____ kg

Stature: _____ cm   Standing reach measurement: _____ cm

	PROTOCOL 7.9.1: ARM SWING	PROTOCOL 7.9.2: NO ARM SWING	PROTOCOL 7.9.3: SINGLE STEP
Trial 1 (cm)			
Trial 2 (cm)			
Trial 3 (cm)			
Greatest effective height jumped (cm)			
Rating			

Interpretation and feedback

First, consider the four steps of interpretation and the three steps of feedback and discussion outlined in Appendix G, and refer to Table 7.12.

Activity 7.10 Standing long jump

AIMS: Assess the power of the legs in projecting the body in a forward direction, interpret the results and provide feedback to a participant.

Background

The standing long jump is a fundamental motor skill for a variety of sports involving high-velocity contractions, including athletics (sprinting, hurdling and jumping), various combat sports, football and ski jumping. It is frequently used as one of the best functional tests to assess ballistic power of the lower extremity.[59] The standing long jump has been shown to have an acceptable between-day reproducibility (mean $\pm$ SD (standard deviation) 0.80 $\pm$ 0.13; ICC (intraclass correlation coefficient) and CV (coefficient of variation) 8.1 $\pm$ 4.1%).[60] However, a greater proportion of the performance measures from the standing long jump have lower ICC and/or higher CV values compared with other common jump tests, probably owing to the somewhat more complex nature of the long jump test.[60]

The standing long jump can be used as a valuable performance test to identify differences of sprinting ability in elite female rugby players[61] and assist prediction of involvement with the ball in recreational youth soccer players.[62]

Protocol summary

The participant stands with toes behind the starting line of a standing long jump mat, swings the arms backwards, crouches, then vigorously swings their arms forwards while jumping as far forwards as possible.

Protocol

1 Follow the pre-exercise test procedures outlined in Appendix B and general methods for neuromuscular strength, power and strength endurance tests described in Table 7.1.

2 Check Appendix C to ensure that there are no contraindications to exercise testing.

3 Measure and record the participant's body mass (see Practical 4, Physique assessment).

4 The participant completes a 5-minute general warm-up which may include light jogging, cycling, jumping rope, etc.

5 Demonstrate the test to ensure correct form.

6 The participant removes their shoes.

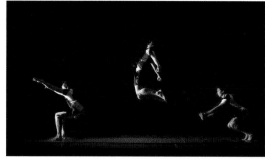

Figure 7.26 Standing long jump
Used with permission from Hart Sport

7 The participant stands with feet parallel to each other and with toes behind the starting line of a standing long jump mat.

8 The participant is then allowed three practice trials, with at least 60 seconds rest before their first measured attempt.

9 When ready, the participant swings the arms backwards, crouches, then vigorously swings their arms forwards while jumping as far forwards as possible (Figure 7.26).

10 The tester watches the landing of the participant's feet very closely, marking the landing point of the back of the foot closest to the starting line.

11 Using a tape measure, measure and record the shortest distance from the landing mark to the starting line to the nearest centimetre.

12 The participant should make at least three attempts with a minimum of 30 seconds rest allocated between each jump.

13 Record results and compare them with Table 7.13 to evaluate performance.

14 Clean and disinfect all equipment (see Appendix A).

Data recording

Participant's name: _____   Date: _____

Age: _____ years   Sex: _____   Body mass: _____ kg

Stature: _____ cm

Jump attempts:

1. _____ cm

2. _____ cm

3. _____ cm

Best jump: _____ cm   Rating: _____

Interpretation

First, consider the four steps of interpretation outlined in Appendix G, and refer to Table 7.13.

Strength endurance

Strength endurance is the ability of a muscle group to execute repeated contractions over a period of time sufficient to cause muscular fatigue. Dynamic strength endurance tests are commonly performed as part of physical fitness testing batteries within the defence force to predict recruit graduation, incumbent performance and injury risk.

TABLE 7.13 Standing long jump reference data		
	FEMALES (cm)	**MALES (cm)**
Very poor	<150	<220
Poor	150–165	220–232
Average	166–173	233–240
Good	174–180	241–251
Excellent	>180	>251
Mean	166	235
Standard deviation	26	23
Minimum	71	150
Maximum	270	310

Based on data from 342 Australian exercise science students (females, $n = 166$) aged 18–30. Very poor $\leq$20th percentile; poor = 21st–40th percentile; average = 41st–60th percentile; good = 61st–80th percentile; excellent $\geq$81st percentile

Activity 7.11 Dynamic strength endurance test (push-up)

AIMS: assess dynamic muscle endurance of the upper body, interpret the results and provide feedback to a participant.

Background

Simple field tests such as the dynamic push-up test may be used to evaluate the endurance of the upper body muscle groups. There are several different test protocols used to assess dynamic muscular endurance. For example, within the literature the push-up test has been performed: (i) in time with a metronome, (ii) with or without rest over a set amount of time (e.g. 15 seconds), (iii) until a set rating of perceived exertion (RPE; see Appendix E; e.g. 12/20), (iv) until technique failure, (v) until volitional fatigue, or (vi) via subjective assessment of push up technique over 5 repetitions, to name but a few.

Dynamic strength endurance tests can predict athletic activity performance, with the push-up test strongly correlated with softball throw distance.[63] At police academy entry, successful graduates were able to perform more push-ups and sit-ups than those failing to graduate, with push-ups the most significant predictor of successful graduation.[64] Indeed, a recent study of over 1500 firefighters found that being able to complete more than 40 push-ups was associated with a significant reduction in incident cardiovascular disease event risk compared with those completing fewer than 10 push-ups.[65] Interestingly, a systematic review concluded that the evidence for fewer push-ups increasing the risk of musculoskeletal injuries is strong in men but limited in women.[66]

Protocol summary

The participant lowers their body until their chin touches a marking cone and pushes back up to a straight arm position as many times as possible.

Protocol

1 Follow the pre-exercise test procedures outlined in Appendix B and general methods for neuromuscular strength, power and strength endurance tests described in Table 7.1.

2 Check Appendix C to ensure that there are no contraindications to exercise testing.

3 The participant completes a 5-minute general warm-up which may include light jogging, cycling, jumping rope, etc.

4 The exercise should be performed on a flat, non-slip surface with a 5 cm high soft sports marker disc or other soft marking cone of the same height, placed where it will be touched by the participant's lowered chin.

5 Demonstrate the test to ensure correct form.

6 Male participants should assume a position with hands shoulder-width apart, back straight, head up, and using the toes as the pivotal point (Figure 7.27a).

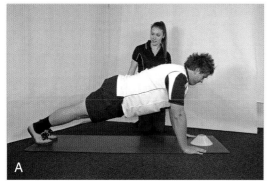
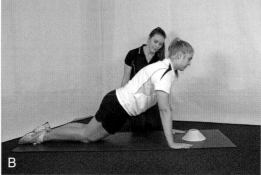

Figure 7.27 a: Push-up start and finish position for males. b: Push-up start and finish position for females

7 Female participants should assume a position with legs together, lower leg in contact with the mat and ankles plantarflexed, back straight, hands shoulder-width apart, and head up (Figure 7.27b). A thin mat (e.g. yoga mat) should be placed under the participant's knees to reduce discomfort.

8 The participant must lower the body until their chin touches the cone; the torso should not touch the mat (Figure 7.28a and b). Where it is not possible for the the torso to avoid touching the mat at the height of the cone, increase the height of the cone as appropriate.

9 For both males and females, the participant's knees, gluteals, back and shoulders must be moving in a straight line at all times and the participant must push up to a straight arm position.

10 Have the participant complete up to three repetitions to ensure correct technique prior to testing.

11 The participant rests for 1 minute.

12 Count down '3, 2, 1, GO' and commence the test.

13 This is a maximal test; therefore, the participant will require verbal encouragement to perform the maximum number of push-ups.

14 The maximum number of push-ups performed consecutively without rest is counted as the score.

15 The tester should discard any repetitions where the participant fails to maintain the appropriate technique – for example, doesn't complete the full range of motion (including touching the chin to the cone and fully extending the elbows), or the lower back is 'sagging' or arching, gluteals are too elevated, or torso is touching the ground.

16 The participant should be immediately cued to correct any technique errors.

17 The tester should provide a warning when two consecutive repetitions are performed incorrectly/ with poor technique.

18 The test is terminated once the participant reaches volitional exhaustion or fails to complete three consecutive repetitions with correct technique.

19 Record the number of successfully completed repetitions and compare it with Table 7.14.

20 Clean and disinfect all equipment (see Appendix A).

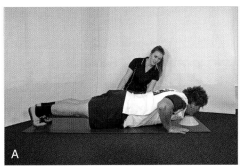
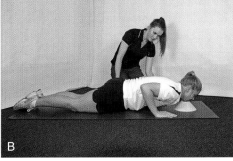

Figure 7.28 a: Lowered push-up technique for males. b: Lowered push-up technique for females

Data recording

Participant's name: _____   Date: _____

Age: _____ years   Sex: _____

Maximal number of push-ups: _____

Rating: _____

Interpretation

First, consider the four steps of interpretation and the three steps of feedback and discussion outlined in Appendix G, and refer to Table 7.14.

TABLE 7.14 Maximal push up reference data

	FEMALES	MALES
Very poor	<13	<31
Poor	13–20	31–40
Average	21–26	41–44
Good	27–33	45–50
Excellent	>33	>50
Mean	24	41
Standard deviation	11	11
Minimum	6	3
Maximum	50	73

Based on data from 374 Australian exercise science students (females, $n = 175$) aged 18–30. Very poor $\leq$20th percentile; poor = 21st–40th percentile; average = 41st–60th percentile; good = 61st–80th percentile; excellent $\geq$81st percentile

Feedback and discussion

First, consider the three steps of feedback and discussion outlined in Appendix G. Feedback regarding neuromuscular strength, power and strength endurance tests should include more than just stating the result and relevant descriptor; it is important to consider the participant and the purpose of the test. For example, the discussion and feedback for a test conducted as part of a health evaluation would be very different to a test conducted to determine and/or monitor athletic performance. Where the test has been conducted on athletes, it is important to consider the extent to which the measure of neuromuscular strength, power and/or strength endurance performed validly corresponds to their specific sport. This should have been the first consideration when selecting a test to measure neuromuscular strength, power and/or strength endurance; however, the relationship of the test to sport-specific performance will need to be succinctly explained to the participant following the test, as this will influence the recommendations provided. For example, if the test has been found to correlate highly with the participant's sporting performance and/or there are specific reference data available for elite athletes within their sport or from previous testing on this participant, then this should be included in the feedback. Where the participant's test result falls below expected values for their age, sex and, where possible, sport, specific recommendations need to be provided to assist the athlete to improve their neuromuscular strength, power and/or strength endurance to maximise athletic performance.

For non-athletic participants, the importance of neuromuscular strength, power and strength endurance measurements to optimise health should be discussed. Similar to athletes, feedback and discussion of the results will depend on the participant, their goals and the purpose of the test; for example, determine risk of dependency in activities of daily living versus monitoring progress of rehabilitation.

Case studies

Case Study 1

Setting: You are working as a strength and conditioning coach for a national sporting institute.

Participant: On the advice of her coach, a 19-year-old female state team basketball player comes to see you for advice about improving her physical performance. You decide to initially assess her

continued

Case studies *(continued)*

vertical jump and reach test, reactive strength and 3-repetition maximum (3RM) leg press. She has the following scores:

Vertical jump and reach test (Activity 7.9: the client takes a single preliminary step with an arm swing prior to take-off from one foot). *Best = 37 cm*

3RM leg press (Activity 7.4: the client performs a 3RM back squat test with a standard 20 kg barbell and Olympic weights). *Best = 1.30 kg/kg body mass*

Reactive strength (Activity 7.7: the client performs a series of box jumps at 15, 30, 45 and 60 cm). *Best = 68 kgm/s and 456 ms*

Interpret the results, and provide and discuss feedback:

_____

_____

_____

_____

_____

_____

How does your answer compare with the worked example provided in the Case Studies and Answers at the back of the manual?

_____

_____

_____

Case Study 2

Setting: You are working as a sport scientist for a research institution, and are approached by the strength and conditioning coach from the regional AFL team.

Task: The coach informs you that he has performed isometric mid-thigh pull tests and countermovement vertical jump tests on players in his team. Both tests were performed on a dual-force plate system allowing for diagnostics of imbalances between the right and left leg. The coach has some results from these tests that he would like to discuss with you. Key points that the coach wants your advice on are as follows:

1 The coach has noticed a 5%–15% difference in the peak force and rate of force development (RFD) achieved with the left and right leg during the isometric mid-thigh pull for some players.

2 The coach has also noticed a 7%–12% difference in the RFD achieved with the right and left leg during the countermovement vertical jump for some players.

What actions and/or further tests would you recommend for these athletes?

_____

_____

_____

_____

continued overpage

Case studies *(continued)*

Interpret the results, and provide and discuss feedback:

_____

_____

_____

_____

_____

_____

How does your answer compare with the worked example in the Case Studies and Answers at the back of the manual?

_____

_____

Case Study 3

Setting: You have been approached by a residential aged care facility to design an exercise program to enhance residents' physical function and reduce their falls risk. Your first client is Dorothy, a 72-year-old female who is underweight and has osteoporosis. She has not done any structured exercise previously. She is worried that she sometimes loses her balance and doesn't know whether she will be able to get up if she falls down. She lives with her husband, who is currently doing a resistance training program.

Task: As part of a home visit, design a brief initial health assessment for this client, choosing from the battery of tests within this practical and Practical 15, Functional measures. Describe and justify the most important measure of neuromuscular strength that you would include in this testing battery.

Within your practical session, partner with another student, who will role-play the client, to conduct this test. Interpret these results according to the four steps of interpretation outlined in Appendix G. Particular reference should be made to how this result will be used to design the client's exercise program.

TEST BATTERY:
Priority test
Name and describe the test:

_____

_____

_____

Justify the test, with specific reference to the case study:

_____

_____

_____

_____

continued

Case studies *(continued)*

Practise completing this test, including data recording and calculations as appropriate. Interpret the results, and provide and discuss feedback:

How does your answer compare with the worked example in the Case Studies and Answers at the back of the manual?

References

[1] Taekema DG, Gussekloo J, Maier AB, Westendorp RGJ, de Craen AJM. Handgrip strength as a predictor of functional, psychological and social health. A prospective population-based study among the oldest old. Age Ageing 2010;39:331–7.

[2] Newton RU, Kraemer WJ. Power. In: Ackland TR, Elliott BC, Bloomfield J, eds. Applied anatomy and biomechanics in sport, 2nd ed. Champaign, IL: Human Kinetics; 2008, Chapter 7, p. 155–76.

[3] Townsend JR, Bender D, Vantrease W, Hudy J, Huet K, Williamson C, et al. Isometric mid-thigh pull performance is associated with athletic performance and sprinting kinetics in division I men and women's basketball players. J Strength Cond Res 2019;33(10):2665–73.

[4] Khamoui AV, Brown LE, Nguyen D, Uribe BP, Coburn JW, Noffal GJ, et al. Relationship between force-time and velocity-time characteristics of dynamic and isometric muscle actions. J Strength Cond Res 2011;25:198–204.

[5] Morin JB, Slawinski J, Dorel S, de Villareal ES, Couturier A, Samozino P, et al. Acceleration capability in elite sprinters and ground impulse: push more, brake less? J Biomech 2015;48:3149–54.

[6] Kawamori N, Nosaka K, Newton RU. Relationships between ground reaction impulse and sprint acceleration performance in team sport athletes. J Strength Cond Res 2013;27:568–73.

[7] Reuter SE, Massy-Westropp N, Evans AM. Reliability and validity of indices of hand-grip strength and endurance. Aust Occup Ther J 2011;58:82–7.

[8] Newman AB, Kupelian V, Visser M, Simonsick EM. Strength, but not muscle mass, is associated with mortality in the health, aging and body composition study cohort. J Gerontol A Biol Sci Med Sci 2006;61:72–7.

[9] Kilgour RD, Vigano A, Trutschnigg B, Lucar E, Borod D, Morais JA. Handgrip strength predicts survival and is associated with markers of clinical and functional outcomes in advanced cancer patients. Support Care Cancer 2013;21:3261–70.

[10] Leong DP, McKee M, Yusuf S; PURE Investigators. Population muscle strength predicts Olympic medal tallies: evidence from 20 countries in the PURE Prospective Cohort Study. PLoS One 2017;12:e0169821.

[11] Whaley MH, Brubaker PH, Otto RM. The ACSM's guidelines for exercise testing and prescription. Baltimore, MD: Lippincott, Williams and Wilkins; 2005.

[12] Massy-Westropp NM, Gill TK, Taylor AW, Bohannon RW, Hill CL. Hand grip strength: age and gender stratified normative data in a population-based study. BMC Res Notes 2011;4:127.

[13] McGuigan MR, Newton MJ, Winchester JB, Nelson AG. Relationship between isometric and dynamic strength in recreationally trained men. J Strength Cond Res 2010;24:2570–3.

[14] Stone MH, Sands WA, Pierce KC, Ramsey MW, Haff GG. Power and power potentiation among strength-power athletes: preliminary study. Int J Sports Physiol Perform 2008;3:55–67.

[15] McGuigan MR, Winchester JB. The relationship between isometric and dynamic strength in college football players. J Sports Sci Med 2008;7:101–5.

[16] Nuzzo JL, McBride JM, Cormie P, McCaulley GO. Relationship between countermovement jump performance and multijoint isometric and dynamic tests of strength. J Strength Cond Res 2008;22:699–707.

[17] Wrigley T, Strauss G. Strength assessment by isokinetic dynamometry. In: Gore CJ, ed. Physiological tests for elite athletes. Champaign, IL: Human Kinetics; 2000, p. 155–99.

[18] Croisier JL, Ganteaume S, Binet J, Genty M, Ferret J-M. Strength imbalances and prevention of hamstring injury in professional soccer players: a prospective study. Am J Sports Med 2008;36:1469–75.

[19] Cameron M, Adams R, Maher C. Motor control and strength as predictors of hamstring injury in elite players of Australian football. Phys Ther Sport 2003;4:159–66.

[20] Oh JH, Yoon JP, Kim JY, Oh CH. Isokinetic muscle performance test can predict the status of rotator cuff muscle. Clin Orthop Relat Res 2010;468:1506–13.

[21] Perry AC, Wang X, Feldman BB, Ruth T, Signorile J. Can laboratory-based tennis profiles predict field tests of tennis performance? J Strength Cond Res 2004;18:136–43.

[22] Wrigley T, Strauss G. Strength assessment by isokinetic dynamometry. In: Gore CJ, eds. Physiological tests for elite athletes. Champaign, IL: Human Kinetics; 2000, p. 155–99.

[23] Coombs R, Garbutt G. Developments in the use of the hamstring/quadriceps ratio for the assessment of muscle balance. J Sports Sci Med 2002;1:56–62.

[24] Beam WC, Bartels RL, Ward RW, Clark RN, Zuelzer WA. Multiple comparisons of isokinetic leg strength in male and female collegiate athletic teams. Med Sci Sport Exerc 1985;17:Abstract #20, 269.

[25] Gilliam TB, Sady SP, Freedson PS, Villanaci J. Isokinetic torque levels for high school football players. Arch Phys Med Rehabil 1979;60:110–14.

[26] Housh TJ, Thorland WG, Tharp GD, Johnson GO. Isokinetic leg flexion and extension strength of elite adolescent female track and field athletes. Res Q Exerc Sport 1984;55:347–50.

[27] Housh TJ, Johnson GO, Marty L, Eischen G, Eischen C, Housh DJ. Isokinetic leg flexion and extension strength of university football players. J Orthop Sports Phys Ther 1988;9:365–9.

[28] Wyatt MP, Edwards AM. Comparison of quadriceps and hamstring torque values during Isokinetic exercise. J Orthop Sports Phys Ther 1981;3:48–56.

[29] Adams GM. Exercise physiology laboratory manual. New York, NY: McGraw-Hill; 2001.

[30] Brockett CL, Morgan DL, Proske U. Predicting hamstring strain injury in elite athletes. Med Sci Sports Exerc 2004;36:379–87.

[31] Debanne T, Laffaye G. Predicting the throwing velocity of the ball in handball with anthropometric variables and isotonic tests. J Sports Sci 2011;29:705–13.

[32] Marques MC, van den Tilaar R, Vescovi JD, Gonzalez-Badillo JJ. Relationship between throwing velocity, muscle power, and bar velocity during bench press in elite handball players. Int J Sports Physiol Perform 2007;2:414–22.

[33] Davis DS, Barnette BJ, Kiger JT, Mirasola JJ, Young SM. Physical characteristics that predict functional performance in Division I college football players. J Strength Cond Res 2004;18:115–20.

[34] Fry AC, Kraemer WJ. Physical performance characteristics of American collegiate football players. J Appl Sport Sci Res 1991;5:126–38.

[35] Pickett CW, Nosaka K, Zois J, Hopkins WG, Blazevich AJ. Maximal upper body strength and oxygen uptake are associated with performance in high-level 200-m sprint kayakers. J Strength Cond Res 2018;32(11):3186–92.

[36] Braith RW, Graves JE, Leggett SH, Pollock ML. Effect of training on the relationship between maximal and submaximal strength. Med Sci Sports Exerc 1993;25:132–8.

[37] Mayhew JL, Prinster JL, Ware JS, Zimmer DL, Arabas JR, Bemben MG. Muscular endurance repetitions to predict bench press strength in men of different training levels. J Sports Med Phys Fitness 1995;35:108–13.

[38] Hunt AP, Orr RM, Billing DC. Developing physical capability standards that are predictive of success on Special Forces selection courses. Mil Med 2013;178:619–24.

[39] Norris CM. Abdominal muscle training in sport. Br J Sports Med 1993;27:19–27.

[40] Jordan MJ, Aagaard P, Herzog W. Lower limb asymmetry in mechanical muscle function: A comparison between ski racers with and without ACL reconstruction. Scand J Med Sci Sports 2015;25:e301–9.

[41] Jordan MJ, Aagaard P, Herzog W. Rapid hamstrings/quadriceps strength in ACL-reconstructed elite Alpine ski racers. Med Sci Sports Exerc 2015;47:109–19.

[42] Baker DG, Newton RU. Adaptations in upper-body maximal strength and power output resulting from long-term resistance training in experienced strength-power athletes. J Strength Cond Res 2006;20:541–6.

[43] Argus CK, Gill ND, Keogh JW. Characterization of the differences in strength and power between different levels of competition in rugby union athletes. J Strength Cond Res 2012;26:2698–704.

[44] Liossis LD, Forsyth J, Liossis C, Tsolakis C. The acute effect of upper-body complex training on power output of martial art athletes as measured by the bench press throw exercise. J Hum Kinet 2013;39:167–75.

[45] Terzis G, Georgiadis G, Vassiliadou E, Manta P. Relationship between shot put performance and triceps brachii fiber type composition and power production. Eur J Appl Physiol 2003;90:10–15.

[46] Cronin JB, Owen GJ. Upper-body strength and power assessment in women using a chest pass. J Strength Cond Res 2004;18:401–4.

[47] Baker D. Comparison of upper-body strength and power between professional and college-aged rugby league players. J Strength Cond Res 2001;15:30–5.

[48] Kipp K, Kiely MT, Geiser CF. Reactive strength index modified is a valid measure of explosiveness in collegiate female volleyball players. J Strength Cond Res 2016;30:1341–7.

[49] Pehar M, Sekulic D, Sisic N, Spasic M, Uljevic O, Krolo A, et al. Evaluation of different jumping tests in defining position-specific and performance-level differences in high level basketball players. Biol Sport 2017;34:263–72.

[50] Leard JS, Cirillo MA, Katsnelson E, Kimiatek DA, Miller TW, Trebincevic K, et al. Validity of two alternative systems for measuring vertical jump height. J Strength Cond Res 2007;21:1296–9.

[51] Walsh MS, Bohm H, Butterfield MM, Santhosam J. Gender bias in the effects of arms and countermovement on jumping performance. J Strength Cond Res 2007;21:362–6.

[52] Roe G, Darrall-Jones J, Till K, Phibbs P, Read D, Weakley J, et al. Between-days reliability and sensitivity of common fatigue measures in rugby players. Int J Sports Physiol Perform 2016;11:581–6.

[53] Mooney MG, Cormack S, O'Brien BJ, Morgan WM, McGuigan M. Impact of neuromuscular fatigue on match exercise intensity and performance in elite Australian football. J Strength Cond Res 2013;27:166–73.

[54] Rowell AE, Aughey RJ, Hopkins WG, Stewart AM, Cormack SJ. Identification of sensitive measures of recovery after external load from football match play. Int J Sports Physiol Perform 2017;12:969–76.

[55] Isaacs LD. Comparison of the Vertec and Just Jump systems for measuring height of vertical jump by young children. Percept Mot Skills 1998;86:659–63.

[56] Menzel HJ, Chagas MH, Szmuchrowski LA, Araujo SR, Campos CE, Giannetti MR. Usefulness of the jump-and-reach test in assessment of vertical jump performance. Percept Mot Skills 2010;110:150–8.

[57] Gabbett TJ, Jenkins DG, Abernethy B. Relative importance of physiological, anthropometric, and skill qualities to team selection in professional rugby league. J Sports Sci 2011;29:1453–61.

[58] Orr R, Pope R, Peterson S, Hinton B, Stierli M. Leg power as an indicator of risk of injury or illness in police recruits. Int J Environ Res Public Health 2016;13:237.

[59] Mackala K, Stodolka J, Siemienski A, Coh M. Biomechanical analysis of standing long jump from varying starting positions. J Strength Cond Res 2013;27:2674–84.

[60] Hebert-Losier K, Beaven CM. The MARS for squat, countermovement, and standing long jump performance analyses: are measures reproducible? J Strength Cond Res 2014;28:1849–57.

[61] Agar-Newman DJ, Klimstra MD. Efficacy of horizontal jumping tasks as a method for talent identification of female rugby players. J Strength Cond Res 2015;29:737–3.

[62] Re AH, Cattuzzo MT, Henrique R dos S, Stodden DF. Physical characteristics that predict involvement with the ball in recreational youth soccer. J Sports Sci 2016;34:1716–22.

[63] Negrete RJ, Hanney WJ, Kolber MJ, Davies GJ, Riemann B. Can upper extremity functional tests predict the softball throw for distance: a predictive validity investigation. Int J Sports Phys Ther 2011;6:104–11.

[64] Shusko M, Benedetti L, Korre M, Eshleman EJ, Farioli A, Christophi CA, et al. Recruit fitness as a predictor of police academy graduation. Occup Med (Lond) 2017;67:555–61.

[65] Yang J, Christophi CA, Farioli A, Baur DM, Moffatt S, Zollinger TW, et al. Association between push-up exercise capacity and future cardiovascular events among active adult men. JAMA Netw Open 2019;2:e188341.

[66] de la Motte SJ, Gribbin TC, Lisman P, Murphy K, Deuster PA. Systematic review of the association between physical fitness and musculoskeletal injury risk: Part 2 Muscular endurance and muscular strength. J Strength Cond Res 2017;31:3218–34.

PRACTICAL 8
STATIC AND DYNAMIC POSTURE

Deirdre McGhee and Margaret Torode

LEARNING OBJECTIVES

- Explain the anatomical basis, purposes, reliability, validity, assumptions and limitations of static and dynamic postural assessments
- Identify and explain the common terminology, processes and equipment required to conduct static and dynamic postural assessments
- Demonstrate the observational skill to identify postures with optimal alignment and malalignment in the upright standing position (static postural assessment) and during movement (dynamic postural assessment)
- Record, analyse and interpret information from static and dynamic postural assessments and determine whether any observed postural malalignment in the upright standing position is fixed (unchangeable) or adjustable (able to be changed)
- Communicate any observed postural malalignments to a participant and interpret their level of postural awareness both in the upright standing position and during movement
- Demonstrate the ability to identify any physical barriers in terms of joint range of motion, muscle flexibility and muscle strength that limit or prevent optimal alignment in the upright standing position and during movement
- Prescribe appropriate exercises to address any physical barriers in terms of joint range of motion, muscle flexibility and muscle strength that would limit further progression of a fixed postural malalignment or address the physical barriers of an adjustable postural malalignment
- Guide movement and posture to improve any adjustable postural alignments identified both in the upright standing position and during movement
- Demonstrate an understanding of functional anatomy by determining the underlying musculoskeletal mechanisms of any identified static and/or dynamic postural malalignment

Equipment and other requirements

- Information sheet and informed consent
- Posture grid rating frame or plumb line
- Full-body mirrors
- Markers/sticker dots
- Small step
- Self-retracting, flexible metal anthropometry tape
- Hand weights
- Swiss balls/Bosu balls

- Barbells
- Dowel sticks

INTRODUCTION

Postural assessment is the observational assessment of the alignment of the segments of the body.[1] It is an essential skill for all exercise professionals.

Static postural assessment is commonly performed in the upright standing position where the alignment of adjacent segments (parts) of the body is observed relative to the line of gravity through the body and the base of support (BoS). Optimal alignment requires the least amount of muscle support and minimises stress on the joints and supporting ligaments because it optimises force distribution.[2] (See Box 8.1 Spinal curvature.)

The postural alignment of adjacent body segments are assessed in static postures and dynamic movements. Movements commonly assessed include activities of daily living (ADLs), movements relevant to the participant's sport and/or work tasks, exercises prescribed by an exercise professional or movements reported to aggravate a participant's symptoms.

Static and dynamic postural assessments have four stages:

- **Stage 1:** observing the postural alignment and summarising whether there is optimal alignment or any segmental malalignment.

- **Stage 2:** communication with the participant to determine whether they are kinaesthetically aware of any postural malalignments. Awareness of postural alignment is necessary prior to any correction or improvement of any postural malalignment.

- **Stage 3:** determining whether any postural malalignments identified are *fixed* (where the skeleton *cannot* move out of that postural malalignment) or *adjustable* (where the skeleton *can* move out of the postural malalignment).

- **Stage 4:** prescription of postural exercises[3] to address physical barriers that may limit the achievement of optimal alignment, and of educational cues that assist to efficiently achieve and maintain optimal postural alignment.

Box 8.1 Spinal curvature

Optimal spinal posture is described as the continuous curvature of cervical lordosis, thoracic kyphosis and lumbar lordosis. Postural assessments of these curvatures are subjectively described as normal (Figure 8.1a), hyper (Figure 8.1b) or hypo. Spinal curvature is objectively measured through sagittal x-rays (Cobb angle) and clinical measures. The thoracic kyphosis and lumbar lordosis Cobb angles are formed by two lines drawn on a sagittal x-ray along the superior or inferior surfaces of two specified vertebral bodies. The normal range of the thoracic kyphosis angle is $20°-50°$ and the lumbar lordosis angle is $20°-70°$ (Figure 8.2).[2] The wide range of Cobb angles (spinal curvatures) considered to be normal is due to variation in the vertebral bodies and surfaces used in each region to form the angles, in different studies. Thoracic kyphosis tends to increase with age.[2]

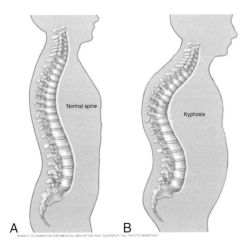

Figure 8.1 a: Normal kyphosis.
b: Hyperkyphosis

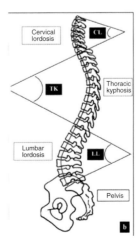

Figure 8.2 Cobb angles in sagittal plane of vertebral column

DEFINITIONS

Anatomical position: the erect position of the body with the face directed forwards, the arms at the side of the body, toes and palms of the hands facing forwards. Used as a reference to describe the relationship of body segments to one another.

Centre of mass: a hypothetical point around which the force of gravity appears to act and at which the combined mass of the body appears to be concentrated. In humans in the anatomical position, it is approximately anterior to the second sacral vertebra. The location changes with every new position of the body and limbs.

Base of support (BoS): refers to the area beneath the person that is in contact with the supporting surface (i.e. in standing it is the feet and any other device in contact with the ground, e.g. crutches or walking sticks). It will vary in different positions (i.e. in sitting it would also include the chair).

Dynamic posture: the alignment of the body segments during movement.

Grid rating frame: a frame designed to provide visual cues of an individual's posture to aid in correcting deviations.

Inclinometer: a device for measuring the angle of inclination of a body part.

Kinaesthetic: a conscious awareness of body position, muscle movement and mass as felt through nerve endings.

Kyphosis: excessive outward curvature of the spine.

Lordosis: excessive inward curvature of the spine.

Plumb line: a line (e.g. string) with a weight at one end (e.g. plumb bob) that is used to determine verticality.

Postural malalignment: differences in alignment between the left and right sides of the body and/or the front and back of the body.

Postural sway: horizontal movement around the centre of gravity.

Scoliosis: excessive lateral curvature of the spine.

Static posture: the alignment of the body while stationary.

Valgus: a deformity involving oblique displacement of part of a limb away from the midline.

Varus: a deformity involving oblique displacement of part of a limb towards the midline.

Static postural assessment

Stability in the upright standing position requires the centre of mass of the body, which is located just anterior to the second sacral vertebra,[2] to remain over the base of support: the feet. In the upright standing position, small oscillations of the body's centre of mass occur in both the anterior–posterior and the medial–lateral direction, referred to as 'postural sway'.[1,4] Postural alignment of the whole body is the sum of the alignment of the adjacent segments (parts). Any malalignment between adjacent segments may lead to a localised impairment (referred to as a primary postural malalignment[2]). It might also be a compensatory malalignment of other adjacent or distant segments in order to maintain the centre of mass over the BoS and the position of the eyes level. Postural malalignments can be caused by many factors including bony deformities, muscle imbalance, joint hypermobility or hypomobility, pain leading to muscle guarding and avoidance postures, excessive body mass, clothing (shoes), ageing, poor postural habits and/or psychological factors such as self-esteem.[4-13] Musculoskeletal pathologies and/or pain may therefore result in local and/or compensatory postural malalignments in more-distant body segments, which can result in changes in the posture of the whole body because body segments are interrelated. Segmental malalignments can also lead to muscular imbalances as the muscles local to the segment adapt over time to the muscle length and strength required to maintain the segment in this position. This is because any persistent muscle activity and positioning can alter the relative length and strength of agonist/antagonist muscles by lengthening one muscle (or muscles) and excessively shortening its opposing muscle(s). As muscle strength is related to muscle length, the relative strength of opposing muscles can also change accordingly.

The force generated by the mass of each segment of the body applies an external moment to the joints within each segment. The location of the body's centre of mass relative to the line of gravity within each body segment/joint defines the direction of these external moments.[2] These are balanced (resisted) by either muscles or non-contractile connective tissues (or both) at each body segment.[2] The location of the line of gravity through the segments/joints of the body in the sagittal plane in the upright standing position and its directional effect are displayed in Table 8.1. The muscle activity in the upright posture with optimal alignment and symmetrical weight-bearing through the lower limbs should be consistent

TABLE 8.1 Location of the line of gravity, the external moment of gravity and the stabilising tissue in the segments/joints of the body[a]

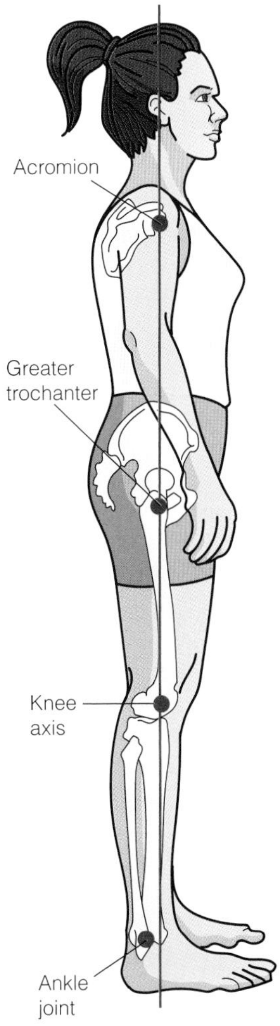

	COLUMN 1 Body segment	COLUMN 2 Line of gravity through segment	COLUMN 3 External moment (force of gravity on segment)	COLUMN 4 Segment stabilised by:
Cervical spine	External auditory meatus in vertical line with acromion process Curvature: lordosis	Cervical flexion	Cervical erector spinae (semispinalis muscle)
	Thoracic spine	Through vertebral bodies Curvature: kyphosis	Thoracic flexion	Thoracic erector spinae, some scapula retraction (slight activity upper trapezius, serratus anterior, middle trapezius, rhomboids major/minor)
	Lumbar spine/pelvis	Through vertebral bodies with anterior superior iliac spine and posterior superior iliac spine level in horizontal plane Curvature: lordosis	Lumbar extension	Lower abdominal wall tension, low level of contraction of rectus abdominis, internal oblique, external oblique, transverse abdominis (support abdominal contents)
	Hips	Slightly posterior to centre of hip joint	Hip extension	Anterior hip joint capsule/ligaments with intermittent iliopsoas activity to prevent creep of the ligaments
	Knees	Slightly anterior to centre of knee joint	Knee extension	Ligaments of the knee, passive joint stability
	Ankle	Slightly anterior to lateral malleolus	Dorsiflexion	Soleus muscle
	Foot	Through talus (even weight bearing between ball and heel of foot)	Flatten longitudinal arches of the foot	Passive (bony alignment and ligaments) and dynamic (extrinsic and intrinsic muscles of the foot) provide stability of longitudinal arches of the foot

Diagram labels: Acromion, Greater trochanter, Knee axis, Ankle joint

[a] Location of the line of gravity through the segments/joints of the body in the sagittal plane in the upright standing position with optimal alignment (columns 1 and 2). The directional effect of the external moment of gravity through each segment/joint (column 3) and the tissue within each segment that resists the force of gravity to stabilise the segment/joint (column 4)

TABLE 8.2 Segmental muscle activity required to maintain optimal alignment in the sagittal plane in the upright standing position

BODY SEGMENT	SEGMENTAL MUSCLE ACTIVITY
Head and cervical spine	Cervical erector spinae
Thoracic spine and scapula	Thoracic erector spinae and scapula retractor muscles (middle trapezius, rhomboids major/minor)
Lumbar spine and pelvis	Rectus abdominis, internal oblique, external oblique, transverse abdominis to support abdominal contents
Hip joint	No activity of gluteus maximus – should be soft to palpation
Knee joint	No activity of quadriceps – should be soft to palpation
Ankle joint	Soleus
Foot	Intrinsic and extrinsic foot muscles to stabilise longitudinal arches of the foot

Note: Muscle activity should only be at a low level of maximal voluntary contraction

with the tissues at each segment/joint. These are used to resist the external moments and to stabilise each segment/joint. This is displayed in Tables 8.1 and 8.2. Passive tissues (ligaments and bony alignment), for example, stabilise the knee joint, therefore the quadriceps muscle should have minimal muscle activity in the erect standing position.[2] The muscle activity required to resist the external moments at each segment/joint is low, requiring a relatively low level of muscle contraction intensity (low percentage of maximal voluntary contraction). Consequently, maintaining optimal alignment in the upright standing position should be very efficient and require a low level of energy expenditure. Although postural sway will affect muscle activity at each segment/joint, it will cause only intermittent bursts of muscle activity.

Fixed postural malalignments cannot be improved as they are due to changes to bone structure; for example, an excessive thoracic kyphosis posture due to anterior wedging of the thoracic vertebral bodies is an example of a fixed postural malalignment. Postural education and exercises can still be prescribed and helpful to the patient, to limit any further progression of the postural malalignment. Adjustable postural malalignments can be improved through variation in muscle activity, to shift the alignment of the centre of mass through the segments of the body. Physical barriers such as restrictions in joint range of motion, muscle flexibility or deficiencies in muscle strength may limit changes to adjustable postural malalignments, to efficiently achieve and maintain optimal alignment of the segments.

Examples of common adjustable postural malalignments and their physical barriers include: (i) knee and hip flexion postural malalignments due to restrictions in knee and hip joint extension range of motion; (ii) excessive thoracic kyphosis angle due to decreased flexibility of the pectoralis minor and major muscles; (iii) excessive lumbar lordosis due to deficient strength of the lower abdominal wall muscles.

Postural exercises aiming to optimise the alignment of adjustable postural malalignments may incorporate joint range of motion, muscle flexibility and muscle-strengthening exercises, as well as education and kinaesthetic awareness of optimal postural alignment.[3]

The spinal curvature within the cervical region is commonly measured at the cervicothoracic junction as the relative location of the head (external auditory meatus) and the upper torso (seventh cervical vertebra or acromion process). A forward head posture, where the head sits forwards relative to the trunk (Figure 8.3), is a common postural malalignment that is subjectively classified as mild, moderate or severe. Although this appears to increase with age, reliable and valid (concurrent) measures and data on this postural malalignment are lacking.[14]

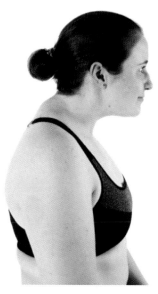

Figure 8.3 Forward head posture

Objective measurement of the specific spinal curvatures is not routinely included in a postural assessment. An exception is where clinical reasoning justifies the time required for an exercise professional to take this measurement. Objective clinical measures of thoracic and lumbar curvature include the use of the Flexicurve ruler (Figure 8.4) or inclinometer (Figure 8.5), which have been strongly correlated to the x-ray Cobb angles.

The interrelationship between pelvic alignment and lumbar lordosis is controversial.[15] There is some evidence to suggest that an anterior pelvic tilt is associated with an increased lordosis (Figure 8.6a) and a posterior pelvic tilt is associated with a decreased lordosis.[16] Pelvic alignment can be measured as the angle formed by a line parallel to the superior surface of the body of S1 and the horizontal, or as the angle formed by a line connecting the posterior superior iliac spine (PSIS) and anterior superior iliac spine (ASIS) with the horizontal (Figure 8.6b and c). The PSIS and ASIS should be approximately in the same horizontal plane.

An excessive lumbar lordosis in the upright standing position can therefore be associated with an excessive anterior tilt of the pelvis and a flexed hip posture owing to the interdependent relationship between the pelvis, hip and lumbar spine in the closed kinetic chain position during upright standing.

Assumptions, limitations and application of postural assessments

The criteria used to classify a posture as 'optimal' is hypothetical and based on research that investigated the postural alignment of participants who had no musculoskeletal pathology or pain.[1] Optimal alignment in the upright standing position is thought to require the least amount of muscular support and is therefore the most efficient, while at the same time minimising any stress on the musculoskeletal system.[4] Normative data constituting optimal posture do not currently exist and there is little evidence to show that a postural abnormality is actually relevant to any musculoskeletal pathology or pain. Postural assessments are therefore only one part of the physical assessment performed by an exercise professional, and clinical reasoning must be used to determine whether any postural abnormalities detected are relevant to the participant's symptoms. Through this clinical reasoning, the exercise professional will determine how much of their exercise prescription and time is targeted at changing the posture of the participant.

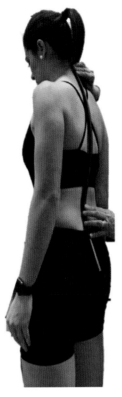

Figure 8.4 Flexicurve ruler

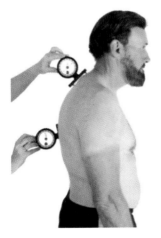

Figure 8.5 Inclinometer measuring thoracic kyphosis

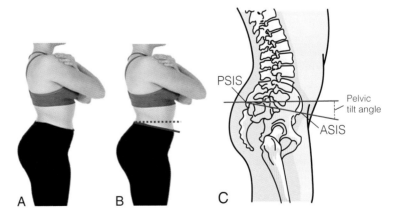

Figure 8.6 a: Increased anterior pelvic tilt and increased lumbar lordosis. b & c: Measuring pelvic alignment

Activity 8.1 Static postural assessment

AIM: perform a static postural assessment of a participant in the upright standing position.

Background

Static postural assessments identify postural deviations or movement compensations. Postural alignment of the whole body is the sum of the alignment of the adjacent parts. Any malalignment between adjacent segments may lead to a localised impairment (referred to as a primary postural malalignment[2]) and/or a compensatory malalignment of other adjacent or distant segments, in order to maintain the centre of mass over the base of support and the position of the eyes level. The challenge for exercise professionals is to determine whether any postural malalignment is a primary or a compensatory abnormality, and whether it is relevant to the participant's symptoms and/or exercise prescription needs.

Protocol summary

Perform the four-stage static postural assessment of a participant by viewing the participant from the side (sagittal plane), behind and in front (coronal plane) – to assess postural alignment and muscle symmetry/activity.

Protocol

1 Work in groups of two, with one person as the participant and the other as an assessor.

2 Ensure that the participant is appropriately dressed, so as to easily view body segments and spinal curvature.

3 Place markers on the external auditory meatus, acromion process, greater trochanter, lateral condyle of the femur and lateral malleolus of the participant (Figure 8.7).

4 Stand the participant in front of the grid rating frame or with a plumb line, that is in line with their lateral malleolus (Figure 8.8).

5 Before each of the following assessments, ask the participant to 'take three steps on the spot and look straight ahead'.

Stage 1: observing and recording static posture

Postural alignment 1: sagittal plane

6 The assessor observes the posture of the participant from side on (sagittal plane) and completes the data-recording sheet by circling either optimal alignment (Option 1), or the appropriate malalignment (Options 2 or 3) for the eight body segments listed.

Postural alignment 2: coronal plane – posterior view

7 The assessor observes the posture of the participant from behind (coronal plane – posterior view). Emphasise to the participant that weight-bearing should be equal on the left and right foot. The assessor completes the data-recording sheet by circling either optimal alignment (Option 1), or the appropriate malalignment (Options 2 or 3) for the eight body segments listed.

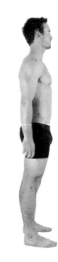

Figure 8.7 Marker placement

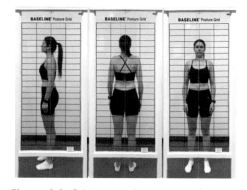

Figure 8.8 Grid rating frame and plumb line (sagittal, posterior and anterior view)

Muscle symmetry/tone/bulk 1: coronal plane – posterior view

8 The assessor observes the posture of the participant from behind (coronal plane – posterior view) and notes the symmetry, activity (tone) and bulk of the muscles listed on the muscle symmetry/tone/bulk data-recording sheet. If good symmetry/tone/bulk (Option 1) is observed, the assessor places a 'tick' in this column. If asymmetry is observed, the assessor records which is the smaller side in Option 2 (e.g. 'asymmetry – left < right'). If unilateral poor tone or hyperactivity is observed, the assessor writes the level of muscle activity and on which side (e.g. 'poor tone – left') in Option 2. If bilateral poor tone or hyperactivity is observed then the assessor records in a similar manner (e.g. 'poor tone – bilateral').

Postural alignment 3: coronal plane – anterior view

9 The assessor observes the posture of the participant from the front (coronal plane – anterior view) and completes the data-recording sheet by circling either optimal alignment (Option 1), or the appropriate malalignment (Options 2 or 3) for the eight body segments listed.

Muscle symmetry/tone/bulk 2: coronal plane – anterior view

10 The assessor observes the posture of the participant from the front (coronal plane – anterior view) and notes the symmetry, activity (tone) and bulk of the muscles listed on the muscle symmetry/tone/ bulk data-recording sheet. If good symmetry/tone/bulk (Option 1) is observed, the assessor places a 'tick' in this column. If asymmetry is observed, the assessor records which is the smaller side in Option 2 (e.g. 'asymmetry – left < right'). if unilateral poor tone or hyperactivity is observed, the assessor writes the level of muscle activity and on which side (e.g. 'poor tone – left') in Option 2. If bilateral poor tone or hyperactivity is observed then the assessor records in a similar manner (e.g. 'poor tone – bilateral').

11 Complete the data-recording sheet 'Summary of postural assessment in the sagittal and coronal planes' by providing a list of any observed malalignments, asymmetries from the previous data-recording sheets and any possible physical barriers that may be limiting the achievement of optimal alignment (e.g. limitations in range of motion, muscle length or muscle strength).

Stage 2: communicating postural malalignments

12 The assessor uses a full-length mirror to show the participant any observed postural malalignments or muscle asymmetries and to determine whether they are kinaesthetically aware of any postural malalignment.

Stage 3: determining whether postural malalignments are fixed or adjustable

13 The assessor will then guide the participant to move out of any postural malalignment observed to correct (optimise) their postural alignment. Some examples of cues that may assist the participant to improve postural malalignments are provided in Table 8.3. This will determine whether the observed postural malalignments are fixed or adjustable.

Stage 4: prescription of postural exercises that address physical barriers

14 Although a postural malalignment may be identified, it is important to consider whether it is relevant to the participant's symptoms and/or exercise goals; that is, should postural change be included in the treatment aims and exercise prescription? Specific exercises should be prescribed to address any identified physical barriers of range of motion, flexibility or strength deficits. Postural education may be needed. If any symptoms are aggravated then the participant should be referred to a physiotherapist. A follow-up assessment should be scheduled to evaluate the effectiveness of the prescribed exercises.

TABLE 8.3 Examples of cues to assist participant to improve (correct) any observed postural malalignment

BODY REGION	CUES
Base of support	Stand up straight with your body weight evenly distributed between your left and right foot and between the balls and heels of your feet.
Knees	Soften the muscles on the front of your thighs.
Centre of mass (pelvis)	Gently draw in your lower abdominal muscles and tuck your bottom in slightly. Your buttock muscles (gluteus maximus) and lower back muscles (lumbar erector spinae) should feel soft to touch.
Sternum	Your breastbone should be facing upwards and forwards.
Head	Eyes look straight ahead.

Data recording

Participant's name: _____   Date: _____

Age: _____ years   Sex: _____

Postural alignment 1: sagittal plane

Circle the observed posture for each segment/joint (row) in either Option 1, 2 or 3.

BODY SEGMENT	OPTION 1 OPTIMAL ALIGNMENT	OPTION 2 MALALIGNMENT	OPTION 3 MALALIGNMENT
Head position/ cervical spine	Head over trunk, normal cervical lordosis	Forward head posture	
Thoracic spine	Sternum facing up and forwards, normal kyphosis	Hyperkyphotic	Hypokyphotic
Lumbar spine	Normal lordosis	Hyperlordosis + bulging abdominal wall	Hypolordosis

continued

Data recording (continued)

BODY SEGMENT	OPTION 1 OPTIMAL ALIGNMENT	OPTION 2 MALALIGNMENT	OPTION 3 MALALIGNMENT
Pelvic alignment	ASIS and PSIS level (normal)	Anterior pelvic tilt	Posterior pelvic tilt
Hips	$0°$ hip extension	Flexed hip (anterior pelvic tilt)	Hyper extended ($>0°$ hip (posterior pelvic tilt)
Knees	$0°$ knee extension	Hyperextended (genu recurvatum)	Flexed left knee
Ankles	Plantargrade	Plantarflexed	Dorsiflexed left ankle

continued overpage

Data recording *(continued)*

BODY SEGMENT	OPTION 1 OPTIMAL ALIGNMENT	OPTION 2 MALALIGNMENT	OPTION 3 MALALIGNMENT
Feet	Normal medial longitudinal arch	Excessively pronated	Excessively supinated

Postural alignment 2: coronal plane – posterior view

Circle the observed posture for each segment/joint (row) in either Option 1, 2 or 3.

BODY SEGMENT	OPTION 1 OPTIMAL ALIGNMENT	OPTION 2 MALALIGNMENT	OPTION 3 MALALIGNMENT
Head position/ cervical spine	Head midline	Left side flexed	Right side flexed
Shoulders	Shoulders level	Left side elevated	Right side elevated
Scapulae	Symmetrical position	Left side elevated	Right side elevated

continued

Data recording *(continued)*

BODY SEGMENT	OPTION 1 OPTIMAL ALIGNMENT	OPTION 2 MALALIGNMENT	OPTION 3 MALALIGNMENT
Coronal spinal curvature	No lateral curvature	Lateral curvature (scoliosis): left side flexed and right rotated thoracolumbar region	Lateral curvature (scoliosis): right side flexed and left rotated in thoracolumbar region
Iliac crests	Iliac crest level	Left side elevated	Right side elevated
Gluteal folds	Gluteal folds level	Left side lower than right and smaller muscle bulk	Right side lower than left and smaller muscle bulk
Knee creases	Knee creases level	Left side elevated	Right side elevated
Calcaneus alignment	Neutral arch and symmetrical weight-bearing between the left and right feet	Left foot excessively pronated (calcaneovalgus)	Right foot excessively supinated (calcaneovarus)

continued overpage

Data recording *(continued)*

Muscle symmetry/tone/bulk 1: coronal plane — posterior view

For each muscle, if good symmetry/tone/muscle bulk is observed then place a tick in each region in Option 1. If asymmetry/lack of tone/hyperactivity/decreased muscle bulk then record details in Option 2.

MUSCLE	OPTION 1 GOOD SYMMETRY/ TONE/BULK	OPTION 2 ASYMMETRY/LACK OF TONE/HYPERACTIVITY/ DECREASED MUSCLE BULK
Upper trapezius		
Triceps		
Thoracic/lumbar erector spinae		
Gluteus maximus		
Hamstrings		
Gastrocnemius/soleus		

Postural alignment 3: coronal plane — anterior view

Circle the observed posture for each segment (row) in either Option 1, 2 or 3.

BODY SEGMENT	OPTION 1 OPTIMAL ALIGNMENT	OPTION 2 MALALIGNMENT	OPTION 3 MALALIGNMENT
Head position/ cervical spine	Head midline	Left side flexed	Right side flexed
Shoulders	Shoulders level, palms facing the lateral aspect of the thigh	Left shoulder elevated (may be accompanied by internal rotation of ipsilateral glenohumeral joint)	Right shoulder elevated (may be accompanied by internal rotation of ipsilateral glenohumeral joint)

continued

Data recording *(continued)*

BODY SEGMENT	OPTION 1 OPTIMAL ALIGNMENT	OPTION 2 MALALIGNMENT	OPTION 3 MALALIGNMENT
Iliac crests	Iliac crests level	Left side elevated	Right side elevated
Hip (as indicated by patella orientation)	Patellae facing directly forwards	Patellae facing medially (hip internal rotation)	Patellae facing laterally (hip external rotation)
Knee	Angle between femur and tibia $<15°$ (knees face straight with feet and knees similar distance apart)	Genu valgum (knock knees)	Genu varum (bow legs)
Feet	Slightly turned out and symmetrical weight-bearing between the left and right feet	Feet pointing medially (hip internal rotation)	Feet pointing laterally (hip external rotation)

continued overpage

Data recording *(continued)*

Muscle symmetry/tone/bulk 1: coronal plane — anterior view

For each muscle, if good symmetry/tone/muscle bulk is observed then place a tick in for Option 1. If asymmetry/lack of tone/hyperactivity/decreased muscle bulk then record details in Option 2.

MUSCLE	OPTION 1 GOOD SYMMETRY/TONE/BULK	OPTION 2 ASYMMETRY/LACK OF TONE/HYPERACTIVITY/DECREASED MUSCLE BULK
Pectoralis major		
Deltoid		
Biceps brachii		
Abdominal wall		
Quadriceps		
Dorsiflexors		

Summary of postural assessment in the sagittal and coronal planes

ASSESSMENT	OBSERVATIONS
Sagittal plane — postural alignment	
Coronal plane — postural alignment	
Muscle symmetry/tone/bulk	
Stage 1: Summary	
Stage 2: Is participant aware of any postural malalignment?	
Stage 3: Are postural malalignments fixed or adjustable?	
Stage 4: Prescription of exercises/strategies to address possible physical barriers (e.g. ROM, muscle length, muscle strength)? Barriers: Exercise prescription/strategies:	

Activity 8.2 Dynamic postural assessment

AIM: to perform a dynamic postural assessment of a participant during various exercises.

Background

Dynamic posture assessments involve observing the posture of the segments of the body during various movements. These movements are commonly activities of daily living, strength and flexibility exercises or movements specific to sport or work tasks. The ability to observe the body as a whole during movement is a specific skill that takes time and practice to develop. Students learn this skill by initially observing body segments (i.e. upper limb, trunk, lower limb) rather than the body as a whole unit, while movements are performed at slow speeds. Movements performed at high speeds can be difficult for even a skilled observer of dynamic posture to analyse. Consequently, they are commonly recorded on a device and replayed at a slower speed for visual (observational) analysis. These recordings can also be used to educate participants on how to improve their dynamic posture and movement quality.

Physical barriers such as restrictions in joint range of motion (ROM), muscle flexibility or deficiencies in muscle strength and motor control may limit the ability of the body to perform a movement with optimal dynamic posture. During this activity, students will practise their observational skills of assessing dynamic posture.

The dynamic postural assessments have the same four stages as the static postural assessment. Five movements referred to as 'test movements' will be assessed to guide students on the principles of dynamic postural analysis, which can then be applied to assess any movement. Each movement that is assessed is organised into a table (data-recording sheet) with four columns.

Column 1: Contains the test movement along with easier and harder versions of the test movement. If the participant performs the test movement correctly according to the criteria in column 2, use a harder version of the test movement. If the test movement is too difficult for the participant to perform, use an easier version of the test movement.

Column 2: Contains the optimal dynamic posture of the body segments (trunk/upper limb/lower limb) that should be observed when the test movement is performed correctly (i.e. with optimal dynamic posture).

Column 3: Contains potential physical deficiencies in strength, flexibility or motor control that may explain why the observed test movement was not performed correctly (i.e. with optimal dynamic posture).

Protocol summary

Perform the four-stage dynamic postural assessment of a participant while they perform five test movements.

Protocol

1 Work in groups of three, with one person acting as the participant and two as assessors.

Stage 1: observing and recording dynamic posture

2 One of the assessors demonstrates the test movement described in column 1 on the data-recording sheet. Ensure that the participant understands the essential components of the test movement prior to attempting the exercise.

3 The participant performs the test movement as the assessors observe the segmental dynamic posture of the trunk/upper limb/lower limb, comparing it with the optimal segmental dynamic posture described in column 2. The assessors cross out (strikethrough) any of the criteria in column 2 they observe to be moving 'non-optimally' (i.e. different to what is written in column 2). Notes explaining what has been observed are added to column 2.

4 If the test movement is too easy for the participant such that the assessors do not highlight or cross out any criteria in column 2, a harder version of the test movement is performed until the participant fails at least one of the criteria in column 2. The assessors circle the version of the test movement used. The participant then performs this version of the test movement as the assessors cross out the criteria in column 2 that they observe to be moving 'non-optimally'.

5 If the test movement is too difficult for the participant to perform, the easier version of the test movement is performed and analysed by the assessors.

Stage 2: communicating postural malalignments

6 Once stage 1 is complete (dynamic posture observed and recorded), the assessors show the participant any dynamic postural malalignment observed and determine whether the participant is kinaesthetically aware of any dynamic postural malalignment.

Stage 3: determining whether postural malalignments are fixed or adjustable

7 The assessor will then guide the participant to move with correct dynamic postural alignment and identify any physical barriers (deficiencies in strength, flexibility or motor control) that may explain why the observed test movement was not performed correctly. If the participant is **able** to perform the movement correctly with the additional guidance from the assessors, it is likely that motor control is the only physical barrier. If they are **still not able** to perform the movement correctly, they are likely to also have physical barriers associated with ROM, flexibility or muscle strength.

8 Using the results of step 7 and participant feedback with questions such as 'What about the movement is difficult?' and 'What do you feel is limiting you from performing the movement correctly?', in conjunction with their prior knowledge of anatomy and biomechanics, the assessors then circle or write in column 3 any physical deficiencies in strength, flexibility or motor control which they believe explains why the test movement was not performed correctly.

9 Examples of participant feedback: 'The movement was too difficult' may indicate a deficiency in muscle strength or motor control. 'I felt tightness in the front of my thigh during the movement' may indicate a deficiency in muscle flexibility.

Stage 4: prescription of postural exercises that address physical barriers

10 Summarise the physical limitations (deficiencies in strength, flexibility or motor control) identified in column 3, which could later be addressed by an appropriate exercise prescription intervention to allow the test movement to be performed with optimal dynamic posture. These should be personalised to address the needs and goals of the participant.

Data recording

Participant's name: _____   Date: _____

Age: _____ years   Sex: _____

Test movement 1: squat

COLUMN 1	COLUMN 2	COLUMN 3
Test movement (easier/harder versions)	What can you see? Optimal segmental dynamic posture requires:	Why is the participant moving non-optimally? Potential physical barriers (strength, flexibility and/or motor control)
Movement: squat full ROM, × 3 reps – performed SLOWLY	*UL/trunk:* • Head in line with trunk, thoracic spine extension and scapulae retraction, which is maintained throughout movement *Trunk:* • Pelvis initiates movement and moves in a trajectory that is backwards and downwards • Trunk is stable with the lumbar spine in a neutral position and the abdominal wall activated throughout the squat movement	*Flexibility deficiency LL (sensation of tightness in this region):* • Hamstrings ($\downarrow$ combined hip and knee flexion ROM, and/or loss of lumbar lordosis) • Gluteus maximus ($\downarrow$ hip flexion ROM, and/or loss of lumbar lordosis) • Vasti group ($\downarrow$ knee flexion ROM) • Soleus ($\downarrow$ ankle dorsiflexion ROM) *Joint ROM deficiency LL (sensation of stiffness in the joint):* • Hip joint stiffness ($\downarrow$ hip flexion ROM, and/or loss of lumbar lordosis)

continued

Data recording *(continued)*

COLUMN 1	COLUMN 2	COLUMN 3
Easier version: Sit to stand (with higher chair or use of UL) *Harder versions:* Load (weighted squat) Impact (jump squat) ROM (sustain at end of range) 	*LL:* ● No hip adduction/internal rotation, knees stay in vertical line with feet (not moving excessively forwards) ● Heels remain on the ground throughout movement Squat ROM: (knee flexion range) ● $<90°$ knee flexion ● $=90°$ knee flexion ● $>90°$ knee flexion	● Knee joint stiffness ($\downarrow$ knee flexion ROM) ● Ankle joint stiffness ($\downarrow$ ankle dorsiflexion ROM) *Strength deficiency LL (sensation of weakness in this region):* ● Gluteus maximus/hamstrings ($<90°$ knee flexion) ● Gluteus medius/minimus (hip adduction/internal rotation or excessive coronal plane movement of trunk or lateral pelvic tilt) ● Vasti group ($\downarrow$ knee flexion ROM or hip adduction/internal rotation) ● Gastrocnemius/soleus ($\downarrow$ ankle dorsiflexion ROM) *Strength deficiency trunk:* ● Abdominals/deep lumbar spine stabilising muscles (excessive coronal plane movement of trunk or excessive erector spinae activity and bulging of the abdominal wall or movement of the vertebral column in sagittal plane) ● UL: scapulae retractors/thoracic extensors (excessive scapulae protraction and elevation when glenohumeral joint flexion is above $90°$) *Motor control:* ● Poor control of hip/knee/ankle alignment (hip adduction/internal rotation) ● Poor control of trunk posture (excessive coronal plane movement of trunk or excessive erector spinae activity and bulging of the abdominal wall or movement of the vertebral column in sagittal plane) ● Poor control of lumbar spine/pelvic alignment at low point of squat movement, and/or loss of lumbar lordosis

LL = lower limbs; ROM = range of motion; UL = upper limbs

continued overpage

Data recording *(continued)*

Test movement 2: lunge

COLUMN 1	COLUMN 2	COLUMN 3
Test movement (easier/harder versions)	*What can you see?* Optimal segmental dynamic posture requires:	*Why is the participant moving non-optimally?* Potential physical barriers (strength, flexibility and/or motor control)
Step lunge: (LL/trunk strength) Feet hip width apart *Movement:* large step forwards (lunge) & return to starting position $\times$ 3 reps – SLOW Standardise foot position: Compare left/right lower limb positions *Easier version:* Supported static lunge with less ROM *Harder versions:* Load: add hand weights	*Trunk:* <ul><li>Head in line with trunk, thoracic spine extension and scapulae retraction, which are maintained throughout movement</li><li>Pelvis (ASIS/PSIS) and shoulders level, trunk upright (no leaning forwards or to either side)</li><li>Trunk is stable with the lumbar spine in a neutral position, abdominal wall activated throughout the squat movement</li><li>No $\uparrow$ in erector spinae activity or $\uparrow$ in lordosis of lumbar spine as step front leg forwards in lunge</li></ul> *Front LL:* <ul><li>Correct hip/knee/ankle alignment throughout – no knee valgus</li><li>Front heel stays on ground throughout movement</li></ul> *Back LL:* <ul><li>Strong gluteus maximus contraction</li><li>Correct hip/knee/ankle alignment</li><li>No rotation (pivot) of foot on ground</li></ul> *Lunge ROM: (distance that back knee reaches to the floor in low point of movement):* <ul><li>Back knee touches floor</li><li>Back knee greater than $\frac{1}{2}$ way to floor</li><li>Back knee less than $\frac{1}{2}$ way to floor</li></ul>	*Flexibility deficiency front lower limb (sensation of tightness in this region):* <ul><li>Hamstrings ($\downarrow$ hip flexion ROM)</li><li>Gluteus maximus ($\downarrow$ hip flexion ROM)</li><li>Vasti group ($\downarrow$ knee flexion ROM)</li><li>Soleus ($\downarrow$ ankle dorsiflexion ROM or heel lifts off ground)</li></ul> *Flexibility deficiency back lower limb (sensation of tightness in this region):* <ul><li>Iliopsoas ($\downarrow$ hip extension ROM)</li><li>Rectus femoris ($\downarrow$ hip extension and knee flexion ROM)</li><li>Soleus ($\downarrow$ ankle dorsiflexion ROM or pivot of foot on ground)</li></ul> *Strength deficiency front LL (sensation of weakness in this region):* <ul><li>Gluteus maximus/hamstrings (lengthen range) ($\downarrow$ hip flexion ROM)</li><li>Gluteus medius/minimus (poor hip/knee/ankle alignment or excessive coronal plane movement of trunk or lateral pelvic tilt)</li><li>Vasti group ($\downarrow$ knee flexion ROM)</li><li>Gastrocnemius/soleus ($\downarrow$ knee flexion and ankle dorsiflexion ROM)</li></ul> *Strength deficiency back LL (sensation of weakness in this region):* <ul><li>Gluteus maximus (weak in shortened range) ($\downarrow$ hip extension ROM)</li><li>Rectus femoris (in shortened range at the hip) ($\downarrow$ hip extension ROM)</li></ul>

continued

Data recording *(continued)*

COLUMN 1	COLUMN 2	COLUMN 3
Stability: step up lunge		<ul><li>Gluteus medius/minimus (poor hip/knee/ankle alignment or excessive coronal plane movement of trunk or lateral pelvic tilt)</li><li>Vasti group ($\downarrow$ knee flexion ROM)</li><li>Gastrocnemius/soleus ($\downarrow$ ankle dorsiflexion ROM)</li></ul>
Impact: jump lunge		*Strength deficiency trunk:* <ul><li>Coronal plane: abdominals/ deep lumbar spine stabiliser muscles (excessive coronal plane movement of trunk/lateral pelvic tilt</li><li>Sagittal plane: abdominals/deep lumbar spine stabiliser muscles (excessive erector spinae activity and bulging of the abdominal wall, and/or increase lumbar lordosis)</li></ul>*Motor control:* <ul><li>Poor control of hip/knee/ankle alignment (hip adduction/ internal rotation)</li><li>Poor control of trunk posture (excessive coronal or sagittal plane movement of trunk/pelvis or excessive erector spinae activity and bulging of the abdominal wall)</li><li>Poor balance throughout movement</li></ul>

ASIS = anterior superior iliac spine; LL = lower limbs; PSIS = posterior superior iliac spine; ROM = range of motion; UL = upper limbs

continued overpage

Data recording *(continued)*

Test movement 3: step down

COLUMN 1	COLUMN 2	COLUMN 3
Test movement (easier/harder versions)	*What can you see?* Optimal segmental dynamic posture requires:	*Why is the participant moving non-optimally?* Potential physical barriers (strength, flexibility and/or motor control)
Movement: start with both feet on the step then step down $\times$ 3 reps – SLOW. Compare left/ right lower limb stepping down	*Trunk:* • Head in line with trunk, trunk upright (no leaning forwards or to either side), trunk stable – neutral position lumbar spine, abdominal wall activated throughout the movement • Pelvis (ASIS/PSIS) and shoulders level *Weight-bearing LL:* • Strong contraction of gluteus maximus and gluteus medius/minimus • No lateral tilt of pelvis • Correct hip/knee/ankle alignment throughout movement – no knee valgus • Heel stays on step throughout movement	*Flexibility deficiency weight-bearing LL (sensation of tightness in this region):* • Soleus ($\downarrow$ ankle dorsiflexion ROM; heel lifts off ground or increased pronation) *Strength weight-bearing LL (sensation of weakness in this region):* • Gluteus medius/minimus (lateral tilt of pelvis, poor hip/knee/ ankle alignment – knee valgus) • Gluteus maximus ($\downarrow$ hip flexion ROM or unsteady (poor balance on the standing leg) • Vasti group ($\downarrow$ knee flexion ROM or poor hip/knee/ankle alignment – knee valgus) • Soleus ($\downarrow$ ankle dorsiflexion ROM or increased pronation)
Easier versions: Trendelenburg test: one leg stance Assisted for step down *Harder versions:* ROM: 1 leg squat Stability: stand on disc Impact: 1 leg hop Load: add hand weights	*Non-weight-bearing LL:* • Correct hip/knee/ankle alignment *Step-down ROM (distance that non-weight-bearing heel or toe reaches to the floor from standing position):* • Toe very near to floor • Toe ½ step height • Toe reaches top of step only	*Strength deficiency trunk:* • Coronal plane: abdominals/ deep lumbar spine stabiliser muscles (excessive coronal plane movement of trunk /lateral pelvic tilt) • Sagittal plane: abdominals/ deep lumbar spine stabiliser muscles (excessive erector spinae activity and bulging of the abdominal wall and/or $\uparrow$ in lumbar lordosis *Motor control:* • Poor balance throughout movement • Poor control of hip/knee/ankle alignment (hip adduction/ internal rotation) • Poor control of trunk posture (excessive coronal or sagittal plane movement of trunk/pelvis or excessive erector spinae activity and bulging of the abdominal wall) • Poor control of lumbar spine/ pelvic alignment at low point of movement 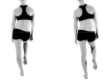

ASIS = anterior superior iliac spine; LL = lower limbs; PSIS = posterior superior iliac spine; ROM = range of motion; UL = upper limbs

continued

Data recording *(continued)*

Test movement 4: bird dog

COLUMN 1	COLUMN 2	COLUMN 3
Test movement (easier/harder versions)	*What can you see?* Optimal segmental dynamic posture requires:	*Why is the participant moving non-optimally?* Potential physical barriers (strength, flexibility and/or motor control)
Bird dog (trunk/LL/UL strength) *Position:* prone kneeling with knees/hands hip width apart, knees under hips, hands under shoulders, scapula retracted and neutral spine re thoracic kyphosis and lumbar lordosis, head in line with trunk	*Trunk:* • Head in line with trunk, trunk stable – neutral position lumbar spine, abdominal wall activated throughout the movement	*Strength deficiency trunk (sensation of weakness in this region):* • Sagittal plane: abdominals/deep lumbar spine stabiliser muscles (excessive erector spinae activity and bulging of the abdominal wall or movement of the vertebral column in sagittal plane) – $\uparrow$ lumbar lordosis or thoracic kyphosis
Movement: lift opposite upper limb and lower limb until they are parallel to ground (hip/knee extension and shoulder flexion/elbow extension). Do not move vertebral column. $\times$ 3 reps – SLOW; compare movement along left diagonal to right diagonal *Easier version:* Move upper limb and lower limb in isolation to each other	• Pelvis (ASIS/PSIS) and shoulders level, no rotation trunk or $\uparrow$ lumbar lordosis or thoracic kyphosis as the UL or LL are moved • No posterior shift of COG, i.e. $\uparrow$ knee flexion of weight-bearing leg as the UL or LL are moved *Non-weight-bearing lower limb:* • Hip extension/knee extension movement with no $\uparrow$ lumbar lordosis *Bird dog (non-weight-bearing) LL ROM: (hip flexion range):* • Hip flexion angle: $= 0°$ • Hip flexion angle: $0–45°$ • Hip flexion angle: $>45°$ *Non-weight-bearing UL:* • Shoulder flexion/elbow extension movement only with no $\uparrow$ thoracic kyphosis *Bird dog UL ROM: (position of arm/forearm relative to the ground):* • Horizontal to ground • ½ way horizontal to ground • Less than ½ way horizontal to ground	• Transverse plane: abdominals/deep lumbar spine stabiliser muscles (excessive rotation of pelvis/trunk) *Strength LL (sensation of weakness in this region):* • Weight-bearing LL – gluteus medius/minimus (rotation trunk or pelvic asymmetry) or $\uparrow$ lumbar lordosis or posterior shift of COG (no $\uparrow$ knee flexion) of weight-bearing leg as the UL or LL are moved) • Non-weight-bearing LL – gluteus maximus/hamstrings ($\downarrow$ hip extension ROM or unstable) • Non-weight-bearing LL – vasti group ($\downarrow$ knee extension ROM) *Strength UL (sensation of weakness in this region):* • Weight-bearing UL – scapular stabilisers – co-contraction serratus anterior/upper and lower trapezius with rhomboids/middle trapezius (poor scapulohumeral rhythm e.g. excessive elevation of scapulae or excessive rotation of pelvis/trunk) • Non-weight-bearing UL – deltoid, latissimus dorsi/teres major with scapular stabilisers – co-contraction serratus anterior/upper and lower trapezius with rhomboids/middle trapezius ($\downarrow$ shoulder flexion ROM)

continued overpage

Data recording *(continued)*

COLUMN 1	COLUMN 2	COLUMN 3
Harder versions: Load: add hand weights Stability: unstable base/on toes instead of knee 		*Flexibility deficiency non-weight-bearing LL* *(sensation of tightness in this region):* • Iliopsoas ($\downarrow$ hip extension ROM) *Flexibility deficiency non-weight-bearing UL* *(sensation of tightness in this region):* • Pectoralis major ($\downarrow$ shoulder flexion ROM) • Latissimus dorsi/teres major ($\downarrow$ shoulder flexion ROM) • Rhomboids/middle trapezius ($\downarrow$ shoulder flexion ROM) *Motor control:* • Poor hip/pelvis/lumbar spine control – $\uparrow$ lumbar lordosis with hip extension and bulging of the abdominal wall • Poor scapulohumeral rhythm/thoracic spine control – $\uparrow$ thoracic kyphosis with shoulder flexion • Poor control of trunk/pelvis in transverse plane – drop of pelvis on non-weight-bearing LL side • Poor balance throughout movement

ASIS = anterior superior iliac spine; COG = centre of gravity; LL = lower limbs; PSIS = posterior superior iliac spine; ROM = range of motion; UL = upper limbs

continued

Data recording *(continued)*

Test movement 5: push up

COLUMN 1	COLUMN 2	COLUMN 3
Test movement (easier/harder versions)	*What can you see?* Optimal segmental dynamic posture requires:	*Why is the participant moving non-optimally?* Potential physical barriers (strength, flexibility and/or motor control)
Position: hands hip width apart and under shoulders, scapula retracted, thoracic spine extension, head in line with trunk, lumbar spine neutral position *Movement:* push-up $\times$ 3 reps – SLOW *Easier version:* Load: wall push-up or incline push-up 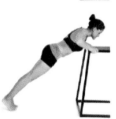 *Harder versions:* Load: on toes, decline pushup Stability: on Swiss ball 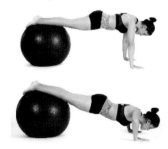	*Trunk:* • Head in line with trunk, trunk stable – neutral position lumbar spine, abdominal wall activated throughout the movement • No ↑ lumbar lordosis or thoracic kyphosis as move UL *UL:* • Even, smooth movement of GHJ horizontal extension/elbow flexion with wrist extension and scapulothoracic joint retraction (no ↑ scapula elevation or thoracic kyphosis) *Push-up ROM (distance of chest to the ground at the low point of the movement):* • Chest to floor • Chest ½ to floor • Chest less than ½ to floor	*Strength deficiency UL (sensation of weakness in this region):* • Serratus anterior (poor scapulohumeral rhythm e.g. excessive winging of scapulae or ↓ ROM chest to floor) • Scapulae stabilisers: co-contraction serratus anterior with rhomboids/middle trapezius (poor scapulohumeral rhythm, e.g. excessive elevation scapula or ↓ ROM chest to floor) • GHJ stabilisers sagittal plane: co-contraction pectoralis major and anterior deltoid with latissimus dorsi/teres major/posterior deltoid (↓ ROM chest to floor or excessive elevation scapula) • Elbow: co-contraction triceps/brachialis (↓ ROM chest to floor – elbow flexion) *Strength deficiency trunk (sensation of weakness in this region):* • Sagittal plane: rectus abdominis/internal oblique/external oblique/deep lumbar spine stabiliser muscles (excessive bulging of the abdominal wall or movement of the vertebral column in sagittal plane – ↑ lumbar lordosis or thoracic kyphosis) *Strength deficiency LL (sensation of weakness in this region):* • Hips: co-contraction gluteus maximus with iliopsoas (↑ lumbar lordosis and anterior pelvic tilt) *Flexibility deficiency UL (sensation of weakness in this region):* • Serratus anterior (↓ ROM chest to floor) • Pectoralis major/minor (↓ ROM chest to floor) • Anterior deltoid (↓ ROM chest to floor)

continued overpage

Data recording *(continued)*

COLUMN 1	COLUMN 2	COLUMN 3
		Motor control: • Poor control lumbar spine control ($\uparrow$ lumbar lordosis and bulging of the abdominal wall) • Poor control scapulohumeral rhythm/thoracic spine control ($\uparrow$ thoracic kyphosis with shoulder movement) • Poor control scapula stabilisers (poor scapulohumeral rhythm, e.g. excessive scapulae protraction or elevation)

GHJ = glenohumeral joint; LL = lower limbs; ROM = range of motion; UL = upper limbs

Case studies

The following case studies are presented as worked examples of postural assessments of common postural abnormalities.

Case Study 1

Setting: A 55-year-old man (BMI: 29 kg/m^2) with mild–moderate osteoarthritis of his left knee has started attending the gym aiming to decrease his body mass after a health check by his GP. He has a 'slight limp' in gait due to decreased left knee extension in stance phase of gait.

Summary of postural assessment in the sagittal and coronal planes

ASSESSMENT	OBSERVATIONS
Sagittal plane – postural alignment	Hip – left: 5° hip flexion Knee – left: 10° knee flexion
Coronal plane – postural alignment	Iliac crests – left: lower than right Gluteal folds – left: lower than right Knee creases – left: lower than right
Muscle symmetry/tone/bulk	Gluteus maximus – left < right Quadriceps – left < right Hamstrings – left < right Gastrocnemius/soleus – left < right

Stage 1: Summary – left knee and hip flexed; muscle atrophy of quadriceps, hamstrings, gluteus maximus and gastrocnemius/soleus.

Stage 2: Is participant aware of any postural malalignment? Participant is unaware of flexed knee and hip posture in standing. He is aware he has a limp when walking.

Stage 3: Are postural malalignments fixed or adjustable? Possibly fixed postural malalignment (fixed knee joint contracture).

Stage 4: Prescription of exercises/strategies to address possible physical barriers (e.g. ROM, muscle length, muscle strength)?

continued

Case studies *(continued)*

BARRIERS: LIMITING KNEE AND HIP JOINT EXTENSION ROM

- decreased flexibility in left hamstrings and gastrocnemius (left knee flexion) or stiffness left knee joint; decreased flexibility left iliopsoas (left hip flexion)
- decreased strength in left quadriceps and gluteus maximus, as well as opposing muscles (hamstrings and gastrocnemius/soleus) = decreased muscle bulk.

Clinical reasoning confirms that postural correction is relevant to the exercise prescription, as it will also allow a normal gait pattern to be achieved, through which physical activity can be increased to achieve the participant's weight loss goal.

EXERCISE PRESCRIPTION/STRATEGIES:

1 *Strength:* strengthening exercises of left quadriceps and gluteus maximus, particularly in their shortened range (to gain strength in any additional extension ROM acquired by the flexibility exercises). Strengthening exercises of opposing muscles are also prescribed (left hamstrings and gastrocnemius) in their lengthened range.

2 *Flexibility:* stretches of left hamstrings and gastrocnemius (and posterior joint capsule) to increase knee extension ROM; stretches of left iliopsoas to increase hip extension ROM.

3 *Postural education:* cues to improve postural alignment of the hip and knees in the upright standing position and during gait in order to use any additional knee and hip extension ROM achieved.

4 *Monitor symptoms:* evaluate whether exercises and/or postural changes aggravate the hip or knee arthritic symptoms and pain. If symptoms are aggravated, recommend referral to physiotherapist for assessment. Evaluate whether the knee and hip extension ROM changes (i.e. it is possible that the postural malalignment is fixed).

Case Study 2

Setting: A 35-year-old woman (BMI: 27 kg/m^2, 8 kg heavier than pre-pregnancy body mass), 6 months post-partum, who wishes to improve her appearance. She feels that she still looks pregnant owing to a sagging abdominal wall.

Summary of postural assessment in the sagittal and coronal planes

ASSESSMENT	OBSERVATIONS
Sagittal plane – postural alignment	Lumbar spine – excessive lordosis, bulging abdominal wall Pelvic alignment – excessive anterior pelvic tilt Hips – flexed in standing due to excessive anterior pelvic tilt
Coronal plane – postural alignment	Feet – symmetrical weight-bearing: greater body mass through forefeet compared with heels
Muscle symmetry/tone/bulk	Lumbar erector spinae – hyperactive in stance (bilateral) Gluteus maximus – decreased muscle mass (bilateral) Hamstrings – hyperactive in stance (bilateral) Abdominal wall – poor tone, no diastasis (separation of linea alba)

Stage 1: Summary – excessive anterior pelvic shift, lumbar lordosis and decreased strength of muscles of anterior abdominal wall (bulging abdominal wall). (NB. increased abdominal adipose tissue can also contribute to increased anterior pelvic tilt (anterior load shifting COM).)

continued overpage

Case studies *(continued)*

Stage 2: Is participant aware of any postural malalignment? Participant can correct both excessive anterior pelvic shift and lumbar lordosis; therefore, it is an adjustable postural malalignment, but she feels she has to contract abdominal muscles a lot to maintain optimal alignment.

Stage 3: Are postural malalignments fixed or adjustable? Participant can correct both excessive anterior pelvic shift and lumbar lordosis. Therefore, she has an adjustable postural malalignment, but she feels she has to contract abdominal muscles a lot and bend her knees to maintain optimal alignment.

Stage 4: Prescription of exercises/strategies to address possible physical barriers (e.g. ROM, muscle length, muscle strength)?

BARRIERS: POSSIBLE BARRIERS LIMITING MAINTENANCE OF OPTIMAL ALIGNMENT OF PELVIC SHIFT AND LUMBAR LORDOSIS EFFICIENTLY:

- decreased strength of internal obliques/external obliques/rectus abdominis/transverse abdominis
- possible decreased flexibility of iliopsoas due to anterior pelvic tilt in closed kinetic chain (flexed hip posture).

Clinical reasoning confirms that postural correction is relevant to the exercise prescription/education as it will also allow optimal alignment to be maintained efficiently.

EXERCISE PRESCRIPTION/STRATEGIES:

1. *Strength:* strengthening of exercises internal oblique/external oblique/rectus abdominis/transverse abdominis particularly in their neutral and shortened range to decrease effort to maintain activation in the upright standing position. Strengthening exercises of gluteus maximus in inner range, e.g. bridging exercise, to assist decreasing anterior pelvic tilt and possibly tight iliopsoas muscle.

2. *Flexibility:* stretches of iliopsoas to decrease resistance to achieve more posteriorly tilted pelvic position (and associated hip extension position) in the upright standing position.

3. *Postural education:* cues to improve postural alignment of the pelvis, lumbar spine and hips in the upright standing position, as well as during dynamic activities such as gait.

4. *Increased physical activity to decrease body mass:* to decrease any increased abdominal adipose tissue that may also be contributing to the increased anterior pelvic tilt by shifting the centre of mass anteriorly.

5. *Monitor symptoms:* evaluate whether exercises and/or postural changes cause any pain in the lumbar spine/pelvic region. If pain occurs, recommend referral to physiotherapist for assessment.

Case Study 3

Setting: A 75-year-old woman (BMI: 20 kg/m^2) with osteopenia is referred by her GP to attend an exercise class to decrease her falls risk. She lives independently and also has an increased thoracic kyphosis, which causes her no problems other than she has some difficulty with activities where her hands are raised above her head.

Summary of postural assessment in the sagittal and coronal planes

ASSESSMENT	OBSERVATIONS
Sagittal plane – postural alignment	Thoracic spine – increased thoracic kyphosis Upper limbs – increased internal rotation glenohumeral joints (bilateral), both scapulae protracted
Coronal plane – postural alignment	
Muscle symmetry/tone/bulk	Thoracic erector spinae – bilateral muscle bulk decreased in erector spinae and scapula retractor muscles

continued

Case studies *(continued)*

Stage 1: Summary – excessive thoracic kyphosis angle, scapulae protraction, glenohumeral joint internal rotation, and decreased strength of thoracic erector spinae and scapula retractor muscles (middle trapezius and rhomboids).

Stage 2: Is participant aware of any postural malalignment? Participant is aware of increased thoracic kyphosis but was not aware of scapulae or shoulder postural malalignments.

Stage 3: Are postural malalignments fixed or adjustable? Participant cannot correct thoracic kyphosis angle but can change protracted position of her scapulae and internal rotation of her glenohumeral joints. Therefore, fixed thoracic kyphosis postural malalignment is due to stiffness of the thoracic spine and wedging thoracic vertebra, but adjustable scapulae protraction postural malalignment.

Stage 4: Prescription of exercises/strategies to address possible physical barriers (e.g. ROM, muscle length, muscle strength)?

BARRIERS: POSSIBLE BARRIERS LIMITING IMPROVEMENT IN SCAPULAE PROTRACTION POSTURE:

- decreased strength of thoracic erector spinae and scapula retractor muscles (middle trapezius and rhomboids), which would also assist to limit any further progression of increased thoracic kyphosis.

Clinical reasoning confirms that postural correction is relevant to the exercise prescription/education as it will limit further progression of the thoracic kyphosis angle and improve the ability to perform activities where her hands are raised above her head.

EXERCISE PRESCRIPTION/STRATEGIES:

1 *Strength:* strengthening exercises of thoracic erector spinae and scapula retractor muscles (middle trapezius and rhomboids) in shortened range to limit further progression of the thoracic kyphosis angle and improve posture of scapulae and glenohumeral joints.

2 *Flexibility:* stretches of pectoralis major/minor and serratus anterior to decrease resistance to achieve more scapulae retraction in the upright standing position.

3 *Postural education:* cues to improve postural alignment of the scapulae and activity of thoracic erector spinae in the upright standing position, as well as during dynamic activities such as activities where her hands are raised above her head.

4 *Monitor symptoms:* evaluate whether exercises and/or postural changes cause any pain in the thoracic spine region. If pain occurs, recommend referral to physiotherapist for assessment.

Case Study 4

Setting: A 55-year-old woman (BMI: 27 kg/m^2) is complaining of mild right lateral hip pain when walking down stairs. You undertake a dynamic postural assessment of her step-down exercise.

Summary of dynamic postural assessment

ASSESSMENT	OBSERVATIONS
Version of test movement performed	Step-down version of the movement off a small step with no upper limb support – with left leg on step and then right leg on step

continued overpage

Case studies *(continued)*

ASSESSMENT	OBSERVATIONS
Non-optimal dynamic alignment	When standing with right leg on step (stepping down with left), patient could not maintain alignment of: <ul><li>trunk in coronal plane or keep pelvis and shoulders level</li><li>poor right hip/knee/ankle alignment (right knee moved into valgus position)</li></ul>
Potential physical barriers	Decreased strength of right gluteus medius and minimus and decreased strength of right gluteus maximus – patient complained that 'the movement was too difficult' Poor awareness of trunk posture – patient was not aware of mal-alignments of their trunk or their right lower limb

Stage 1: Summary – When standing with right leg on step (stepping down with left), patient could not maintain alignment of:

- trunk in coronal plane or keep pelvis and shoulders level;
- poor right hip/knee/ankle alignment (right knee moved into valgus position).

Stage 2: Participant aware of any postural malalignment? Participant was not aware of trunk or lower limb malalignment but felt more unstable and weaker standing on the right lower limb and stepping down with the left foot compared with standing on the left lower limb and stepping down with the right foot.

Stage 3: Are postural malalignments fixed or adjustable? Participant could correct trunk and right lower limb alignment if they held onto a handrail when they stood on right leg. Confirmed as an adjustable *dynamic postural* malalignment.

Stage 4: Prescription of exercises/strategies to address possible physical barriers (e.g. ROM, muscle length, muscle strength)

BARRIERS:

Decreased strength of right gluteus medius and minimus to control pelvic alignment; decreased strength of right gluteus maximus to eccentrically control hip flexion; poor awareness of trunk and lower limb posture.

EXERCISE PRESCRIPTION/STRATEGIES:

1 *Strength:* strengthening exercises of right gluteus medius and minimus and maximus with hip in extension.

2 *Postural education:* cues to improve postural alignment of the trunk and right lower limbs during step down movement.

3 *Monitor symptoms:* evaluate whether exercises and/or postural changes improve right hip pain.

PRACTICAL 9
FLEXIBILITY

Tania Brancato Best, Sally Lark and Tina Skinner

LEARNING OBJECTIVES

- Identify and explain the common terminology, processes and equipment required to conduct accurate and safe measures of flexibility
- Identify and describe the limitations, contraindications or considerations that may require the modification of flexibility assessments, and make appropriate adjustments for relevant populations or participants
- Explain the scientific rationale, purposes, reliability, validity, assumptions and limitations of common flexibility assessments
- Conduct appropriate pre-assessment procedures, including explaining the test and obtaining informed consent and a focused medical history, and performing a pre-exercise risk assessment
- Identify the need for guidance or further information from an appropriate health professional, and recognise when to cease a test
- Select and conduct appropriate protocols for safe and effective flexibility assessments
- Record, analyse and interpret information from flexibility assessments and convey the results, including the validity and limitations of the assessments, through relevant verbal and/or written communication with the participant or involved professional
- Integrate knowledge of and skills in flexibility assessment with other study areas of exercise science, in particular the physiology that underpins common exercise contraindications

Equipment and other requirements

- Information sheet and informed consent form
- Adult Pre-exercise Screening System (APSS) form
- Goniometer and/or inclinometer
- Massage table
- Self-retracting, flexible metal anthropometry tape
- Cleaning and disinfecting equipment (see Appendix A)

INTRODUCTION

Healthy human movement requires a flexible musculoskeletal system that can perform activities of daily living (ADLs), employment and leisure. By measuring range of motion (ROM) about a joint, we are making an indirect judgment about the flexibility of structures, such as soft tissues (fascia, ligaments, tendons and muscles) that surround the joint. Reference ROM data exist for most joints of the body, though there is some minor variation in reported ROM across studies and populations.[1-3] These reference ranges assist health professionals in determining whether a participant has 'normal', reduced or excessive ROM – essential information for prescribing exercise programs. A lack of flexibility may reduce the body's capacity to engage in ADLs. Research is yet to conclusively prove that this may also increase the risk of injury.[4] Alternatively, for participants with excessive flexibility (often labelled 'hypermobility'), studies suggest there may be an increased risk of injury.[5] The potential issues associated with flexibility outside of the reference ROM highlights the need for assessments that identify participants across the flexibility spectrum.

Reference ROM data for apparently healthy populations differ depending on the level of maturation (often simplified to 'years of age') and sex of the participant. Across the lifespan, a person's flexibility is the greatest and most varied during childhood and adolescence, reaches a plateau in adulthood and declines with advancing age.[3,6,7] Sex differences also exist, with females typically demonstrating greater flexibility than males following the onset of puberty.[6,8] Therefore, when assessing flexibility, the ROM measured is considered 'normal flexibility' when appropriate for the specific joint, age and sex of the participant. Variations may exist for target populations such as high-performing athletes, who may achieve different ROM values as a result of their individual sporting requirements (e.g. gymnastics).[7] There are other situations where laxity of joints naturally occurs (e.g. during pregnancy to allow relaxation of the pelvic girdle for expansion of the cervix and pelvic opening for delivery of the baby).[9] This laxity ($>10\%$) is measurable at other joints of the body and is associated with the release of hormones during pregnancy such as relaxin[9] and cortisol.[10]

The effect of hormones on joint laxity involves a complicated interplay between sex hormones, which are altered by exercise and age. In its most simplistic view, testosterone decreases joint laxity and oestrogen increases it. The oestrogen receptor sites on ligaments, tendons and muscles[11] enable oestrogen to block the androgen receptors to testosterone, thereby increasing joint laxity. Indeed, greater ligament and tendon laxity in females has been proposed to explain why females have more anterior cruciate ligament injuries than males.[12] Pre-pubertal injury rates are not different between boys and girls, but, after the age of 12, females experience more sprains.[6,13] Prepubescent boys and girls (8–10-year-olds) also report less tibiofemoral joint stiffness compared with post-pubescent individuals, irrespective of height and mass.[6,13] So it is not unreasonable to assume sex hormones play a role in joint laxity and injury rates.

Oestrogens have a direct effect on collagen and collagen synthesis. High oestrogen concentrations, such as those seen in young women not using contraception, positively influence collagen morphology and biomechanical properties.[14] When oestrogen concentrations are low, such as when taking a contraceptive, or in post-menopausal women not on hormone replacement therapy, collagen synthesis rate and tensile strength decrease, increasing the laxity of the joint. Although oestrogen enhances collagen synthesis, the ligaments of females have significantly lower stress and strain properties[15] compared with males, which is why there is increased joint laxity when androgen receptors to testosterone are blocked.

Several studies have examined the potential link between hormone changes through the menstrual cycle and increased laxity in women. Although increased muscle extensibility has been fairly consistently observed at ovulation when oestrogen levels are at their highest,[16–18] the results of other studies reporting the relationship between sex hormones and joint laxity have been equivocal and appear to be influenced by exercise and training. For example, in 2005 Beynnon and colleagues[19] recorded a greater degree of ankle and knee laxity in females compared with males; however, this was not attributed to higher levels of oestrogen or progesterone.

DEFINITIONS

Abnormal end feel: an end feel that occurs during a range of motion assessment that is outside the normal range of motion expected and/or uncharacteristic for the joint being tested, e.g. capsular early in the range, unexpected bone on bone, spasm, springy block or empty.

Active range of motion (AROM): involves the participant voluntarily moving their limb through the pain-free range of motion available at the joint in a specific direction.

Anatomical position: a common position for participants to be asked to stand during flexibility assessments. The erect position of the body with the face directed forwards, the arms at the side, and toes and palms of the hands facing forwards. Used as a reference in describing the relation of body parts to one another.

Creep: increases in range of motion occurring with repeated assessment, due to the test itself 'stretching' the non-contractile tissues surrounding the joint.

Hypermobility: more specifically known as benign joint hypermobility syndrome (BJHS), is the presence of an excessive range of motion throughout the body and associated symptoms.[20]

Inter-tester reliability: also known as between-tester reliability, is the amount of agreement (reliability) between two different testers measuring the same parameter on the same individual.

Intra-tester reliability: also known as within-tester reliability, is the amount of agreement (reliability) from the same tester measuring the same parameter on different occasions.

Laxity: increased range of motion in a specific direction at a specific joint, often the result of a ligamentous injury.

Normal end feel: an end feel that occurs within the expected normal range of motion with a quality that is characteristic for the joint being tested e.g. capsular, bone on bone or soft tissue approximation.

Passive range of motion (PROM): involves the tester moving the participant's relaxed limb through the pain-free range of motion available at the joint in a specific direction.

Proprioceptive neuromuscular facilitation (PNF): a stretching technique that utilises various combinations of lengthening (stretching), contraction movements and static holds of the muscles within the area being targeted.

Range of motion (ROM): the arc of movement through which a joint can move or be moved, usually expressed in degrees and measured from the anatomical position.

Soft tissue approximation (STA): the arc of movement through which a joint can move or be moved.

RELIABILITY AND VALIDITY

The flexibility assessments in this practical are based on the key assumption that ROM measures using external anatomical landmarks are a valid representation of the movement that occurs internally about the joints. The limitations in flexibility assessments include: (1) repeatability discrepancies due to the test itself stretching the joint across multiple measures (known as 'creep'), (2) tester differences in repeated ROM measures with approximately 77% intra-tester reliability and 64% inter-tester reliability,[21–24] (3) moderate concurrent validity for several measures of flexibility, including the sit and reach test with the passive straight leg raise ($R^2 = 0.63$),[25] (4) the need for standard flexibility assessment protocols that ensure that factors such as the measuring device used and participant positioning are identical between test–retest measures;[3,26,27] and (5) the fact that there is only moderate evidence that hamstring flexibility, as measured by performance on a sit-and-reach test or active straight-leg raise test assessed with goniometry, and ankle flexibility, assessed with goniometry, are associated with risk of musculoskeletal injury.[28]

General methods for conducting flexibility tests are outlined in Box 9.1 and contraindications for flexibility testing are provided in Box 9.2.[29,30]

Box 9.1 General methods for flexibility tests

Pre-Test Requirements

1. Conduct an appropriate participant history and physical examination for the presence of injury (e.g. swelling, redness, pain, heat and loss of function). Any participant displaying symptoms of injury should receive first aid and referral to a health practitioner as appropriate.

2. Through participant history, aim to identify participants who are pregnant and/or hypermobile, and modify or exclude flexibility tests as appropriate.

3. Participants should be informed that tests of flexibility may require the removal of clothing that obscures the joint/s being assessed and that the tests may elicit mild discomfort (stretching sensation); however, at no time should assessments cause pain.

> **Box 9.1 General methods for flexibility tests** *(continued)*
>
> **Test Requirements**
>
> 1 An appropriate warm-up and stretching protocol should be performed to help ensure a safe and reliable testing session. ACSM advocate the following warm-up: walking ($\approx$4.5 km/h) or pedalling on a cycle ergometer at 50 rpm with a work rate of 0.5 kpm for 5 minutes.[29] It is also recommended that adequate stretches be included for the areas being tested to ensure the participant is achieving a maximum ROM during testing. The tester should guide the participant through these stretches.
>
> 2 Ensure that participants conduct all flexibility assessments in a slow and controlled manner (no fast or jerky movements) aiming for a gradual, pain-free increase in ROM.

> **Box 9.2 Contraindications for flexibility testing**
>
> Tests of flexibility are generally safe for most individuals to perform. However, there are certain populations where flexibility assessment would be considered a contraindication. Flexibility assessment of a participant may be contraindicated for the following reasons[30]:
>
> - A bony block limits joint motion
> - Recent fracture or incomplete bony union
> - Acute inflammatory or infectious process (heat or swelling), or when soft tissue healing could be disrupted in the restricted tissues or surrounding region
> - Sharp, acute pain with joint movement or muscle elongation
> - A haematoma or other indication of tissue trauma
> - Joint hypermobility (see Activity 9.1)
> - Shortened soft tissue provides necessary joint stability in lieu of normal structural stability or neuromuscular control
> - Shortened soft tissue enables a patient with paralysis or severe muscle weakness to perform specific functional skills otherwise not possible
>
> **NOTE:** Most of these contraindications for flexibility testing may be considered relative if the benefits of testing outweigh the perceived risks. A decision regarding whether to waive the risks should be made in consultation with the treating medical practitioner and the participant.

Activity 9.1 Beighton scoring system

AIMS: conduct the Beighton Scoring System test, interpret the results and provide feedback to a participant.

Background

The Beighton Scoring System is a test used to determine whether a participant has excessive ROM throughout the body. It was first described by Beighton and colleagues[8] and has since been incorporated into the more comprehensive Beighton Criteria,[20] the new standard for determining benign joint hypermobility syndrome (BJHS). If the measured ROM about a joint is more than the expected 'normal' range for the participant's age and sex, they are considered to have excessive flexibility at that joint. There are many causes of excessive ROM – for example, a past history of injury causing joint laxity, occupational and sporting activities, or congenital factors such as hypermobility (the lay term for BJHS).[20,26] Where hypermobility is suspected, the Beighton Scoring System should be used to inform flexibility assessments, exercise prescription and/or referral to additional health professionals, as appropriate.[3]

Protocol summary

The participant performs nine simple tests of ROM to determine whether they are considered to have excessive ROM throughout the body.

Protocol

1 Follow the pre-test procedures outlined in Appendix B and the general methods for flexibility tests described in Box 9.1 (excluding the stretches, as stretching can be contraindicated in populations requiring assessment with the Beighton Scoring System).[31]

2 Check Box 9.2 to ensure that there are no contraindications to flexibility testing.

3 The participant should perform all actions within the Beighton Scoring System unassisted where possible.

4 The Beighton Scoring System involves taking the participant through nine basic tests and recording ROM observations using binary notations (0 and 1) (Figure 9.1). If a participant is able to achieve the ROM stipulated in a test within the Beighton Scoring System, then they receive a score of 1. If the participant is unable to achieve the ROM, a score of 0 is recorded.

Data recording
Participant's name: _____   Date: _____
Age: _____ years   Sex: _____
Sum of Beighton Scoring System test: _____ / 9
Excessive ROM throughout the body (score $\geq$4/9): Y / N

Interpretation

First, consider the four steps of interpretation outlined in Appendix G. If a score $\geq$4/9 is achieved, the participant is considered to have excessive ROM throughout the body.[20] In apparently healthy populations, if a participant is found to have excessive ROM at a specific joint, stretching would not usually be indicated for that movement at that joint.[31] However, in athletic populations where excessive ROM may be required to optimise performance, stretching may still be indicated in the presence of excessive flexibility.[7] It is important to note that, once hypermobility is identified, further ROM testing and referral to a medical practitioner and/or other allied health professionals may be warranted to ensure the best care for the participant.

Evidence for the influence of general joint hypermobility, as determined from the Beighton Scoring System test, on function and the risk of injury is mixed. For example, studies found there was no significant difference in Beighton scores between athletes with and without a history of ankle sprain,[32] nor was it associated with radiographic ankle and foot osteoarthritis and symptoms.[33] However, female athletes with general joint hypermobility demonstrated increased midfoot loading and increased risk for medial collapse of the foot.[34] Although general joint hypermobility does not appear to predict postoperative knee stability and function[35] following an anterior cruciate ligament reconstruction, it was a risk factor for posterior laxity after posterior cruciate ligament reconstruction.[36] Finally, adults, but not children, with general joint hypermobility had lower knee function (knee-related quality of life, pain, symptoms, ability to perform activities of daily living and sport/recreation) and hamstring:quadriceps ratio compared with those without general joint hypermobility, regardless of age and knee pain.[37]

BEIGHTON TEST	IS THE PARTICIPANT ABLE TO:	SCORE		
1	Place hands flat on the floor with straight legs and feet together	No Yes	0 1	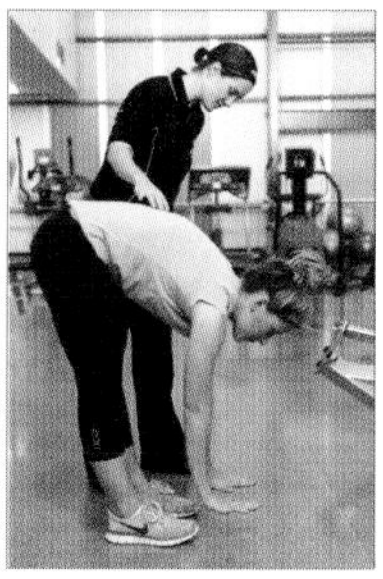
2	Hyperextend left knee (bending knee backwards >0° extension)	No Yes	0 1	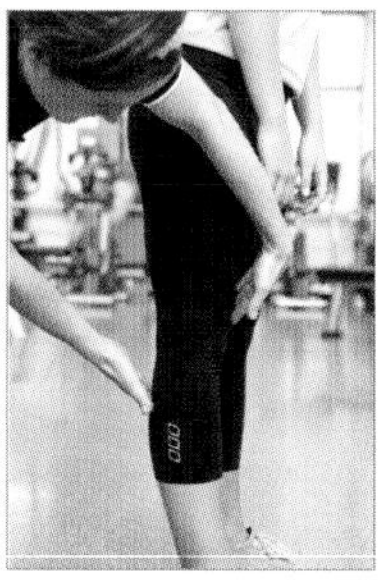
3	Hyperextend right knee (bending knee backwards >0° extension)	No Yes	0 1	
4	Hyperextend left elbow (bending elbow backwards >0° extension)	No Yes	0 1	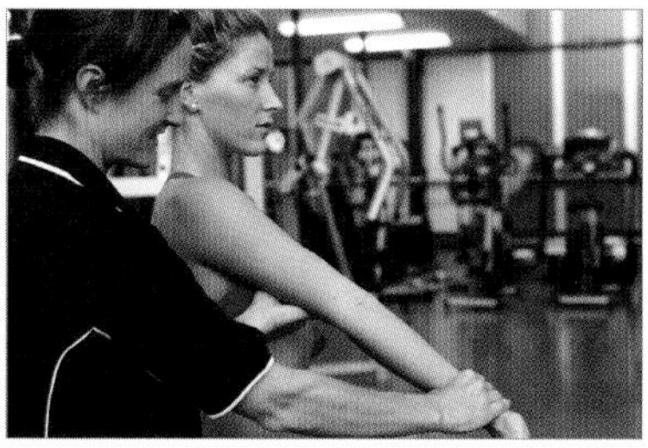
5	Hyperextend right elbow (bending elbow backwards >0° extension)	No Yes	0 1	
6	Touch the left thumb to the forearm	No Yes	0 1	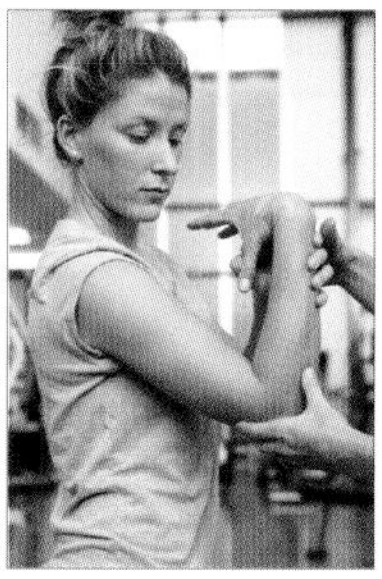
7	Touch the right thumb to the forearm	No Yes	0 1	
8	Bend left little finger backwards past 90°	No Yes	0 1	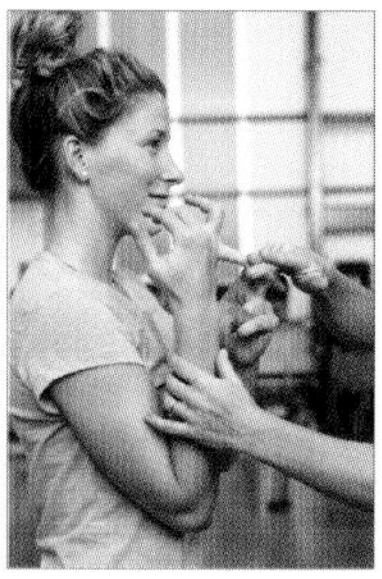
9	Bend right little finger backwards past 90°	No Yes	0 1	

Figure 9.1 Beighton Scoring System Protocol

Adapted from Beighton et al[8]

Activity 9.2 Sit and reach test

AIMS: conduct the sit and reach test, interpret the results and provide feedback to a participant.

Background

The sit and reach test is a widely used functional measure of low back, gluteal, hip and hamstring flexibility. Poor low back, hip and hamstring flexibility may potentially contribute to the development of muscular low back pain, which affects 60%–85% of the developed world.[38]

The major limitation of the sit and reach test is that there is no distinction or discrimination between the joints being tested (i.e. low back, gluteals, hips and hamstrings). The standard sit and reach test (Protocol 9.2.1) does not account for discrepancies in limb lengths (i.e. long upper limb and short lower limb overestimates performance, and vice versa). However, the introduction of the modified sit and reach test (Protocol 9.2.2) does account for limb length by establishing individual 'zero' points for the participant. The chair sit and reach test (Protocol 9.2.3) allows the test to be conducted with participants who are unable to comfortably perform tests on the floor, while maintaining a strong correlation ranging between 0.76 and 0.81 with hamstring flexibility.[39]

> **Note:** No version of the sit and reach test should be used for individuals with diagnosed osteoporosis of the lumbar spine due to the increased risk of sustaining a vertebral fracture with forward bending.

Protocol 9.2.1: Standard sit and reach test

1 Follow the pre-test procedures outlined in Appendix B and the general methods for flexibility tests described in Box 9.1 (excluding the stretches, as stretching can be contraindicated in populations requiring assessment with the Beighton Scoring System).[31]

2 Check Box 9.2 to ensure that there are no contraindications to flexibility testing.

3 The sit and reach box should be placed against a wall with a thin mat (e.g. a yoga mat) extended out from the box.

4 Demonstrate the test to ensure the correct form.

5 The participant should remove their shoes, sit on the mat facing the sit and reach box and straighten their legs. The soles of the participant's feet should be placed firmly against the sit and reach box feet, with the inner edges of the feet 15 cm apart.

6 The fingertips of the participant's hand should be kept parallel (i.e. the tester should watch closely to ensure that one hand does not slide forwards and reach further than the other during the test). The tester asking the participant to place one hand directly on top of the other may assist in ensuring the fingertips stay parallel during the reach.

7 The participant is instructed to slowly reach forwards with both hands gliding along the measuring tape on the sit and reach box so that the metal block is pushed as far as possible. The maximum reach position should be held momentarily.

8 The tester should closely observe to ensure that the participant does not jerk or bounce their movement forwards, or 'flick' the metal block further than the distance the fingers reached. If this occurs, the test should be repeated.

9 To assist with the attempt, the participant should be instructed to exhale and drop the head between the arms when reaching, similar to a 'dive' position (Figure 9.2a and b).

10 Testers should closely observe the participant's knees during the test to confirm they stay soft but extended at $180°$ throughout the test. If the participant's knees hyperextend ($>180°$) or flex

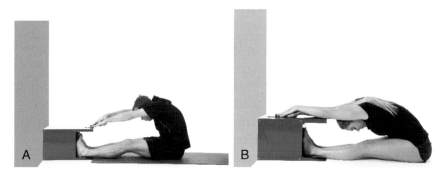

Figure 9.2 a: Standard sit and reach protocol with greater contribution of lower back to the movement. b: Standard sit and reach protocol with greater contribution of hamstring to the movement

Used with permission from Baseline

($<180°$), inform the participant that the test will not be valid and needs to be repeated. The tester should not press down on the participant's knees.

11 Observe the position of the participant at their most distant point reached to subjectively identify whether their ROM is limited by their low back, gluteal, hip and/or hamstring muscles.

12 The objective score is the most distant point reached at the proximal end of the metal block by the fingertips on both hands.

13 If the participant is not flexible enough to reach the sit and reach box, extend a tape measure from the fingertips to the sit and reach box to obtain a valid measure.

14 Record the distance reached to the nearest 0.5 of a cm.

15 Record your subjective observation of the ROM-limiting joint (i.e. low back, gluteal, hips and/or hamstrings).

16 The participant performs three trials, with a minimum of 5 seconds rest between each trial.

Data recording

Participant's name: _____   Date: _____

Age: _____ years   Sex: _____

Trial 1: _____ cm   Trial 2: _____ cm

Trial 3: _____ cm   Best: _____ cm

Adjusted best[a]: _____ · _____ cm

Percentile (Table 9.1): _____

Rating (Table 9.1): _____

Subjective ROM-limiting joint: _____

[a] The sit and reach reference data were derived from tests conducted on a sit and reach box where the toes = 0 cm. If using a sit and reach box where the measuring tape does not align the '0 cm' with the location of the toes, calculate an 'adjusted best' result for a valid comparison to the reference data.

Interpretation

First, consider the four steps of interpretation outlined in Appendix G and, using the 'adjusted best' result as appropriate, refer to Table 9.1. The sit and reach reference data were derived from tests conducted on a sit and reach box where the toes = 0 cm. For example, if the participant reached 6 cm

TABLE 9.1 Standard sit and reach test reference data		
	FEMALES (cm)	MALES (cm)
Very poor	<-20.0	<-23.0
Poor	-20.0 to -9.0	-23.0 to -5.2
Average	-8.9 to 5.4	-5.1 to 4.6
Good	5.5 to 13.5	4.7 to 11.6
Excellent	>13.5	>11.6

Reaching one's toes $= 0$ cm. Based on data from 172 Australian exercise science students (females, $n = 81$) aged 18–25 years. Very poor $<$20th percentile; poor $=$ 20th–40th percentile; average $=$ 41st–60th percentile; good $=$ 61st–80th percentile; excellent $>$80th percentile

further than the start of their toes then the participant would have a score of 6 cm. If the participant is 7 cm short of reaching their toes the score is -7 cm. If using a sit and reach box where the measuring tape does not align the '0 cm' with the location of the toes, this should be accounted for in the calculation of the 'adjusted best' result for a valid comparison to the reference data. For example, if using a sit and reach box where the foot line has the toes at 23 cm and the participant reaches to the 29 cm line, then the participant would have a score of $29 - 23$ cm $= 6$ cm. If the participant reached to the 12 cm line on the same sit and reach box, then the participant would have a score of $12 - 23$ cm $= -11$ cm.

In addition to the objective sit and reach data measured in centimetres, it is important to collect subjective information – that is, information from the body that cannot be easily measured but can be observed and recorded. Figure 9.2a and b contains images of two participants completing the sit and reach test. Subjective observation of the position reveals differences in the flexibility of the low back, gluteal, hips and hamstrings. The first participant has tight hamstrings and achieves most of his ROM by curving his thoracic spine and stretching through his shoulder joint. The second participant demonstrates a far greater contribution of the hamstring to the movement. This subjective information can be combined with the objective measure of flexibility to provide more detailed feedback to the participant.

Protocol 9.2.2: Modified sit and reach test

1 Follow the pre-test procedures outlined in Appendix B and the general methods for flexibility tests described in Box 9.1 (excluding the stretches, as stretching can be contraindicated in populations requiring assessment with the Beighton Scoring System).[31]

2 Check Box 9.2 to ensure that there are no contraindications to flexibility testing.

3 Place a thin mat parallel to the wall.

4 Demonstrate the test to ensure the correct form.

5 The participant should remove their shoes, sit on the mat with their buttocks, shoulder and head in contact with a wall, and straighten their legs so they are soft but extended at 180°.

6 Place the sit and reach box firmly against the soles of the participant's feet, with the inner edges of the feet 15 cm apart.

> **Note:** As the box is not against the wall the tester may need to apply pressure against the box so it doesn't shift during the test.

7 Keeping the buttocks, shoulders and head in contact with the wall, the participant stretches their arms towards the sit and reach box.

8 Record the distance passively reached by the tips of the fingers to the nearest 0.1 cm with the buttocks, shoulders and head in contact with the wall (this is the relative zero point). If the participant is unable to reach the sit and reach box, use an additional ruler to extend the distance able to be measured to find the relative zero point. Record the distance reached (Figure 9.3).

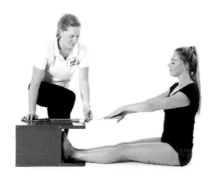

Figure 9.3 Modified sit and reach test start position
Used with permission from Baseline

9 The fingertips of the participant's hand should be kept parallel (i.e. the tester should watch closely to ensure that one hand does not slide forwards and reach further than the other during the test). The tester asking the participant to place one hand directly on top of the other may assist in ensuring the fingertips stay parallel during the reach.

10 The participant is then instructed to slowly reach forwards with both hands gliding along the tape of the sit and reach box so that the metal block is pushed as far as possible. The maximum reach position should be held momentarily.

11 The tester should closely observe to ensure that the participant does not jerk or bounce their movement forwards, or 'flick' the metal block further than the distance the fingers reached. If this occurs, the test should be repeated.

12 To assist with the attempt, the participant should be instructed to exhale and drop the head between the arms when reaching forwards, similar to a 'dive' position (see Figure 9.2a and b).

13 The tester should closely observe the participant's knees during the test to confirm they stay soft but extended at $180°$ throughout the test. If the participant's knees hyperextend ($>180°$) or flex ($<180°$), inform the participant that the test will not be valid and needs to be repeated. The tester should not press down on the participant's knees.

14 Observe the position of the participant at their most distant point reached so as to identify subjectively whether their ROM is limited by their low back, gluteal, hip and/or hamstring muscles.

15 Record the most distant point reached at the proximal end of the metal block by the fingertips on both hands.

16 Record the distance reached to the nearest 0.1 cm.

17 Record your subjective observation of the ROM-limiting joint (i.e. low back, gluteal, hips and/or hamstrings).

Data recording

Participant's name: _____   Date: _____

Age: _____ years   Sex: _____

Relative zero point: _____ cm

Trial 1: _____ cm   Trial 2: _____ cm   Trial 3: _____ cm

Best: _____ cm   Best − relative zero point: _____ cm

Percentile (Table 9.2): _____

Rating (Table 9.2): _____

Subjective ROM-limiting joint: _____

Interpretation

First, consider the four steps of interpretation outlined in Appendix G, and using the 'best − relative zero point' result, refer to Table 9.2. Also refer to the interpretation section from Protocol 9.2.1: Standard sit and reach test for subjective interpretation of the flexibility of the low back, gluteal, hips and hamstrings.

TABLE 9.2 Modified sit and reach test reference data		
	FEMALES (cm)	**MALES (cm)**
Very poor	$<$10.4	$<$14.5
Poor	10.4–16.3	14.5–17.4
Average	16.4–27.6	17.5–28.2
Good	27.7–39.4	28.3–43.0
Excellent	$>$39.4	$>$43.0

Based on data from 109 Australian exercise science students (females, $n = 55$) aged 18–25 years. Very poor $<$20th percentile; poor $=$ 20th–40th percentile; average $=$ 41st–60th percentile; good $=$ 61st–80th percentile; excellent $>$80th percentile

Protocol 9.2.3: Chair sit and reach test

1 Follow the pre-test procedures outlined in Appendix B and the general methods for flexibility tests described in Box 9.1 (excluding the stretches, as stretching can be contraindicated in populations requiring assessment with the Beighton Scoring System).[31]

2 Check Box 9.2 to ensure that there are no contraindications to flexibility testing.

3 Ensure that a stable chair is placed firmly against the wall.

4 Demonstrate the test to ensure the correct form.

5 The participant carefully sits on the front edge of the chair. Ensure that the participant's position on the chair is stable and that they will not tip forwards during the test.

6 One leg is bent so the knee is at 90° with the foot flat on the floor. The other leg is extended with the knee at 180° in front of the corresponding hip; the heel is placed on the floor and the foot is dorsiflexed at 90° (Figure 9.4a).

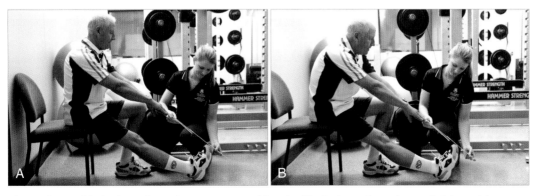

Figure 9.4 a: Chair sit and reach test start position. b: Chair sit and reach test finish position
Used with permission from Baseline

7 The participant should complete two practice trials on both legs to decide which leg is preferred (the one resulting in the best score).

> **Note:** Depending on the aim of the test it may be appropriate to conduct testing on both legs. However, for the purpose of this test, only the preferred leg will be used for scoring purposes.

8 The fingertips of the participant's hand should be kept parallel (i.e. the tester should watch closely to ensure that one hand does not slide forwards and reach further than the other during the test). The tester asking the participant to place one hand directly on top of the other may assist in ensuring the fingertips stay parallel during the reach.

9 The participant is instructed to slowly reach forwards with both hands reaching along the outstretched leg as far as possible. The maximum reach position should be held momentarily (see Figure 9.4b).

10 The tester should closely observe to ensure that the participant does not jerk or bounce their movement forwards. If this occurs, the test should be repeated.

11 To assist with the attempt, the participant should be instructed to exhale and drop the head between the arms when reaching, similar to a 'dive' position (see Figure 9.2).

12 Testers should closely observe the participant's outstretched knee during the test to confirm it stays soft but extended at $180°$ throughout the test. If the participant's knee hyperextends ($>180°$) or flexes ($<180°$), inform the participant that the test will not be valid and needs to be repeated. The tester should not press down on the participant's knee.

13 The score obtained is the distance between the distal aspect of the fingertips and the toes, measured using a straight-edged ruler. If the participant reaches past the toes, the measure is recorded as a positive number. If the participant fails to reach the toes, the measure is recorded as a negative number. If the participant reaches their toes exactly, the measure is recorded as zero.

14 Observe the position of the participant at their most distant point reached to subjectively identify whether their ROM is limited by their low back, gluteal, hips and/or hamstrings.

15 Record the distance reached to the nearest 0.1 of a cm.

16 Record your subjective observation of the ROM-limiting joint (i.e. low back, gluteal, hips and/or hamstrings).

Data recording

Participant's name: _____   Date: _____

Age: _____ years   Sex: _____

Extended leg: right / left

Trial 1: _____ cm   Trial 2: _____ cm   Trial 3: _____ cm

Best: _____ cm   Percentile (Table 9.3): _____

Rating (Table 9.3): _____

Subjective ROM-limiting joint: _____

Interpretation

First, consider the four steps of interpretation outlined in Appendix G and, using the 'best' result, refer to Table 9.3.[40] Also refer to the interpretation section from Protocol 9.2.1: Standard sit and reach test for subjective interpretation of the flexibility of the low back, gluteal, hips and hamstrings.

TABLE 9.3 Chair sit and reach test reference data (cm)

MALES	AGE (YEARS)				
PERCENTILE	60–64	65–69	70–74	75–79	80+
10th	−2.0	−16.0	−18.0	−19.7	−28.0
30th	2.0	−5.4	−6.0	−11.0	−13.0
50th	6.5	2.0	0	−3.0	−4.0
70th	10.7	7.0	6.0	2.1	1.0
90th	20.4	16.0	15.0	9.9	7.0
FEMALES					
10th	−5.4	−4.6	−9.0	−7.3	−13.2
30th	3.0	1.0	0	0.7	−2.0
50th	6.0	6.0	4.0	3.8	0
70th	12.7	10.9	10.0	6.3	5.9
90th	20.8	18.8	17.6	15.0	12.1

Based on data from 1088 older, functionally independent, community-dwelling adults from Taipei City (females, $n = 498$) aged 60–92 years. The majority of participants were currently unemployed and in the habit of exercising three times per week. For 590 male participants, scores ranged from −42.0 to 34.0 cm, with a total mean score of −2.3 cm. For 498 female participants, scores ranged from −31.0 to 30.0 cm, with a total mean score of 4.9 cm. Very poor <20th percentile; poor = 20th–40th percentile; average = 41st–60th percentile; good = 61st–80th percentile; excellent >80th percentile
Adapted from: Chen et al[40]

Activity 9.3 Thomas test

AIMS: conduct the Thomas test, interpret the results and provide feedback to a participant.

Background

The Thomas test, also known as the Hugh Owen Thomas test or rectus femoris contracture test, determines the ROM about the anterior hip and knee and assesses the length of the rectus femoris, psoas major, iliacus, tensor fasciae latae and the iliotibial band. Participants with poor anterior hip ROM may have an increased risk of lower limb injury, particularly in athletic populations.[41,42]

Protocol summary

The Thomas test involves the participant lying supine on a plinth with the leg to be tested hanging over the edge; hip extension, hip abduction and/or external rotation, and knee flexion are observed.

Protocol

1 Follow the pre-test procedures outlined in Appendix B and the general methods for flexibility tests described in Box 9.1 (excluding the stretches, as stretching can be contraindicated in populations requiring assessment with the Beighton Scoring System).[31]

2 Check Box 9.2 to ensure that there are no contraindications to flexibility testing

3 Demonstrate the test to ensure correct form.

4 Participants commence this test by lying supine on a plinth, with their bottom at the very end of the plinth. The participant grasps one knee with both hands and brings the knee towards the chest. The tester should ensure that the lumbar spine, while flattening against the plinth, does not become lordotic.

5 The participant gently lowers the free leg, ensuring the knee is hanging unobstructed (Figure 9.5a).

6 The tester then observes the position of the hip and knee of the free leg from the lateral view (i.e. on the side of the free leg). In a normal hip, the femur will remain in contact with the plinth and the knee angle will be $\leq 90°$ in its relaxed state.

7 The tester then observes the position of the hip and knee of the free leg from the end of the plinth. In a normal hip, the femur will remain parallel to the long axis of the body (see Figure 9.5a) – that is, not abducted and/or externally rotated (see Figure 9.5b).

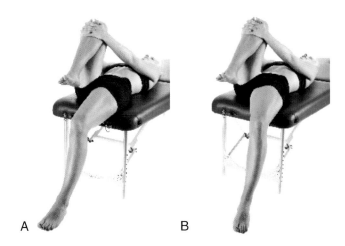

Figure 9.5 a: Thomas test with the femur parallel to the long axis of the body. b: Thomas test with the femur abducted and externally rotated

8 The participant then extends the knee and the tester observes to see whether the position of the femur has changed (to differentiate between iliopsoas and rectus femoris tightness).

9 Assist the participant to return the free leg back to the plinth.

10 Repeat the test on the contralateral side.

11 Clean and disinfect all equipment (see Appendix A).

Data recording

Participant's name: _____   Date: _____

Age: _____ years   Sex: _____

Right leg:

The femur remained in full contact with the plinth: Y / N

The femur remained parallel to the long axis of the body i.e. not abducted and/or externally rotated: Y / N

The knee angle was $\leq 90°$: Y / N

Straightening the leg identified tightness in (circle as appropriate): iliopsoas or rectus femoris

Left leg:

The femur remained in full contact with the plinth: Y / N

The femur remained parallel to the long axis of the body, i.e. not abducted and/or externally rotated: Y / N

The knee angle was $\leq 90°$: Y / N

Straightening the leg identified tightness in (circle as appropriate): iliopsoas or rectus femoris

Interpretation

First, consider the four steps of interpretation outlined in Appendix G. This test provides an indication of the length of the anterior structures of the hip and knee (i.e. hip flexors, hip abductors and knee extensors). When using the Thomas test, a result of 'no' for one or more of the three observed measures (i.e. femur position – elevation, abduction/external rotation and knee angle) is considered 'restricted'. It is important to note that this test may provide false-negative results for participants with poor lumbopelvic stability. These participants lack the control required to flatten the lumbar spine against the plinth. Subsequently, these participants become excessively lordotic through their lumbar spine, resulting in the femur remaining in full contact with the plinth and not necessarily because their hip flexor ROM is within the normal range. Advanced testing procedures which assist in reducing false-negative results can be found in Hattam and Smeatham.[43]

Activity 9.4 Back scratch test

AIMS: conduct the back scratch test, interpret the results and provide feedback to a participant.

Background

The back scratch test, also known as the zipper test or over under test, determines the functional range about the upper body (shoulder). The ROM at the shoulder is important for activities of daily living such as combing one's hair, putting on overhead garments, reaching one's back pocket and reaching for a seat belt. Poor shoulder ROM may have an increased risk of neck, upper back and shoulder injury, especially with advancing age.[30] This test is part of the Senior Fitness Test battery,[44] which is designed to test the functional fitness of older adults. This test is a relative contraindication for participants with benign joint hypermobility or a history of upper limb and/or neck pathologies.

Protocol summary

The back scratch test involves the participant attempting to touch or overlap the middle fingers of both hands behind the back, with one hand reaching over the shoulder, and one up the middle of the back. The distance between extended middle fingers ($+$ or $-$) is measured.

Protocol

1 Follow the pre-test procedures outlined in Appendix B and the general methods for flexibility tests described in Box 9.1 (excluding the stretches, as stretching can be contraindicated in populations requiring assessment with the Beighton Scoring System).[31]

2 Check Box 9.2 to ensure that there are no contraindications to flexibility testing.

3 Demonstrate the test to ensure the correct form.

4 The participant commences this test by performing two practice trials on each side to determine their preferred position (this should be the hand over the shoulder that produces the best score).

5 Ask the participant to stand and place their preferred hand over the same shoulder, palmar surface against the skin/clothing and fingers extended, and gently reach down the middle of the back as far as possible.

> **Note:** The elbow is pointed up.

6 Instruct the participant to gently place the other arm around the back of their lower back/waist with the dorsal surface against the skin/clothing, reaching up the middle of the back as far as possible in an attempt to touch or overlap the extended middle fingers of both hands.

7 Check to see whether the middle fingers are directed towards each other as best as possible.

8 Without moving the participant's hands, ask the participant to move their middle fingers to the alignment that produces the best result.

9 Ensure that the participant does not grab/pull their fingers or clothing to assist with the movement.

10 Stop the test immediately should the participant feel any pain.

11 Remind the participant to continue breathing as they stretch and to avoid any bouncing or rapid movements.

12 The tester then observes the position of the participant's middle fingers. If the tips of the middle fingers touch then the score equals zero. If the tips of the middle fingers do not reach each other, use a measuring tape to record the distance between middle fingers as a negative ($-$) score (Figure 9.6a). If the tips of the middle fingers reach past each other, use a measuring tape to record the distance of overlap between the middle fingers as a positive ($+$) score (see Figure 9.6b).

13 Record scores to the nearest 0.1 cm.

14 Administer two trials, recording the results.

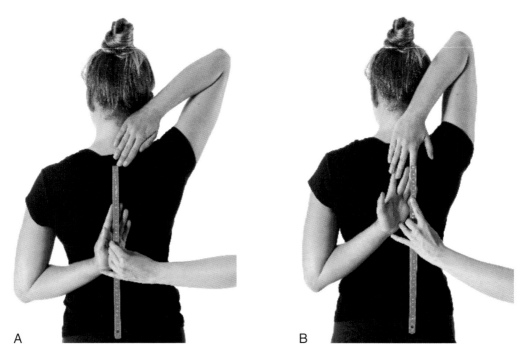

A   B

Figure 9.6 a: Back scratch test negative result. b: Back scratch test positive result

Data recording

Participant's name: _____   Date: _____

Age: _____ years   Sex: _____

Hand over shoulder (right or left): _____

Trial 1: _____ cm   Trial 2: _____ cm   Best: _____ cm

Percentile (Table 9.4): _____

Rating (Table 9.4): _____

At risk for loss of functional mobility (Table 9.4): (Y / N): _____

Interpretation

First, consider the four steps of interpretation outlined in Appendix G, and refer to Table 9.4.[45] This test provides an indication of the functional reach of the upper extremities (i.e. shoulder flexion, extension, abduction, adduction, internal and external rotation). When measuring the back scratch test, a result of ≤ -10.2 cm for men and ≤ -5.1 cm for women is considered at risk for loss of functional mobility.

TABLE 9.4 Back scratch test reference data (cm)							
MALES	**AGE (YEARS)**						
PERCENTILE	**60–64**	**65–69**	**70–74**	**75–79**	**80–84**	**85–89**	**90–94**
At risk	≤ -10.16	≤ -10.16	≤ -10.16	≤ -10.16	≤ -10.16	≤ -10.16	≤ -10.16
25th	< -16.51	< -19.05	< -20.32	< -22.86	< -24.13	< -25.40	< -26.67
50th	-16.51 to 0	-19.05 to -2.54	-20.32 to -2.54	-22.86 to -5.08	-24.13 to -5.08	-25.4 to -7.62	-26.67 to -10.16
75th	>0.0	>2.54	>2.54	>5.08	>5.08	>7.62	>10.16
FEMALES							
At risk[a]	≤ -5.08	≤ -5.08	≤ -5.08	≤ -5.08	≤ -5.08	≤ -5.08	≤ -5.08
25th	< -7.62	< -8.89	< -10.16	< -12.70	< -13.97	< -17.78	< -20.32
50th	-7.62 to 3.81	-8.89 to 3.81	-10.16 to 2.54	-12.70 to 1.27	-13.97 to 0	-17.78 to -2.54	-20.32 to -2.54
75th	>3.81	>3.81	>2.54	>1.27	>0	>-2.54	>-2.54

[a]At risk = at risk for loss of functional mobility. Based on data from 7183 older, functionally-independent, community-dwelling adults, who were ambulatory without regular use of an assisted device from 265 test sites across the United States (females, $n = 5048$) aged 60–94 years.
Above average = $>$75th percentile; average = 50th percentile; below average = $<$25th percentile
Adapted from: Jones and Rikli[45]

Activity 9.5 Weight-bearing lunge test

AIMS: conduct the weight-bearing lunge test, interpret the results and provide feedback to a participant.

Background

The weight-bearing lunge test determines the ROM about the talocrural (ankle) joint in the direction of dorsiflexion. Participants with poor ankle ROM, particularly in dorsiflexion, may have an increased risk of lower limb injury, particularly in athletic populations.[46]

Protocol summary

The weight-bearing lunge test involves a simple repetitive movement to determine the maximum weight-bearing dorsiflexion present at the talocrural joint. A tape measure is used as the measure of ROM in this test.

Protocol

1 Follow the pre-test procedures outlined in Appendix B and the general methods for flexibility tests described in Box 9.1 (excluding the stretches, as stretching can be contraindicated in populations requiring assessment with the Beighton Scoring System).[31]

2 Check Box 9.2 to ensure that there are no contraindications to flexibility testing.

3 Demonstrate the test to ensure the correct form.

4 The participant should remove their shoes.

5 The participant commences this test by facing a wall with one foot (test leg) aligned in front of the other and hands placed on the wall for support.

6 There should be approximately 10 cm from the wall to the great toe on the front foot and approximately 30 cm from the heel of the front foot to the toes of the back foot.

> **Note:** The heel of the back foot does not need to maintain contact with the floor.

7 The participant then bends the front knee, aiming to gently touch the patella to the wall without lifting the heel off the ground (Figure 9.7).

8 If the participant's patella cannot touch the wall without the heel lifting off the ground, ask the participant to move the front foot closer to the wall in small increments, until this is achieved.

9 Alternatively, if the participant's patella is able to touch the wall easily without the heel lifting off the ground, move the front foot further away from the wall in small increments.

10 The participant's front knee should be tracking over the second toe throughout this test.

11 The tester should palpate using two fingers gently touching the side of the calcaneus to ensure that the heel is in full contact with the ground.

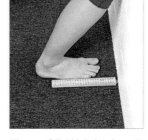

Figure 9.7 Weight-bearing lunge test

12 When the front foot is at the maximal distance from the wall while the heel remains in contact with the ground and the patella is in contact with the wall, use a ruler or measuring tape to measure the perpendicular distance between the wall and tip of the great toe.

13 Repeat the test on the contralateral side.

Data recording

Participant's name: _____   Date: _____

Age: _____ years   Sex: _____

Right ankle:

Trial 1: _____ cm   Trial 2: _____ cm   Best: _____ cm

Restricted ($<$9–10 cm): Y / N

Left ankle:

Trial 1: _____ cm   Trial 2: _____ cm   Best: _____ cm

Restricted ($<$9–10 cm): Y / N

Interpretation

First, consider the four steps of interpretation outlined in Appendix G. This test provides an indication of the length of the posterior structures (calf muscles and joint structures) that cross the talocrural joint. When measuring the weight-bearing lunge test, a result <9–10 cm is considered restricted. It is important to note that this test may provide false-negative results for participants of above average height; that is, tall participants often achieve >9–10 cm owing to the length of their tibia, and not necessarily because their talocrural dorsiflexion is within the normal range. Advanced testing procedures using goniometers which assist in reducing false-negative results can be found in the article by Hoch and colleagues.[47]

Activity 9.6 Goniometer and inclinometer joint ROM measurements

AIMS: conduct joint ROM tests with a goniometer and inclinometer, interpret the results and provide feedback to a participant.

Background

There are numerous instruments available to measure joint ROM. The following descriptions focus on the two most common and cost-effective devices: the lever arm goniometer and the inclinometer, as shown in Figure 9.8. The goniometer has an intra-tester reliability of ±4.0°,[24] which includes ±2.0° of instrument error (see Practical 1, Test accuracy, reliability and validity).[27] The inclinometer has an intra-tester reliability of 0.6–1.5°,[48–50] which includes ±2.0° of instrument error.

Figure 9.8 Lever arm goniometers (A and B) and an inclinometer (C)

Used with permission from Baseline

Lever-arm goniometer

The lever-arm goniometer has two arms joined together at a pivot point (see Figure 9.8). Around the pivot point on one of the arms a 360° scale is visible. The pivot point is placed at the axis of rotation, otherwise referred to as the fulcrum point, which is usually positioned over the joint line. The original angle is determined by then aligning the stationary lever arm with the closest proximal bony landmark and the movable lever arm with the closest distal bony landmark (Figure 9.9a). The participant is then instructed to move their limb through a particular motion and, once complete, the lever arms are repositioned to the same bony landmarks to determine the end range angle (see Figure 9.9b).

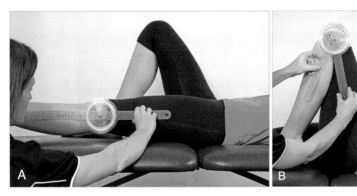

Figure 9.9 a: Positioning of goniometer for original angle. b: Positioning of goniometer for end range angle

The total ROM at this joint is calculated as:

$$\text{Total joint ROM} = \text{end of range angle} - \text{original angle}$$

For the example provided in Figure 9.9a and b, the total joint ROM for the knee is calculated as:

$$\text{Total joint ROM} = \text{end of range angle} - \text{original angle}$$
$$= 135^0 - 0^0$$
$$= 135^0$$

Inclinometer

The bubble inclinometer is a circular column of coloured fluid contained between two discs of plastic (see Figure 9.10a). The top piece of plastic is moveable, circular and imprinted with a 360^0 scale. It is connected at the centre point to a shaped base which is ideal for placement on either curved or flat surfaces. The simplicity of using the inclinometer is that the fluid level is always set on 0^0 in the neutral position, so the ROM can be read directly from the angle to which the fluid moves (see Figure 9.10b). The inclinometer is situated on the limb itself, therefore it is not necessary to align over the joint line with the proximal or distal bony landmarks (Figure 9.11).

> **Note:** It is not possible to measure rotation with the inclinometer in the transverse plane.

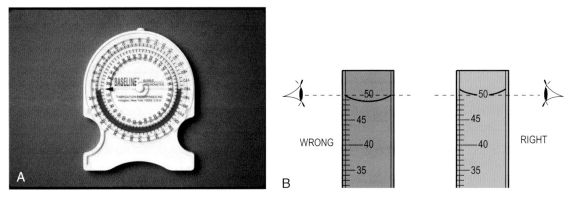

Figure 9.10 a: Start inclinometer dial at zero. b: Reading an inclinometer
Part a: Used with permission from: Baseline.

Protocol summary

These joint ROM tests involve measuring body and limb ROM in various positions using goniometers and inclinometers.

Protocol

Knowledge of surface anatomy and proficiency in the use of the measuring devices are required to ensure that these tests are conducted accurately and with clinically reliable and concurrently valid results.

1 Follow the pre-test procedures outlined in Appendix B and the general methods for flexibility tests described in Box 9.1 (excluding the stretches, as stretching can be contraindicated in populations requiring assessment with the Beighton Scoring System).[31]

2 Check Box 9.2 to ensure that there are no contraindications to flexibility testing.

Figure 9.11 Knee flexion with an inclinometer
Used with permission from 66Fit

3 Planes of movement listed in Tables 9.5–9.12 are described relative to the standing neutral position (i.e. standard plane of movement for the limb, unless stated otherwise).

TABLE 9.5 Cervical ranges of joint motion measured using a goniometer, tape measure or inclinometer

MEASUREMENT	POSITION OF PARTICIPANT	PLANE AND JOINT MOVEMENT	GONIOMETER PIVOT POINT ALIGNMENT	PROXIMAL ARM ALIGNMENT (OR POSITION OF TAPE MEASURE)	DISTAL ARM ALIGNMENT (OR POSITION OF TAPE MEASURE)	MEASUREMENT WITH INCLINOMETER
Flexion	Seated	Sagittal plane Chin to chest without slumping the shoulders forwards	Centre of the ear	Parallel to the floor (0–180° axis line)	Aligned with the inferior nasal border	Place at the vertex (crown) of the head in the direction of movement, set to zero
Extension	Seated	Sagittal plane Tip head back without arching the back	Centre of the ear	Parallel to the floor (0–180° axis line)	Aligned with the inferior nasal border	Place at the vertex (crown) of the head in the direction of movement, set to zero
Lateral flexion	Seated	Frontal plane Move ear towards the shoulder, take care not to raise the shoulder or rotate the head	C6–C7	Centrally down the spine (perpendicular with the floor)	Occipital protuberance ≈C1	Place on the head, vertex aligned in the direction of head movement
Rotation	Seated	Transverse plane Turn and look over the shoulder, take care not to move the upper torso	Vertex of the head	Acromion process	Centre of the nose	Can be measured in the supine position Inclinometer is placed on the forehead in the direction of movement

Used with permission from 66Fit

TABLE 9.6 Thoracolumbar ranges of joint motion measured using a goniometer, tape measure or inclinometer

MEASUREMENT	POSITION OF PARTICIPANT	PLANE — JOINT MOVEMENT	GONIOMETER PIVOT POINT ALIGNMENT	PROXIMAL ARM ALIGNMENT (OR POSITION OF TAPE MEASURE)	DISTAL ARM ALIGNMENT (OR POSITION OF TAPE MEASURE)	MEASUREMENT WITH INCLINOMETER
Flexion	Standing	Sagittal plane Bending forwards, hands reaching to floor	–	Spinous process of C7 (indicated by coloured dot). Note: Tape measure is the preferred measuring technique	Spinous process of S2 (indicated by coloured dot)	Positioned longitudinally with the superior aspect of the inclinometer over the C7 spinous process. Note: Avoid including cervical movement in the measurement
Extension	Standing Hands on hips	Sagittal plane Bending backwards	–	Spinous process of C7 (indicated by coloured dots) Note: Tape measure is the preferred measuring technique	Spinous process of S2 (indicated by coloured dots)	Positioned longitudinally with the superior aspect of the inclinometer over the C7 spinous process Note: Avoid including cervical movement in the measurement
Lateral Flexion	Standing	Frontal plane Bending sideways, hand reaching to floor	–	Spinous process of C7 (indicated by coloured dots)	Spinous process of S2 (indicated by coloured dots)	Positioned longitudinally over the mid-shaft of the humerus with arm in contact with the thigh

continued

TABLE 9.6 Thoracolumbar ranges of joint motion measured using a goniometer, tape measure or inclinometer (continued)

MEASUREMENT	POSITION OF PARTICIPANT	PLANE – JOINT MOVEMENT	GONIOMETER PIVOT POINT ALIGNMENT	PROXIMAL ARM ALIGNMENT (OR POSITION OF TAPE MEASURE)	DISTAL ARM ALIGNMENT (OR POSITION OF TAPE MEASURE)	MEASUREMENT WITH INCLINOMETER
Rotation	Seated with arms crossed, thumbs on chin and fingers on upper trapezius to lock in head and shoulder position	Transverse plane Turn upper torso to look over your shoulder, take care not to move hips off chair, or move head independently of the shoulders	Vertex of the head	Acromion process	Centre of the nose	–

Note: The C7 spinous process can be located by flexing the neck (chin to chest motion) and selecting the most prominent spinous process that is visible on the posterior surface of the neck, at the base of the neck. The S2 spinous process can be located by first palpating the posterior superior iliac spines, drawing an imaginary line between the two landmarks and then selecting the spinous process which exists at the intersection of this line and the sacrum. The thoracic and lumbar spine are typically measured together owing to the functionality of spinal movement and the practicality of measuring this ROM
Used with permission from 66Fit

TABLE 9.7 Shoulder ranges of joint motion measured using a goniometer, tape measure or inclinometer

MEASUREMENT	POSITION OF PARTICIPANT	PLANE – JOINT MOVEMENT	GONIOMETER PIVOT POINT ALIGNMENT	PROXIMAL ARM ALIGNMENT (OR POSITION OF TAPE MEASURE)	DISTAL ARM ALIGNMENT (OR POSITION OF TAPE MEASURE)	MEASUREMENT WITH INCLINOMETER
Flexion	Standing or seated with the arm able to swing freely	Sagittal plane/ cardinal axis Thumbs facing forwards, raise the arm up forwards of the body	The centre of the head of the humerus	Aligned with midline of lateral trunk or the iliac crest can work well	Midline of upper arm	Place longitudinally mid-way on midline of the upper arm in the direction of movement Ensure dial is facing laterally for reading
Extension	Standing	Sagittal plane/ cardinal axis From the neutral position, extend the straight arm backwards	The centre of the head of the humerus	Aligned with midline of lateral trunk or the iliac crest can work well	Midline of upper arm	Place longitudinally mid-way on midline of the upper arm in the direction of movement Ensure dial is facing laterally for reading

continued overpage

TABLE 9.7 Shoulder ranges of joint motion measured using a goniometer, tape measure or inclinometer (continued)

MEASUREMENT	POSITION OF PARTICIPANT	PLANE — JOINT MOVEMENT	GONIOMETER PIVOT POINT ALIGNMENT	PROXIMAL ARM ALIGNMENT (OR POSITION OF TAPE MEASURE)	DISTAL ARM ALIGNMENT (OR POSITION OF TAPE MEASURE)	MEASUREMENT WITH INCLINOMETER
Abduction (lateral flexion)	Standing	Frontal plane Thumbs facing upwards, raise the straight arm laterally away from the body towards the head	The centre of the head of the humerus on the anterior of the body	The medial end of the clavicle on front of the body	Aligned to the centre of the elbow crease	Place longitudinally on the midline of the upper arm in the direction of movement
Medial rotation	Supine (passive)	About the transverse plane Upper arm is abducted 90° and elbow bent to 90° (perpendicular to the floor) Lower the forearm and palm towards the floor	Olecranon Stationary and move-able arm aligned	Aligned vertically	Aligned along the ulnar	Place longitudinally on the midline of the superior surface (same side as dorsum of the hand) of the forearm
Lateral rotation	Supine (passive)	About the transverse plane Lower the dorsal surface of the hand backwards towards the floor	Olecranon Stationary and move-able arm aligned	Aligned vertically	Aligned along the ulnar	Place longitudinally on the midline of the inside (same as palmar surface) of forearm
Horizontal abduction	Seated	Transverse plane arm is abducted 90° laterally move the straight arm posteriorly	Placed on top of the acromion	Aligned to mid-neck line; however, logistically will sit just behind	Aligned along the upper arm to the head of the radius	Can be measured in the supine position Inclinometer is placed longitudinally on the midline of the upper arm in the direction of movement

In clients with extreme hypertrophy of the biceps, the passive ROM should be measured to ensure that the biceps do not increase in size/volume with activation, restricting the ROM
Used with permission from 66Fit

				PROXIMAL ARM ALIGNMENT (OR POSITION OF TAPE MEASURE)	DISTAL ARM ALIGNMENT (OR POSITION OF TAPE MEASURE)	
TABLE 9.8 Elbow ranges of joint motion measured using a goniometer, tape measure or inclinometer						
MEASUREMENT	**POSITION OF PARTICIPANT**	**PLANE — JOINT MOVEMENT**	**GONIOMETER PIVOT POINT ALIGNMENT**			**MEASUREMENT WITH INCLINOMETER**
Flexion	Seated or standing with arm in neutral position	Sagittal plane Move palmar surface towards the shoulder	Lateral epicondyle	Lateral midline of the upper arm towards the centre of head of the humerus	Lateral midline of the forearm	Along the midline of the forearm on the dorsal surface Ensure the dial is facing laterally for ease of reading
Hyper-extension	Seated or standing	Sagittal plane Easier to measure hyperextension with arm in 90° shoulder flexion, palmar surface facing up	Lateral epicondyle	Lateral midline of the upper arm towards the centre of head of the humerus	Lateral midline of the forearm	Along the midline of the forearm on the anterior surface Ensure the dial is facing later-ally for ease of reading
Supination	Seated or standing	About the transverse plane axis Elbow is flexed to 90°, fingers making a light fist, thumb extended and palmar surface facing medially. Move the dorsal surface of the hand inferiorly so palm is facing up	Base of third metacarpal	Aligned vertically	Along the thumb	Horizontally across the palmar surface of the hand and perpendicular to the floor
Pronation	Seated or standing	About the transverse plane axis Elbow is flexed to 90°, fingers making a light fist, thumb extended, and palmar surface facing medially Move the palmar surface inferiorly so the palm faces the floor	Base of third metacarpal	Aligned vertically	Along the thumb	Horizontally across the dorsal surface of the hand and perpendicular to the floor

Used with permission from 66Fit

TABLE 9.9 Wrist ranges of joint motion measured using a goniometer, tape measure or inclinometer

MEASUREMENT	POSITION OF PARTICIPANT	PLANE AND JOINT MOVEMENT	GONIOMETER PIVOT POINT ALIGNMENT	PROXIMAL ARM ALIGNMENT (OR POSITION OF TAPE MEASURE)	DISTAL ARM ALIGNMENT (OR POSITION OF TAPE MEASURE)	MEASUREMENT WITH INCLINOMETER
Flexion	Seated or standing	Sagittal plane Keeping the hand flat and fingers together, flex the wrist downwards	At the styloid process of the ulna	Along the ulna	Aligned along the little finger	Longitudinally on the dorsum of the hand
Extension	Seated or standing	Sagittal plane Keeping the hand flat, flex the wrist upwards	At the styloid process of the ulna	Along the ulna	Aligned along the little finger	Longitudinally on the dorsum of the hand
Ulnar deviation (adduction)	Seated or standing	Transverse plane Keeping the hand flat and fingers together, flex the wrist laterally	Centre of the wrist joint	Along the midline of the forearm	Along the middle finger	Position the forearm vertically in neutral pronation/supination Dial positioned along midline of the third metacarpal
Radial deviation (abduction)	Seated or standing	Transverse plane Keeping the hand flat and fingers together, flex the wrist medially	Centre of the wrist joint	Along the midline of the forearm	Along the middle finger	Position the forearm vertically in neutral pronation/supination Dial positioned along midline of the third metacarpal

The wrist is not measured from the anatomical neutral stance. The starting position for testing wrist/hand ROM is with the elbow flexed $90°$, hand and wrist flat with the palmar surface face down

TABLE 9.10 Hip ranges of joint motion measured using a goniometer, tape measure or inclinometer

MEASUREMENT	POSITION OF PARTICIPANT	PLANE AND JOINT MOVEMENT	GONIOMETER PIVOT POINT ALIGNMENT	PROXIMAL ARM ALIGNMENT (OR POSITION OF TAPE MEASURE)	DISTAL ARM ALIGNMENT (OR POSITION OF TAPE MEASURE)	MEASUREMENT WITH INCLINOMETER
Flexion	Supine	Sagittal plane Lift the entire leg, bending the knee as you go to release the hamstring tension at insertion for true hip flexion End of range once the extended contralateral limb starts to lift	The greater trochanter	Along the midline of the torso towards the armpit	Along the ITB band (lateral midline of the femur)	Placed longitudinally on the front midline of the femur, approximately middle of the limb

continued

TABLE 9.10 Hip ranges of joint motion measured using a goniometer, tape measure or inclinometer *(continued)*

MEASUREMENT	POSITION OF PARTICIPANT	PLANE AND JOINT MOVEMENT	GONIOMETER PIVOT POINT ALIGNMENT	PROXIMAL ARM ALIGNMENT (OR POSITION OF TAPE MEASURE)	DISTAL ARM ALIGNMENT (OR POSITION OF TAPE MEASURE)	MEASUREMENT WITH INCLINOMETER
Extension	Prone, standing, or side-lying	Sagittal plane Lift the entire leg with the knee supported beneath. If standing move straight leg backwards, ensure standing vertical	The greater trochanter	Along the midline of the torso towards the armpit	Along the ITB (lateral midline of the femur)	Placed longitudinally on the midline of the hamstrings approximately middle of the limb
Abduction	Supine	Transverse plane	Intersection point of the vertical line of the ASIS and horizontal line of the greater trochanter	Aligned with ASIS	Along the front midline of the femur	Can be done in the standing position (frontal plane) Inclinometer placed longitudinally on the ITB midway down the limb Abduct the leg with end of range obtained once the torso starts to move in the opposite direction
Adduction	Supine	Transverse plane Move the leg towards the midline behind the flexed contralateral limb	Intersection point of the vertical line of the ASIS and horizontal line of the greater trochanter	Aligned with ASIS	Along the front midline of the femur	Can be done in the standing position (frontal plane) Inclinometer placed longitudinally on the ITB midway down the limb Move the leg medially in front of the contralateral limb
Medial rotation	Prone, knee $\approx 90°$; or seated, hips and knees $\approx 90°$, feet free of the floor	About the transverse plane Move the lower limb and foot lateral (causes medial rotation at the hip)	Centre of knee joint	Arm vertical	Along the tibial shaft	For the prone position, place longitudinally on the medial surface midline, mid-way down the lower leg

continued overpage

TABLE 9.10 Hip ranges of joint motion measured using a goniometer, tape measure or inclinometer (continued)

MEASUREMENT	POSITION OF PARTICIPANT	PLANE AND JOINT MOVEMENT	GONIOMETER PIVOT POINT ALIGNMENT	PROXIMAL ARM ALIGNMENT (OR POSITION OF TAPE MEASURE)	DISTAL ARM ALIGNMENT (OR POSITION OF TAPE MEASURE)	MEASUREMENT WITH INCLINOMETER
Lateral rotation	Prone, knee ≈90°; or seated, hips and knees ≈90°, feet free of the floor	About the transverse plane Move the lower limb and foot medial (causes lateral rotation at the hip)	Centre of knee joint	Arm vertical	Along the tibial shaft	For the prone position, place longitudinally on the lateral surface mid-line, mid-way down the fibula

ASIS = anterior superior iliac spine; ITB = iliotibial band
Used with permission from 66Fit

TABLE 9.11 Knee ranges of joint motion measured using a goniometer, tape measure or inclinometer

MEASUREMENT	POSITION OF PARTICIPANT	PLANE AND JOINT MOVEMENT	GONIOMETER PIVOT POINT ALIGNMENT	PROXIMAL ARM ALIGNMENT (OR POSITION OF TAPE MEASURE)	DISTAL ARM ALIGNMENT (OR POSITION OF TAPE MEASURE)	MEASUREMENT WITH INCLINOMETER
Flexion (1)	Prone Limited by quadriceps muscle length	Sagittal plane Move the foot and lower leg towards the buttocks	At knee joint line	Along lateral midline of the thigh or aligned with greater trochanter	Lateral midline of lower leg	Placed longitudinally on the midline of the posterior surface, on the lower half of the limb so movement is not impeded
Flexion (2)	Supine Release tension of quadriceps at hip origin	Sagittal plane ≈45° hip flexion straight leg raise position Move the foot towards the buttocks while maintaining the initial hip flexion	At knee joint line	Along lateral midline of the thigh or aligned with greater trochanter	Lateral midline of lower leg	Placed longitudinally on the midline of the tibial shaft
Hyperextension	Supine	Sagittal plane Lift the lower leg by supporting the Achilles tendon Take care as only small degree of movement	At knee joint line	Along lateral midline of the thigh or aligned with greater trochanter	Lateral midline of lower leg	Place longitudinally on the tibial shaft

Used with permission from 66Fit

TABLE 9.12 Ankle ranges of joint motion measured using a goniometer, tape measure or inclinometer

MEASUREMENT	POSITION OF PARTICIPANT	PLANE AND JOINT MOVEMENT	GONIOMETER PIVOT POINT ALIGNMENT	PROXIMAL ARM ALIGNMENT (OR POSITION OF TAPE MEASURE)	DISTAL ARM ALIGNMENT (OR POSITION OF TAPE MEASURE)	MEASUREMENT WITH INCLINOMETER
Dorsiflexion	Seated or lying with feet not touching the floor/bed and ankle at 90°	Sagittal plane Flex the foot upwards towards the head	Lateral malleolus	Along the fibular shaft	On the lateral foot surface towards the 5th metatarsal	Longitudinally on the dorsal surface
Plantarflexion	Seated or lying with feet not touching the floor/bed and ankle at 90°	Sagittal plane Flex the foot towards the floor	Lateral malleolus	Along the fibular shaft	On the lateral foot surface towards the 5th metatarsal	Longitudinally on the dorsal surface Can be done as a continuation of movement after dorsiflexion as zero was already set
Inversion	Seated or lying with feet not touching the floor/bed and ankle at 90°	About the transverse plane Invert the foot medially Take care not to cause rotation at the hips	Anterior ankle between the malleoli	Along the tibia shaft	Along the shaft of the second metatarsal	Place horizontally across the cuneiforms of the foot
Eversion	Seated or lying with feet not touching the floor/bed and ankle at 90°	About the transverse plane Evert the sole of the foot laterally Take care not to cause rotation at the hips	Anterior ankle between the malleoli	Along the tibia shaft	Along the shaft of the second metatarsal	Place horizontally across the cuneiforms of the foot

Used with permission from 66Fit

4 Ensure that seated measurements start with good upright posture.

5 For standing measurements, ensure that the participant is standing in the anatomical position.

> **Note:** The wrist is not measured from the anatomical neutral stance. The starting position for testing wrist/hand ROM is with the elbow flexed 90°, hand and wrist flat with the palmar surface face down.

6 The joint to be measured should be isolated to avoid the use of ancillary muscles.

7 All joint ROM measurements outlined in Tables 9.5–9.12 are carried out with the standard lever arm goniometer and inclinometer.

8 Align the central pivot point of the goniometer over the axis of rotation/joint line and align the arms with the distal joint bony landmarks.

9 Hold the inclinometer using the thumb and forefinger spanning across the base of the instrument; hold it securely against the body part/limb to be measured.

10 Ensure that the inclinometer is set to zero at the start of the movement and that the final ROM measure is read from the bottom of the meniscus at eye level so as to minimise parallax error (see Figure 9.10b).

11 When the measuring device is positioned, ask the participant to move their limb in the desired direction.

12 When full active ROM has been achieved by the participant, ensure that the placement of the measuring device remains correct, then measure and record the degrees of movement observed.

13 Subjectively observe and record whether the end feel is bone on bone, capsular, ligamentous, soft tissue approximation or muscular. It can be difficult to differentiate the muscular and capsular end feels. One way to tell the difference is to conduct a proprioceptive neuromuscular facilitation (PNF) technique (i.e. hold/relax) at the end of the available range; increasing range indicates a muscular feel (i.e. not capsular). It is often the case that more than one muscle or structure contributes to the end feel of a joint ROM.

14 Clean and disinfect all equipment (see Appendix A).

Interpretation

First, consider the four steps of interpretation outlined in Appendix G. 'Normal' values for ROM of each joint have been described in Table 9.13 for most joints or body segments.[51–53] The minimum ROM required to complete common functional activities of daily living (e.g. walking, eating) has been provided for various joints (Table 9.13). Compare the recorded ROM and the subjectively observed end feel to the 'normal' ROM, functional ROM and end feel in Table 9.13 to determine whether the participant has normal, reduced or excessive flexibility. Record your findings in the 'Interpretation' column in Table 9.13.

TABLE 9.13 Full range of joint motion reference data

JOINT	ACTION	'NORMAL' ROM (°)	FUNCTIONAL ROM (°)	'NORMAL' END FEEL	RECORDED ROM (°)	RECORDED END FEEL	INTERPRETATION
Cervical	Flexion	50		Muscular			
	Extension	70		Bone on bone			
	Lateral flexion	45		Muscular			
	Rotation	70		Muscular			
Thoracic and lumbar spine	Flexion	10 cm	Sitting: 56%–66% of lumbar flexion Lifting from the floor: 95% of lumbar flexion	STA			
	Extension	10 cm		Bone on bone or muscular			
	Lateral flexion	45		STA or muscular			
	Rotation	70		Muscular or bone on bone			

continued

TABLE 9.13 Full range of joint motion reference data *(continued)*

JOINT	ACTION	'NORMAL' ROM (°)	FUNCTIONAL ROM (°)	'NORMAL' END FEEL	RECORDED ROM (°)	RECORDED END FEEL	INTERPRETATION
Shoulder	Flexion	180	Eating: 35 Drinking: 45 Combing hair: 110	SL and LL: muscular			
	Extension	45		Bone on bone			
	Abduction	180	Eating: 25 Drinking: 35 Combing hair: 100	STA or bone on bone			
	Medial rotation	90	Eating: 20 Drinking: 25 Combing hair: 45	Capsular			
	Lateral rotation	90		Capsular			
	Horizontal abduction	30		SL and LL: muscular			
	Horizontal adduction	135		STA			
Elbow	Flexion	145	Eating: 130 Drinking: 130 Opening a door: 60	STA			
	Extension	5		Bone on bone			
Forearm[a]	Pronation	80		Muscular or bone on bone			
	Supination	90		Muscular			
Wrist	Flexion	90	Eating: 5 Drinking: 5	Muscular, bone on bone or ligamentous			
	Extension	70	Eating: 40 Drinking: 40	Muscular, bone on bone or ligamentous			
	Abduction	25		Bone on bone			
	Adduction	65		Bone on bone			

continued overpage

TABLE 9.13 Full range of joint motion reference data (continued)

JOINT	ACTION	'NORMAL' ROM (°)	FUNCTIONAL ROM (°)	'NORMAL' END FEEL	RECORDED ROM (°)	RECORDED END FEEL	INTERPRETATION
Hip	Flexion	120	Sitting: 90 Stairs: 65 Walking: 30	SL: STA LL: muscular			
	Extension	15	Stairs: 5 Walking: 10	Muscular			
	Abduction	45		Muscular			
	Adduction	20		Muscular			
	Medial rotation	35		Capsular			
	Lateral rotation	45		Capsular			
Knee	Flexion	135	Sitting: 95 Stairs: 105 Walking: 65	STA or muscular			
	Hyperextension	5		Capsular			
Ankle	Plantaflexion	45^b	Walking: 30 Walking downstairs: 30	Bone on bone or muscular			
	Dorsiflexion	15^c	Sitting: 10 Walking: 15 Walking downstairs: 35	Muscular or capsular			
Foot	Inversion	30		Bone on bone, muscular or capsular			
	Eversion	15		Bone on bone or muscular			

LL = long lever; SL = short lever; STA = soft tissue approximation
^{a} Not covered in above Tables.
^{b} Plantarflexion is at maximum ROM at 2 years of age (62°) and decreases over the course of the lifespan.
^{c} Ankle dorsiflexion is at maximum ROM at birth/neonate (59°) and decreases over the course of the lifespan.[2]
Adapted from: Schultz et al,[1] Capuano-Pucci et al,[51] Soames,[2] Mian et al[52] and Mak et al[53]

Normal flexibility interpretation

If the measured ROM about a joint is within the expected 'normal' range for the participant's sex, the participant is considered to have normal flexibility (at that joint). However, the following flexibility changes across the lifespan should be considered with respect to what is considered a 'normal' ROM:

Pre-pubertal:

- No difference in pre-pubertal ROM between girls and boys.

Young adult:

- Increased ROM in young adults compared with pre-pubertal girls and boys owing to sex hormones.
- Decrease in lateral lumbar flexion ROM of ~2.0° per decade of life after 30 years in women.[54,55]

Older adult

- ROM decreases with increasing age, explaining 50%–60% variability.
- ROM maintenance is dependent on physical activity levels.
- ROM decreases to a greater extent in females compared with males.
- Decrease in ROM is joint specific and dependent on habitual use of the joint ROM:
  - shoulder and trunk ROM are most affected
  - elbow and knee ROM are better preserved.[56]
- There is no age-related influence on creep of tissues.
- Change in integrity and contribution of passive and active elements with increasing age due to:
  - increased quantity of inter- and intra-muscular collagen
  - stiffer collagen through cross-linking.
- Increased stiffness in passive tissues is due to increased collagen content and irreversible cross-linking.
- Change in posture is due to changes in osseous anatomy and alignment:
  - kyphosis affecting cervical ROM
  - pronounced forward head extension[57]
  - decreased height and width of cervical vertebrae[58]
  - decreased height and stenosis of intervertebral space and spinal canal.[58]

Reduced flexibility interpretation

If the measured ROM about a joint is less than the expected 'normal' range, the participant is considered to have reduced flexibility (at that joint). In apparently healthy populations the main cause of reduced ROM is often musculotendinous tightness. Several other anatomical structures such as ligament, joint capsule, adipose tissue and bone may also limit ROM about a joint. Distinguishing between these structures is outside the scope of this practical.

Although the evidence is mixed, there are several studies that have reported increased risk of injury with reduced flexibility. Weight-training participants with subacromial impingement syndrome had significantly decreased internal and external rotation active ROM compared with participants without subacromial impingement syndrome.[59] Competitive female swimmers aged 8–11 years, but not older swimmers,[60] experienced shoulder pain and disability with reduced shoulder flexion. Whereas hip internal rotation, abduction and extension were not associated with the risk or presence of groin pain,[61] there was strong evidence that total rotation of both hips below 85° measured at pre-season was a risk factor for groin pain development. Australian Football League players with low hip flexor/quadriceps flexibility and high stiffness of the lower-limb and hamstring, but not static hamstring flexibility, had an increased hamstring injury risk.[62] Finally, of all the measured performance factors, only reduced ankle dorsiflexion range was associated with patellar tendinopathy in volleyball players.[63]

Excessive flexibility interpretation

If the measured ROM about a joint is more than the expected 'normal' range, participants are considered to have excessive flexibility (at that joint). There are many causes of excessive ROM – for example, previous history of injury which has led to joint laxity, occupational or sporting movements which have increased ROM over time, or congenital factors such as excessive ROM throughout the body.

Consistent with reduced flexibility, the evidence for the relationship between excessive flexibility and risk of injury is varied. For example, hyper hip abduction, and lower back and hamstring flexibility among young dancers (10–11 years old), and hyper ankle dorsiflexion for adolescent dancers

(12–14 years old), predicted patellofemoral pain syndrome. However, for 15–16-year-old dancers, patellofemoral pain syndrome was predicted by limited ankle plantar-flexion (odds ratio (OR) $= 1.060$), and limited hip internal rotation (OR $= 1.063$).[64] Furthermore, according to self-reported history of low back and lower extremity injuries, ballet dancers have a greater risk of injury if they reach a turnout position that is greater than their available bilateral passive hip external rotation ROM.[65]

Feedback and discussion

First, consider the three steps of feedback and discussion outlined in Appendix G. Before providing feedback, check whether the participant is currently, or has previously, participated in sport or activities that may have influenced the results. For example, the flexibility of a female rhythmic gymnast would be influenced by her participation in the sport; therefore the feedback and discussion of the results may need to be adjusted accordingly.

Using the results from ROM tests to make judgments in relation to a participant's flexibility is an essential skill for exercise professionals. For example, simply informing a participant they have 135° of knee flexion is insufficient. It is important to highlight the degree of reduced or excessive flexibility, and discuss whether this has resulted in any issues or causes for concern for the participant when performing ADLs. Additional explanations such as how this result compares with published reference ROM tables, and the meaning of ROMs for the participant's health, wellbeing or sporting performance, are also required. If the ROM assessment justifies the addition of stretching exercises into the participant's exercise program, provide feedback and discuss this in relation to their exercise prescription, and whether stretching is appropriate for single or multiple joints.

Normal flexibility feedback and discussion

In apparently healthy populations with normal ROM, stretching programs are still recommended to maintain current joint flexibility.[29]

Reduced flexibility feedback and discussion

Flexibility assessments which show a reduced ROM due to musculotendinous tightness directly inform exercise prescription, such as stretching. For example, if an apparently healthy participant with no injury history is unable to achieve normal knee flexion (135°) and the restriction is felt in the quadriceps, the ROM assessment justifies the addition of quadriceps stretching into the participant's exercise program.

Excessive flexibility feedback and discussion

Where excessive ROM throughout the body is suspected, the Beighton Scoring System should be used as a means of pre-screening, as well as being useful for informing appropriate flexibility assessments, exercise prescription and/or referral to additional health professionals. In apparently healthy populations, if a participant were found to have excessive ROM at a specific joint, stretching would usually not be indicated for that movement at that joint.

In athletic populations where excessive ROM may be required to optimise performance, stretching may still be indicated in the presence of excessive flexibility.

Reduced or excessive ROM that has a direct link to sporting or occupational performance, or ADLs that have a muscular end feel, should be prioritised when designing your intervention. That being said, not every reduced ROM you measure needs to be acted upon given the limited evidence to suggest that flexibility training will reduce injury rates. Furthermore, you should consider the specificity and sensitivity of the measure. For example, you measure a 65-year-old participant's dorsiflexion to be 20°, limited by posterior calf stretch; normal dorsiflexion ROM is 25° and functional ROM for walking is 15°. You measure this ROM with a goniometer, which has a measurement error of $\pm 4°$. Taking all these factors into account, increasing dorsiflexion ROM would be considered a low priority for this participant.

Any reduced or excessive ROM that has a negative impact on sporting or occupational performance, or ADLs, requires an intervention. If during the assessment you determine that the reduced or excessive ROM end feel is not due to impaired muscular strength or flexibility, refer to a medical practitioner in the first instance. For example, a 50-year-old carpet layer reports knee stiffness after squatting at work, which is affecting his ability to complete a full 8-hour work day. You measure his knee flexion at $105°$, limited by medial knee pain deep in the joint; normal dorsiflexion ROM is $120°–140°$ and functional ROM for sitting is $90°$. You measure this ROM with an inclinometer, which has a measurement error of $\pm0.6–1.2°$. Taking all these factors into account, including the participant reporting a negative impact on their work capacity, further investigation via referral to a medical practitioner is warranted as the ROM is not limited by muscular strength or flexibility.

Case studies

Case Study 1

Setting: You are a new sport scientist at the New Zealand Institute of Sport and have a special interest in the association between ROM and performance. The athletes will commence pre-season fitness screening in the coming weeks and you have been asked for your input into the best flexibility protocols to use. The results from these tests, and the feedback you will provide to the coaching staff, will directly influence the type of training programs that individual athletes will receive over the coming year.

Participant: A client is an 18-year-old female swimmer who has just joined the Institute. As she enters the testing room, you observe that when she stands still her knees curve backwards $\approx10°$ from neutral (genu recurvatum, commonly known as hyperextended knees) and her elbows hyperextend. Her coach reports that her diving technique needs work, particularly that her shoulder position entering the water has an anterior drop.

Your task: Design a pre-season fitness screening for this swimmer, choosing from the battery of tests within this practical. Describe and justify the two most important flexibility tests that you would prioritise including in this testing battery. Conduct these tests on your partner and interpret the results according to the four steps of interpretation outlined in Appendix G. Particular reference should be made to how these results may impact her swimming performance.

TEST BATTERY:

Priority test 1

Name and describe the test.

_____

_____

_____

Justify the test, with specific reference to the case study.

_____

_____

_____

_____

continued overpage

Case studies (continued)

Practise completing this test, including data recording and calculations as appropriate.

Interpret the results, and provide feedback.

Priority test 2:

Name and describe the test.

Justify the test, with specific reference to the case study.

Practise completing this test, including data recording and calculations as appropriate.

Interpret the results, and provide feedback.

How do your answers compare with the worked example provided at the end of this manual?

continued

Case studies *(continued)*

Case Study 2

Setting: You are working as an Accredited Exercise Scientist at a fitness centre and are in charge of supervision of the gym floor for the day. You are tasked with monitoring the technique of the patrons who are exercising independently and providing advice, feedback and exercise prescription as necessary.

Client: A 55-year-old 'fly in, fly out' mine worker who completes 12-hour shifts for 3 weeks at a time and then returns home for a 7-day rest. Until recently he has never exercised regularly in his life; however, last month he purchased a gym membership at your centre to utilise during his week away from work. As he bends over to pick up a 5 kg dumbbell, you observe his movements are stiff, particularly in his hip and low back. After approaching the client and initiating a conversation, you learn more about the hard physical labour of his job, the fact that he has no history of musculoskeletal injury and also that he has never performed any flexibility exercises such as stretching.

Task: Select a measure of flexibility from the battery of tests within this practical that can be efficiently incorporated into the last 10 minutes of his next gym session. Describe and justify the most important flexibility test that you would use. Conduct this test and interpret the results according to the four steps of interpretation outlined in Appendix G. Particular reference should be made to how these results may impact his ability to pick things up off the floor.

TEST BATTERY:

Priority test

Name and describe the test.

_____

_____

_____

Justify the test, with specific reference to the case study.

_____

_____

_____

_____

Practise completing this test, including data recording and calculations as appropriate.

_____

_____

_____

_____

Interpret the results, and provide feedback.

_____

_____

_____

_____

How do your answers compare with the worked example provided at the end of this manual?

_____

_____

References

[1] Schultz DJ, Houglan PA, Perrin DH. Examination of musculoskeletal injuries. Champaign, IL: Human Kinetics; 2005.

[2] Soames R. Joint motion: clinical measurement and evaluation. Edinburgh, Scotland: Churchill Livingstone; 2003.

[3] Soucie JM, Wang C, Forsyth A, Funk S, Denny M, Roach KE, et al; Hemophilia Treatment Center N. Range of motion measurements: reference values and a database for comparison studies. Haemophilia 2011;17:500–7.

[4] Yeung SS, Yeung EW, Gillespie LD. Interventions for preventing lower limb soft-tissue running injuries. Cochrane Database Syst Rev 2011:CD001256.

[5] Pacey V, Nicholson LL, Adams RD, Munn J, Munns CF. Generalized joint hypermobility and risk of lower limb joint injury during sport: a systematic review with meta-analysis. Am J Sports Med 2010;38:1487–97.

[6] Quatman CE, Ford KR, Myer GD, Paterno MV, Hewett TE. The effects of gender and pubertal status on generalized joint laxity in young athletes. J Sci Med Sport 2008;11:257–63.

[7] Alter MJ. Science of flexibility. Champaign, IL: Human Kinetics; 2004.

[8] Beighton P, Solomon L, Soskolne CL. Articular mobility in an African population. Ann Rheum Dis 1973;32:413–18.

[9] Vollestad NK, Torjesen PA, Robinson HS. Association between the serum levels of relaxin and responses to the active straight leg raise test in pregnancy. Man Ther 2012;17:225–30.

[10] Marnach ML, Ramin KD, Ramsey PS, Song SW, Stensland JJ, An KN. Characterization of the relationship between joint laxity and maternal hormones in pregnancy. Obstet Gynecol 2003;101:331–5.

[11] Liu SH, al-Shaikh R, Panossian V, Yang RS, Nelson SD, Soleiman N, et al. Primary immunolocalization of estrogen and progesterone target cells in the human anterior cruciate ligament. J Orthop Res 1996;14:526–33.

[12] Price MJ, Tuca M, Cordasco FA, Green DW. Nonmodifiable risk factors for anterior cruciate ligament injury. Curr Opin Pediatr 2017;29:55–64.

[13] Aronson P, Rijke A, Hertel J, Ingersoll CD. Medial tibiofemoral-joint stiffness in males and females across the lifespan. J Athl Train 2014;49:399–405.

[14] Hansen M, Kongsgaard M, Holm L, Skovgaard D, Magnusson SP, Qvortrup K, et al. Effect of estrogen on tendon collagen synthesis, tendon structural characteristics, and biomechanical properties in postmenopausal women. J Appl Physiol (1985) 2009;106:1385–93.

[15] Chandrashekar N, Mansouri H, Slauterbeck J, Hashemi J. Sex-based differences in the tensile properties of the human anterior cruciate ligament. J Biomech 2006;39:2943–50.

[16] Bell DR, Myrick MP, Blackburn JT, Shultz SJ, Guskiewicz KM, Padua DA. The effect of menstrual-cycle phase on hamstring extensibility and muscle stiffness. J Sport Rehabil 2009;18:553–63.

[17] Bowerman SJ, Smith DR, Carlson M, King GA. A comparison of factors influencing ACL injury in male and female athletes and non-athletes. Phys Ther Sport 2006;7:144–52.

[18] Pollard CD, Braun B, Hamill J. Influence of gender, estrogen and exercise on anterior knee laxity. Clin Biomech (Bristol, Avon) 2006;21:1060–6.

[19] Beynnon BD, Bernstein IM, Belisle A, Brattbakk B, Devanny P, Risinger R, et al. The effect of estradiol and progesterone on knee and ankle joint laxity. Am J Sports Med 2005;33:1298–304.

[20] Grahame R, Bird HA, Child A. The revised (Beighton 1998) criteria for the diagnosis of benign joint hypermobility syndrome (BJHS). J Rheumatol 2000;27:1777–9.

[21] Kim PJ, Peace R, Mieras J, Thoms T, Freeman D, Page J. Interrater and intrarater reliability in the measurement of ankle joint dorsiflexion is independent of examiner experience and technique used. J Am Podiatr Med Assoc 2011;101:407–14.

[22] Nadeau S, Kovacs S, Gravel D, Piotte F, Moffet H, Gagnon D, et al. Active movement measurements of the shoulder girdle in healthy subjects with goniometer and tape measure techniques: a study on reliability and validity. Physiother Theory Pract 2007;23:179–87.

[23] Menadue C, Raymond J, Kilbreath SL, Refshauge KM, Adams R. Reliability of two goniometric methods of measuring active inversion and eversion range of motion at the ankle. BMC Musculoskelet Disord 2006;7:60.

[24] Mayerson NH, Milano RA. Goniometric measurement reliability in physical medicine. Arch Phys Med Rehabil 1984;65:92–4.

[25] Ayala F, Sainz de Baranda P, De Ste Croix M, Santonja F. Reproducibility and criterion-related validity of the sit and reach test and toe touch test for estimating hamstring flexibility in recreationally active young adults. Phys Ther Sport 2012;13:219–26.

[26] Clarkson HM. Musculoskeletal assessment, joint motion and muscle testing. Philadelphia, PA: Lippincott, Williams and Wilkins; 2013.

[27] Loder RT, Browne R, Bellflower J, Kayes K, Wurtz D, Loder AJ. Angular measurement error due to different measuring devices. J Pediatr Orthop 2007;27:338–46.

[28] de la Motte SJ, Lisman P, Gribbin TC, Murphy K, Deuster PA. A systematic review of the association between physical fitness and musculoskeletal injury risk: part 3 – flexibility, power, speed, balance, and agility. J Strength Cond Res 2019;33(6):1723–35.

[29] American College of Sports Medicine. ACSM's guidelines for exercise testing and prescription, 10th ed. Baltimore, MD: Lippincott, Williams and Wilkins; 2018.

[30] Imagama S, Hasegawa Y, Wakao N, Hirano K, Muramoto A, Ishiguro N. Impact of spinal alignment and back muscle strength on shoulder range of motion in middle-aged and elderly people in a prospective cohort study. Eur Spine J 2014;23:1414–19.

[31] Russek LN. Hypermobility syndrome. Phys Ther 1999;79:591–9.

[32] Halabchi F, Angoorani H, Mirshahi M, Pourgharib Shahi MH, Mansournia MA. The prevalence of selected intrinsic risk factors for ankle sprain among elite football and basketball players. Asian J Sports Med 2016;7:e35287.

[33] Golightly YM, Hannan MT, Nelson AE, Hillstrom HJ, Cleveland RJ, Kraus VB, et al. Relationship of joint hypermobility with ankle and foot radiographic osteoarthritis and symptoms in a community-based cohort. Arthritis Care Res (Hoboken) 2019;71(4):538–44.

[34] Foss KD, Ford KR, Myer GD, Hewett TE. Generalized joint laxity associated with increased medial foot loading in female athletes. J Athl Train 2009;44:356–62.

[35] Kim SJ, Moon HK, Kim SG, Chun YM, Oh KS. Does severity or specific joint laxity influence clinical outcomes of anterior cruciate ligament reconstruction? Clin Orthop Relat Res 2010;468:1136–41.

[36] Kim SJ, Chang JH, Oh KS. Posterior cruciate ligament reconstruction in patients with generalized joint laxity. Clin Orthop Relat Res 2009;467:260–6.

[37] Juul-Kristensen B, Hansen H, Simonsen EB, Alkjaer T, Kristensen JH, Jensen BR, et al. Knee function in 10-year-old children and adults with generalised joint hypermobility. Knee 2012;19:773–8.

[38] Sahar T, Cohen MJ, Ne'eman V, Kandel L, Odebiyi DO, Lev I, et al. Insoles for prevention and treatment of back pain. Cochrane Database Syst Rev 2007;4:CD005275.

[39] Jones CJ, Rikli RE, Max J, Noffal G. The reliability and validity of a chair sit-and-reach test as a measure of hamstring flexibility in older adults. Res Q Exerc Sport 1998;69:338–43.

[40] Chen HT, Lin CH, Yu LH. Normative physical fitness scores for community-dwelling older adults. J Nurs Res 2009;17:30–41.

[41] VandenBerg C, Crawford EA, Enselman ES, Robbins CB, Wojtys EM, Bedi A. Restricted hip rotation is correlated with an increased risk for anterior cruciate ligament injury. Arthroscopy 2017;33:317–25.

[42] Tainaka K, Takizawa T, Kobayashi H, Umimura M. Limited hip rotation and non-contact anterior cruciate ligament injury: a case–control study. Knee 2014;21:86–90.

[43] Hattam P, Smeatham A. Special tests in musculoskeletal examination. Edinburgh: Elsevier; 2010.

[44] Rikli RE, Jones CJ. Senior fitness test manual. Champaign, IL: Human Kinetics; 2012.

[45] Jones CJ, Rikli RE. Measuring functional fitness of older adults. J Act Ageing 2002;March-April:25–30.

[46] Hadzic V, Sattler T, Topole E, Dervisevic E. Risk factors for ankle sprain in volleyball players: a preliminary analysis. Isokinet Exerc Sci 2009;17:155–60.

[47] Hoch MC, McKeon PO. Normative range of weight-bearing lunge test performance asymmetry in healthy adults. Man Ther 2011;16:516–19.

[48] Lewis JS, Valentine RE. Clinical measurement of the thoracic kyphosis. A study of the intra-rater reliability in subjects with and without shoulder pain. BMC Musculoskelet Disord 2010;11:39.

[49] Boyd BS. Measurement properties of a hand-held inclinometer during straight leg raise neurodynamic testing. Physiotherapy 2012;98:174–9.

[50] Konor MM, Morton S, Eckerson JM, Grindstaff TL. Reliability of three measures of ankle dorsiflexion range of motion. Int J Sports Phys Ther 2012;7:279–87.

[51] Capuano-Pucci D, Rheault W, Aukai J, Bracke M, Day R, Pastrick M. Intratester and intertester reliability of the cervical range of motion device. Arch Phys Med Rehabil 1991;72:338–40.

[52] Mian OS, Thom JM, Narici MV, Baltzopoulos V. Kinematics of stair descent in young and older adults and the impact of exercise training. Gait Posture 2007;25:9–17.

[53] Mak MK, Levin O, Mizrahi J, Hui-Chan CW. Joint torques during sit-to-stand in healthy subjects and people with Parkinson's disease. Clin Biomech (Bristol, Avon) 2003;18:197–206.

[54] Intolo P, Milosavljevic S, Baxter DG, Carman AB, Pal P, Munn J. The effect of age on lumbar range of motion: a systematic review. Man Ther 2009;14:596–604.

[55] Troke M, Moore AP, Maillardet FJ, Cheek E. A normative database of lumbar spine ranges of motion. Man Ther 2005;10:198–206.

[56] Medeiros HB, de Araujo DS, de Araujo CG. Age-related mobility loss is joint-specific: an analysis from 6,000 flexitest results. Age (Dordr) 2013;35:2399–407.

[57] Quek J, Pua YH, Clark RA, Bryant AL. Effects of thoracic kyphosis and forward head posture on cervical range of motion in older adults. Man Ther 2013;18:65–71.

[58] Yukawa Y, Kato F, Suda K, Yamagata M, Ueta T. Age-related changes in osseous anatomy, alignment, and range of motion of the cervical spine. Part I: Radiographic data from over 1,200 asymptomatic subjects. Eur Spine J 2012;21:1492–8.

[59] Kolber MJ, Hanney WJ, Cheatham SW, Salamh PA, Masaracchio M, Liu X. Shoulder joint and muscle characteristics among weight-training participants with and without impingement syndrome. J Strength Cond Res 2017;31:1024–32.

[60] Tate A, Turner GN, Knab SE, Jorgensen C, Strittmatter A, Michener LA. Risk factors associated with shoulder pain and disability across the lifespan of competitive swimmers. J Athl Train 2012;47:149–58.

[61] Tak I, Engelaar L, Gouttebarge V, Barendrecht M, Van den Heuvel S, Kerkhoffs G, et al. Is lower hip range of motion a risk factor for groin pain in athletes? A systematic review with clinical applications. Br J Sports Med 2017;51:1611–21.

[62] Hrysomallis C. Injury incidence, risk factors and prevention in Australian Rules Football. Sports Med 2013;43:339–54.

[63] Malliaras P, Cook JL, Kent P. Reduced ankle dorsiflexion range may increase the risk of patellar tendon injury among volleyball players. J Sci Med Sport 2006;9:304–9.

[64] Steinberg N, Tenenbaum S, Hershkovitz I, Zeev A, Siev-Ner I. Lower extremity and spine characteristics in young dancers with and without patellofemoral pain. Res Sports Med 2017;25:166–80.

[65] Coplan JA. Ballet dancer's turnout and its relationship to self-reported injury. J Orthop Sports Phys Ther 2002;32:579–84.

PRACTICAL 10
$\dot{V}O_2$max

Jeff Coombes and David Pyne

LEARNING OBJECTIVES

- Understand the scientific rationale, purpose, reliability, validity, assumptions and limitations of $\dot{V}O_2$max testing
- Identify and explain the common terminology, processes and equipment required to conduct an accurate and safe $\dot{V}O_2$max test
- Identify and describe contraindications and considerations that may require modification of the $\dot{V}O_2$max tests, and appropriate adjustments for relevant populations or participants
- Describe the principles and rationale for the calibration of equipment used in $\dot{V}O_2$max testing and recognise and adjust incorrectly calibrated equipment
- Conduct appropriate pre-assessment procedures, including explaining the test, obtaining informed consent and performing a pre-exercise risk assessment
- Identify the need for guidance or further information from an appropriate health professional, recognise when medical supervision is required, and when to cease a test
- Select and conduct an appropriate $\dot{V}O_2$max test, including instructing the participant and assistants on the correct use of equipment
- Calculate $\dot{V}O_2$max from expired gas fractions and ventilation data
- Record, analyse and interpret information from a $\dot{V}O_2$max test and convey the results, including the validity and limitations of the assessments, through relevant verbal and/or written communication to a participant or other professional

Equipment and other requirements

- Information sheet and informed consent form
- Adult Pre-exercise Screening System (APSS) form
- Programmable motorised treadmill or cycle ergometer
- Metabolic system and associated components (mouthpiece set-up, ventilation tubing, calibration equipment – including gases)
- Thermometer (temperature) and hygrometer (humidity)
- Body mass scales
- Heart rate monitor set (e.g. transmitter, receiver, chest strap)
- Stopwatch
- Rating of perceived exertion (RPE) chart (see Appendix E)
- Sphygmomanometer on stand with various size arm cuffs (with size indicators)
- Stethoscope

- Alcohol wipes
- Calculator and/or laptop/personal computer
- Bucket and mop
- Paper towel and tissues
- Sports tape/Micropore tape and nose clip
- Cleaning and disinfecting equipment (see Appendix A)

INTRODUCTION

The $\dot{V}O_2$max test is the criterion method for assessing cardiorespiratory fitness. The laboratory-based test is mainly used in sports science or research settings, although they are becoming more frequently incorporated into clinical settings. Exercise physiology laboratory environments are likely to contain the equipment needed, but more importantly can support the ongoing maintenance necessary to ensure the validity and reliability of a single test or series of tests. For example, the test is widely used in the Australian academies and institutes of sport across many different individual and team sports. In clinical exercise testing a cardiopulmonary exercise test (commonly referred to as a 'CPET') combines electrocardiogram (ECG) (see Practical 19, Data analysis) and expired gas analysis for potential determination of $\dot{V}O_2$max during a graded exercise test (GXT). The ability to understand, conduct, and interpret a $\dot{V}O_2$max test, and convey the outcomes to an athlete or coach, is a core skill of exercise and sports science professionals.

Physiological background

$\dot{V}O_2$max describes the highest rate at which energy is provided via aerobic metabolism. This rate is dependent on two main factors:

1 the capacity of the pulmonary, cardiac, vascular and cellular mechanisms to transport oxygen to the aerobic machinery within the muscles, and

2 the capacity to utilise oxygen within the working muscles.

The Fick principle is used to understand the factors that influence $\dot{V}O_2$max:

$$\dot{V}O_2\text{max} = \text{cardiac output} \times \text{arterial} - \text{venous oxygen difference}$$

or

$$\dot{V}O_2\text{max} = (\text{heart rate} \times \text{stroke volume}) \times (\text{arterial oxygen content} - \text{venous oxygen content})$$

Athletes who participate in sports that demand sustained effort in excess of 2 minutes, especially when utilising a large muscle mass to perform high, continuous work rates (e.g. rowing, running, cycling, triathlon), generally possess a high $\dot{V}O_2$max value.

The relationship between $\dot{V}O_2$max and health outcomes is well recognised. Low levels of cardiorespiratory fitness are associated with a higher risk of cardiovascular disease and all-cause mortality.[1] Importantly, improvements in $\dot{V}O_2$max are associated with a reduced risk of mortality.[2]

Heredity plays a large role in determining $\dot{V}O_2$max values, but improvements of $\approx 25\%$ after weeks to months of aerobic exercise training have been recorded in healthy, young, untrained adults.[3] Although a high $\dot{V}O_2$max is a good predictor of aerobic performance in trained individuals, the ability to sustain high work rates at a percentage of $\dot{V}O_2$max (i.e. the lactate threshold) is generally a better predictor of endurance performance.[4] Practical 12 describes the measurement of the lactate threshold.

$\dot{V}O_2$max is often referred to as maximal oxygen consumption or maximal oxygen uptake. Other terms are also commonly used to describe this physiological characteristic such as cardiorespiratory fitness, maximum aerobic power, exercise capacity, work capacity, functional capacity and aerobic capacity, and combinations of these (e.g. functional aerobic capacity). Some of these terms (exercise capacity, work capacity and functional capacity) should not be used when referring to a $\dot{V}O_2$max value. They are more appropriate for other values such as the peak power output on a maximal cycle ergometer test, or the time on test during a maximal treadmill protocol. $\dot{V}O_2$ is a rate measure (volume of oxygen per minute) and therefore aerobic power is the preferred term. The term 'aerobic power' should not be confused with the use of 'power' to refer to the work rate that an individual is exercising at (e.g. watts on a cycle ergometer).

A further distinction is the term $\dot{V}O_2$peak. This descriptor might be used when the individual undergoing the test is believed to have not attained their maximal value (i.e. when there is no clear plateauing of oxygen consumption). Another common mistake is for an individual to complete a submaximal test and be assigned a '$\dot{V}O_2$max value'. This outcome should be conveyed as the person's 'predicted' or 'estimated' $\dot{V}O_2$max.

DEFINITIONS

Absolute contraindication: a reason or criterion that makes it inadvisable to conduct or continue the test. Undertaking or continuing the test could place the participant at a higher risk of an untoward event (e.g. injury or medical condition) occurring as a result of the test. See Appendix C.

Cardiopulmonary exercise testing (CPET): combines electrocardiogram (ECG) stress testing with measures of gas exchange during a graded exercise test.

Cardiorespiratory fitness: ability of the circulatory and respiratory systems to supply oxygen and support the energy demands during sustained physical activity. Also known as aerobic fitness or aerobic endurance.

Exercise capacity: the maximum amount of physical exertion that a person can sustain (e.g. peak power output on a maximal cycle ergometer test or total distance covered during a treadmill graded exercise test).

$F_E O_2$: oxygen fraction (e.g. 0.1655 or 16.55%) of expired gas ventilation.

$F_I O_2$: oxygen fraction (e.g. 0.2093 or 20.93%) of inspired gas ventilation.

Functional capacity: an individual's capacity to function in a specific situation. In an exercise test, the term functional capacity is usually synonymous with exercise capacity.

Graded exercise test: Multistage exercise test (usually on treadmill or cycle ergometer) in which exercise intensity is progressively increased (graded) through levels that bring the participant to a volitional fatigue level.

Indirect calorimetry: determining the heat equivalent produced by a participant by measuring the amount of oxygen consumed.

Maximum aerobic power: synonym for $\dot{V}O_2max$.

Relative contraindication: a reason or criterion that needs to be considered in deciding whether to conduct, modify or continue the test. Factors such as the risk versus benefit, availability of medical support, qualifications, knowledge and experience of the tester and access to medical support need to be considered. See Appendix C.

Steady state: the body in a state that is characterised by stable or mildly fluctuating physiological characteristics (e.g. heart rate) or systems (e.g. $\dot{V}O_2max$).

V_E: volume of expired gas.

V_I: volume of inspired gas.

$\dot{V}O_2max$: abbreviation for maximal oxygen uptake, this is a measure of cardiorespiratory fitness that describes the ability of the circulatory and respiratory systems to supply oxygen and support the energy demands during sustained physical activity.

$\dot{V}O_2peak$: reflects the highest (submaximal) $\dot{V}O_2$ value attained during a graded exercise test when a plateau in oxygen consumption is not observed.

CONDUCTING A $\dot{V}O_2$MAX TEST

A $\dot{V}O_2max$ test is usually conducted using a commercially available metabolic cart. However, for understanding the underlying principles of the measurements, the use of a Douglas bag for the collection of expired air is recommended.[5] It is then possible to visualise the gas volumes, making it easier to explain and understand expired fractions and minute ventilation.

Contraindications to exercise testing

It is not always appropriate to conduct exercise tests. Appendix C provides absolute and relative contraindications to exercise testing. Sometimes the decision to undertake the exercise test is made in the days before the scheduled visit to the laboratory, but occasionally on the same day after an assessment by testing staff.

Selecting the protocol

A graded exercise test (GXT) to volitional exhaustion is the gold standard test to measure $\dot{V}O_2$max in a motivated participant who is well prepared. An important step in measuring $\dot{V}O_2$max is selection of the protocol. There are many protocols available that vary with the mode, duration and intensity of each increment in the exercise test. The purpose of the test, exercise history of the participant, likely capacity and limitations of the participant, availability of equipment and facilities, and the specific requirements of the participant, coach, team or organisation. All need to be considered during protocol selection.

MEASURING EXERCISE THRESHOLDS DURING THE $\dot{V}O_2$MAX TEST

There is often the desire to determine submaximal thresholds (e.g. ventilatory or blood lactate thresholds) during the $\dot{V}O_2$max test.[6] In this situation, a protocol is selected that has the individual at a steady state for longer periods during each stage. For example, it is common to use 3–5-minute stages when determining an exercise threshold in a sports science setting. The derived threshold values are then used to prescribe exercise and training intensities.

RAMP VERSUS EXTENDED STAGE PROTOCOLS

Historically, protocols employ stages between 2 and 5 minutes duration. These are known as *extended stage protocols*. In a CPET the standard[7] or modified Bruce[8] protocols are commonly used. Both use 3-minute stages, with the modified version containing two extra initial stages at lower intensities. In this setting it may be more appropriate to determine an exercise threshold (e.g. ventilatory threshold) rather than attempt to measure $\dot{V}O_2$max. Recently, the use of shorter stages (e.g. $\leq$1 minute) has been popular and these are known as *ramp protocols*. The ramp approach avoids large and sometimes unequal increments in work rate, allowing for a more uniform physiological response. Ramp protocols with 1-minute stages will be used in this practical.

MODE OF TESTING

In a sports science test the mode (or type) of exercise, and therefore the choice of equipment/ergometer, should reflect the athlete's primary sporting activity, movement patterns and muscle mass recruitment. Ideally, such testing should be performed in the field, but often this is not possible or the precision of measurement is somewhat compromised compared with laboratory testing. Thus, much effort has gone into designing laboratory methods and equipment for specific sports (e.g. treadmill, kayak, rowing, cross-country ski and cycle ergometers). Reference $\dot{V}O_2$max values are available for numerous sports[6] and the general population[9] and care should be taken to ensure specificity of mode when interpreting $\dot{V}O_2$max values. The majority of individuals will attain a higher $\dot{V}O_2$ when performing a treadmill protocol given the larger muscle mass used and less local (e.g. leg muscle) fatigue.[10] When testing a participant who is not an athlete, a treadmill is the preferred test mode owing to the likelihood that it will elicit a higher $\dot{V}O_2$max value compared with other modes (e.g. cycling). An exception to this would be if the person does a lot of cycling and no or hardly any running. When testing a clinical or older participant, a cycle ergometer may be preferred for safety reasons or if there are gait issues or joint pain exacerbated by activity on the treadmill.

TEST DURATION

In well-prepared athletes, the actual test duration is not a major concern (e.g. total test time 8 min vs 20 min)[11] and elite male cyclists can complete either 1-minute or 5-minute stages and attain similar $\dot{V}O_2$max values with both protocols.[12] Tests using longer 4- or 5-minute stages can extend the overall test duration to 30–40 minutes depending on the protocol used and the fitness of the individual. In less-trained individuals, tests should be of sufficient length (e.g. around 10 minutes[13]) to permit the participant's adjustment to each progressive work rate, but short enough so that factors such as lactate accumulation, heat load or muscle soreness do not force termination of the test before $\dot{V}O_2$max is achieved. In deconditioned individuals, test duration may only be a few minutes.

WARM-UP

When testing athletes, a warm-up specific to the test mode should be used. This process typically includes a few minutes of low-intensity exercise (e.g. workload of the first stage of the test) and several shorter but higher intensity, faster, but not maximal efforts. In non-athletes the first few stages of the test often serve as the warm-up.

ATHLETE PROTOCOLS

When testing athletes, it is often appropriate to start at a higher work rate than that suggested in the protocols used in this practical. For example, in the cycling protocol (see Table 10.1),[14] a female cyclist might start at stage 4 (100 watts) and a male cyclist at stage 6 (150 watts).[6] In runners a protocol with fewer grade increments and greater increases in speed is preferable.

TABLE 10.1 Cycle ergometer protocol modified from Myers et al[14,a]		
STAGE	**TIME (min)**	**WORK RATE (watts)[b]**
1	1	100
2	1	125
3	1	150
4	1	175
5	1	200
6	1	225
7	1	250
8	1	275
9	1	300
10	1	325
11	1	350
12	1	375
13	1	400
14	1	425
15	1	450
16	1	475

[a] If participant completes stage 16 then the work rate is increased by 25 W every minute
[b] Self-selected cadence

Expired air gas sampling

The two approaches currently used by metabolic systems to sample expired air are either 'breath-by-breath' or a 'mixing chamber'. As the name suggests, 'breath-by-breath' analysis involves sampling each expired breath, whereas a 'mixing chamber' samples the expired air that is collected in a chamber (or Douglas bag) via a ventilation tube, for a specified interval. This practical will assume a mixing chamber approach is available.

Software considerations

Different metabolic systems have unique customised software for processing, analysing and displaying data often in real-time or near real-time. Most systems allow the user to define the variables displayed during the test and provided in summary reports. These are important considerations as they can influence the interpretation of test results. Important parameters that are normally user defined in the software include the sampling interval and the averaging technique (see below).

SAMPLING INTERVALS AND AVERAGING TECHNIQUES

The sampling interval of the expired air by the gas analysers in the metabolic system may need to be chosen prior to conducting the test. If a 'breath-by-breath' system is being used, the sampling interval is defined by either the number of breaths or a time interval. If a mixing chamber is used, a time-sampling interval (sometimes called an 'epoch') is used. A short interval (e.g. 5 s) can lead to greater variability between subsequent $\dot{V}O_2$ values, whereas a longer interval (e.g. 1 minute) may make it harder to determine whether there is a $\dot{V}O_2$ plateau.[15] A 30-second sampling interval is common when 1-minute stages are being used. In deconditioned individuals where the test may only last for a few minutes, a shorter sampling interval (e.g. 15 s) would be more appropriate, although this depends on the averaging technique being used.

The averaging technique refers to approaches such as either (a) taking an average from each interval or (b) using a 'rolling average' where the $\dot{V}O_2$ values are calculated continuously at specified time intervals (e.g. if '30-second intervals with 10-second rolling averages' are used then the system is using the previous 30 seconds of gas collection to provide a $\dot{V}O_2$ value every 10 seconds). The rolling average technique has been suggested as the optimal approach in a CPET.[10] For testing highly trained participants, taking an average from each interval is commonly used; for less-trained participants, a rolling average approach is recommended. In this practical a 30-second interval with the $\dot{V}O_2$ value averaged from this interval will be used.

Calibration

It is important that the room or laboratory space used for testing has a controlled environment (e.g. air conditioning). Prior to the test, calibration of the gas analysers and volume/flow device are vital steps to ensure accuracy of the test. Ideally, the analysers should be calibrated with three precision gases that span the physiological and environmental range (e.g. for F_EO_2 between 0.14 and 0.21, for F_ECO_2 between 0.001 and 0.05) and the volume/flow device at three different rates (L/min) that span the likely measurement range (5–200 L/min). However, some systems do not allow for this number of calibration steps. It is therefore common for the calibration of the O_2 and CO_2 gas analysers to involve just one or two different gas mixtures.[6] This modification is likely to influence the accuracy of the test. Further information regarding calibration is detailed in Practical 1.

Additional measures

Submaximal gas exchange and work rate data from the $\dot{V}O_2$max test can be used to assess additional parameters of aerobic function. Some of these measures have been used as surrogate markers of cardiorespiratory fitness including ventilatory threshold, $\dot{V}O_2$-work rate slope and measures of $\dot{V}O_2$ kinetics. Examples of $\dot{V}O_2$ kinetics measures are the $V_E/\dot{V}CO_2$ slope and the oxygen uptake efficiency slope (OUES). The OUES is derived from the relationship between $\dot{V}O_2$ and the log of minute ventilation during incremental exercise.[16] The logarithmic transformation of minute ventilation creates a linear relationship with a steeper slope or higher OUES representing a more efficient oxygen uptake, whereas a lower OUES indicates that more ventilation is required for given oxygen uptake.[17]

Verification

Given the possible 'electronic drift' in various measuring devices during the test, it is important to check the magnitude of the drift immediately after the test. This process is usually achieved by having the metabolic system sample the calibration gases and then recording the concentrations provided by the analysers. A criterion threshold (or value) should be used to either accept or disregard the $\dot{V}O_2$max test based on the amount of drift. For this practical an absolute value of 0.1% for each of the two analysers will be used. Further information regarding verification is detailed in Practical 1, Test accuracy, reliability and validity.

Validity

$\dot{V}O_2$max during large muscle mass exercise such as running or cycling is considered a valid (concurrent) measure of integrated cardiopulmonary muscle oxidative function. However, this validity depends on reaching an unambiguous $\dot{V}O_2$-work rate plateau while exercising to volitional exhaustion. In well-prepared, highly motivated individuals (e.g. athletes) this is usually not a concern. However, participants who are test naïve, less motivated and/or have one or more clinical condition may stop exercising before $\dot{V}O_2$max is reached. In this situation a $\dot{V}O_2$peak value is usually assigned. It has been argued that this approach may be problematic.[18] For example, if this value is used to assess the efficacy of an exercise training program in non-athletes (e.g. a clinical population), it is likely that an inaccurate baseline value (i.e. due to test naïvity) will yield an overestimate of the improvement in '$\dot{V}O_2$max'. This overestimation will be due to participants likely doing better on a second test because of improved confidence and experience. Potential solutions to these issues are using a familiarisation visit or a verification test. A familiarisation visit is where the protocol is replicated to allow the participant to become familiar with the environment and allow for any learning effect.[19] A verification test may require a participant to first undertake a $\dot{V}O_2$max test and then approximately 20 minutes later have $\dot{V}O_2$ measured during a supramaximal constant load test ($\approx 110\%$ of the work rate achieved during the initial $\dot{V}O_2$max test).[18] This approach would be more suitable for younger, fitter participants.

Reliability

For young, healthy participants who are accustomed to exercising to volitional exhaustion, the $\dot{V}O_2$max test is highly reproducible, irrespective of the exercise test protocol or pacing strategy.[20] In participants with clinical conditions the reliability of estimates can be worse. For example, in people with multiple sclerosis the day-to-day variation from test to retest dictated that a change of more than 10% in $\dot{V}O_2$max is required to be interpreted as a real change (see Practical 1, Test accuracy, reliability and validity).[21]

Limitations

A major limitation of the $\dot{V}O_2$max test is that it is complex and challenging for both the participant and the testing staff. The test relies on having specialised well-maintained equipment, competent operators and highly motivated participants. Further, a participant may stop the test early (e.g. due to a musculoskeletal limitation, discomfort or lack of motivation) and therefore a valid $\dot{V}O_2$max result may not be obtained.

Assumptions

- When an individual is exercising at $\dot{V}O_2$max, they are at their maximal cardiac output and maximal arterial–venous oxygen difference.
- The Fick principle is concurrently valid at a maximal work rate (technically only valid during steady state).[22]
- The metabolic system is accurately measuring the three parameters (V_E, $\dot{V}O_2$, $\dot{V}CO_2$) that are used to calculate $\dot{V}O_2$max.
- The concentrations of different gases in the inspired air remain constant during a test.

Activity 10.1 $\dot{V}O_2$max test

AIMS: to conduct a $\dot{V}O_2$max test, interpret the results and provide feedback/discuss with a participant.

Background

$\dot{V}O_2$max will be measured using indirect calorimetry on a treadmill and/or cycle ergometer using the protocols in Tables 10.1 and 10.2. These protocols are suitable for younger, healthier individuals. Tables 10.3 and 10.4 contain protocols more suitable for clinical populations and/or older individuals.

TABLE 10.2 Treadmill protocol (Bruce Ramp)[7a]			
STAGE	**TIME (min)**	**GRADIENT (%)**	**SPEED (km/h)**
1	1	0	1.6
2	1	5	2.1
3	1	10	2.7
4	1	10	3.4
5	1	11	3.7
6	1	12	4.0

continued

TABLE 10.2 Treadmill protocol (Bruce Ramp)[7,a] (continued)

STAGE	TIME (min)	GRADIENT (%)	SPEED (km/h)
7	1	12	4.2
8	1	13	5.0
9	1	14	5.4
10	1	14	6.1
11	1	15	6.6
12	1	16	6.7
13	1	16	7.2
14	1	17	7.7
15	1	18	8.0
16	1	18	8.5

[a] If participant completes stage 16 then the gradient is increased by 1% every minute

TABLE 10.3 Individualised cycle ergometer protocol suitable for clinical populations and/or older individuals[a]

STAGE	TIME (min)	WORK RATE (watts)[b]
1	1	25
2	1	50
3	1	75
4	1	100
5	1	125
6	1	150
7	1	175
8	1	200
9	1	225
10	1	250
11	1	275
12	1	300
13	1	325
14	1	350
15	1	375
16	1	400

[a] The warm-up consists of 4 minutes at an RPE of 10 (on a 6–20 scale; see Appendix E). If participant completes stage 16 then the work rate is increased by 25 W every minute
[b] Self-selected cadence. Avoid slow cadences that may cause localised muscle fatigue at higher work rates

TABLE 10.4 Individualised treadmill protocol suitable for clinical populations and/or older individuals[a]

STAGE	TIME (min)	GRADIENT (%)	SPEED (km/h)
1	1	0	Fast walking speed
2	1	1	Fast walking speed
3	1	2	Fast walking speed
4	1	3	Fast walking speed + 1 km/h
5	1	4	Fast walking speed + 1 km/h
6	1	5	Fast walking speed + 1 km/h
7	1	6	Fast walking speed + 2 km/h
8	1	7	Fast walking speed + 2 km/h
9	1	8	Fast walking speed + 2 km/h
10	1	9	Fast walking speed + 3 km/h
11	1	10	Fast walking speed + 3 km/h
12	1	11	Fast walking speed + 3 km/h
13	1	12	Fast walking speed + 4 km/h
14	1	13	Fast walking speed + 4 km/h
15	1	14	Fast walking speed + 4 km/h
16	1	15	Fast walking speed + 5 km/h

[a] Fast walking speed is determined by the participant during the warm-up by asking them to adjust (or the tester adjusting) the treadmill speed. The warm-up consists of 2 minutes at 4 km/h with 0% gradient followed by 2 minutes during which the participant selects their fast walking speed at 0% gradient. During the first 2 minutes the participant should confirm that the 4 km/h is slower than their fast walking speed. If it isn't then slow the treadmill to 3 km/h and ask again. Continue to slow the treadmill if needed. If participant completes stage 16 then the gradient is increased by 1% every minute

The data-recording sheet is designed for sampling expired air gas concentrations every 30 seconds. Although the metabolic system will provide the $\dot{V}O_2$ values, this practical also requires you to manually calculate $\dot{V}O_2$ using data collected by the system during the test. This sequence will promote an understanding of the general principles of the calculations, and with data interpretation and troubleshooting if there is a technical issue.

Protocol summary

A participant completes a graded exercise test to volitional exhaustion on a treadmill and/or cycle ergometer while their expired air is analysed to determine $\dot{V}O_2$max.

Protocol

Test preparation (prior to the participant's arrival)

1 Initial metabolic system set-up:

   a Prior to the start of the test it will be necessary to switch the metabolic system/analysers/pumps on so they are given adequate time to warm up. The system's manual should be consulted to check the time required, but analysers using zirconium fuel cells should be left on all the time. Most pumps need to be switched on ≈30 minutes before testing.

2 Prepare solutions for post-test clean-up (see Appendix A).

3 Prepare mouthpiece/respiratory valve.

4 Place a chair near the treadmill for the participant to sit on after the test if needed.

5 Have all data collection forms ready for completion and ascertain the variables on the data-recording sheet collected via the computer during the test or manually recorded during the test.

6 If a programmable cycle ergometer or treadmill is used, ensure that the correct protocol is entered (Tables 10.1 and 10.2 are suitable for younger healthier individuals and Tables 10.3 and 10.4 for clinical/older individuals).

7 Measure and enter relevant environmental data into the metabolic system software on the computer, e.g. temperature, humidity and barometric pressure.

8 Calibrate analysers and volume/flow devices according to the instructions in the manual or laboratory procedures (see Practical 1, Test accuracy, reliability and validity).

9 Ensure familiarity with test termination criteria (see Appendix F).

Pre-test (with participant present)

1 Follow the pre-exercise test procedures outlined in Appendix B.

2 Check Appendix C to ensure there are no contraindications to exercise testing.

3 Measure the height and body mass of the participant (see Practical 4, Physique assessment) and record the values.

4 Enter participant details into the computer (e.g. name, sport (if applicable), group (if applicable), date of birth, sex, body mass).

5 Estimate the participant's age-predicted maximal heart rate (HRmax) using $208 - (0.7 \times age)$.[23]

6 Have the participant place their water bottle and towel in close proximity to the cycle ergometer/treadmill.

7 Fit the heart rate monitor and record the heart rate (see Practical 3, Cardiovascular health).

8 Measure and record blood pressure in the exercising posture (e.g. standing or sitting) (see Practical 3) — the blood pressure provides a baseline measure and is used to determine whether the participant has exceeded the criteria for a contraindication to exercise (see Appendix C).

9 Consult the exercise protocol to determine whether a warm-up is included (e.g. the first few minutes are at a low-intensity).[a] If the protocol does not contain a warm-up, the participant should complete a 5-minute warm-up. In the interest of time the warm-up can be done during the test preparation.

10 If using a treadmill, provide treadmill safety precautions to the participant (see Appendix D). An assessment of their ability to walk/jog safely should be conducted prior to starting the test.

11 Provide details of the test, including the protocol, hand signals the participant can use during the test, and explanation of the rating of perceived exertion (RPE) (see Appendix E), test termination and safety (see Appendix F).

12 Encourage the participant to push themselves to their maximum capacity (volitional exhaustion) for valid test results.

Test

1 With the participant on the treadmill or cycle ergometer, fit the headpiece and mouthpiece.

> **Note:** If a mask that covers the mouth and nose is being used, ensure there are no gaps between the face and mask by blocking the valve and checking suction.

---

[a] For clinical populations or older individuals a shorter warm-up is recommended as a longer warm-up may lead to considerable fatigue prior to the test. See Tables 10.3 and 10.4 for warm-up protocols for clinical populations or older individuals.

2 Place the nose tape (e.g. Micropore™ tape) and nose clip on the participant. Ask the participant to check carefully for leaks by attempting to breathe in and out of the nose with the mouth closed; reposition the nose clip if necessary.

3 The participant should start exercising at the intensity specified for stage 1.

4 Once this intensity is reached the test should be started via a countdown – '3, 2, 1, go'. Most software programs require you to click 'start test' on the computer keyboard or touchscreen.

5 Your primary responsibility during the test is the safety of the participant.

6 During the test, monitor closely the power output and cadence (cycle ergometer), or speed and gradient (treadmill) and overall test time even though you may be using a programmable piece of equipment. The tester should assume a position that allows these parameters to be observed along with viewing of the participant's performance, posture, position and facial expressions. For the treadmill protocol, the tester (or assistant) may need to move towards the rear of the treadmill, put their hand behind the participant's back, and provide verbal encouragement if they are tending to move to the back of the treadmill.

7 Manually record any data that is not being automatically recorded and saved by the computer.

8 Heart rate and RPE are recorded at the end of each minute.

9 Encourage the participant to exercise until volitional exhaustion by focusing on completion of each stage. As a guide, the most vigorous verbal encouragement is often required when the respiratory exchange ratio (RER) is greater than ≈1.05.

10 During the test it may be necessary to prematurely stop the test – see Appendix F for more detail and criteria.

11 At volitional exhaustion, prioritise the safety and wellbeing of the participant. Then record the participant's heart rate at volitional exhaustion as the maximum heart rate (sometimes referred to as the peak heart rate).

12 Record the work rate (cycle ergometer) or gradient and speed (treadmill) at volitional exhaustion.

Post-test

1 At the completion of the test the participant's wellbeing is paramount. When exercise stops, reduce the work rate immediately to as little as 3 km/h (treadmill) with no incline or 25–50 W (cycle ergometer) so that after terminating the test a cool-down can start as soon as possible. Monitoring the heart rate during recovery will help to determine the length of the cool-down. Keep the participant on the treadmill or cycle ergometer and encourage them to start the cool-down as soon as practicable.

2 Click 'end test' (or similar) on the computer or touchscreen. Save the test.

3 Remove the headpiece and nose clip. Be careful not to spill saliva from the mouthpiece and ventilation tube. A wad of tissues placed into the mouthpiece can be a useful temporary 'plug'. A bucket should be available to place the mouthpiece and tubes in to avoid saliva spilling onto the floor.

4 Provide the participant with their own water bottle and towel.

5 Ensure the participant has an adequate cool-down – heart rate should return to at least 50% of HRmax. In some situations you may wish to measure the RPE, blood pressure (BP) and heart rate during recovery (e.g. 1 and 5 minutes post-test). It is good practice to keep observing the participant at all times. If they walk away from the treadmill or cycle ergometer, ensure they are steady on their feet.

6 Verify the calibration of gas analysers to ensure that there was minimal drift during the test (see Practical 1, Test accuracy, reliability and validity). Accept the test results if the drift is less than 0.1% (absolute) in each of the two analysers.

7 Shut down the metabolic system and computer.

8 Clean and disinfect all equipment (see Appendix A), including the ergometer/treadmill, as sweat can cause corrosion of mechanical and electronic components.

Data recording: $\dot{V}O_2$max (cycle ergometer) data sheet

Participant's name: _____   Date: _____

Age: _____ years   Sex: _____   Body mass: _____ kg

Stature: _____ m

Age-predicted maximal heart rate[b]: _____ bpm

Protocol (e.g. Bruce ramp): _____

Testing location: _____

Supervising staff: _____   Sport (if applicable): _____

STAGE	TIME (min: s)	WORK RATE (watts)[a]	V_E[b] (L/min)	F_EO_2 (fraction)	F_ECO_2 (fraction)	HR (bpm)	RPE (6–20)	METABOLIC SYSTEM $\dot{V}O_2$ (mL/kg/min)	CALCULATED[c] $\dot{V}O_2$ (mL/kg/min)
1	0:30								
	1:00								
2	1:30								
	2:00								
3	2:30								
	3:00								
4	3:30								
	4:00								
5	4:30								
	5:00								
6	5:30								
	6:00								
7	6:30								
	7:00								
8	7:30								
	8:00								
9	8:30								
	9:00								
10	9:30								
	10:00								

[a] Refer to Table 11.1 to convert from kgm/min or kpm/min to watts
[b] Depending on the system and the position of the flow-measuring device (e.g. this will be V_E if the flow volume is collected on the expired side)
[c] Calculate $\dot{V}O_2$ manually for some of the completed 30-second intervals

continued overpage

[b] $208 - (0.7 \times \text{age})$. This is more accurate than $220 - \text{age}$.

Data recording: $\dot{V}O_2$max (cycle ergometer) data sheet (continued)

STAGE	TIME (min: s)	WORK RATE (watts)[a]	V_E[b] (L/min)	F_EO_2 (fraction)	F_ECO_2 (fraction)	HR (bpm)	RPE (6–20)	METABOLIC SYSTEM $\dot{V}O_2$ (mL/kg/min)	CALCULATED[c] $\dot{V}O_2$ (mL/kg/min)
11	10:30								
	11:00								
12	11:30								
	12:00								
13	12:30								
	13:00								
15	14:30								
	15:00								
16	15:30								
	16:00								

[a] Refer to Table 11.1 to convert from kgm/min or kpm/min to watts
[b] Depending on the system and the position of the flow-measuring device (e.g. this will be V_E if the flow volume is collected on the expired side)
[c] Calculate $\dot{V}O_2$ manually for some of the completed 30-second intervals

Maximum heart rate: _____ bpm

Maximum work rate[c]: _____ watts

Plateau criteria: $<$150 mL/min/body mass (kg) $= <$ _____ mL/kg/min

Circle: $\dot{V}O_2$max or $\dot{V}O_2$peak $=$ _____ mL/kg/min

Data recording: $\dot{V}O_2$max (treadmill) data sheet

Participant's name: _____   Date: _____

Age: _____ years   Sex: _____   Body mass: _____ kg

Stature: _____ m

Age-predicted maximal heart rate[d]: _____ bpm

Protocol (e.g. Bruce Ramp): _____

Testing location: _____

Supervising staff: _____   Sport (if applicable): _____

continued

---

[c] From a completed stage.
[d] 208 − (0.7 × age). This is more accurate than 220 − age.

Data recording: $\dot{V}O_2$max (treadmill) data sheet *(continued)*

STAGE	TIME (min: s)	TREADMILL		V_E OR $V^{a,b}$ (L/min)	F_EO_2 (fraction)	F_ECO_2 (fraction)	HR (bpm)	RPE (6–20)	METABOLIC SYSTEM $\dot{V}O_2$ (mL/kg/min)	CALCULATED^b $\dot{V}O_2$ (mL/kg/min)
		GRADIENT (%)	SPEED (km/h)							
1	0:30									
	1:00									
2	1:30									
	2:00									
3	2:30									
	3:00									
4	3:30									
	4:00									
5	4:30									
	5:00									
6	5:30									
	6:00									
7	6:30									
	7:00									
8	7:30									
	8:00									
9	8:30									
	9:00									
10	9:30									
	10:00									
11	10:30									
	11:00									
12	11:30									
	12:00									
13	12:30									
	13:00									

continued overpage

Data recording: $\dot{V}O_2$max (treadmill) data sheet *(continued)*

STAGE	TIME (min: s)	TREADMILL		V_E OR $V^{a,b}$ (L/min)	F_EO_2 (fraction)	F_ECO_2 (fraction)	HR (bpm)	RPE (6–20)	METABOLIC SYSTEM $\dot{V}O_2$ (mL/kg/min)	CALCULATED[b] $\dot{V}O_2$ (mL/kg/min)
		GRADIENT (%)	SPEED (km/h)							
14	13:30									
	14:00									
15	14:30									
	15:00									
16	15:30									
	16:00									

[a] Depending on the system and the position of the flow-measuring device (e.g. this will be V_E if the flow volume is collected on the expired side)
[b] Calculate $\dot{V}O_2$ manually for the last two completed 30-second intervals

Maximum heart rate: _____ _____ bpm

Maximum work rate[e]: _____ watts

Plateau criteria: <150 mL/min/body mass $= <$ _____ mL/kg/min

Circle: $\dot{V}O_2$max or $\dot{V}O_2$peak $=$ _____ mL/kg/min

Data analysis

Manual calculation of $\dot{V}O_2$max

The following sequence of steps is a simplified approach to calculating oxygen uptake ($\dot{V}O_2$) at different intensities. More detail can be located in Box 10.1 and in a publication from the Australian Institute of Sport.[6]

For the last six completed 30-second intervals, manually calculate the $\dot{V}O_2$ and enter these values into the data table (final column).

Each calculation requires three steps:

1 calculate F_EN_2 = the fraction of expired nitrogen

2 calculate V_ESTPD = the volume of expired air at standard temperature pressure dry

3 $\dot{V}O_2$ = the volume of oxygen consumed and used.

[e] From a completed stage.

Box 10.1 Gas calculation

To understand the manual calculation of $\dot{V}O_2$, it is helpful to know three different ways gas volumes are expressed. These variations are needed because the volume of a gas changes depending on temperature and pressure.

ATPS: Ambient Temperature and Pressure Saturated with water vapour. When an expired gas from an individual is measured outside of the body in a laboratory under normal room conditions the volume is referred to as ATPS (e.g. V_IATPS = volume of inspired gas at ATPS). This means that the measured gas has not been standardised but is dependent on the temperature of the room, the barometric pressure in the room *and* assumes that the gas is saturated with water vapour.

BTPS: Body Temperature and Pressure Saturated with water vapour. Refers to the volume of the gas when it is in the body (at body temperature). We do not measure gas volumes while they are in the body but convert gas volumes measured outside the body (ATPS) to reflect what the gas volume would be inside the body. Metabolic systems often provide V_E on the screen/printout as a BTPS value. This means the volume is assumed to be at 37°C (body temperature).

STPD: Standard Temperature and Pressure Dry. To allow for comparisons of volumes measured at different temperatures and pressures and under varying humidity the ATPS and BTPS volumes are converted to STPD. The temperature is standardised at 0°C, the pressure is 760 mmHg (sea level) and the humidity is 0% (absence of water vapour).

CALCULATING $\dot{V}O_2$ WHEN V_I IS MEASURED

To calculate $\dot{V}O_2$ requires the measurement of the volume either of expired (V_E) or inspired (V_I) gas per minute. Most metabolic systems measure V_I by having the flow/volume measuring device on the inspired side of the circuit. This set-up can be determined by examining the mouthpiece, valves and flow/volume measuring device. In this situation it is necessary to measure the relative humidity, temperature and barometric pressure of the room. This information is entered into the metabolic system when setting it up. The metabolic system then standardises the inspired volumes and provides them as V_ISTPD on the screen/printout.

With V_ISTPD provided, V_E can be calculated using the Haldane transformation formula (step 2 in the manual calculation of $\dot{V}O_2$). This transformation is based on the assumption that the volume of nitrogen exhaled must equal the volume of nitrogen inhaled because nitrogen is inert and neither used nor produced in the body.

For these calculations, from each of the last six completed 30-second intervals from the data-recording sheet you need:

1 F_EO_2 = fraction of expired oxygen

2 F_ECO_2 = fraction of expired carbon dioxide

3 V_ISTPD = volume of inspired oxygen at standard temperature pressure dry.

STEP 1

$$F_EN_2 = 1 - (F_EO_2 + F_ECO_2)$$

$$= 1 - (\underline{\hspace{2cm}} + \underline{\hspace{2cm}})$$

$$= \underline{\hspace{3cm}}$$

STEP 2

$$V_E STPD = V_I STPD \times \frac{0.7904^f}{F_E N_2}$$

$$= \underline{\hspace{3cm}} \times 0.7904$$

$$= \underline{\hspace{3cm}}$$

STEP 3

$$\dot{V}O_2 = \text{volume of oxygen inspired} - \text{volume of oxygen expired}$$

$$= (V_I STPD \times 0.2093^g) - (V_E STPD \times F_E O_2)$$

$$= (\underline{\hspace{1.5cm}} \times \underline{\hspace{1.5cm}}) - (\underline{\hspace{1.5cm}} \times \underline{\hspace{1.5cm}})$$

$$= \underline{\hspace{1cm}} \times \frac{1000}{\text{body mass}}$$

$$= \underline{\hspace{1cm}} \text{mL/kg/min}$$

Interpretation

First, consider the four steps of interpretation outlined in Appendix G.

1. Valid or invalid test?

First a decision should be made regarding the concurrent validity of the test (i.e. did the test generate a $\dot{V}O_2$ value that is representative of a person's maximal aerobic power?). An example of an invalid test is when the participant stops due to a musculoskeletal issue (e.g. a muscle cramp during the test). However, there are many situations when it is difficult to decide whether a test should be deemed valid (e.g. participant is clearly uncomfortable with the mouthpiece) and established criteria should be used to determine test validity. It is suggested that if the participant has crossed the ventilatory threshold and indicated that they were at volitional exhaustion then the test is typically classified as valid.

2. $\dot{V}O_2$max or $\dot{V}O_2$peak?

If the test is deemed valid then the next decision is whether the value should be called $\dot{V}O_2$max or $\dot{V}O_2$peak. For an individual to be at $\dot{V}O_2$max there should be a plateau in oxygen consumption with an increase in work rate. This relationship is shown in Figure 10.1. If a $\dot{V}O_2$ plateau is not evident then the value should be reported as $\dot{V}O_2$peak.

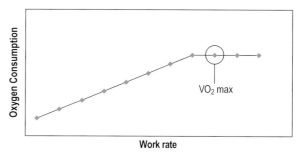

Figure 10.1 Plateau in oxygen consumption with an increase in work rate

There has been much debate around the criteria for determining a plateau in $\dot{V}O_2$ and whether additional supplementary criteria are needed to validate the achievement of $\dot{V}O_2$max. For the purpose of this manual these issues will not be discussed further; however, a number of investigators have explored this debate.[18,22,24–26] Determining whether there is a plateau in oxygen consumption with an increased work rate depends on a number of factors including the interval for sampling the expired gas, the duration of the stages, and the $\dot{V}O_2$max of the participant. The following criteria are recommended for a protocol with 1-minute stages and 30-second intervals where the participant is young and relatively healthy.[27]

Plateau criteria = using data from the 30-second epochs, if the work rate has increased and the

$$\dot{V}O_2 \text{ increase is} < \frac{150\text{mL } O_2/\text{min}}{\text{Body mass}}$$

---

f The fraction of nitrogen in dry atmospheric air, assumed as 79.04%/100.
g The fraction of oxygen in dry atmospheric air, assumed as 20.93%/100.

The following example in Figure 10.2 shows how this can be determined. The participant's body mass is 65 kg, therefore:

$$\text{Plateau criteria} < \frac{150}{65} \rightarrow < 2.5 \text{ mL/kg/min}$$

Note that in this example the $\dot{V}O_2$ value provided at a time point reflects data collected during the previous 30 seconds (e.g. at 5 minutes the $\dot{V}O_2$ of 53.5 mL/kg/min reflects data collected between 4.5 and 5.0 minutes). As the exercise protocol used during this example has increments every minute, determining a plateau in $\dot{V}O_2$ between two consecutive 30-second epochs requires a comparison of the value reported on the minute (e.g. 5.0 minutes = 53.5 mL/kg/min) and 30 seconds later (e.g. 5.5 minutes = 58.8 mL/kg/min). This scenario reflects when there has been an increase in intensity during the test. During this time (between 4.5 and 5.5 minutes), the difference between the $\dot{V}O_2$ values (58.8 − 53.5 = 5.3 mL/kg/min) is greater than the plateau criteria (2.5 mL.kg/min); therefore this is not a plateau. However, between 6.5 and 7.5 minutes there is a plateau (as well as between 7.5 and 8.5 and between 8.5 and 9.5 minutes). Therefore, the plateau criteria have been met, which means the derived value (see below for how you calculate this value) can be called $\dot{V}O_2$max.

Then $\dot{V}O_2$max or $\dot{V}O_2$peak can be circled on the data-recording sheet.

subject:	Matthew					
mass:	65.0 kg					
height:	196.0 cm					
age:	22.0 yrs					
gender:	Male					
Time	V_I	F_EO_2	F_ECO_2	V_E	VO_2	VO_2
minutes	stpd	%	%	btps	1/min	mL/kg/min
0.000	−215.13	19.31	2.47	−261.692		−3.058
0.500	46.38	18.83	2.77	56.292	0.904	13.910
1.000	41.41	17.00	3.45	49.531	1.674	25.751
1.500	43.78	15.94	4.00	52.029	2.275	35.004
2.000	44.19	15.85	4.45	52.639	2.318	35.655
2.500	54.79	15.79	4.48	65.358	2.895	44.536
3.000	57.98	16.00	4.53	69.373	2.917	44.873
3.500	56.57	16.00	4.81	67.729	2.840	43.690
4.000	56.27	15.61	4.73	67.275	3.052	46.959
4.500	67.92	15.89	4.77	81.414	3.470	53.386
5.000	70.52	16.03	4.58	84.732	3.479	53.517
5.500	84.08	16.38	4.46	101.216	3.822	58.807
6.000	85.63	16.59	4.45	103.202	3.697	56.871
6.500	84.57	16.63	4.32	114.029	4.038	62.124
7.000	102.83	16.89	4.18	124.173	4.098	63.051
7.500	112.33	17.09	3.99	135.767	4.238	65.193
8.000	129.69	17.36	3.80	156.896	4.515	69.454
8.500	135.53	17.61	3.68	164.086	4.360	67.074
9.000	150.35	17.77	3.51	182.110	4.592	70.645
9.500	162.42	17.95	3.34	196.778	4.655	71.613
10.000	52.64	18.11		63.770	1.425	21.917

Annotations to the right of the VO₂ column:
- 5.3 / 5.3: In these two epochs, there has been an increase in work rate and the $\dot{V}O_2$ has increased by ≥ 2.5 mL/kg/min
- 2.1 / −2.4 / 1.0: In these three epochs, there has been an increase in work rate but the $\dot{V}O_2$ has not increased by ≥2.5 mL/kg/min. This indicates a plateau in oxygen consumption

Figure 10.2 Determining whether the $\dot{V}O_2$ data has met the criteria of a plateau. In this example the criteria have been met, which means the value can be called $\dot{V}O_2$max

3. How to calculate $\dot{V}O_2$max or $\dot{V}O_2$peak value

There are different approaches to selecting/calculating the $\dot{V}O_2$max/$\dot{V}O_2$peak value. For this activity the two highest consecutive 30-second values will be averaged to obtain the $\dot{V}O_2$max/$\dot{V}O_2$peak value. When calculating the $\dot{V}O_2$max/$\dot{V}O_2$peak value, it is important to take into account if one of the values is an outlier (i.e. disproportionately greater than the other). This discrepancy may be caused by a slight malfunction in the metabolic system. To determine whether the higher value is an outlier, the plateau criteria value (calculated during step 2 above) is used. If the highest value is greater than the second highest value plus the plateau criteria value then it is deemed an outlier. You then replace this outlier (higher value) with the next highest value from the adjacent 30-second interval, and then use the average of these two as the $\dot{V}O_2$max/$\dot{V}O_2$peak value.

> **Note**: You do not continue to check if these values are disproportionately different – this is only done once. This process is based on the assumption that the value replaced is due to a measurement error.

Then you can record the relative value (mL/kg/min) on the data-recording sheet.

In the example in Figure 10.2, this will be a $\dot{V}O_2$max value and the two highest consecutive values are 71.6 and 70.6 mL/kg/min. The difference between these values (1.0 mL/kg/min) is less than the plateau criteria value (2.5 mL/kg/min) therefore these two values are used to obtain their average (71.1 mL/kg/min).

Note: This approach of averaging consecutive 30-second intervals after checking for an outlier is based on the protocol that has 1-minute stages and 30-second sampling intervals using a mixing chamber system with young healthy adults. In other situations, different approaches may be advisable based on the equipment, participant, exercise protocol and whether there may be a specific question being addressed (e.g. investigating $\dot{V}O_2$ kinetics).
The following two recommendations illustrate this:

1 With participants who are less fitness level, older or who have chronic disease, use shorter sampling intervals (e.g. 10 or 15 seconds) and select the two highest consecutive $\dot{V}O_2$ values after checking for an outlier.

2 In highly-trained individuals, use a 30-second sampling interval but select the highest $\dot{V}O_2$ value from one 30-second sampling interval after checking that it is not an outlier.
The protocol to select the $\dot{V}O_2$max/$\dot{V}O_2$peak value should be clearly described in the clinic or laboratory manual to ensure consistency.

4. Comparing with reference values

$\dot{V}O_2$max/$\dot{V}O_2$peak is usually reported as a volume per minute relative to body mass (mL/kg/min). The majority of $\dot{V}O_2$max tests are for athletes and the use of reference values is generally of little use for their sport-specific feedback. However, where a comparison is needed, Table 10.5 (treadmill) and Table 10.6 (cycle ergometer) can be used to give age- and sex-specific reference percentile values and qualitative descriptors (in the Tables' footers).

TABLE 10.5 Treadmill $\dot{V}O_2$max reference data (mL/kg/min)						
	AGE (years)					
PERCENTILE[a]	20–29	30–39	40–49	50–59	60–69	70–79
Men						
95	66.3	59.8	55.6	50.7	43.0	39.7
75	55.2	49.2	45.0	39.7	34.5	30.4
50	48.0	42.4	37.8	32.6	28.2	24.4
25	40.1	35.9	31.9	27.1	23.7	20.4
5	29.0	27.2	24.2	20.9	17.4	16.3
Women						
95	56	45.8	41.7	35.9	29.4	24.1
75	44.7	36.1	32.4	27.6	23.8	20.8
50	37.6	30.2	26.7	23.4	20	18.3
25	30.5	25.3	22.1	19.9	17.2	15.6
5	21.7	19	17	16	13.4	13.1

[a] The following terms may be used as descriptors for the percentile rating: superior ($\geq$95); excellent (75–94.9); good (50–74.9); below average (25–49.9); poor (5–24.9) and very poor (<5)
Obtained from the FRIEND Registry for men and women who were considered free from known CVD[9]

TABLE 10.6 Cycle ergometer $\dot{V}O_2$max reference data (mL/kg/min)

PERCENTILE[a]	AGE (YEARS)					
	20–29	30–39	40–49	50–59	60–69	70–79
Men						
95	58.5	44.7	41.9	37.4	32.4	34.0
75	49.5	35.0	31.8	29.3	25.5	22.5
50	41.9	30.1	27.1	24.8	22.4	19.5
25	34.7	26.2	22.9	22.1	19.7	17.1
5	25.5	19.3	18.9	18.1	15.3	14.4
Women						
95	45.2	33.2	29.3	25.0	22.0	19.2
75	37.1	25.1	22.6	20.1	18.3	16.5
50	31.0	21.6	19.4	17.3	16.0	14.8
25	23.2	17.9	16.5	15.3	14.4	13.2
5	17.1	14.4	13.5	12.8	12.2	11.3

[a] The following terms may be used as descriptors for the percentile rating: superior ($\geq$95); excellent (75–94.9); good (50–74.9); below average (25–49.9); poor (5–24.9) and very poor ($<$5)
Obtained from the FRIEND Registry for men and women who were considered free from known CVD[28]

Note: These reference data are from a multi-institutional registry (Fitness Registry and the Importance of Exercise; FRIEND) collating data from over 7700 maximal cardiopulmonary exercise tests.[9,28] For sport-specific reference data, refer to Physiological Tests for Elite Athletes.[6]

Feedback and discussion

First, consider the three steps of feedback and discussion outlined in Appendix G. If the participant is an athlete then it is likely that feedback needs to be provided to their coach, preferably in the presence of the athlete. It would be unusual to compare an athlete's value with reference scores from the general population. The interpretation is made in the context of their previous test value, their current training and the purpose of the test. Any subsequent discussion would be related to these issues.

Feedback to a non-athlete could use the reference values in Tables 10.5 and 10.6 depending on whether it is a treadmill or cycle ergometer test for comparative purposes, or any test scores obtained from a previous test. It may be useful to also provide additional data from the test, such as maximum heart rate and work rate. These values could be especially useful for exercise intensity prescription. Feedback should mention the importance of increased cardiorespiratory fitness to reduce the risk of cardiometabolic disease and all-cause mortality. A discussion on what types of exercise will improve $\dot{V}O_2$max should discuss the benefits that higher-intensity aerobic exercise have on $\dot{V}O_2$max.

Case study

Setting: You are working as a sports scientist for Cycling Australia.

Task: You have been asked by the coach to perform a $\dot{V}O_2$max on a junior cyclist who has been recovering from injury and has not been training for 6 months. Before the injury her $\dot{V}O_2$max was measured at 67 mL/kg/min. Using the data below, (1) manually calculate the $\dot{V}O_2$ at the last 30-second stages, (2) complete the data sheet determining whether it is a max or a peak test and (3) interpret the results and provide feedback to Rachel and her coach.

Data Recording: $\dot{V}O_2$max (cycle ergometer) Data Sheet

PARTICIPANT:

Participant's name: _Rachel Smith_   Date: _12/10/2021_

Age: _20_ years   Sex: _Female_   Body mass: _61_ kg

Stature: _1.72_ m

Age-predicted maximal heart rate[h]: _194_ bpm

Protocol (e.g. Bruce ramp): _Modified Myers_

Sport (if applicable): _Cycling_

STAGE	TIME (min: s)	WORK RATE (watts)	V_E^a (L/min)	F_EO_2 (fraction)	F_ECO_2 (fraction)	HR (bpm)	RPE(6–20)	METABOLIC SYSTEM $\dot{V}O_2$ (mL/kg/min)	CALCULATED[b] $\dot{V}O_2$ (mL/kg/min)
1	0:30	25	14.37	0.1598	0.0399			12.1	
	1:00		15.95	0.1587	0.0390	72	6	13.8	
2	1:30	50	22.12	0.1606	0.0397			18.3	
	2:00		21.36	0.1602	0.0395	90	6	17.9	
3	2:30	75	29.43	0.1723	0.0338			18.2	
	3:00		28.65	0.1609	0.0376	103	7	23.8	
4	3:30	100	33.04	0.1631	0.0401			25.7	
	4:00		34.88	0.1637	0.0403	119	7	26.7	
5	4:30	125	35.28	0.1648	0.0399			26.3	
	5:00		37.91	0.1663	0.0409	131	9	27.0	
6	5:30	150	46.06	0.1670	0.0408			32.2	
	6:00		46.80	0.1687	0.0404	148	11	31.2	
7	6:30	175	54.11	0.1677	0.0416			37.0	
	7:00		58.94	0.1708	0.0401	163	13	36.9	

continued

[h] 208 − (0.7 × age). This is more accurate than 220 − age.

Case studies (continued)

STAGE	TIME (min: s)	WORK RATE (watts)	$V_E{}^a$ (L/min)	F_EO_2 (fraction)	F_ECO_2 (fraction)	HR (bpm)	RPE (6–20)	METABOLIC SYSTEM $\dot{V}O_2$ (mL/kg/min)	CALCULATED^b $\dot{V}O_2$ (mL/kg/min)
8	7:30	200	68.13	0.1715	0.0391			42.0	
	8:00		68.92	0.1729	0.0386	174	15	40.7	
9	8:30	225	78.44	0.1734	0.0381			45.6	
	9:00		86.07	0.1759	0.0371	18.5	17	46.1	

^{a} Depending on the system and the position of the flow-measuring device (e.g. this will be V_E if the flow volume is collected on the expired side)
^{b} Calculate $\dot{V}O_2$ manually for the last two completed 30-second intervals

Maximum heart rate = _____ bpm

Maximum work rate^i = _____ watts

Plateau criteria: <150 mL/min/body mass =

Circle: $\dot{V}O_2$max or $\dot{V}O_2$peak =

References

[1] Ross R, Blair SN, Arena R, Church TS, Despres JP, Franklin BA, et al; American Heart Association PhysicaCommittee of the Council on L, Cardiometabolic H, Council on Clinical C, Council on E, Prevention, Council on C, Stroke N, Council on Functional G, Translational B, Stroke C. Importance of assessing cardiorespiratory fitness in clinical practice: a case for fitness as a clinical vital sign: a scientific statement from the American Heart Association. Circulation 2016;134:e653–99.

[2] Lee DC, Artero EG, Sui X, Blair SN. Mortality trends in the general population: the importance of cardiorespiratory fitness. J Psychopharmacol 2010;24:27–35.

[3] Bouchard C. Genomic predictors of trainability. Exp Physiol 2012;97:347–52.

[4] Jacobs RA, Rasmussen P, Siebenmann C, Diaz V, Gassmann M, Pesta D, et al. Determinants of time trial performance and maximal incremental exercise in highly trained endurance athletes. J Appl Physiol 2011;111:1422–30.

[5] Douglas CG. A method for determining the total respiratory exchange in man. J Physiol 1911;42:17–18.

[6] Australian Institute of Sport. Physiological tests for elite athletes. Champaign, IL: Human Kinetics; 2013.

[7] Bruce RA, Blackman JR, Jones JW, Strait G. Exercise testing in adult normal subjects and cardiovascular patients. Pediatrics 1963;21(Suppl.):742–56.

[8] Bruce RA, Kusumi F, Hosmer D. Maximal oxygen intake and nomographic assessment of functional aerobic impairment in cardiovascular disease. Am Heart J 1973;85:546–62.

[9] Kaminsky LA, Arena R, Myers J. Reference standards for cardiorespiratory fitness measured with cardiopulmonary exercise testing: data from the Fitness Registry and the Importance of Exercise National Database. Mayo Clin Proc 2015;90: 1515–23.

[10] Myers J, Arena R, Franklin B, Pina I, Kraus WE, McInnis K, et al. Recommendations for clinical exercise laboratories: a scientific statement from the American Heart Association. Circulation 2009;119:3144–61.

[11] Withers RT, Van der Ploeg G, Finn JP. Oxygen deficits incurred during 45, 60, 75 and 90-s maximal cycling on an air-braked ergometer. Eur J Appl Physio 1993;67:185–91.

[12] Martin DT. Australian Institute of Sport Cycling Physiologist, personal communication, 2012.

[13] Buchfuhrer MJ, Hansen JE, Robinson TE, Sue DY, Wasserman K, Whipp BJ. Optimizing the exercise protocol for cardiopulmonary assessment. J Appl Physiol 1983;55:1558–64.

[14] Myers J, Buchanan N, Walsh D, Kraemer M, McAuley P, Hamilton-Wessler M, et al. Comparison of the ramp versus standard exercise protocols. J Am Coll Cardiol 1991;17:1334–42.

[15] Astorino TA. Alterations in VOmax and the VO plateau with manipulation of sampling interval. Clin Physiol Funct Imaging 2009;29:60–7.

^{i} From a completed stage.

[16] Baba R, Nagashima M, Goto M, Nagano Y, Yokota M, Tauchi N, et al. Oxygen uptake efficiency slope: a new index of cardiorespiratory functional reserve derived from the relation between oxygen uptake and minute ventilation during incremental exercise. J Am Coll Cardiol 1996;28:1567–72.

[17] Akkerman M, van Brussel M, Hulzebos E, Vanhees L, Helders PJ, Takken T. The oxygen uptake efficiency slope: what do we know? J Cardiopulm Rehabil Prev 2010;30:357–73.

[18] Poole DC, Jones AM. Measurement of the maximum oxygen uptake VO_2max: VO_2peak is no longer acceptable. J Appl Physiol (1985) 2017;122:997–1002.

[19] Edgett BA, Bonafiglia JT, Raleigh JP, Rotundo MP, Giles MD, Whittall JP, et al. Reproducibility of peak oxygen consumption and the impact of test variability on classification of individual training responses in young recreationally active adults. Clin Physiol Funct Imaging 2018;38:630–8.

[20] Chidnok W, Dimenna FJ, Bailey SJ, Burnley M, Wilkerson DP, Vanhatalo A, et al. VO_2max is not altered by self-pacing during incremental exercise. Eur J Appl Physiol 2013;113:529–39.

[21] Langeskov-Christensen M, Langeskov-Christensen D, Overgaard K, Moller AB, Dalgas U. Validity and reliability of VO(2)-max measurements in persons with multiple sclerosis. J Neurol Sci 2014;342:79–87.

[22] Howley ET, Bassett DR, Jr., Welch HG. Criteria for maximal oxygen uptake: review and commentary. Med Sci Sports Exerc 1995;27:1292–301.

[23] Tanaka H, Monahan KD, Seals DR. Age-predicted maximal heart rate revisited. J Am Coll Cardiol 2001;37:153–6.

[24] Hawkins MN, Raven PB, Snell PG, Stray-Gundersen J, Levine BD. Maximal oxygen uptake as a parametric measure of cardiorespiratory capacity. Med Sci Sports Exerc 2007;39:103–7.

[25] Noakes TD. Maximal oxygen uptake: "classical" versus "contemporary" viewpoints: a rebuttal. Med Sci Sports Exerc 1998;30:1381–98.

[26] Poole DC, Wilkerson DP, Jones AM. Validity of criteria for establishing maximal O_2 uptake during ramp exercise tests. Eur J Appl Physiol 2008;102:403–10.

[27] Taylor HL, Buskirk E, Henschel A. Maximal oxygen intake as an objective measure of cardio-respiratory performance. J Appl Physiol 1955;8:73–80.

[28] Kaminsky LA, Imboden MT, Arena R, Myers J. Reference standards for cardiorespiratory fitness measured with cardiopulmonary exercise testing using cycle ergometry: data from the Fitness Registry and the Importance of Exercise National Database (FRIEND) Registry. Mayo Clin Proc 2017;92:228–33.

PRACTICAL 11
SUBMAXIMAL TESTS FOR CARDIORESPIRATORY FITNESS

Jeff Coombes and Chris Askew

LEARNING OBJECTIVES

- Explain the scientific rationale, purposes, reliability, validity, assumptions and limitations of common submaximal tests for cardiorespiratory fitness
- Identify and explain the common terminology, processes and equipment required to conduct accurate and safe submaximal tests for cardiorespiratory fitness
- Identify and describe contraindications or considerations that may require the modification of submaximal tests for cardiorespiratory fitness, and make appropriate adjustments for populations or participants
- Describe the principles and rationale for the calibration of equipment commonly used in submaximal tests for cardiorespiratory fitness
- Conduct appropriate pre-assessment procedures, including explaining the test, obtaining informed consent and a focused medical history, and performing a pre-exercise risk assessment
- Identify the need for guidance or further information from an appropriate health professional, and recognise when medical supervision is required before or during an assessment and when to cease a test
- Select and conduct appropriate submaximal tests for cardiorespiratory fitness, including instructing participants on the correct use of equipment
- Record, analyse and interpret information from a submaximal test for cardiorespiratory fitness and convey the results, including the validity and limitations of the assessment, through relevant verbal and/or written communication with the participant or relevant professional

Equipment and other requirements

- Information sheet and informed consent form
- Adult Pre-exercise Screening System (APSS) form
- Heart rate monitor set (e.g. transmitter, receiver, chest strap)
- Stopwatch
- Sphygmomanometer on stand with various size arm cuffs (with size indicators)
- Stethoscope
- Alcohol wipes
- Cycle ergometer (e.g. Monark)
- Motorised treadmill

- 30 cm step (measuring tape to ensure that height is correct)
- Chester step test audio track (e.g. CD, digital track)
- Audio player (e.g. CD player, smartphone)
- Rating of perceived exertion chart (see Appendix E)
- Calculator
- Cleaning and disinfecting equipment (see Appendix A)

INTRODUCTION

The widely accepted gold standard measure of cardiorespiratory fitness is maximal oxygen uptake, or $\dot{V}O_2$max. The direct measurement of $\dot{V}O_2$max requires expensive, sophisticated equipment and technical expertise. Furthermore, participants are required to exercise to their limit and exert maximal effort. This leads to a small degree of medical risk associated with high-intensity exercise for some individuals. A recent study reported a fivefold increased risk of sudden cardiac death and 3.5-fold increased risk of acute myocardial infarction during or shortly after vigorous physical activity.[1]

Various submaximal tests have been developed to estimate $\dot{V}O_2$max, and these tests will be the focus of this practical. The equipment needed for submaximal tests is less complex, less expensive, easier to use and is often suitable for field assessments. Furthermore, the tests require moderate–vigorous-intensity exercise (i.e. most submaximal protocols require the test to stop when 80%–85% HRmax is achieved) and are therefore associated with reduced medical risk compared with maximal tests.[2] For this reason, medical supervision is usually not required.[2] To better understand maximal aerobic power, students should familiarise themselves with Practical 10, which addresses the direct measurement of $\dot{V}O_2$max, including the physiological determinants of $\dot{V}O_2$max.

As a measure of cardiorespiratory fitness, $\dot{V}O_2$max provides a prognostic indicator of health. Poor $\dot{V}O_2$max is a strong predictor of all-cause mortality[3] and the development of cardiovascular disease.[4] In athletes, $\dot{V}O_2$max is used as a marker of endurance performance and is typically measured to evaluate the effectiveness of a training period. In most settings, direct or indirect estimates of a person's $\dot{V}O_2$max can be used to prescribe exercise intensity and direct exercise prescription.

Important outcomes of submaximal tests are the various physiological data and other indices that can be measured during the test. These include the rating of perceived exertion (RPE; see Appendix E), blood pressure (BP) and heart rate that may be collected at different stages, and observations regarding the individual's capacity to undertake exercise. In many cases, this information can be more valuable (e.g. for the purpose of exercise prescription) than the estimated $\dot{V}O_2$max value itself. It is important to keep this in mind when conducting a submaximal test.

This practical will cover the use of three submaximal test protocols to estimate $\dot{V}O_2$max. These protocols have been selected to provide students with an opportunity to practise the skills associated with conducting a submaximal test using a range of exercise modalities and data analysis approaches. Some submaximal exercise tests incorporate single-stage protocols where nomograms or a formula are used to estimate $\dot{V}O_2$max based on the participant characteristics and their response to the test. Most submaximal tests, including the tests in this practical, use multi-stage protocols and assume a linear relationship between heart rate, work rate and oxygen consumption to estimate $\dot{V}O_2$max.

It is expected that you will have completed a unit of study in the discipline of exercise physiology and are aware of the principles of force, work and power, and how these are measured in the context of exercise. You will also have an understanding of a graded exercise test to volitional exhaustion and the normal changes in oxygen consumption and heart rate during incremental exercise (see Practical 10, $\dot{V}O_2$max).

The ability to estimate $\dot{V}O_2$max accurately from a submaximal test is one of the key skills in which graduates from exercise science programs are expected to be competent. Indeed, our profession is unique in having this skill. It is important that you not only aim to be proficient in the practical skills of conducting a submaximal test, but you also develop an understanding of the physiological principles that underpin the estimation of $\dot{V}O_2$max. This would lead to the ability to select the most appropriate protocol for individuals and/or design your own test protocols if needed.

Other methods of assessing or estimating cardiorespiratory fitness not covered in this practical include:

- graded submaximal exercise test with indirect calorimetry (analysis of expired air)
- exercise capacity tests such as the multi-stage shuttle run test (MSRT, see Practical 16, Exercise capacity) that use formulae to estimate $\dot{V}O_2$max
- non-exercise tests that estimate $\dot{V}O_2$max based on prediction models that may include factors such as resting heart rate and waist circumference.[5]

DEFINITIONS

Absolute contraindication: a reason or criterion that makes it inadvisable to conduct or continue the test. Undertaking or continuing the test could place the participant at a higher risk of an untoward event (e.g. injury or medical condition) occurring as a result of the test. See Appendix C.

Cardiorespiratory fitness: ability of the circulatory and respiratory systems to supply oxygen and support the energy demands during sustained physical activity. Also known as aerobic fitness or aerobic power.

Concurrent validity: in this practical, it is the ability of the submaximal test to estimate $\dot{V}O_2$ max.

Relative contraindication: a reason or criterion that needs to be considered in deciding whether to conduct, modify or continue the test. Factors such as the risk versus benefit, availability of medical support, qualifications, knowledge and experience of the tester and access to medical support need to be considered. See Appendix C.

Reliability: the ability of a measure to provide consistent/repeatable data.

$\dot{V}O_2$ max or maximal oxygen uptake: is a measure of cardiorespiratory fitness that describes the ability of the circulatory and respiratory systems to supply oxygen and support the energy demands during sustained physical activity.

ASSUMPTIONS AND LIMITATIONS

Most submaximal protocols are based on the key assumption of a linear relationship between heart rate, work rate and oxygen consumption. This relationship is stronger when the exercise intensity is below the anaerobic/ventilatory threshold. It is important that a steady-state heart rate is achieved at each work rate throughout the tests as $\dot{V}O_2$ max is estimated by extrapolating submaximal heart rate responses to a predicted maximum work rate or power output. This is often based on an age-predicted maximum heart rate (HRmax), and the subsequent estimation of $\dot{V}O_2$ max from the established relationships between power output (e.g. work rate on a cycle ergometer) and oxygen consumption. The physiological basis for the estimation of $\dot{V}O_2$ max from submaximal tests is also based on a number of other assumptions, including:

- a steady-state heart rate is obtained for a given work rate and is consistent within and between days
- the maximal work rate is indicative of $\dot{V}O_2$ max
- the maximal heart rate for a given age is uniform and the equation used to estimate it is accurate
- mechanical efficiency (i.e. $\dot{V}O_2$ at a given work rate) is the same for everyone
- the heart rate is not being altered by medications, fatigue or any other stimulant/depressant.

Most submaximal protocols require a significant fitness level to complete the test, which may make them unsuitable for older or deconditioned individuals. Conversely, some protocols will not elicit a sufficient heart rate stimulus for highly fit individuals. For step tests, special care needs to be taken to avoid a fall when participants have poor balance.

VALIDITY AND RELIABILITY

The concurrent validity of submaximal exercise test is mainly affected by the underlying physiological assumptions, detailed previously, that may vary considerably between individuals and populations. Many submaximal tests are specific to the population for which the test was developed. This should be considered when choosing a test. Concurrent validity and reliability also rely on consistent test and pre-test procedures (e.g. standardised instructions in relation to prior physical activity, test familiarisation, caffeine intake and food). As an example, in the situation where an individual has an elevated heart rate because they were running to get to the test on time, this will probably influence their heart rate response and potentially invalidate the test. Other factors that will affect accuracy include familiarisation with the test and set-up of the treadmill/ergometer (e.g. seat too low), the environment and the actions of the person during the test (talking, gripping handrails/handle bars tightly). An invalid test can have significant consequences, particularly when the test is being used to guide exercise prescription. Appendix B outlines pre-test procedures, including instructions to the participant that should be adhered to for all tests. Specific details on the accuracy and reliability of the selected tests are provided in the respective sections below (see also Practical 1, Test accuracy, reliability and validity).

Activity 11.1 YMCA cycle ergometer test

AIMS: conduct the YMCA cycle ergometer submaximal test, interpret the results and provide feedback to a participant.

Background

The YMCA cycle ergometer test is recognised as one of the most robust submaximal protocols.[6] First described in 1989,[7] the test estimates $\dot{V}O_2$max from the participant's heart rate response to a series of incremental submaximal work rates. It then extrapolates this to a predicted maximal heart rate, and a corresponding estimated maximum work rate and estimated $\dot{V}O_2$max. A cross-validation study in 102 individuals reported that the YMCA test accurately estimated $\dot{V}O_2$max (mean difference 1.3 mL/kg/min).[6] Good reliability was shown in 35 participants who completed two YMCA tests.[8] There was no significant difference between the estimated $\dot{V}O_2$max from the two tests (40.6 $\pm$ 5.2 vs 41.0 $\pm$ 6.9 mL/kg/min), with a reliability coefficient of 0.62.[8] These validity and reliability studies used the ACSM metabolic equations to estimate $\dot{V}O_2$ at submaximal workloads. Recently, new equations have been developed for cycling[9] and walking/running[10] using objectively measured $\dot{V}O_2$max values from the FRIEND registry. These have been shown to provide better estimates of $\dot{V}O_2$ and may therefore improve the concurrent validity and reliability of the YMCA test.[9,10]

Protocol summary

The protocol uses a Monark cycle ergometer with the participant completing three or more consecutive $\geq$3-minute stages that are designed to raise the heart rate to $\geq$110 bpm and <85% of the age-predicted HRmax during two consecutive work rates.

Protocol

Test preparation (prior to participant's arrival)

1 Prepare solutions for post-test clean-up (see Appendix A).

2 Have all data collection forms ready for completion

3 Ensure familiarity with test termination criteria (see Appendix F).

Pre-test (with participant present)

1 Follow the pre-exercise test procedures outlined in Appendix B.

2 Check Appendix C to ensure that there are no contraindications to exercise testing.

3 Weigh the participant (see Practical 4, Physique assessment) and record the values.

4 Calculate 85% of the participant's age-predicted HRmax [0.85 $\times$ (208 − (0.7 $\times$ age))].[11,a]

5 Have the participant place their water bottle and towel in close proximity to the cycle ergometer.

6 Establish seat height (when the participant's leg is stretched vertically, with the ball of the foot on the pedal, the leg should be slightly bent at about 5° flexion). Seat height can affect mechanical efficiency. Some ergometers have numbered holes on the seat posts and handlebars; record these settings for retest purposes.

---

[a]The formula 220 − age is often used to estimate maximal heart rate. However, the formula used throughout this manual has been shown to be more accurate.

7 Fit the heart rate monitor and record heart rate while participant is in the exercising position (see Practical 3, Cardiovascular health).

8 Measure and record blood pressure in the exercising posture (i.e. sitting on the cycle ergometer), (see Practical 3) – the blood pressure provides a baseline measure and is used to determine whether the participant has exceeded the criteria for a contraindication to exercise (see Appendix C).

9 Provide details of the test, including the protocol, hand signals the participant can use during the test, explanation of the rating of perceived exertion (RPE) (see Appendix E), test termination and safety (see Appendix F).

10 Ask the participant to remain silent during the test unless they experience discomfort. They can indicate an RPE by pointing at the chart. Inform them that talking may increase the heart rate and affect the results of the test.

11 Ask the participant if they have any questions prior to the commencement of the test.

Test

1 If the participant is unfamiliar with cycling it is recommended that a 3-minute cycle at the intensity of the first stage be implemented prior to beginning the test. If this is needed then allow the heart rate to return to approximately the pre-cycling value before commencing the test. If the participant is familiar with cycling, then no warm-up or test-familiarisation is needed as the first stage of the protocol acts as a warm-up.

2 Ask the participant to cycle at 50 rpm at the first resistance of 0.5 kp (150 kpm/min or 25 W).

3 Start the stopwatch once the participant is cycling at the required cadence and resistance.

4 Continually monitor cadence as participants have a tendency to cycle faster than the requested cadence, which invalidates the test.

5 Record heart rate at the end of each minute throughout the test.

6 The rating of perceived exertion (RPE) should be recorded at the end of each stage. The participant can indicate an RPE by pointing at the chart.

7 Blood pressure should be measured and recorded at the end of each stage, between the 2nd and 3rd minutes (start taking blood pressure 2 minutes after the stage has started – after recording the 2nd minute heart rate). If the stage needs to be continued to the 4th minute, take and record the blood pressure again between the 3rd and 4th minutes.

8 Continue at each stage measuring HR and blood pressure each minute until a steady-state heart rate has been achieved.

9 Blood pressure should be re-measured and recorded in the event of a hypotensive or hypertensive response (see Practical 3, Cardiovascular health).

10 After 3 minutes at stage 1, compare the 2nd and 3rd minute heart rates to establish whether a steady state has been achieved:

   a if they differ by ≤ 5 bpm, go to stage 2 of the test protocol (refer to Figure 11.1 – based on the participant's heart rate after the 3rd minute; Table 11.1 may be needed to determine work rate if this information is not provided on the Monark bike)

   b if they differ by > 5 bpm, continue on that stage until two successive minute heart rate recordings differ by ≤ 5 bpm. Then go to stage 2 (refer to Figure 11.1 – based on the participant's final minute heart rate).

11 At the end of the next stages, use the same criteria as the first stage (i.e. only move to the next stage after 3 minutes if the last two successive minute heart rates differ by ≤ 5 bpm).

12 During the next stages, obtain and record heart rate, RPE and blood pressure values as in stage 1.

13 The workloads for the 3rd and (if required) 4th stages are obtained from Figure 11.1 by following the column vertically.

14 A minimum of three stages must be completed.

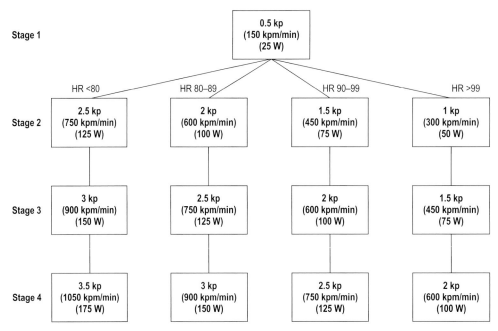

Figure 11.1 Guide to setting work rates for the YMCA test. HR = heart rate

TABLE 11.1 Relationships between force and power on a Monark cycle ergometer							
	RESISTANCE	FORCE	POWER		RESISTANCE	FORCE	POWER
kg or kp	N	kgm/min or kpm/min	W	kg or kp	N	kgm/min or kpm/min	W
0.5	5	150	25	3.5	35	1050	175
1.0	10	300	50	4.0	40	1200	200
1.5	15	450	75	4.5	45	1350	225
2.0	20	600	100	5.0	50	1500	250
2.5	25	750	125	5.5	55	1650	275
3.0	30	900	150	6.0	60	1800	300

kg = kilogram; kgm/min = kilogram metres per minute[a]; kp = kilopond; kpm/min = kilopond metres per minute[a]; N = newtons; W = watts
[a]For the purpose of this practical, kilogram metres per minute are the same as kilopond metres per minute. Note that some sources will interchange the use of these terms.
Note: Values are based on cycle cadence of *50* revolutions per minute. For Monark cycle ergometers, the power output (watts) is the product of resistance (kg) and pedal cadence (rpm); e.g. 2 kg × 50 rpm = 100 W
Used with permission from Monark

15 Continue the test until at least two stages (work rates) have corresponding steady-state heart rate values ≥110 bpm and <85% of the age-predicted HRmax. Progress to the 4th stage if required.

> **Note:** The participant must complete at least three stages.

16 The test should not exceed 16 minutes and should be stopped if the heart rate exceeds 85% of the age-predicted HRmax or if other test termination criteria are met (see Appendix F).

17 After the final stage, or if the test is terminated, the participant cools down by cycling with a light resistance (e.g. 0.5 kp) at a self-selected cadence for 3 minutes.

18 Heart rate and RPE should be monitored during the cool-down to provide an indication of appropriate recovery. It is not necessary for these values to have returned to pre-test levels but there should be significant decreases compared with the end of the test. If the participant experiences a hypertensive response, monitor blood pressure during recovery.

19 Clean and disinfect all equipment (see Appendix A).

Data analysis

1 Identify the two stages when the heart rates were in the required zone ($\geq$110 bpm and $<$85% of the age-predicted HRmax).

2 For the work rates at these two stages, use the cycle ergometry metabolic equation (Table 11.2)[2,9,10] to calculate $\dot{V}O_2$ and record the values.

3 Calculate the slope (m) of the HR and $\dot{V}O_2$ relationship using the equation on the data-recording sheet.

4 $\dot{V}O_2$max is then estimated from the equation provided on the data-recording sheet.

5 Use Table 11.3[12] to determine percentile and rating and provide feedback to the participant.

TABLE 11.2 Metabolic equations for the estimation of $\dot{V}O_2$ (mL/kg/min) during cycle ergometry, treadmill walking and running, and stepping	
Cycle ergometry: males	$1.76 \times$ (work rate $\times$ 6.12/kg of body mass) $+ 3.5$
Cycle ergometry: females	$1.65 \times$ (work rate $\times$ 6.12/kg of body mass) $+ 3.5$
Treadmill walking and running[10]	speed $\times$ [0.17 + (grade $\times$ 0.79)] $+ 3.5$
Stepping[2]	$3.5 + (0.2 \times$ steps/min) $+ [1.33 \times (1.8 \times$ step height $\times$ steps/min)]

Work rate in watts (150 kpm/min = 25 W); speed in m/min where 1 km/h = 16.7 m/min; grade in % expressed as a decimal; step height in m

TABLE 11.3 Cycle ergometer $\dot{V}O_2$max reference data (mL/kg/min)						
	AGE (YEARS)					
PERCENTILE[a]	20–29	30–39	40–49	50–59	60–69	70–79
Men						
95	58.5	44.7	41.9	37.4	32.4	34.0
75	49.5	35.0	31.8	29.3	25.5	22.5
50	41.9	30.2	27.1	24.8	22.4	19.5
25	34.7	26.2	22.9	22.1	19.7	17.1
5	25.5	19.3	18.9	18.1	15.3	14.4
Women						
95	45.2	33.2	29.3	25.0	22.0	19.2
75	37.1	25.1	22.6	20.1	18.3	16.5
50	31.0	21.6	19.4	17.3	16.0	14.8
25	23.2	17.9	16.5	15.3	14.4	13.2
5	17.1	14.4	13.5	12.8	12.2	11.3

[a] The following terms may be used as descriptors for the percentile rating: superior ($\geq$95); excellent (75–94.9); good (50–74.9); below average (25–49.9); poor (5–24.9) and very poor ($<$5)
Obtained from the FRIEND Registry for men and women who were considered free from known CVD[12]

Data recording

Participant's name: _____   Date: _____

Age: _____ years   Sex: _____   Body mass: _____ kg

Seat height: _____

Baseline HR: _____ bpm   Baseline BP: _____ mmHg

Age-predicted HRmax[a]: _____ bpm   85% HRmax: _____ bpm

Stage	Minute	Work rate (kpm/min)	$\dot{V}O_2$ (mL/kg/min)	Heart rate (bpm)	RPE	BP (mmHg)
1	1					
	2					
	3					
	4 (if necessary)					
2	1					
	2					
	3					
	4 (if necessary)					
3	1					
	2					
	3					
	4 (if necessary)					
4 (if necessary)	1					
	2					
	3					
	4 (if necessary)					

$\dot{V}O_2$ at 2nd-last work rate: _____ mL/kg/min

$\dot{V}O_2$ at last work rate: _____ mL/kg/min

$$Slope(m) = \frac{(\dot{V}O_2 \text{ at last stage} - \dot{V}O_2 \text{ at 2nd last stage})}{(\text{final heart rate at last stage} - \text{final heart rate at 2nd last stage})}$$

$$= \underline{\hspace{4cm}}$$

Estimated $\dot{V}O_2$max (mL/kg/min) = m (HRmax − final heart rate at last work rate[b])

$+\dot{V}O_2$ at last work rate[b]

$$= \underline{\hspace{4cm}} \text{mL/kg/min}$$

Percentile: _____   Rating: _____

[a]208 − (0.7 age). This is more accurate than 220 − age.[11]
[b]Where steady state HR in final minute values that is ≥110 bpm and <85% of the age predicted HRmax.

Activity 11.2 Bruce treadmill test

AIMS: conduct the Bruce treadmill submaximal test, interpret the results and provide feedback to a participant.

Background

The standard Bruce protocol was first developed by Robert Bruce and published in 1963.[13] It is most commonly used in clinical exercise stress test settings, with participants exercising to volitional exhaustion while the electrical activity of the heart is monitored using electrocardiography (ECG) (see Practical 16, Exercise capacity). When used as a submaximal test, it uses the same principle as the YMCA test by estimating $\dot{V}O_2max$ from the participant's heart rate response to a series of submaximal work rates, and this is then extrapolated to their predicated maximal heart rate.

Although the Bruce protocol is well validated (concurrent) as a standard protocol for maximal exercise testing, little evidence about the validity of its use for submaximal exercise testing exists. One recent study in 60 participants found that estimated $\dot{V}O_2max$ differed from a 'true $\dot{V}O_2max$' by around 2 mL/kg/min (ICC = 0.62, CV of 10% and TEM of 1.5 mL/kg/min).[14] It appears that the reliability of the test has not yet been reported in the scientific literature.

Protocol summary

The participant completes two or more consecutive stages that are designed to raise the heart rate to $\geq$110 bpm and <85% of the age-predicted HRmax for two consecutive work rates.

Protocol

Test preparation (prior to the participant's arrival)

1 Prepare solutions for post-test clean-up (see Appendix A).

2 Have all data collection forms ready for completion.

3 Ensure familiarity with test termination criteria (see Appendix F).

Pre-test (with participant present)

1 Follow the pre-exercise test procedures outlined in Appendix B.

2 Check Appendix C to ensure that there are no contraindications to exercise testing.

3 Calculate 85% of the participant's age-predicted HRmax $[0.85 \times (208 - (0.7 \times age))]$.[11]

4 Have the participant place their water bottle and towel in close proximity to the treadmill.

5 Fit the heart rate monitor and record the heart rate (see Practical 3, Cardiovascular health).

6 Measure and record the blood pressure in the exercising posture (i.e. standing on the treadmill) (see Practical 3) – the blood pressure provides a baseline measure and is used to determine whether the participant has exceeded the criteria for a contraindication to exercise (see Appendix C).

7 Provide treadmill safety precautions to the participant (see Appendix D). An assessment of their ability to walk/jog safely should be conducted prior to starting the test.

8 Provide details of the test, including the protocol, hand signals the participant can use during the test, and explanation of the rating of perceived exertion (RPE) (see Appendix E), test termination and safety (see Appendix F).

9 Ask the participant to remain silent during the test unless they experience discomfort. They can indicate an RPE by pointing at the chart. Inform them that talking may increase the heart rate and affect the results of the test.

Protocol

1 If the participant is unfamiliar with walking on a treadmill, it is recommended that a 3-minute walk at the intensity of the first stage be implemented prior to the test. If this is needed then allow the heart rate to return to approximately the pre-walking value before commencing the test.

2 If the participant is familiar with walking on a treadmill, then no warm-up or test-familiarisation is needed as the first stage of the protocol acts as a warm-up.

3 Ask the participant to walk on the treadmill at the grade and speed of the first stage.

4 Start the stopwatch when the treadmill reaches the appropriate speed and grade.

5 During the test it may be necessary to prematurely stop the test – see Appendix F for more detail and criteria.

6 Record heart rate at the end of each minute.

7 RPE should be recorded at the end of each stage.

8 Blood pressure should be measured and recorded at the end of each stage, between the 2nd and 3rd minutes (start taking blood pressure 2 minutes after the stage has started – after recording the 2nd-minute heart rate). If the stage needs to be continued to the 4th minute, take the blood pressure again between the 3rd and 4th minutes.

9 Blood pressure should be re-measured in the event of a hypotensive or hypertensive response.

10 After 3 minutes on stage 1, compare the 2nd- and 3rd-minute heart rates to ensure that a steady-state heart rate has been achieved:

   a If they differ by ≤ 5 bpm, go to stage 2 (from Table 11.4).

   b If the 2nd- and 3rd-minute heart rates differ by >5 bpm, continue on that stage until two successive heart rate recordings differ by ≤ 5 bpm, then go to stage 2.

TABLE 11.4 Standard Bruce treadmill protocol

STAGE	TIME (min)	SPEED (kph)	GRADE (%)
1	3	2.7	10
2	3	4	12
3	3	5.4	14
4	3	6.7	16
5	3	8.0	18

11 During the next stages, move to the following stage after 3 minutes only if the last two successive minute heart rates differ by ≤ 5 bpm.

12 During the next stages, repeat points 6–8 (above) to obtain heart rate, RPE and blood pressure values as in stage 1.

13 Continue the test until at least two work rates have corresponding steady-state heart rate values ≥ 110 bpm and $<85\%$ of the age-predicted HRmax.

14 The test should not exceed 16 minutes and should be stopped if the heart rate exceeds 85% of the age-predicted HRmax or if other test termination criteria are met (see Appendix F).

15 After the final stage the participant cools down by walking at a slow pace (e.g. 2.7 kph at 0% grade) for 3 minutes.

16 Heart rate and RPE should be monitored during the cool-down to provide an indication of appropriate recovery. It is not necessary for these values to have returned to pre-test levels, but there should be significant decreases compared with the end of the test. If the participant experienced a hypertensive response, monitor blood pressure during recovery.

17 Clean and disinfect all equipment (see Appendix A).

Data analysis

1 Identify the last two stages when the heart rates were in the required zone ($\geq$110 bpm and $<$85% of the age-predicted HRmax).

2 For these two stages, use the appropriate metabolic equation (see Table 11.2) to calculate $\dot{V}O_2$ and record the values.

3 Calculate the slope (m) of the HR and $\dot{V}O_2$ relationship using the equation on the data-recording sheet.

4 $\dot{V}O_2$max is then estimated from the equation provided on the data-recording sheet.

5 Use Table 11.5[15] to determine percentile and rating and provide feedback to the participant.

TABLE 11.5 Treadmill $\dot{V}O_2$max reference data (mL/kg/min)

PERCENTILE[a]	AGE (years)					
	20–29	30–39	40–49	50–59	60–69	70–79
Men						
95	66.3	59.8	55.6	50.7	43.0	39.7
75	55.2	49.2	45.0	39.7	34.5	30.4
50	48.0	42.4	37.8	32.6	28.2	24.4
25	40.1	35.9	31.9	27.1	23.7	20.4
5	29.0	27.2	24.2	20.9	17.4	16.3
Women						
95	56	45.8	41.7	35.9	29.4	24.1
75	44.7	36.1	32.4	27.6	23.8	20.8
50	37.6	30.2	26.7	23.4	20	18.3
25	30.5	25.3	22.1	19.9	17.2	15.6
5	21.7	19	17	16	13.4	13.1

The following terms may be used as descriptors for the percentile rating: superior ($\geq$95); excellent (75–94.9); good (50–74.9); below average (25–49.9); poor (5–24.9) and very poor ($<$5)

Obtained from the FRIEND Registry for men and women who were considered free from known CVD[9]

Data recording

Participant's name: _____   Date: _____

Age: _____ years   Sex: _____   Body mass: _____kg

Baseline HR: _____ bpm   Baseline BP: _____ mmHg

Age-predicted HRmax[a]: _____ bpm   85% HRmax: _____ bpm

Stage	Minute	$\dot{V}O_2$ (mL/kg/min)	Heart rate (bpm)	RPE	BP (mmHg)
1	1				
	2				
	3				
	4 (if necessary)				
2	1				
	2				
	3				
	4 (if necessary)				
3 (if necessary)	1				
	2				
	3				
	4 (if necessary)				
4 (if necessary)	1				
	2				
	3				
	4 (if necessary)				

$\dot{V}O_2$ at 2nd-last stage: _____ mL/kg/min

$\dot{V}O_2$ at last stage: _____ mL/kg/min

$$\text{Slope(m)} = \frac{(\dot{V}O_2 \text{ at last stage} - \dot{V}O_2 \text{ at 2nd last stage})}{(\text{final heart rate at last stage} - \text{final heart rate at 2nd last stage})}$$

$$= \underline{\hspace{4cm}}$$

Estimated $\dot{V}O_2$max (mL/kg/min) = m (HRmax − final heart rate at last stage)
$+\dot{V}O_2$ at last stage

$$= \underline{\hspace{3cm}} \text{mL/kg/min}$$

Percentile: _____   Rating: _____

[a]208 − (0.7 × age). This is more accurate than 220 − age.[11]

Activity 11.3 Chester step test

AIMS: conduct the Chester step test, interpret the results and provide feedback to a participant.

Background

Step protocols were some of the first exercise tests used. They provide a simple, effective and ecologically valid (concurrent) method of submaximally assessing cardiorespiratory fitness. The limited requirements for space and equipment (step, heart rate monitor, perceived exertion scale and, in some cases, an audio device) make the test portable and attractive for field testing. A step test protocol developed at University College, Chester has been used in a variety of situations (e.g. testing fire brigades, airport fire fighters and ambulance workers).[16] The test estimates $\dot{V}O_2$max from the participant's heart rate response to a series of submaximal work rates. It then extrapolates this to a predicted maximal heart rate, and a corresponding estimated $\dot{V}O_2$max. The stepping speed increases every 2 minutes. An audio recording with guided verbal instructions and the metronome sound for pacing is available in a number of commercial health and fitness assessment packages. The test has been highly correlated ($r = 0.92$) with directly measured $\dot{V}O_2$max during a treadmill test and has a standard error of the estimate of 3.9 mL/kg/min. Reliability from repeated measures on separate days was also excellent, with a mean difference of -0.7 mL/kg/min (limits of agreement: 4.5 mL/kg/min) between measures (see Practical 1, Test accuracy, reliability and validity).[16]

Protocol summary

The participant steps up and down on a step with a set height at a rate that increases every 2 minutes (following the audio recording) until 80% of the age-predicted maximal heart rate is reached.

Protocol

Test preparation (prior to the participant's arrival)

1 Choose the step height:

15 cm – for participants over 40 years of age who do little or no regular physical exercise

20 cm – for participants under 40 years of age who do little or no regular physical exercise

25 cm – for participants over 40 years of age who regularly exercise and are accustomed to moderately vigorous exertion

30 cm – for participants under 40 years of age who regularly exercise and are accustomed to moderately vigorous exertion.

2 Prepare solutions for post-test clean-up (see Appendix A).

3 Have all data collection forms ready for completion.

4 Ensure familiarity with test termination criteria (see Appendix F).

Pre-test (with participant present)

1 Follow the pre-exercise test procedures outlined in Appendix B.

2 Check Appendix C to ensure that there are no contraindications to exercise testing.

3 Calculate 80% of the participant's age-predicted HRmax [$0.8 \times (208 - (0.7 \times age))$].[11]

4 Have the participant place their water bottle and towel in close proximity to the step.

5 Fit the heart rate monitor and record the heart rate (see Practical 3, Cardiovascular health).

6 Measure and record blood pressure in the exercising posture (i.e. standing) (see Practical 3) – the blood pressure provides a baseline measure and is used to determine whether the participant has exceeded the criteria for a contraindication to exercise (see Appendix C).

7 Explain the protocol (including the collection of rating of perceived exertion data – see Appendix E), hand signals they can use during the test, test termination and safety (see Appendix F).

8 Ask the participant to remain silent during the test unless they experience discomfort. They can indicate an RPE by pointing at the chart. Inform them that talking may increase the heart rate and affect the results of the test.

9 Ask the participant whether they have any questions.

Protocol

1 Start the audio track and have the participant(s) listen to the instructions.

2 When instructed by the audio track, the participant commences stepping at 15 steps/min for 2 min (level 1).

3 The step rate then increases by 5 steps/min to 20 steps/min for a further 2 min (level 2).

4 The test follows this incremental pattern until the participant either reaches 80% of their age-predicted maximal heart rate or completes level 5 (35 steps/min).

5 HR and RPE should be recorded at the end of each level. The person should point at the RPE chart rather than talking.

6 Blood pressure is measured during each level between the 1st and 2nd minutes. If the tester is around the same height as the participant then they should stand on a step about half the height of the actual step while taking the blood pressure. The participant keeps stepping during the whole protocol.

7 The maximum test duration is 10 minutes (level 5).

8 The test may also be stopped if other test termination criteria are met (see Appendix F).

9 Once the test is completed, the participant cools down by walking slowly within observation of the tester for 3 minutes.

10 Heart rate and RPE should be monitored during the cool-down to provide an indication of appropriate recovery. It is not necessary for these values to have returned to pre-test levels but there should be significant decreases compared with the end of the test. If the participant experienced a hypertensive response, monitor blood pressure during recovery.

11 Clean and disinfect all equipment (see Appendix A).

Data analysis

1 Use the metabolic equation for stepping (see Table 11.2) to calculate $\dot{V}O_2$ for each stage completed and record the values.

2 Plot the HR at the end of each stage against the $\dot{V}O_2$ of that stage on the graph paper (Figure 11.2) using a cross to increase accuracy, rather than a point.

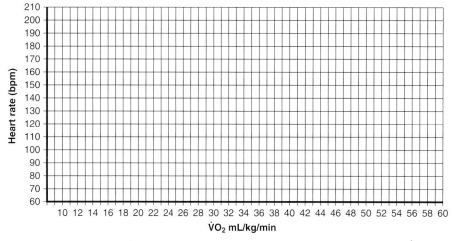

Figure 11.2 Graph for plotting heart rate at the end of each stage against $\dot{V}O_2$ for the Chester step test

3 Draw a visual line of best fit between the crosses, projecting the line up to the participant's age-predicted maximal heart rate.

4 Then drop a vertical line to intersect with the x-axis and record the $\dot{V}O_2$ value at this point as the person's estimated $\dot{V}O_2$max.

Data recording

Participant's name: _____   Date: _____

Age: _____ years   Sex: _____   Body mass: _____ kg

Baseline HR: _____ bpm   Baseline BP: _____ mmHg

Age-predicted HRmax[a]: _____ bpm   80% HRmax: _____ bpm

Step height: _____ cm

STEP LEVEL	1	2	3	4	5
Heart rate (bpm)					
RPE					
Blood pressure (mmHg)					

$\dot{V}O_2$ at stage 1 _____ $\dot{V}O_2$ at stage 4 _____

$\dot{V}O_2$ at stage 2 _____ $\dot{V}O_2$ at stage 5 _____

$\dot{V}O_2$ at stage 3 _____

Estimated $\dot{V}O_2$max: _____ mL/kg/min

Percentile: _____   Rating (use Table 11.3): _____

[a]$208 - (0.7 \times \text{age})$. This is more accurate than $220 - \text{age}$.[11]

Interpretation of submaximal tests

First, consider the four steps of interpretation outlined in Appendix G. Due to the large number of assumptions and limitations with submaximal testing, you should first determine whether the protocol has been followed and the result looks appropriate. Assessing the validity of the result would include comparing the value against the reference $\dot{V}O_2$max value based on the person's age, sex and mode (see Tables 11.3 and 11.5), and what you may expect for a $\dot{V}O_2$max value if you are aware of the activity level of the participant. For a step test, use the cycle ergometer reference values (Table 11.3). If you are not confident in the validity of the test, it still should have provided useful information regarding the individual's responses and their capacity to undertake exercise. This can be valuable for exercise prescription.

If you are confident that the protocol has been followed and the estimated $\dot{V}O_2$max value appears valid, then use Tables 11.3 or 11.5 to find the percentile and an associated rating. The value will probably fall between two percentiles. You can roughly estimate what percentile this is. For example, if you are testing a 20-year-old male on a treadmill and his estimated $\dot{V}O_2$max is 33 mL/kg/min, the 5th percentile is 29 mL/kg/min and the 25th percentile is 40.1 mL/kg/min, you could estimate that it would be around the 15th percentile. It is usually more useful to calculate the exact percentile using the steps below. It is recognised that this assumes that there is a linear relationship between the percentiles and

$\dot{V}O_2$max – which is likely not to be the case. However, providing a specific percentile rather than a range will usually be more understandable by the participant.

Using the example of 33 mL/kg/min for a 20-year-old male, this falls between the 5th (29 mL/kg/min) and 25th (40.1 mL/kg/min) percentiles:

1 Calculate the amount that the value (mL/kg/min) is away from the lowest percentile value

$= 33 - 29 = 4$ mL/kg/min

2 Calculate the value (mL/kg/min) between the two percentile values

$= 40.1 - 29 = 11.1$ mL/kg/min

3 Calculate the ratio of these two values

$= 4/11.1 = 0.36$

4 Calculate the percentile range that this value is between

$= 25 - 5 = 20$

5 Calculate what value along this range the ratio (calculated in step 3) provides

$= 0.36 \times 20 = 7.2$

6 Add this to the lowest percentile to get the exact percentile

$= 5 + 7.2 = 12.2$ (round up/down to closest integer $= 12$).

Therefore, an estimated $\dot{V}O_2$max for a 20-year-old male of 33 mL/kg/min is at the 12th percentile. The qualitative rating for this is 'poor'.

Enter the estimated or calculated percentile, and the associated qualitative rating, on the data-recording sheet.

Feedback and discussion

First, consider the three steps of feedback and discussion outlined in Appendix G. The term 'cardiorespiratory fitness' is not easily understood by most lay individuals. For this reason, when explaining the results it is suggested to use terms such as 'aerobic fitness' to describe the measure. This can be in association with a lay definition such as *'measures the fitness of your heart and lungs during exercise'*.

Feedback regarding submaximal tests should include more than just stating the estimated $\dot{V}O_2$max and the relevant descriptor. The following example explains how a participant can understand more about the test they have just completed, the relevance of the result and how the data can be used.

*'You just completed a fitness test which provides an estimate of your aerobic fitness or $\dot{V}O_2$max. This is a measure of **the fitness of your heart and lungs during exercise** and is a very good indicator of your overall health. Your score is 57 mL/kg/min and this places you in the 60th percentile, meaning that it is better than 60% of men your age. This is classified as 'good'. I will be able to use information from this test for your exercise prescription. As your goal is to improve your aerobic fitness, I will write you a program that aims to move you into the 'excellent' category. We also have your heart rate, blood pressure and exertion rating scores that we can use to inform your exercise prescription. These will enable us to prescribe and monitor an exercise intensity that suits you. Also, when we re-test you we can see if these values have improved.'*

If the protocol was not followed and/or you are not confident in the accuracy of the estimated $\dot{V}O_2$max value, then the following feedback would be appropriate.

'You just completed a fitness test, which can provide us with an estimate of your aerobic fitness. The value obtained does not appear to be accurate, which could be due to a number of reasons. For example, the activity you were doing before the test may have impacted on your heart rate response during the test. Nevertheless, the test has provided us with some useful information such as your heart rate, blood pressure and rating of exertion during the test. I will be able to use this for your exercise prescription. When we next test you our goal will be for you to have a lower exertion while doing the same exercise as you did today.'

If a participant has a value that is below average, poor or very poor and you are confident that it is accurate, then you should inform them of the important relationship between low fitness and increased risk of poor health and premature death.

A discussion should focus on what can be done to maintain and/or improve the participant's cardio-respiratory fitness. Referring to exercise and physical activity guidelines will be helpful in this situation.

Case studies

Case Study 1

Setting: You are an exercise science student completing practicum hours within an on-campus health and fitness centre. The university offers a personal training program for medical students. As part of the program, clients receive a baseline fitness test that includes the YMCA cycle ergometer test. This is followed by 8 weeks of supervised exercise training and a post-training fitness test that is the same as the baseline test.

Task: Matthew is an undergraduate medical student who has completed the APSS and ticked 'No' to all questions on stage 1 and stated that his current weekly physical activity is 20 minutes/week. He recognises that he needs to start exercising but has never been involved in a structured program previously. The following are data from his YMCA cycle ergometer test.

Participant's name: _Matthew Venestanakos_   Date of Birth: _9/11/1997_   Sex: _Male_

Age: _23 years_   Body mass: _80 kg_   Seat height: _9_

Baseline HR: _58_ bpm   Baseline BP: _114/72_ mmHg   Age-predicted HRmax: _192_ bpm

85% HRmax: _163_ bpm

Stage	Minute	Work rate (kpm/min)	$\dot{V}O_2$ (mL/kg/min)	Heart rate (bpm)	RPE	BP (mmHg)
1	1			71		
	2	150		78		
	3			79	8	134/82
	4 (if necessary)					
2	1			109		
	2	750		115		
	3			119	9	148/84
	4 (if necessary)					
3	1			127		
	2	900		133		
	3			137	12	160/84
	4 (if necessary)					
4 (if necessary)	1					
	2					
	3					
	4 (if necessary)					

Use the test data to calculate the estimated $\dot{V}O_2$max for the participant. What is the percentile and rating? What feedback would you give the participant?'

continued overpage

Case studies *(continued)*

Case Study 2

Setting: You work for a corporate wellness company. One of your company's clients is a large multinational technology organisation that wants to offer their employees fitness testing. The fitness test includes a Bruce submaximal $\dot{V}O_2$max test.

Task: Alice is a Senior Executive of the organisation; she states that she wants the fitness test because she is concerned that her sedentary lifestyle has impacted on her health. She completes the APSS and ticks 'no' to all questions on stage 1, stating that her current weekly physical activity is 40 minutes/week.

Participant's name: *Alice Sullivan*

Date of Birth: *14/11/1978*   Sex: *Female*

Age: *42* years   Baseline HR: *74* bpm   Baseline BP: *124/82* mmHg

Age-predicted HRmax: *178* bpm   85% HRmax: *151* bpm

Stage	Minute	$\dot{V}O_2$ (mL/kg/min)	Heart rate (bpm)	RPE	Stage
1	1		96		
	2		98		
	3		102	10	140/80
	4 (if necessary)				
2	1		139		
	2		141		
	3		148	16	150/80
	4 (if necessary)		150	17	82
3 (if necessary)	1				
	2				
	3				
	4 (if necessary)				
4 (if necessary)	1				
	2				
	3				
	4 (if necessary)				

Use the test data to calculate the estimated $\dot{V}O_2$max for the participant. What is the percentile and rating? What feedback would you give the participant?

Case Study 3

Setting: You own an exercise physiology business that has won a contract to provide fitness testing services to ambulance workers. The fitness test includes a Chester step test to estimate $\dot{V}O_2$max.

Task: Rahaf is a trainee ambulance worker who has completed the APSS and ticked 'no' to all questions on stage 1. She states her current weekly physical activity is 200 minutes/week. During the test the participant reached 80% HRmax prior to the completion of the fifth stage and the test was stopped then.

Participant's name: *Rahaf Mohammed*   Date of Birth: *22/01/1998*   Sex: *Female*

Age: *22* years   Baseline HR: *64* bpm   Baseline BP: *124/82* mmHg

Age-predicted HRmax: *193* bpm   80% HRmax: *154* bpm

Step height: *30* cm

continued

Case studies *(continued)*

STEP LEVEL	1	2	3	4	5
Heart rate (bpm)	*95*	*111*	*125*	*143*	
RPE	*8*	*10*	*13*	*15*	
Blood pressure (mmHg)	*132/84*	*146/84*	*160/86*	*172/86*	

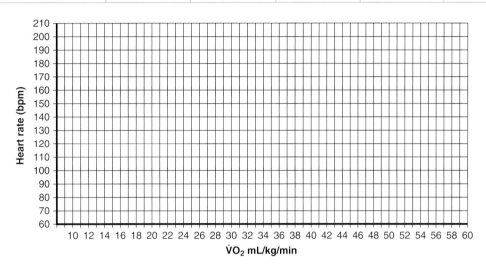

Plot the graph for heart rate at each stage, and calculate the $\dot{V}O_2$ at stage 5, and hence the estimated $\dot{V}O_2$max for the participant. What is the percentile and rating? What feedback would you give the participant?

References

[1] Dahabreh IJ, Paulus JK. Association of episodic physical and sexual activity with triggering of acute cardiac events: systematic review and meta-analysis. *JAMA* 2011;305:1225–33.

[2] American College of Sports Medicine. ACSM's guidelines for exercise testing and prescription, 10th ed. Baltimore, MD: Lippincott, Williams & Wilkins; 2018.

[3] Kodama S, Saito K, Tanaka S, Maki M, Yachi Y, Asumi M, et al. Cardiorespiratory fitness as a quantitative predictor of all-cause mortality and cardiovascular events in healthy men and women: a meta-analysis. JAMA 2009;301:2024–35.

[4] Church TS, LaMonte MJ, Barlow CE, Blair SN. Cardiorespiratory fitness and body mass index as predictors of cardiovascular disease mortality among men with diabetes. Arch Intern Med 2005;165:2114–20.

[5] Nes BM, Janszky I, Vatten LJ, Nilsen TI, Aspenes ST, Wisloff U. Estimating $\dot{V}O_2$peak from a nonexercise prediction model: the HUNT Study, Norway. Med Sci Sports Exerc 2011;43:2024–30.

[6] Beekley MD, Brechue WF, deHoyos DV, Garzarella L, Werber-Zion G, Pollock ML. Cross-validation of the YMCA submaximal cycle ergometer test to predict $\dot{V}O_2$max. Res Q Exerc Sport 2004;75:337–42.

[7] Golding LA, Myers CR, Sinning WE. Y's way to physical fitness, 3rd ed. Champaign, IL: Human Kinetics; 1989.

[8] Kidd J. 2018. Validity and reliability of the YMCA submaximal cycle test using an electrically braked ergometer. https://commons.lib.jmu.edu/honors201019/602.

[9] Kokkinos P, Kaminsky LA, Arena R, Zhang J, Myers J. A new generalized cycle ergometry equation for predicting maximal oxygen uptake: the Fitness Registry and the Importance of Exercise National Database (FRIEND). Eur J Prev Cardiol 2018:2047487318772667.

[10] Kokkinos P, Kaminsky LA, Arena R, Zhang J, Myers J. New generalized equation for predicting maximal oxygen uptake (from the Fitness Registry and the Importance of Exercise National Database). Am J Cardiol 2017;120:688–92.

[11] Tanaka H, Monahan KD, Seals DR. Age-predicted maximal heart rate revisited. J Am Coll Cardiol 2001;37:153–6.

[12] Kaminsky LA, Imboden MT, Arena R, Myers J. Reference standards for cardiorespiratory fitness measured with cardiopulmonary exercise testing using cycle ergometry: data from the Fitness Registry and the Importance of Exercise National Database (FRIEND) Registry. Mayo Clin Proc 2017;92:228–33.

[13] Bruce RA, Blackman JR, Jones JW, Strait G. Exercise testing in adult normal subjects and cardiovascular patients. Pediatrics 1963;21(Suppl):742–56.

[14] Strom CJ, Pettitt RW, Krynski LM, Jamnick NA, Hein CJ, Pettitt CD. Validity of a customized submaximal treadmill protocol for determining $\dot{V}O_2$max. Eur J Appl Physiol 2018;118:1781–87.

[15] Kaminsky LA, Arena R, Myers J. Reference standards for cardiorespiratory fitness measured with cardiopulmonary exercise testing: data from the Fitness Registry and the Importance of Exercise National Database. Mayo Clin Proc 2015;90:1515–23.

[16] Sykes K, Roberts A. The Chester step test – a simple yet effective tool for aerobic capacity. Physiotherapy. 2004;90:183–8.

PRACTICAL 12
LACTATE THRESHOLD

David Bishop, Tina Skinner and Nick Jamnick

LEARNING OBJECTIVES

- Identify and explain the common terminology, processes and equipment required to conduct accurate and safe tests of the lactate threshold

- Identify and describe the limitations, contraindications or considerations that may require the modification of assessment of the lactate threshold, and make appropriate adjustments for relevant populations or participants

- Explain the scientific rationale, purpose, reliability, validity, assumptions and limitations of assessing the lactate threshold

- Recognise and adjust incorrectly calibrated equipment used in the assessment of the lactate threshold

- Conduct appropriate pre-assessment procedures, including explaining the test and obtaining informed consent and a focused medical history, and performing a pre-exercise risk assessment

- Identify the need for guidance or further information from an appropriate health professional, and recognise when medical supervision is required before or during an assessment of the lactate threshold, and when to cease a test

- Select and conduct appropriate protocols for safe and effective assessment of the lactate threshold, including instructing clients on the correct use of equipment

- Record, analyse, and interpret information from an assessment of the lactate threshold and convey the results, including the validity and limitations of the assessments, through relevant verbal and/or written communication with the participant or involved professional

Equipment and other requirements

- Information sheet and informed consent form
- Adult Pre-exercise Screening System (APSS) form
- Programmable motorised treadmill, a cycle ergometer and/or a rowing ergometer
- Metabolic system and associated components (mouthpiece set-up, breathing tubes, calibration equipment – including gases)
- Nose clip
- Body mass scales
- Heart rate monitor set (e.g. transmitter, receiver, chest strap)
- Rating of perceived exertion (RPE) chart (see Appendix E)
- Paper towels
- Spray bottle with diluted bleach (bleach:water, 1:10)
- Sports tape/micropore tape
- Non-latex gloves of appropriate size (S, M, L)

- Alcohol swabs
- Lancets
- Lactate analyser
- Lactate analyser strips/cassettes
- Sharps container
- Band aids/finger cots
- Sterile cotton wool balls/swabs
- Tissues
- Bench surface protection paper
- Biohazard waste container
- Cleaning and disinfecting equipment (see Appendix A)

Personal protective equipment/immunisations

- Laboratory coat
- Protective eyewear (i.e. safety glasses)
- Covered footwear (no thongs, sandals or open-toed shoes)
- Hepatitis B and tetanus immunisations (recommended)

INTRODUCTION

While the frequency and duration of training sessions form a critical component of an effective training stimulus, training at the correct intensity is arguably the most important factor in any exercise training program. If exercise training is performed at intensities that are too low[1] or too high,[2] training benefits will be compromised. Due to the individual variability that exists amongst participants, it is especially important that training intensities are individually determined. Assigning a common training speed or heart rate to a training group is likely to be optimal for only a small percentage of participants. Assessment of blood lactate concentrations has been suggested to provide appropriate markers of training intensities. Indeed, training at the lactate threshold has been recommended,[3,4] with a blood lactate concentration of 4.0 mmol/L suggested to represent the optimum training intensity to improve aerobic fitness in male runners.[5,6] The sampling of blood (for the analysis of lactate) during progressive/incremental exercise to volitional exhaustion can allow researchers and sport scientists to identify a 'break-point', where non-linear increases in blood lactate concentrations (relative to work rate) occur. There are a number of 'lactate inflection' or 'lactate threshold' points that can be quantified using blood lactate data collected during an incremental test. Expired gas analysis is often used in conjunction with blood lactate testing to determine the percentage of $\dot{V}O_2max$ (maximal oxygen consumption) that coincides with these lactate thresholds. The lactate threshold can distinguish endurance performance in athletes with similar $\dot{V}O_2max$ values.[7,8] A shift in the percentage of $\dot{V}O_2max$ at a lactate threshold can indicate changes in aerobic 'fitness'. In addition, the heart rate or intensity (e.g. velocity or power) associated with a lactate threshold can be used to prescribe training.

During an incremental test to volitional exhaustion, lactate levels suddenly increase at a specific 'critical work rate', reflecting a threshold phenomenon. Regardless of the method used for its determination, there is strong evidence that the work intensity at the 'lactate threshold' can predict endurance performance.[5] For example, a 'lactate threshold' has been proposed to occur at the work rate preceding the first increase in lactate concentration (i) above a resting level[9,10] or (ii) of ≥ 1 mmol/L.[11–13] In contrast, fixed blood lactate concentrations of (i) 2 mmol/L[14] or (ii) 4 mmol/L[15] (the so-called 'onset of blood lactate accumulation'; OBLA[16]), have been proposed. Furthermore, other thresholds such as the individual anaerobic threshold (IAT), which is determined from exercise and recovery lactate measurements, can be calculated from blood lactate responses to incremental exercise. Although several different methods of calculating a certain threshold from lactate concentrations during incremental exercise exist, there has been limited comparison between the models in their ability to predict performance or prescribe the optimal training intensity. For the purpose of this practical, reference will predominantly be made to the two lactate parameters that are commonly used by sport scientists in institutes and academies of sport throughout Australia: the lactate transition 1 (LT1) and the lactate transition 2 (LT2)[17] (Figure 12.1). In some individuals (especially if unfit, or if the increments selected for the lactate threshold test are too large), the determination of only one transition may be possible.

Determination of lactate thresholds can be completed via visual, subjective inspection, or by using various curve-fitting procedures such as logarithmic transformations or polynomial curve-fitting such as the Dmax (Figure 12.2) or modified Dmax methods (Figure 12.3).[18] Specific software has been developed to calculate the lactate threshold using the modified Dmax method; however, this will not be used within this practical.

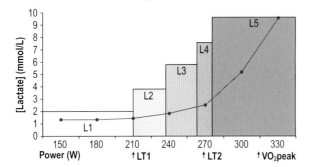

Figure 12.1 Power output–lactate curve. In red is a power output–lactate curve derived from a kayak athlete who has medalled at both Olympic and world championships, with the various terminology to be used in this practical. LT1 = 'lactate transition 1', LT2 = 'lactate transition 2'. L1 to L5 refer to training intensities described later in this practical

Source: David Bishop, Victoria University

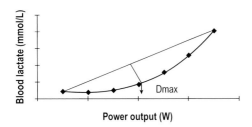

Figure 12.2 Dmax method

Adapted from: Tanner and Bourdon[18]

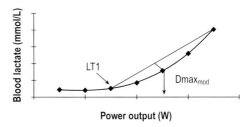

Figure 12.3 Modified Dmax method

Adapted from: Tanner and Bourdon[18]

DEFINITIONS

Absolute contraindication: a reason or criterion that makes it inadvisable to conduct or continue the test. Undertaking or continuing the test could place the participant at a higher risk of an untoward event (e.g. injury or medical condition) occurring as a result of the test. See Appendix C.

Cardiorespiratory fitness: ability of the circulatory and respiratory systems to supply oxygen and support the energy demands during sustained physical activity. Also known as aerobic fitness or aerobic endurance.

Lactate transition 1 (LT1): the power output or speed preceding the first increase in lactate concentration of more than 0.4 mmol/L[a] above the resting level.[19,20]

Lactate transition 2 (LT2): the power output or speed preceding the first increase in lactate concentration of more than 1.0 mmol/L above the resting level.[13,17]

Dmax method: the method used to find the point on the curve at the maximal distance from the line connecting the starting power output or speed and the finishing work rate.[21]

Modified Dmax method: the method used to find the point on the curve at the maximal distance from the line connecting the LT1 and the finishing work rate.[22]

Relative contraindication: a reason or criterion that needs to be considered in deciding whether to conduct, modify or continue the test. Factors such as the risk versus benefit, availability of

---

[a] A value of 0.4 mmol/L is used as it is twice the technical error of measurement when measuring lactate concentration in the laboratory.[20] This allows greater confidence that the 'inflection' observed is 'real' and not due to random variation.

medical support, qualifications, knowledge and experience of the tester and access to medical support need to be considered. See Appendix C.

Steady state: the body in a state that is characterised by stable or mildly fluctuating physiological characteristics (e.g. heart rate) or systems (e.g. $\dot{V}O_2max$).

$\dot{V}O_2max$: abbreviation for maximal oxygen uptake, this is a measure of cardiorespiratory fitness that describes the ability of the circulatory and respiratory systems to supply oxygen and support the energy demands during sustained physical activity.

$\dot{V}O_2peak$: the highest (submaximal) $\dot{V}O_2$ value attained during a graded exercise test when a plateau in oxygen consumption is not observed.

General methods for lactate threshold testing

In general, the determination of LT1 and LT2 involves taking serial blood lactate measurements, plotting these against the work rate and noting where there are changes in lactate concentration. An important step in measuring the various lactate thresholds is the selection of the protocol. There are many protocols available across different modes of testing and they are defined by the mode, starting work rate, and duration and intensity of each increment (e.g. Tables 12.1, 12.2 and 12.3[23]). The protocol selection should always consider the purpose of the test and the sex and fitness of the individual. In a sports science setting the exercise mode should reflect the muscle mass and movement patterns used in the sport. Ideally, such testing should be performed in the field but often this is not possible. Hence much effort has gone into designing laboratory methods and equipment that approximate field conditions (e.g. by using treadmills, kayak, rowing and cycle ergometers).

As lactate breakpoints are most useful when used by coaches for prescribing training intensities, the testing conditions must closely mimic the training environment (i.e. runners should be tested on a treadmill; cyclists should be tested on a cycle ergometer; rowers should be tested on a rowing ergometer). Running at a slight gradient (1%) on the treadmill is thought to be a more realistic representation of running on flat ground because it compensates for the wind resistance normally encountered by a runner, but not experienced on the treadmill.[24,25]

Each increment needs to be a minimum of 3 minutes in duration as this allows time for the blood lactate concentration to reach equilibrium. Incremental tests to determine lactate parameters therefore usually contain 3- to 5-minute stages, with each work period progressively increasing in intensity. There

TABLE 12.1 Lactate threshold treadmill protocol

			SPEED (km/h)			
			UNTRAINED		TRAINED	
STAGE	TIME (min)	% GRADE	Male	Female	Male	Female
1	4	1	6.0	6.0	8	6
2	4	1	7.5	7.0	10	8
3	4	1	9.0	8.0	12	10
4	4	1	10.5	9.0	14	12
5	4	1	12.0	10.0	16	14
6	4	1	13.5	11.0	18	16
7	4	15	15.0	12.0	20	18
8	4	15	16.5	13.0	22	20

Source: David Bishop, Victoria University

TABLE 12.2 Lactate threshold cycle protocol

STAGE	TIME (min)	POWER (W)			
		UNTRAINED		TRAINED	
		Male	Female	Male	Female
1	4	50	50	100	65
2	4	75	70	140	100
3	4	100	90	180	135
4	4	125	110	220	170
5	4	150	130	260	205
6	4	175	150	300	240
7	4	200	170	340	275
8	4	225	190	380	310

Source: David Bishop, Victoria University

TABLE 12.3 Lactate threshold rowing protocol

STAGE	TIME (min)	POWER (W)			
		RECREATIONALLY ACTIVE		TRAINED	
		Male	Female	Male	Female
1	4	110	110	150	130
2	4	130	125	175	155
3	4	150	140	200	180
4	4	170	155	225	205
5	4	190	170	250	230
6	4	210	185	275	255
7	4	Max	Max	Max	Max

Adapted from: Rice[23]

is not a standard incremental protocol, as starting work rate and increments may vary depending on the requirements of the sport and the fitness of the participant. At the end of each work period, there is often a short pause (e.g. 30 to 60 seconds) during which a blood sample is collected (from the ear lobe or fingertip), and blood lactate concentration is subsequently measured. Heart rate and oxygen consumption ($\dot{V}O_2$) are usually measured during exercise depending on the aims of the test. Discontinuous protocols such as this are used for most testing modes where blood is not easily sampled owing to the movements required (e.g. treadmill running and rowing), although a continuous protocol without breaks is sometimes used with cycling, where body position does not change greatly. Participants should complete seven, or preferably eight, stages (but generally not more than ten stages). A minimum of six stages is required for the valid determination of the LT2, and therefore the protocol (starting work rate and increments) should be adjusted accordingly. An individual lactate curve can then be obtained (see Figure 12.1).

> **Note:** When using a cycle ergometer, the participant should use their preferred cadence, which can be determined during the warm-up. Initial work rate and stage increments will need to be carefully considered for each individual.

Validity and reliability

The concurrent validity of LT1 as a determinant of the transition between purely aerobic and the minimal reliance on anaerobic metabolism (i.e. lactate metabolism) is well accepted.[26,27] The 'standard' to confirm the validity of LT2 derived from an exercise test is the maximal lactate steady state (MLSS), which represents the intensity where blood lactate appearance and disappearance is in equilibrium.[28] The validity of the LT2 derived from an incremental exercise test is dependent on the method chosen to calculate the LT and the stage length of the exercise test (see Practical 1, Test accuracy, reliability and validity).[29] The modified Dmax, calculated during a 4-minute stage exercise test where participants complete seven to nine stages, is a valid criterion for establishing the LT2 in cycle ergometry. Similar results have been reported in men for cycling; however, in women the modified Dmax may overestimate the power output sustainable at the MLSS and the mean power output achieved during 40 km time trial performance.[30] For rowing, it has been reported that the modified Dmax, determined during an incremental test consisting of up to six stages of ≥7 minutes, can validly determine the MLSS.[31] There appears to be no research investigating the concurrent validity of the modified Dmax determined during treadmill running to establish the MLSS.

There is a high test–retest reliability of the modified Dmax established during treadmill running (cross-validation (CV) = 1.2%–5.8%).[32,33] There appears to be no research investigating the reliability of modified Dmax method in cycle and rowing ergometry.

Activity 12.1 Lactate threshold test

AIMS: to conduct a lactate threshold test, interpret the results and provide feedback/discuss with a participant.

Background

The following protocol will detail lactate threshold testing, on a cycle ergometer, treadmill or rowing ergometer. It is recommended that gas analysis is incorporated into the protocol for the determination of $\dot{V}O_2$max and the subsequent percentage of $\dot{V}O_2$max at the lactate threshold; details of $\dot{V}O_2$max testing procedures are outlined in Practical 10, $\dot{V}O_2$max. Blood lactate collection and analysis can be conducted using a number of different methods, including portable hand-held analysers, which are used most commonly for performance testing in the field and in laboratories, and benchtop analysers, which require the collection of blood into capillary tubes and further preparation of the sample for subsequent analysis. This method is most commonly used in clinical and research settings, and consequently this practical will describe the use of portable analysers owing to the widespread use of these devices in practical settings throughout Australia. (Please refer to the manufacturer's guidelines for the specific instructions for each different model of analyser.)

Protocol summary

A participant completes a lactate threshold test comprising seven to eight incremental 4-minute stages separated by 1-minute rests, until volitional exhaustion on a treadmill, cycle or rowing ergometer.

Protocol

Pre-test requirements

1 Review all the safety, cleaning and disposing of contaminated items and blood spill procedures outlined in Practical 2, Blood analysis.

2 If a computer is to be used, ensure that it is switched on and that the protocol to be used is programmed into the bike/treadmill/rower (if possible).

3 Follow the instructions outlined in Practical 10 for preparation and protocols for sampling expired air.

4 Measure and record relevant environment data (e.g. temperature, humidity, and barometric pressure).

5 Follow the calibration/verification recommendations for the portable lactate analyser. The portable analysers generally require the insertion of a check strip prior to testing. Peel a check strip packet to the line indicated and insert it into the strip inlet of the analyser, without touching the chip located on the end of the strip. Check that the analyser displays the correct calibration value before beginning the incremental test; if it does not, repeat the procedure. If it still doesn't provide a value in the correct range, the device should not be used and will need to be serviced.

6 Arrange all lactate-testing equipment and consumables on bench surface protection paper on a table/bench (Figure 12.4). Location of the lactate collection workspace should be within close but safe proximity to the ergometer/ treadmill.

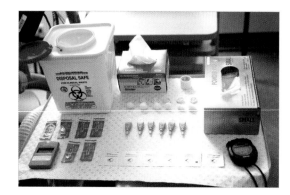

Figure 12.4 Pre-test set-up of blood collection consumables

Used with permission from Lactate Pro

Participant preparation

1 Follow the pre-exercise test procedures outlined in Appendix B.

2 Check Appendix C to ensure that there are no contraindications to exercise testing.

3 Measure and record body mass (see Practical 4, Physique assessment).

4 Enter the participant's details, including name, age (for calculation of age-predicted maximum heart rate (HR)) and sex, body mass and other details as appropriate.

Blood collection

1 Revise the procedure for determining the likelihood of fainting and putting the participant at ease, and the collection of blood (outlined in Practical 2).

2 Thoroughly wash your hands and put the gloves on.

3 Ensure that you are wearing the additional personal protective equipment required for blood collection as outlined in Practical 2.

4 Peel open a lactate strip foil packet to half way (the line indicated on the packet), ensuring you do not touch the strip.

5 Massage the participant's finger/ear to encourage increased blood flow.

6 Clean the finger/ear with an alcohol swab and dry with sterile cotton wool or tissue.

> **Note:** If alcohol contaminates the sample you will not obtain an valid test result.

7 Insert the lactate strip into the analyser (Figure 12.5) until a beep is heard. Remove the foil packet but do not throw it away.

> **Note:** For most portable analysers, if the strip is inserted into the analyser more than 60 seconds prior to blood collection the analyser will go into sleep mode. If this occurs use the original packaging to grasp the lactate strip and remove and re-insert the strip into the analyser prior to blood collection. DO NOT attempt to sample blood whilst the analyser is in sleep mode.

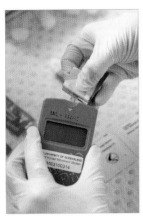

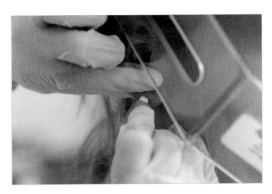

Figure 12.6 Lancet ear puncture technique

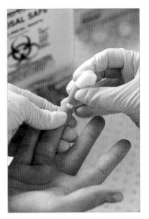

Figure 12.5 Inserting the
lactate strip into the analyser

Used with permission from
Lactate Pro

Figure 12.7 Lancet finger
puncture technique

8 Grasp the participant's ear or finger gently and puncture it with a lancet (Figures 12.6 and 12.7).

9 Wipe off the first droplet of blood with sterile cotton ball/wool or tissue.

> **Note:** If sweat contaminates the sample you will not obtain a valid test result.

10 If blood flow is inadequate, gently massage the participant's finger/ear until a droplet of blood forms.

11 Without allowing the droplet of blood to run, touch the tip of the lactate strip to the beaded drop of blood on the finger/ear until the lactate analyser beeps (Figures 12.8 and 12.9).

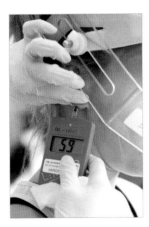

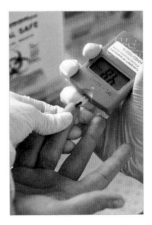

Figure 12.8 Blood collection procedure
for ear prick

Used with permission from Lactate Pro

Figure 12.9 Blood collection procedure for
finger prick

Used with permission from Lactate Pro

> **Note:** Avoid touching the lactate strip to the skin. The strip should not be placed on top or underneath the blood droplet, but directly in line of the flow to encourage the blood to be drawn up towards the analyser. The required amount of blood is 5 μL, which is visible in the lactate strip and achieved when the blood collected forms a 'U' shape.

12 Place a small sterile cotton ball or tissue over the ear or finger to stop blood from running and apply tape or a finger cot to secure it in place (Figures 12.10 and 12.11).

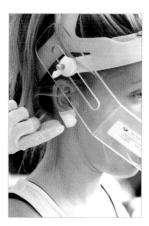

Figure 12.10 Application of cotton ball and tape to ear following blood collection

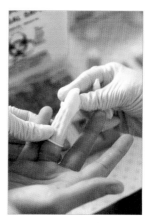

Figure 12.11 Application of cotton ball and finger cot to finger following blood collection

13 The lactate analyser will count down a number of seconds before displaying the lactate concentration (Figure 12.12).

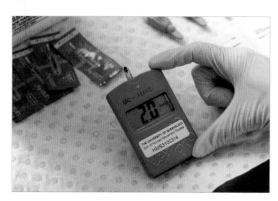

Figure 12.12 Blood lactate reading in mmol/L

Used with permission from Lactate Pro

14 Record the reading displayed on the analyser. If the lactate analyser reads 'Lo' (low) record this as 0.8 mmol/L.

> **Note:** If the display clears before the value is recorded, reinsert the strip and read the number on the screen.

15 Grasp the lactate strip with the foil packet and dispose of the sampling consumables into the biohazardous waste bin.

> **Note:** Lancets are to be placed in the sharps bin.

Test protocol

1 Attach a HR monitor and record the resting HR as per the protocol outlined in Practical 3, Cardiovascular health.

2 Have the participant place their water bottle and towel in close proximity to the cycle ergometer/ treadmill.

3 Measure and record blood pressure in the exercising posture (e.g. standing or sitting) – the blood pressure provides a baseline measure and is used to determine whether the participant has exceeded the criteria for a contraindication to exercise (see Appendix C).

4 If using a treadmill, provide treadmill safety precautions to the participant (see Appendix D). An assessment of their ability to walk/jog safely should be conducted prior to starting the test.

5 Provide details of the test, including the protocol, hand signals the participant can use during the test, explanation of the rating of perceived exertion (RPE) (see Appendix E), test termination and safety (see Appendix F).

6 The participant should complete a 5-minute warm-up.

7 Fit the headpiece and nose clip to the participant (see Practical 10, $\dot{V}O_2$max).

8 Encourage the participant to push themselves to his/her maximum capacity (volitional exhaustion) for valid test results.

9 The participant should start exercising at the intensity required for stage 1 (see Tables 12.1–12.3).

Note: The drag factor for the rowing ergometer must also be set prior to the start of the test (Table 12.4).

TABLE 12.4 Rowing ergometer drag factor settings	
CATEGORY	**DRAG FACTOR**
Junior female	100
Lightweight female	100
Heavyweight female	110
Junior male	125
Lightweight male	125
Heavyweight male	130

Adapted from: Rice[23]

10 Once this intensity is reached, the test should be started via a countdown – '*3, 2, 1, START*'.

Note: Most software programs for $\dot{V}O_2$max require you to click 'start test' on the computer (Figure 12.13).

11 Record speed/power every minute; expired O_2, CO_2 and volume of inspired (V_I) or expired air (V_E)[b] should be recorded every minute on the computer. Measure and record RPE within the final 15 seconds of each stage and heart rate in the final 30 seconds of each stage.

12 During each work rate, indicate to the participant how much time remains and check on their ability to continue.

13 If the treadmill, rower, or bike cannot be programmed then the intensity will need to be manually changed by the assessor or participant for each stage.

14 Stop the belt at the end of the 4-minute stage, giving the participant prior warning with a countdown over the final 5 seconds.

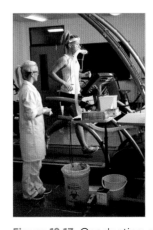

Figure 12.13 Conducting a lactate threshold test

[b] This will depend on the system and the placement of the volume/flow device. See Practical 10 for more details.

> **Note:** If conducting the test on a treadmill, consider safety procedures when slowing or stopping the belt (see Appendix D). Ensure that the participant doesn't stop before the 4 minutes is completed.

15 Immediately upon stopping, blood should be drawn from either the ear lobe or a finger, as described earlier, for the analysis of lactate.

> **Note:** If measuring $\dot{V}O_2$, the participant may remove the nose clip and mouthpiece during the 1-minute rest, though the headset should remain in place.

16 For continuous cycling protocols, the blood sample should be collected in the final 30 seconds of each stage without the participant stopping exercise.

17 All equipment should be in place 30 seconds before the start of the next stage; the treadmill should be started at least 15 seconds before the start of the next stage to allow it to reach the required speed.

18 Repeat the blood collection procedures following completion of each stage throughout the test.

19 The test is terminated when the participant presses the emergency stop button, indicates that they are unable to continue or meets the test termination criteria (see Appendix F), at which point the tester stops the treadmill belt or indicates to the participant to stop cycling. For the rowing ergometer test, participants are required to finish the final maximal effort stage for the test to be valid.

20 At the end of the test, collect an immediate post-exercise blood sample, regardless of how many minutes they have completed at that stage.

21 Ensure the participant has an adequate cool-down – heart rate should return to at least 50% of HRmax. In some situations you may wish to measure the RPE, BP and heart rate during recovery (e.g. 1 and 5 minutes post-test). It is good practice to keep an eye on a participant as they walk away from the treadmill, cycle or rowing ergometer to ensure they are steady on their feet.

22 Verify gas analysers to ensure that there was minimal drift during the test (see Practical 1, Test accuracy, reliability and validity). Accept the test results if the drift is less than 0.1% (absolute) in each of the two analysers.

23 Save and exit the computer program. Shut down the computer and monitor, and turn off the power and pump switches on the analysers.

24 Clean and disinfect all equipment (see Appendix A).

Data recording

Participant's name: _____   Date: _____

Age: _____ years   Sex: _____   Body mass: _____ kg

Training status (untrained/recreationally active, trained): _____

Resting HR: _____ bpm

Age-predicted HRmax[c]: _____ bpm   Baseline [La⁻]: _____ mmol/L

continued

---

[c] Age-predicted maximum heart rate $= 208 - (0.7 \times \text{age})$.

Data recording *(continued)*

Laboratory conditions

Temperature: _____ °C   Humidity: _____ %

Barometric pressure: _____ mmHg

Protocol

Date: _____   Testing location: _____

Supervising staff: _____   Sport: _____

Protocol mode (treadmill, cycle or rowing): _____

Drag factor (if completing a rowing lactate threshold test; see Table 12.4): _____

Initial workload (W for ergometers or speed/grade for treadmill) according to training status (see Table 12.1, 12.2 or 12.3): _____

Stage	Time (min)	Workload: power (W)ᵃ or speed (kph) and grade (%)	Absolute $\dot{V}O_2$ (L/min)	Relative $\dot{V}O_2$ (mL/kg/min)	HR (bpm)	RPE	[La⁻] (mmol/L)
1	1						
	2						
	3						
	4						
	5						
2	6						
	7						
	8						
	9						
	10						

continued overpage

Data recording *(continued)*

Stage	Time (min)	Workload: power (W)[a] or speed (kph) and grade (%)	Absolute $\dot{V}O_2$ (L/min)	Relative $\dot{V}O_2$ (mL/kg/min)	HR (bpm)	RPE	(La⁻) (mmol/L)
3	11						
	12						
	13						
	14						
	15						
4	16						
	17						
	18						
	19						
	20						
5	21						
	22						
	23						
	24						
	25						

continued

Data recording *(continued)*

Stage	Time (min)	Workload: power (W)[a] or speed (kph) and grade (%)	Absolute $\dot{V}O_2$ (L/min)	Relative $\dot{V}O_2$ (mL/kg/min)	HR (bpm)	RPE	[La−] (mmol/L)
6	26						
	27						
	28						
	29						
	30						
7	31						
	32						
	33						
	34						
	35						
8	36						
	37						
	38						
	39						
	40						

continued overpage

Data recording (continued)

Stage	Time (min)	Workload: power (W)[a] or speed (kph) and grade (%)	Absolute $\dot{V}O_2$ (L/min)	Relative $\dot{V}O_2$ (mL/kg/min)	HR (bpm)	RPE	(La$^-$) (mmol/L)
9	41						
	42						
	43						
	44						
	45						
10	46						
	47						
	48						
	49						
	50						

[a] If using a Monark bike, the work rate will be displayed in kiloponds (kp) or kilopond metres (kpm). To convert to watts, refer to Table 11.1

1　Record the maximum/peak work rate and heart rate.

　Maximum/peak work rate: _____ W or kph and % grade

　Maximum/peak HR = _____ bpm

2　Determine whether the test was valid, calculate $\dot{V}O_2$max/peak and confirm whether the test determined a true $\dot{V}O_2$max (see Practical 10, $\dot{V}O_2$max for formulae and examples).

　Circle: Valid or Invalid $\dot{V}O_2$max/peak test

　Plateau criteria: $<$150 mL/min/body mass $= <$ _____ mL/kg/min

　Circle: $\dot{V}O_2$max or $\dot{V}O_2$peak = _____ mL/kg/min

3　Plot lactate and HR against work rate (Figure 12.14).

4　Plot $\dot{V}O_2$ and HR against work rate (Figure 12.15).

continued

Data recording *(continued)*

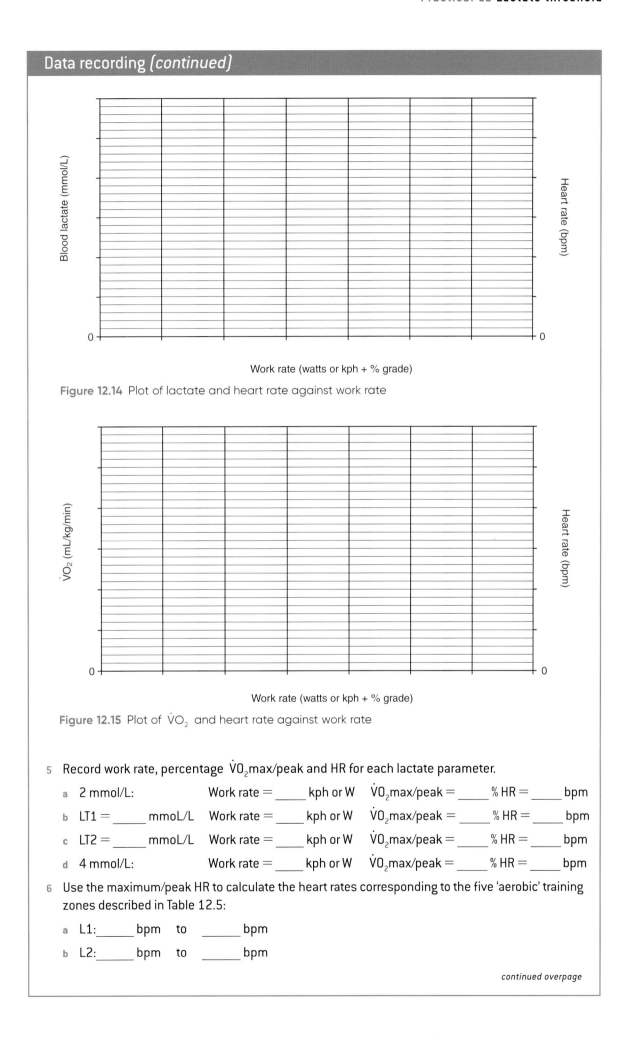

Figure 12.14 Plot of lactate and heart rate against work rate

Figure 12.15 Plot of $\dot{V}O_2$ and heart rate against work rate

5 Record work rate, percentage $\dot{V}O_2$max/peak and HR for each lactate parameter.

  a 2 mmol/L: Work rate = _____ kph or W $\dot{V}O_2$max/peak = _____ % HR = _____ bpm

  b LT1 = _____ mmoL/L   Work rate = _____ kph or W $\dot{V}O_2$max/peak = _____ % HR = _____ bpm

  c LT2 = _____ mmoL/L   Work rate = _____ kph or W $\dot{V}O_2$max/peak = _____ % HR = _____ bpm

  d 4 mmol/L: Work rate = _____ kph or W $\dot{V}O_2$max/peak = _____ % HR = _____ bpm

6 Use the maximum/peak HR to calculate the heart rates corresponding to the five 'aerobic' training zones described in Table 12.5:

  a L1: _____ bpm to _____ bpm

  b L2: _____ bpm to _____ bpm

continued overpage

Data recording *(continued)*

  c L3:_____ bpm   to   _____ bpm

  d L4:_____ bpm   to   _____ bpm

  e L5:_____ bpm   to   _____ bpm

TABLE 12.5 Description of the five 'aerobic' training zones

TRAINING ZONE	HEART RATE (% HRmax)	EFFORT (min)	BLOOD LACTATE (mmol/L)	RATE OF PERCEIVED EXERTION (RPE)
L1 (recovery)	65%–75%	>30	<2.0	Easy (<11)
L2 (extensive endurance)	75%–80%	60–240	2.0–2.5	Light (11–12)
L3 (intensive endurance)	80%–85%	30–120	2.5–3.5	Somewhat hard (13–14)
L4 (threshold training)	85%–92%	10–40	3.5–5.0	Hard (15–16)
L5 (interval training)	92%–100%	2–5	>5.0	Very hard (17–19)

Adapted from: Bourdon[22]

Interpretation, feedback and discussion

First, consider the four steps of interpretation and the three steps of feedback and discussion outlined in Appendix G. You should now provide feedback to the participant and/or their coach as appropriate regarding their lactate threshold results, and how they can use these results to guide their training. It is important to explain initially what the lactate threshold and the work rate represent (i.e. a work rate that is sustainable for a reasonably long period of time), that there is an equivalent HR, speed/W and RPE that reflect the same point, and how these values can be used to guide training (e.g. aerobic versus lactate threshold training) and competition (dependent on duration, but one can generally maintain a pace at or slightly above the lactate threshold). If gas analysis is also performed, the $\dot{V}O_2$max/peak should be reported, as well as the $\dot{V}O_2$ (mL/kg/min) and percentage $\dot{V}O_2$max/peak at the lactate threshold.

As a guide, the lactate threshold (e.g. LT2) usually occurs between 50% and 90% of $\dot{V}O_2$max; typically, the LT2 in trained individuals occurs at a higher percentage of $\dot{V}O_2$max. Below are some general guidelines for values of LT2:

- 50%–60% $\dot{V}O_2$max in untrained individuals
- 60%–80% $\dot{V}O_2$max in trained individuals
- 80%–90% of $\dot{V}O_2$max in elite, endurance-trained athletes.

Lactate threshold results are best used as an indication of changes in aerobic fitness, as a consequence of training, rather than making comparisons between participants. If an individual's LT2 is higher following training, this normally indicates an improved potential for endurance events. The LT2 has been associated with cycling performance for ≈55 minutes, half-marathon speed for trained runners, marathon speed for elite runners, and there is also a strong correlation with 2000 m rowing performance.[34]

The lactate threshold results can also be used to help prescribe training. When working with athletes, it is common for testers to use five 'aerobic' training intensities (see Table 12.5), based on the LT1 and LT2 described in Figure 12.1.

Case study

Setting: You are a practicum placement student at an elite sports institute. The national rowing team is visiting the institute for a training camp to begin their season and, during this time, the physiology department will be conducting lactate threshold and $\dot{V}O_2$max tests. You will be assisting the team's physiologist with the testing.

Task: Calculate the lactate threshold for a rower and provide feedback to the coach on their $\dot{V}O_2$max and lactate thresholds.

DATA COLLECTION SHEET

Participant: _Jack Harris_   Age: _23_ years   Sex: _Male_   Body mass: _71_ kg

Training status (untrained/recreationally-active, trained): _Trained_

Resting HR: _61_ bpm   Age-predicted HRmax[d]: _192_ bpm   Baseline [La⁻]: _1.3 mmol/L_

LABORATORY CONDITIONS

Temperature: _21.4_ °C   Humidity: _59 %_   Barometric pressure: _764.7_ mmHg

PROTOCOL

Date: _14.12.19_   Testing location: _Queensland Academy of Sport_

Supervising staff: _Jane Lai_   Sport: _Rowing_

Protocol mode (treadmill, cycle or rowing): _Rowing_

Drag factor (if completing a rowing lactate threshold test; see Table 12.4): _125_

Initial workload (W for ergometers or speed/grade for treadmill) according to training status (see Table 12.1, 12.2 or 12.3): _150 W_

Stage	Time (min)	Power (W)	Absolute $\dot{V}O_2$ (L/min)	Relative $\dot{V}O_2$ (mL/kg/min)	HR (bpm)	RPE	(La⁻) (mmol/L)
1	1	150	1.25	17.60			
			1.32	18.59			
	2		1.39	19.58			
			1.44	20.28			
	3		1.50	21.13			
			1.56	21.97			
	4		1.60	22.54	115	7	
			1.62	22.82			
	5						1.3

continued overpage

---

[d] Age-predicted maximum heart rate $= 208 - (0.7 \times \text{age})$.

Case studies (continued)

Stage	Time (min)	Power (W)	Absolute $\dot{V}O_2$ (L/min)	Relative $\dot{V}O_2$ (mL/kg/min)	HR (bpm)	RPE	[La$^-$] (mmol/L)
2	6	175	1.40	19.72			
			1.45	20.42			
	7		1.61	22.68			
			1.70	23.94			
	8		1.79	25.21			
			1.88	26.48			
	9		1.95	27.46	127	8	
			1.97	27.75			
	10						1.8
3	11	200	1.74	24.51			
			1.89	26.62			
	12		1.99	28.15			
			2.12	29.86			
	13		2.27	31.97			
			2.40	33.80			
	14		2.52	35.49	141	10	
			2.54	35.77			
	15						2.3
4	16	225	2.22	31.27			
			2.40	33.80			
	17		2.61	36.76			
			2.79	39.30			
	18		2.92	41.13			
			3.09	43.52			
	19		3.20	45.07	159	13	
			3.22	45.35			
	20						3.0

continued

Case studies (continued)

Stage	Time (min)	Power (W)	Absolute $\dot{V}O_2$ (L/min)	Relative $\dot{V}O_2$ (mL/kg/min)	HR (bpm)	RPE	[La⁻] (mmol/L)
5	21	250	2.90	40.85			
			3.14	44.23			
	22		3.29	46.34			
			3.47	48.87			
	23		3.65	51.41			
			3.83	53.94			
	24		3.96	55.77	173	15	
			3.98	56.06			
	25						4.3
6	26	275	3.55	50.00			
			3.70	52.11			
	27		3.82	53.80			
			3.95	55.63			
	28		4.07	57.32			
			4.21	59.30			
	29		4.38	61.69	185	16	
			4.40	61.97			
	30						6.7
7	31	MAX	3.90	54.93			
			4.01	56.48			
	32		4.13	58.17			
			4.20	59.15			
	33		4.32	60.85			
			4.40	61.97			
	34	294 W	4.45	62.68	198	19	
			4.47	62.96			
	35						9.4

Using the above data:

1 Record the maximum/peak work rate and heart rate.

Maximum/peak work rate: _____ W or kph and % grade

Maximum/peak HR = _____ bpm

continued overpage

Case studies *(continued)*

2 Determine whether the test was valid, calculate $\dot{V}O_2$max/peak and confirm whether the test determined a true $\dot{V}O_2$max (see Practical 10, $\dot{V}O_2$max for formulae and examples).
Circle: Valid or Invalid $\dot{V}O_2$max/peak test

Plateau criteria: $<$150 mL/min/body mass $= <$ _____ mL/kg/min

Circle: $\dot{V}O_2$max or $\dot{V}O_2$peak $=$ _____ mL/kg/min

3 Plot lactate and HR against work rate.

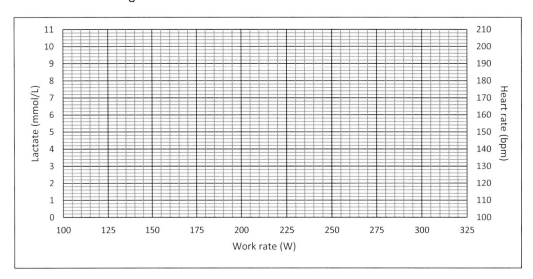

4 Plot $\dot{V}O_2$ and HR against work rate.

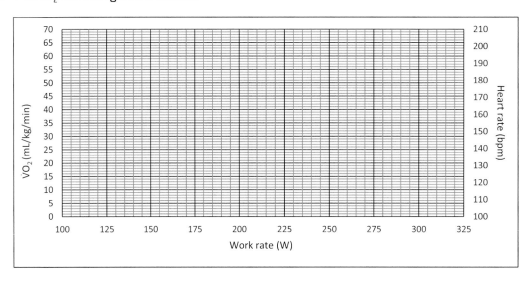

5 Record work rate, percentage $\dot{V}O_2$max/peak and HR for each lactate parameter.

a 2 mmol/L: Work rate $=$ _____ kph or W

$\dot{V}O_2$max/peak $=$ _____ %   HR $=$ _____ bpm

continued

Case studies *(continued)*

b LT1 = _____ mmoL/L Work rate = _____ kph or W $\dot{V}O_2$max/peak = _____ % HR = _____ bpm

c LT2 = _____ mmoL/L Work rate = _____ kph or W $\dot{V}O_2$max/peak = _____ % HR = _____ bpm

d 4 mmol/L: Work rate = _____ kph or W $\dot{V}O_2$max/peak = _____ % HR = _____ bpm

6 Use maximum/peak HR to calculate the heart rates corresponding to the five 'aerobic' training zones described in Table 12.5:

L1:_____ bpm to _____ bpm

L2:_____ bpm to _____ bpm

L3:_____ bpm to _____ bpm

L4:_____ bpm to _____ bpm

L5:_____ bpm to _____ bpm

7 Interpret the results and provide feedback to Jack and his coach.

References

[1] Davies CT, Knibbs AV. The training stimulus. The effects of intensity, duration and frequency of effort on maximum aerobic power output. Int Z Angew Physiol 1971;29:299–305.

[2] Jeukendrup AE, Hesselink MK, Snyder AC, Kuipers H, Keizer HA. Physiological changes in male competitive cyclists after two weeks of intensified training. Int J Sports Med 1992;13:534–41.

[3] Coen B, Schwarz L, Urhausen A, Kindermann W. Control of training in middle-distance and long-distance running by means of the individual anaerobic threshold. Int J Sports Med 1991;12:519–24.

[4] Foster C, Fitzgerald DJ, Spatz P. Stability of the blood lactate–heart rate relationship in competitive athletes. Med Sci Sports Exerc 1999;31:578–82.

[5] Faude O, Kindermann W, Meyer T. Lactate threshold concepts: How valid are they? Sports Med 2009;39:469–90.

[6] Walsh ML, Banister EW. Possible mechanisms of the anaerobic threshold – a review. Sports Med 1988;5:269–302.

[7] Coyle EF, Feltner ME, Kautz SA, Hamilton MT, Montain SJ, Baylor AM, et al. Physiological and biomechanical factors associated with elite endurance cycling performance. Med Sci Sports Exerc 1991;23:93–107.

[8] Coyle EF, Coggan AR, Hopper MK, Walters TJ. Determinants of endurance in well-trained cyclists. J Appl Physiol (1985) 1988;64:2622–30.

[9] Weltman A, Snead D, Seip R, Schurrer R, Levine S, Rutt R, et al. Prediction of lactate threshold and fixed blood lactate concentrations from 3200-m running performance in male runners. Int J Sports Med 1987;8:401–6.

[10] Ivy JL, Withers RT, Vanhandel PJ, Elger DH, Costill DL. Muscle respiratory capacity and fiber type as determinants of the lactate threshold. J Appl Physiol 1980;48:523–7.

[11] Amann M, Subudhi AW, Foster C. Predictive validity of ventilatory and lactate thresholds for cycling time trial performance. Scand J Med Sci Sports 2006;16:27–34.

[12] Bishop D, Jenkins DG, Mackinnon LT. The relationship between plasma lactate parameters, W-peak and 1-h cycling performance in women. Med Sci Sports Exerc 1998;30:1270–5.

[13] Farrell PA, Wilmore JH, Coyle EF, Billing JE, Costill DL. Plasma lactate accumulation and distance running performance. Med Sci Sports Exerc 1979;11:338–44.

[14] Kindermann W, Simon G, Keul J. Significance of the aerobic-anaerobic transition for the determination of work load intensities during endurance training. Eur J Appl Physiol Occup Physiol 1979;42:25–34.

[15] Heck H, Mader A, Hess G, Mucke S, Muller R, Hollmann W. Justification of the 4-mmol/l lactate threshold. Int J Sports Med 1985;6:117–30.

[16] Sjodin B, Jacobs I. Onset of blood lactate accumulation and marathon running performance. Int J Sports Med 1981;2:23–6.

[17] Coyle EF, Coggan AR, Hemmert MK, Walters TJ. Glycogen usage and performance relative to lactate threshold. Med Sci Sports Exerc 1984;16:120–1.

[18] Tanner RK, Bourdon P. Clarification of nomenclature and terms of reference. Laboratory Standards Assistance Scheme. Canberra, ACT: Australian Institute of Sport; 2004.

[19] Australian Institute of Sport. ADAPT [Software program]. Canberra, ACT: Sports Sciences Division, AIS; 1995.

[20] White R, Yaeger D, Stavrianeos S. Determination of blood lactate concentration: reliability and validity of a lactate oxidase-based method. Int J Exerc Sci 2009;2:83–93.

[21] Cheng B, Kuipers H, Snyder AC, Keizer HA, Jeukendrup A, Hesselink M. A new approach for the determination of ventilatory and lactate thresholds. Int J Sports Med 1992;13:518–22.

[22] Bourdon O. Blood lactate thresholds: concepts and applications. In: Tanner RK, Gore CJ, eds. Physiological tests for elite athletes. Champaign, IL: Human Kinetics; 2013, pp. 77–102.

[23] Rice T. Information for athletes, NTC scientists, and pathways programs: 7×4 minute step test protocol. Rowing Australia. Canberra, ACT: Australian Institute of Sport; 2016.

[24] Jones AM, Doust JH. A 1% treadmill grade most accurately reflects the energetic cost of outdoor running. J Sports Sci 1996;14:321–7.

[25] Mooses M, Tippi B, Mooses K, Durussel J, Maestu J. Better economy in field running than on the treadmill: evidence from high-level distance runners. Biol Sport 2015;32:155–9.

[26] Rusko H, Luhtanen P, Rahkila P, Viitasalo J, Rehunen S, Harkonen M. Muscle metabolism, blood lactate and oxygen uptake in steady state exercise at aerobic and anaerobic thresholds. Eur J Appl Physiol 1986;55:181–6.

[27] Beaver WL, Wasserman K, Whipp BJ. Improved detection of lactate threshold during exercise using a log-log transformation. J Appl Physiol 1985;59:1936–40.

[28] Beneke R. Methodological aspects of maximal lactate steady state-implications for performance testing. Eur J Appl Physiol 2003;89:95–9.

[29] Jamnick NA, Botella J, Pyne DB, Bishop DJ. Manipulating graded exercise test variables affects the validity of the lactate threshold and $\dot{V}O_2$peak. PloS One 2018;13(7):e0199794.

[30] Hoffmann SM, Skinner TL, van Rosendal SP, Osborne MA, Emmerton LM, Jenkins DG. The efficacy of the lactate threshold: a sex-based comparison. J Strength Cond Res 2020;34(11):3190–8.

[31] Bourdon PC, Woolford SM, Buckley JD. Effects of varying the step duration on the determination of lactate thresholds in elite rowers. Int J Sports Physiol Perform 2018;13:687–93.

[32] Chalmers S, Esterman A, Eston R, Norton K. Standardization of the Dmax method for calculating the second lactate threshold. Int J Sports Physiol Perform 2015;10:921–6.

[33] Camargo Alves JC, Segabinazi Peserico C, Nogueira GA, Machado FA. The influence of the regression model and final speed criteria on the reliability of lactate threshold determined by the Dmax method in endurance-trained runners. Appl Physiol Nutr Metab 2016;41:1039–44.

[34] Ingham SA, Whyte GP, Jones K, Nevill AM. Determinants of 2,000 m rowing ergometer performance in elite rowers. Eur J Appl Physiol 2002;88:243–6.

PRACTICAL 13
HIGH-INTENSITY EXERCISE

Tina Skinner, Martyn Binnie and David Jenkins

LEARNING OBJECTIVES

- Identify and explain the common terminology, processes and equipment required to conduct accurate and safe measures of high-intensity exercise
- Identify and describe the limitations, contraindications or considerations that may require the modification of high-intensity exercise assessments, and make appropriate adjustments for relevant populations or participants
- Explain the scientific rationale, purposes, reliability, validity, assumptions and limitations of common high-intensity exercise assessments
- Recognise and adjust incorrectly calibrated equipment used in high-intensity exercise assessments
- Conduct appropriate pre-assessment procedures, including explaining the test and obtaining informed consent and a focused medical history, and performing a pre-exercise risk assessment
- Identify the need for guidance or further information from an appropriate health professional, and recognise when medical supervision is required before or during an assessment and when to cease a test
- Select and conduct appropriate protocols for safe and effective high-intensity exercise assessments, including instructing clients on the correct use of equipment
- Record, analyse and interpret information from high-intensity exercise assessments and convey the results, including the validity and limitations of the assessments, through relevant verbal and/or written communication with the participant or involved professional

Equipment and other requirements

- Information sheet and informed consent form
- Adult Pre-exercise Screening System (APSS) form
- Programmable motorised treadmill or cycle ergometer
- Electronic timing gates (i.e. timing lights) or stopwatch (see Box 13.1)
- Metabolic system and associated components (mouthpiece set-up, breathing tubes, calibration equipment – including gases)
- Nose clip
- Body mass scales
- Marker cones
- Calculator
- Tissues

> **Box 13.1 Stopwatch versus timing lights**
>
> The method of timing within several of the tests mentioned within this practical will vary depending on equipment available, with the most common methods being stopwatch or timing lights. Using a stopwatch is often the most practical method and is often the choice of coaches for the majority of sessions. It is usually only at set periods in the season (3–4 times per year) that squads will use timing lights to get benchmark data. Where a stopwatch is used, the timers need to position themselves perpendicular to the most important splits. Standing further away will reduce parallax error. Having at least two testers with stopwatches timing the sprint, with the average time across stopwatches recorded, will further optimise accuracy.

- Spray bottle with diluted bleach (bleach: water, 1:10)
- Sports tape/Micropore tape
- Non-latex gloves of appropriate size (S, M, L)
- Masking tape
- Cleaning and disinfecting equipment (see Appendix A)

INTRODUCTION

Many sports require participants to exercise at intensities above their maximal aerobic power ($\dot{V}O_2max$), either in a single effort (as in sprint events in athletics, swimming or cycling) or multiple sprints where each bout is separated by a limited recovery period. Irrespective of the duration and number, sprints are comprised of three phases: acceleration, maximal speed and speed maintenance. The relative importance of each phase is largely dependent on the duration of the sprint. The test/s used to assess high-intensity exercise performance needs to closely match the sport-specific demands on the athlete/s. For example, assessing high-intensity exercise performance with a football player will require a different test to that used to assess the performance of a 400 m runner; the average distance most players in the football codes sprint is <20 m and this means that acceleration (rather than maximal speed and speed maintenance) is important. In contrast, maximal speed and speed maintenance will be relatively more important for a 400 m runner.

Sprint duration aside, many athletes, particularly those in team and racket sports, engage in repeated bouts of high-intensity exercise – with each bout separated by a relatively brief (and often incomplete) recovery.

A number of tests are available to assess an athlete's capacity for high-intensity exercise and those that are included in this practical represent some of the more accepted, less invasive means of assessing high-intensity exercise performance. The practical is divided into four sections according to the capacities and skills being assessed:

- Section 1: tests of work capacity and peak power
- Section 2: tests of running speed and acceleration
- Section 3: tests of agility and change of direction speed
- Section 4: tests of repeated high-intensity exercise performance.

DEFINITIONS

Agility: the ability to rapidly change direction and position in response to a stimulus.

Average power output: average of the total power generated during the duration of the test (e.g. 30 seconds for the Wingate test).

Maximal accumulated oxygen deficit: difference between the predicted supramaximal oxygen consumption (predicted from the exercise intensity-oxygen consumption relationship) and the measured oxygen consumption assessed during exhaustive supramaximal exercise. It is an indirect measure of anaerobic capacity.

Peak power output (PPO): highest mechanical power generated during the test. It is usually observed during the first 3 to 5 seconds and is a measure of anaerobic power (work per unit of time).

Supramaximal exercise: any exercise performed at intensities greater than that intensity which corresponds to $\dot{V}O_2$max.

Total work: total work accomplished over the duration of the test (e.g. 30 seconds for the Wingate test). It is calculated by multiplying the average power output by the duration of the test and provides a measure of anaerobic capacity.

Physiological background

Muscle contraction is dependent on energy derived from the hydrolysis of adenosine triphosphate (ATP). Resting concentrations of ATP within the muscle are relatively low. For exercise to be maintained beyond just a couple of seconds, ATP has to be continually resynthesised.

The three energy systems that resynthesise ATP during exercise are the:

1 phosphagen system (also referred to as the immediate, alactic, ATP-PCr, ATP-PC or ATP-CP system)

2 glycolytic system (also referred to as the lactic, lactic acid or anaerobic glycolysis system)

3 aerobic system (also referred to as the oxidative system).

The phosphagen system uses energy stored as phosphocreatine (PCr) to resynthesise ATP. A muscle cell's reserves of PCr are used up rapidly in response to all-out exercise. Energy derived from the splitting of PCr is highest at the onset of a sprint but thereafter falls rapidly at a rate proportional to the remaining PCr concentrations. It is important to note that complete resynthesis of PCr may take several minutes following a sprint lasting ≈30 seconds; the relative contribution of each of the energy systems to subsequent sprints therefore changes as the number of sprints increases. As the contribution of the phosphagen system falls with repeated sprints, there is a greater involvement of anaerobic glycolysis and aerobic metabolism to support ATP resynthesis.

Energy derived from the glycolytic system during a sprint also begins at the onset of high-intensity exercise and as the contribution of PCr to the energy yield decreases during high-intensity exercise, energy from the glycolytic system increases. However, the capacity for this system to support ATP resynthesis is also limited and the decrease in muscle pH is believed to be responsible, at least in part, for the decline in the rate of ATP resynthesis during all-out exercise. The decline in the contribution of energy from PCr and glycolysis during high-intensity exercise is accompanied by a greater involvement of the aerobic energy system. Although aerobic metabolism makes a relatively minor contribution to ATP resynthesis during very brief duration high-intensity exercise (e.g. <10 seconds), it becomes more important during single sprints lasting longer than 30 seconds and also during repeated sprints where the recovery duration is too brief for complete resynthesis of PCr and the recovery of muscle pH to resting levels. The contribution of the three energy systems to ATP production and resynthesis is summarised in Figure 13.1.

Although the rate of energy released by the aerobic energy system during high-intensity exercise can be estimated using indirect calorimetry (i.e. analysis of expired air), the contribution of energy from PCr and glycolysis during high-intensity exercise is not as easily estimated. Researchers have used muscle and blood metabolites, ergometric tests of speed and power and the quantification of the deficit in oxygen consumption during short-duration, maximal-intensity exercise to determine the relative contribution of the anaerobic energy systems to exercise. This practical will focus on ergometric assessments to determine (1) work capacity and peak power, (2) speed and acceleration, (3) agility and change of direction and (4) repeat sprint ability.

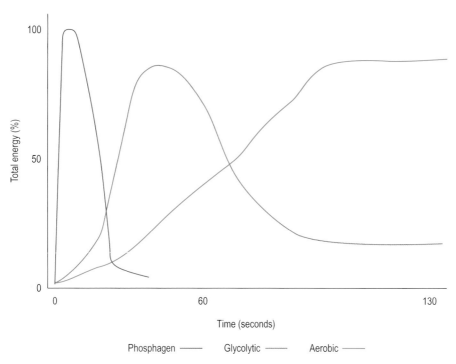

Figure 13.1 Relative contributions of the energy systems during maximal–intensity exercise

Validity and reliability

It is important to ensure the validity and reliability of the results gained from performance testing to provide meaningful comparisons within and between individuals or participant groups (see Practical 1, Test accuracy, reliability and validity). This may be especially pertinent in tests of high-intensity exercise, which require maximal and exhaustive effort from the participant. Various factors may influence both the concurrent validity and the reliability of test measures, and consideration must be given to minimise their influence. First, an appropriate test selection for the competence and experience of your targeted participant group is required. Where possible, familiarisation trials should be used to minimise the influence of a learning effect between repeat trials, or pacing strategies during exhaustive tests. The delivery of verbal encouragement and other factors, such as music, that may impact participant motivation must also be controlled.

Other common pre-test controls include:

- A break of at least 12 h from any prior high-intensity activity.
- Avoid caffeine at least 6 hours pre-test.
- No food or drink in the 2 h prior to each test other than water, which is also allowed ad libitum throughout testing.
- Control time of day and ambient temperature for repeat trials (within-participant).

Repeat trials can be conducted on a representative population to provide a greater understanding of the precision to which you can interpret the results. This typically involves a test–retest on at least 10 participants within a 7-day period to provide a measure of the expected variance in the results due to errors from the equipment and the biological variation of the participant.

SECTION 1: TESTS OF WORK CAPACITY AND PEAK POWER

Activity 13.1 Wingate test

AIMS: determine peak power, work capacity and fatigue index over a 30-second effort, interpret the results and provide feedback to a participant.

Background

The Wingate test is a 30-second all-out sprint, most commonly completed on a wind-braked and/or mechanically braked cycle ergometer. A power versus time curve is obtained from the results (as shown in Figure 13.2), providing data to calculate peak power output, mean power output and total work. Peak power is the highest power output elicited in the test at any given time point (Figure 13.2, point A); the mean power is the average power output across the 30 second period. The total work is the area under the power versus time curve. The Wingate test has been shown to have predictive validity in various athletic populations; for example, increases in peak power and/or mean power output predicts improvements in 1500 m time in elite speed skaters.[1]

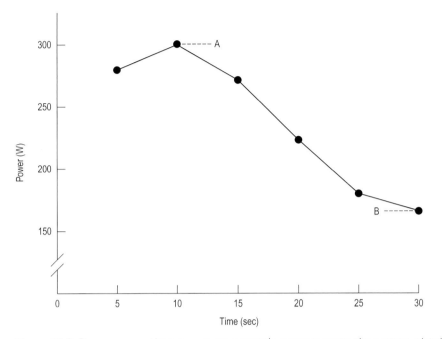

Figure 13.2 Power versus time curve: an example power versus time curve obtained from a Wingate anaerobic test using a Monark cycle ergometer. 'A' represents peak power output while 'B' is the end power output

Protocol summary

The participant is safely secured on a cycle ergometer and cycles as fast as possible for 30 seconds, with the number of pedal revolutions in each 5-second period recorded.

Protocol

Equipment set-up

A cycle ergometer is required for this activity. The cycle ergometer may need to be stabilised during the test. This can be achieved by weighting the floor supports (i.e. position free weight plates or an assistants' body mass). If using a Monark cycle ergometer, a stopwatch and recording sheet will be required. Ergometers with a computer-based interface may automatically time the test and log the data, in which case stopwatches, etc. will not be necessary.

Pre-test

1 Follow the pre-exercise test procedures outlined in Appendix B.

2 Check Appendix C to ensure that there are no contraindications to exercise testing.

3 Measure and record the participant's body mass (see Practical 4, Physique assessment).

4 Calculate the required resistance setting:

$$\text{Resistance (kp)} = 0.075 \times \text{body mass (kg)}$$

a The resistance selection will also depend on factors such as anaerobic fitness, sex and age of the participant. With well-trained athletes who regularly engage in sprint and power activities, resistance can be set as high as 0.10 kp per kg of body mass.[2]

5 Apply the correct resistance setting to the ergometer. This may require adding or removing weights (mechanically braked ergometers), varying airflow (air-braked ergometers) or editing torque factors in computer-controlled ergometers (electromagnetically braked).

6 Position the participant on the cycle ergometer and adjust the seat (the knee should be slightly bent (5°) when the pedal is at the furthest point from the seat in the crank cycle) and handlebars (such that the participant is comfortable).

7 Have the participant complete a 5-minute warm-up on the cycle ergometer at a comfortable work rate (e.g. 50 W). Conclude the warm-up with a practice of the stationary start to the test, as described below. Allow at least 1 minute of recovery between the practice start and the actual test.

Test

1 When ready to begin, ensure the participant's feet are secured to the pedals before assuming the starting position (stationary and seated position with the pedals at a 45° angle and the strongest foot forward) (Figure 13.3). The participant remains seated throughout the test.

2 If using a computer-based system, follow the instructions to commence data collection. If using a Monark ergometer, the number of pedal revolutions in each 5-second period needs to be recorded. This may be automated using a magnetic counter or counted and recorded manually. An assistant may be necessary to maximise accuracy if manually counting and recording pedal revolutions, as well as to ensure that there is no drift in the resistance during the test.

3 Ask the participant whether they have any questions.

4 Instruct the participant to cycle as hard and fast as possible for the full 30 seconds.

5 Using the commands 'three, two, one, GO!' the participant begins pedalling as fast as possible.

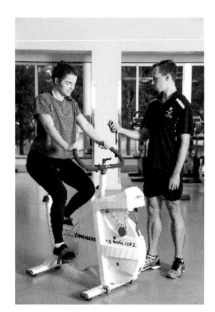

Figure 13.3 Wingate test

6 Within 2–3 seconds the resistance should be applied and the stopwatch started when the required resistance is achieved. The participant is encouraged to cycle as hard and fast as possible for the full 30 seconds.

7 Inform the participant of the elapsed time at 10-second intervals and count down the last 5 seconds ('twenty-six, twenty-seven, twenty-eight, twenty-nine, thirty' – do **not** say 'stop').

8 This is a maximal test; therefore, the participant will require verbal encouragement to cycle as fast as possible for the full 30 seconds.

Post-test

1 After the test, the participant should pedal comfortably at a low resistance for 3–5 minutes to recover.

2 On completion of the test, the participant's wellbeing needs to be the main focus as the 30-second test is extremely stressful, particularly for non-athletes.

   a If the participant feels dizzy or lightheaded, have them lie down and raise their legs.

   b If the participant is nauseous, which sometimes occurs a few minutes following test completion, ensure that a biological waste bag is readily available to contain and dispose of vomit.

3 If using a computer-based system, follow the instructions to obtain the peak power, mean power and total work completed. If using a Monark ergometer, use the formulae below to calculate peak power, mean power and total work.

4 Clean and disinfect all equipment (see Appendix A).

Data recording

Wingate test revolutions counted per 5-second period

Participant's name: _____ Date: _____

Age: _____ years   Sex: _____   Body mass: _____kg

TIME (S)	REVS ($n=$)
0–5 s	
5–10 s	
10–15 s	
15–20 s	
20–25 s	
25–30 s	
Total revs	

Calculations for Monark ergometers

Taking into account the following:

1 revolution of the Monark cranks $=$ 6 m travelled by the flywheel

$$1 \text{ kp} = 1 \text{ kg} \times \text{gravity } (9.81 \text{ m/s}^2)$$

$$1 \text{ W} = 1 \text{ J/s}$$

1 Peak power is usually obtained in the first 5-second interval of the Wingate test and is expressed as follows:

Peak power (W) $=$ force (kp) $\times$ distance / time (s)

$$= [(\underline{\hspace{1cm}} \text{ kg} \times 9.81) \times (\underline{\hspace{1cm}}\text{rev} \times 6 \text{ m})] / 5 \text{ s}$$

$$= \underline{\hspace{1.5cm}}$$

Percentile (according to Table 13.1) $= \underline{\hspace{1.5cm}}$

2 Relative peak power (W/kg) $=$ Peak power (W) / body mass (kg)

$$= \underline{\hspace{1.5cm}}$$

Percentile (according to Table 13.1) $= \underline{\hspace{1.5cm}}$

3 Total work (J) $=$ force (kp) $\times$ total distance (m)

$$= (\underline{\hspace{1cm}} \text{ kg} \times 9.81) \times (\underline{\hspace{1cm}} \text{ total revs} \times 6 \text{ m})$$

$$= \underline{\hspace{1.5cm}}$$

4 Mean power (W) $=$ total work (J) / 30 s

$$= \underline{\hspace{1.5cm}}$$

Percentile (according to Table 13.2) $= \underline{\hspace{1.5cm}}$

5 Relative mean power (W/kg) $=$ mean power (W) / body mass (kg)

$$= \underline{\hspace{1.5cm}}$$

Percentile (according to Table 13.2) $= \underline{\hspace{1.5cm}}$

6 Fatigue index (%) $=$ [peak power (W) $-$ lowest power (W)] / peak power (W) $\times$ 100

TABLE 13.1 Peak power and relative peak power normative data

	PEAK POWER (W)		RELATIVE PEAK POWER (W/kg)	
PERCENTILE	MALES (W)	FEMALES (W)	MALES (W/kg)	FEMALES (W/kg)
95	867	602	11.1	9.3
90	822	560	10.9	9.0
85	807	530	10.6	8.9
80	777	527	10.4	8.8
75	768	518	10.3	8.6
70	757	505	10.2	8.5
65	744	493	10.0	8.3
60	721	480	9.8	8.1
55	706	464	9.5	7.8
50	689	449	9.2	7.6
45	678	447	9.0	7.2
40	671	432	8.9	7.0
35	662	418	8.6	7.0
30	656	399	8.5	6.9
25	646	396	8.3	6.8
20	618	376	8.2	6.6
15	594	362	7.4	6.4
10	570	353	7.1	6.0
5	530	329	6.6	5.7

Based on data from physically active men ($n = 62$) and women ($n = 68$) aged 18–28 years. Very poor $\leq$20th percentile; poor = 21st–40th percentile; average = 41st–60th percentile; good = 61st–80th percentile; excellent $\geq$81st percentile
Adapted from: Maud and Schultz[3]

TABLE 13.2 Mean power and relative mean power normative data

	MEAN POWER (W)		RELATIVE MEAN POWER (W/kg)	
PERCENTILE	MALES (W)	FEMALES (W)	MALES (W/kg)	FEMALES (W/kg)
95	677	483	8.6	7.5
90	662	470	8.2	7.3
85	631	437	8.1	7.1
80	618	419	8.0	7.0
75	604	414	7.9	6.9
70	600	410	7.8	6.8

continued

TABLE 13.2 Mean power and relative mean power normative data (continued)

PERCENTILE	MEAN POWER (W)		RELATIVE MEAN POWER (W/kg)	
	MALES (W)	FEMALES (W)	MALES (W/kg)	FEMALES (W/kg)
65	592	402	7.7	6.7
60	577	391	7.6	6.6
55	575	386	7.5	6.5
50	565	381	7.4	6.4
45	553	377	7.3	6.3
40	548	367	7.2	6.2
35	535	361	7.1	6.1
30	530	353	7.0	6.0
25	521	347	6.8	5.9
20	496	337	6.6	5.7
15	485	320	6.4	5.6
10	471	306	6.0	5.3
5	453	287	5.6	5.1

Based on data from physically active men ($n = 60$) and women ($n = 69$) aged 18–28 years. Very poor ≤20th percentile; poor = 21st–40th percentile; average = 41st–60th percentile; good = 61st–80th percentile; excellent ≥81st percentile
Adapted from: Maud and Schultz[3]

Note: Lowest power is ideally measured in the final 5-second interval of the Wingate test and is expressed as follows:

Lowest power (W) = force (kp) $\times$ distance / time (s)

$\qquad$ = [(_____ kg $\times$ 9.81) $\times$ (_____ rev $\times$ 6 m)] / 5 s

$\qquad$ = _____

Fatigue index = _____
Percentile (according to Table 13.3) = _____

TABLE 13.3 Fatigue index normative data

PERCENTILE	FATIGUE INDEX (%)	
	MALES (%)	FEMALES (%)
5	55	48
10	52	47
15	47	44
20	46	43
25	45	42
30	43	40
35	42	39

continued overpage

TABLE 13.3 Fatigue index normative data *(continued)*

PERCENTILE	FATIGUE INDEX (%)	
	MALES (%)	FEMALES (%)
40	40	38
45	39	38
50	38	35
55	37	34
60	35	33.7
65	34	31
70	31	29
75	30	28
80	29.5	26
85	27	25
90	23	25
95	21	20

Based on data from physically active men ($n = 52$) and women ($n = 50$) aged 18–28 years. Very poor ≤20th percentile; poor = 21st–40th percentile; average = 41st–60th percentile; good = 61st–80th percentile; excellent ≥81st percentile
Adapted from: Maud and Schultz[3]

Interpretation

First, consider the four steps of interpretation outlined in Appendix G, and refer to Tables 13.1–13.3.[3] Given its duration (30 seconds), performance in the Wingate test is underpinned by a combination of acceleration during the first 5 seconds and 'speed-endurance' (or speed maintenance) for at least the final 15 seconds. Energy derived from PCr supports the high power output that occurs in the first 5 seconds up to approximately 15 seconds; energy derived from anaerobic glycolysis becomes more important for the remainder of the test. Those who perform the Wingate test well are individuals with a strong 'anaerobic capacity' – that is, their muscles are adept at deriving energy through glycolysis in the absence of oxygen, and they also have developed resistance to the fatigue that has been partially attributed to the reduction in pH levels. To improve the glycolytic system and thus perform better on tests such as the Wingate test, training should involve a number of maximal sprints that last 20–40 s, with 'incomplete' recovery periods between each sprint. In other words, repeating sprints while still fatigued and with minimal PCr stores will most effectively elicit the necessary adaptations to the skeletal muscle, which will transfer into improved total work and mean power output.

Activity 13.2 Maximal accumulated oxygen deficit (MAOD)

AIMS: to estimate the contribution of the anaerobic energy systems during high-intensity exercise,[4] interpret the results and provide feedback to a participant.

Background

The MAOD is primarily used in research or a sports science setting as an indirect measure of anaerobic capacity. It has been found to be a valid (concurrent) indicator of anaerobic capacity, revealing differences among groups of aerobically and anaerobically trained athletes and significant correlations with other existing anaerobic capacity measures.[5]

The relationship between oxygen uptake ($\dot{V}O_2$) and work rate (speed/grade or power output) is near linear until the point of maximal oxygen consumption (i.e. $\dot{V}O_2$max), where a plateau is often observed. A theoretical estimation of oxygen consumption for a given supramaximal work rate can be calculated by extrapolating this linear relationship beyond the point of $\dot{V}O_2$max. The difference between actual and predicted oxygen consumption during a supramaximal (e.g. $>100\%$ $\dot{V}O_2$max) exercise bout can be used as the estimate of energy derived from anaerobic energy sources – that is, the MAOD (Figure 13.4).

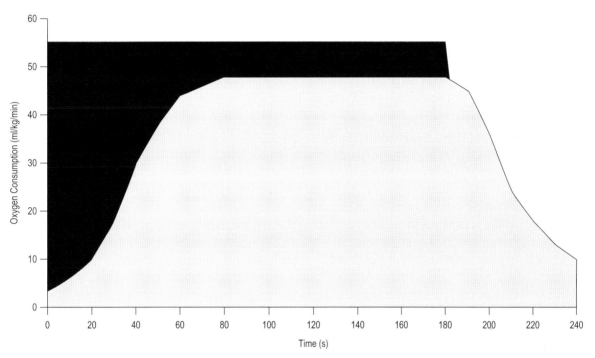

Figure 13.4 Measured oxygen consumption (grey shaded area) during cycle ergometry at 325 watts ($\approx$115% $\dot{V}O_2$max) to volitional exhaustion. Volitional exhaustion occurred at 180 seconds. Predicted oxygen demand was 55 mL/kg/min for the 75 kg participant cycling at this work rate, with a $\dot{V}O_2$max of 48 mL/kg/min. MAOD is calculated to be 38 mL/kg and is shown as the difference between oxygen demand and actual oxygen consumption (black shaded area)

Source: Adrian Gray, University of New England

Determining MAOD requires at least two separate testing sessions. The first is required to construct a linear relationship between work rate (power output or treadmill speed/grade) and oxygen consumption. Individual differences and variation over time result in varying relationships; therefore, this needs to be established each time MAOD is to be determined. The second testing session involves supramaximal exercise to volitional exhaustion. $\dot{V}O_2$max also needs to be determined to calculate MAOD; this can be either performed in isolation according to the protocol outlined in Practical 10, $\dot{V}O_2$max or included within testing session 1 if time is limited.

Protocol summary

The participant completes three tests (i.e. work rate determination, supramaximal exercise to volitional exhaustion and a $\dot{V}O_2$max test) on separate days to calculate MAOD.

MAOD testing session 1

Construction of a linear relationship between work rate and oxygen uptake.

Protocol

The purpose of this session is to establish a relationship between oxygen consumption and work rate. To record the data necessary to calculate a work rate–oxygen consumption regression equation, between 8 and 10 submaximal exercise bouts ideally need to be completed at discrete progressive intensities. The duration of these bouts should be sufficient to obtain a plateau in oxygen consumption. At lower intensities (below anaerobic threshold), exercise bouts lasting 3–6 minutes are typically sufficient; however, at higher intensities (above anaerobic threshold) 8–10 minutes may be required owing to the continued slow increase in oxygen consumption.[6] Indeed, the duration of these bouts has been found to influence the final MAOD result, with longer bouts resulting in higher MAOD estimates.[7] Oxygen consumption during the final minute of exercise at each work rate is recorded.

Time constraints may limit not only the number of discrete submaximal bouts used to generate the work rate–oxygen consumption regression equation, but also whether discrete, separate work rates are used at all. Although not ideal, an acceptable relationship may be derived from a continuous exercise test such as a $\dot{V}O_2$max test. A separate $\dot{V}O_2$max test is preferred to calculate MAOD using $\dot{V}O_2$max (mL/kg/min) and maximum/peak power output (W or kph) data; however, depending on the purpose of the test, converting the MAOD testing session 1 into a $\dot{V}O_2$max test (see Practical 10, $\dot{V}O_2$max) may be done if time is limited. Tables 13.4 and 13.5 show the intensities and durations that can be used to generate the data necessary for a work rate–oxygen consumption regression to be calculated. It is important to recognise that the integrity of the regression is critical to the estimation of the MAOD; unreliable work rate or oxygen consumption data will lead to an invalid regression equation, and oxygen deficit will be either over- or underestimated (see Practical 1, Test accuracy, reliability and validity).

TABLE 13.4 Cycle ergometer protocol to determine work rate–oxygen consumption regression equation relationship

BOUT	EXERCISE DURATION (min)	RECOVERY DURATION (min)	CADENCE (rpm)	POWER OUTPUT	
				WATTS (W)	KILOPONDS (kp)
1	3–10	5–10	70	35	0.5
2	3–10	5–10	70	70	1.0
3	3–10	5–10	70	105	1.5
4	3–10	5–10	70	140	2.0
5	3–10	5–10	70	175	2.5
6	3–10	5–10	70	210	3.0
7	3–10	5–10	70	245	3.5
8	3–10	5–10	70	280	4.0
9	3–10	5–10	70	315	4.5
10	3–10	5–10	70	350	5.0

Source: Adrian Gray, University of New England

TABLE 13.5 Treadmill protocol to determine work rate–oxygen consumption relationship

BOUT	EXERCISE DURATION (min)	RECOVERY DURATION (min)	WORK RATE	
			SPEED (km/h)	GRADE (%)
1	3–10	5–10	8	1
2	3–10	5–10	9	1
3	3–10	5–10	10	1
4	3–10	5–10	11	1
5	3–10	5–10	12	1
6	3–10	5–10	13	1
7	3–10	5–10	14	1
8	3–10	5–10	15	1
9	3–10	5–10	16	1
10	3–10	5–10	17	1

Source: Adrian Gray, University of New England

Test preparation (prior to the participant's arrival)

1 Initial metabolic system set-up:

   a Prior to the start of the test, switch the metabolic system/analysers/pumps on so they are given adequate time to warm up. The system's manual should be consulted to check the time required, but analysers using zirconium fuel cells should be left on all the time. Most pumps need to be switched on ≈30 min before testing.

2 Prepare solutions for post-test clean-up (see Appendix A).

3 Prepare the mouthpiece/respiratory valve.

4 Have all data collection forms ready for completion and ascertain the variables on the data-recording sheet collected via the computer during the test or manually recorded during the test.

5 Measure and enter relevant environmental data into the metabolic system software on the computer (e.g. temperature, humidity and barometric pressure).

6 Calibrate analysers and volume/flow devices according to the instructions in the manual or laboratory procedures (see Practical 1, Test accuracy, reliability and validity).

7 Ensure familiarity with test termination criteria (see Appendix F).

8 Pre-test (with participant present).

9 Follow the pre-exercise test procedures outlined in Appendix B.

10 Check Appendix C to ensure that there are no contraindications to exercise testing.

11 Measure the height and body mass of the participant (see Practical 4, Physique assessment) and record the values.

12 Enter the participant details into the computer (e.g. name, sport (if applicable), group (if applicable), date of birth, sex, body mass).

13 Estimate the participant's age-predicted maximal heart rate (HRmax) using $208 - (0.7 \times age)$.[8]

14 Have the participant place their water bottle and towel in close proximity to the cycle ergometer/treadmill.

15 Fit the heart rate monitor and record the heart rate (see Practical 3, Cardiovascular health).

16 Measure and record blood pressure in the exercising posture (e.g. standing or sitting; see Practical 3) – the blood pressure provides a baseline measure and is used to determine whether the participant has exceeded the criteria for a contraindication to exercise (see Appendix C).

17 If using a treadmill, provide treadmill safety precautions to the participant (see Appendix D). An assessment of their ability to walk/jog safely should be conducted prior to starting the test.

18 Provide details of the test, including the protocol, hand signals the participant can use during the test, explanation of the rating of perceived exertion (RPE) (see Appendix E), test termination and safety (see Appendix F).

19 The participant should complete a 5-minute warm-up. In the interest of time this can be done while the metabolic system is being calibrated and pre-testing data are being entered. The metabolic system should be set to record every 30 seconds.

Test

1 Encourage the participant to push themselves to his/her maximum capacity (volitional exhaustion) for valid test results.

2 With the participant on the treadmill or cycle ergometer, fit the headpiece and mouthpiece.[a]

3 Place the nose tape (e.g. Micropore tape) and nose clip on the participant. Ask the participant to check carefully for leaks by attempting to breathe in and out of the nose with the mouth closed; reposition the nose clip if necessary.

4 Commence the first 3–10-minute exercise bout at the required work rate on a cycle ergometer (see Table 13.4) or treadmill (see Table 13.5).

5 Once this intensity is reached, the test should be started via a countdown – '3, 2, 1, starting now'. Most software programs require you to click 'start test' on the computer keyboard or touchscreen.

6 Your primary responsibility during the test is the safety of the participant.

7 During the test, monitor closely the power output and cadence (cycle ergometer), or speed and gradient (treadmill) and overall test time, even though you may be using a programmable piece of equipment. The tester should assume a position that allows these to be observed along with viewing of the participant's performance, posture, position and facial expressions. For the treadmill protocol, the tester (or assistant) may need to move towards the rear of the treadmill and put their hand behind the participant's back and provide verbal encouragement if they are tending to move to the back of the treadmill.

8 Manually record any data that are not being automatically recorded and saved by the computer.

9 During the test, it may be necessary to prematurely stop the test – see Appendix F for more detail and criteria.

10 After 3 minutes, check the $\dot{V}O_2$ data to see whether a steady state has been achieved (i.e. a plateau has been reached; see Practical 10, $\dot{V}O_2$max). If so, the work rate should be either lowered (if recovery periods are separating each bout) or increased immediately to the next work rate. If $\dot{V}O_2$ is still increasing slowly, exercise should continue until steady state is achieved before the work rate is adjusted.

11 Record the steady-state work rate and $\dot{V}O_2$ from the final minute of each work bout (see Practical 10) in the data-recording sheet.

12 Repeat procedures for each of the 8–10 subsequent work rates.

13 If using discrete exercise bouts, the participant may remove the nose clip and mouthpiece between bouts, though the headset should remain in place.

---

[a] If a mask that covers the mouth and nose is being used, ensure that there are no gaps between the face and mask by blocking the valve and checking suction.

14 All equipment should be in place 30 seconds before the next stage; if using a treadmill it should be increased at least 15 seconds before the start of the next stage to allow it to reach the desired speed.

15 On completion of each exercise bout, the participant's wellbeing needs to be the main focus as some work rates may be stressful, particularly for non-athletes.

Post-test

1 At the completion of the test the participant's wellbeing is paramount. When exercise stops, reduce the work rate immediately to as little as 3 km/h (treadmill) with no incline, or 25–50 W (cycle ergometer), so that after terminating the test a cool-down can start as soon as possible. Monitoring the heart rate during recovery will help to determine the length of the cool-down. Keep the participant on the treadmill or cycle ergometer and encourage them to start the cool down as soon as possible.

2 Click 'end test' (or similar) on the computer or touchscreen. Save the test.

3 Remove the headpiece and nose clip. Be careful not to spill saliva from the mouthpiece and ventilation tube. A wad of tissues placed into the mouthpiece can be a useful temporary 'plug'. A bucket should be available to place the mouthpiece and tubes in to avoid saliva spilling onto the floor.

4 Provide the participant with their water bottle and towel.

5 Ensure the participant has an adequate cool-down – the heart rate should return to at least 50% of HRmax. In some situations you may wish to measure the RPE, BP and heart rate during recovery (e.g. 1 and 5 minutes post-test). It is good practice to keep observing the participant at all times. If they walk away from the treadmill or cycle ergometer, ensure that they are steady on their feet.

6 Verify gas analysers to ensure that there was minimal drift during the test (see Practical 1, Test accuracy, reliability and validity). Accept the test results if the drift is less than 0.1% (absolute) in each of the two analysers.

7 Shut down the metabolic system and computer.

8 Clean and disinfect all equipment (see Appendix A), including the ergometer/treadmill, as sweat can cause corrosion of mechanical and electronic components.

Data analysis

Plot $\dot{V}O_2$ (y-axis) against work rate (x-axis) on Figure 13.5. Add a linear 'trendline' or 'line of best fit' with the y-intercept at 5 mL/kg/min. Using a constant y-intercept of 5 mL/kg/min improves the concurrent

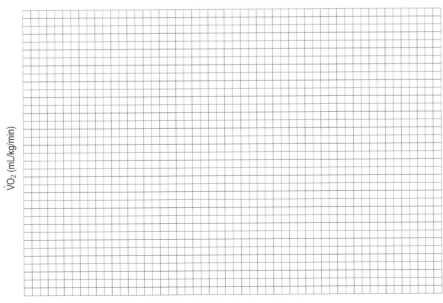

work rate (W or km/h)

Figure 13.5 Plot $\dot{V}O_2$ (y-axis) against work rate (x-axis) on this graph. Add a linear 'trendline' or 'line of best fit' with the y-intercept at 5 mL/kg/min

validity and reliability of MAOD measures.[7] Follow the instructions below to determine the slope of the trendline, and substitute the slope (m) to establish the linear regression equation. Alternatively, this plot and linear regression may be performed using data analysis software (e.g. Microsoft Excel or SPSS). Follow software-specific instructions to produce the plot and linear regression equation.

Data recording

Participant's name: _____ Date: _____

Age: _____ years   Sex: _____   Body mass: _____ kg

EXERCISE BOUT	WORK RATE (W FOR CYCLE ERGOMETRY) (km/h AND % GRADE FOR TREADMILL)	STEADY STATE $\dot{V}O_2$ (mL/kg/min)
Resting	0	5 (given)
1		
2		
3		
4		
5		
6		
7		
8		
9		
10		

Determining the linear regression equation

The trendline generated in Figure 13.5 shows the relationship between oxygen consumption and work rate. The relationship is assumed to be linear and therefore expressed in the form:

$$y = mx + c$$

where $y = \dot{V}O_2$ (mL/kg/min), m = slope, x = work rate (W) and c = resting $\dot{V}O_2$ (mL/kg/min) (the y-intercept).

Given that $\dot{V}O_2$ (mL/kg/min) is shown on the y-axis, work rate (W or km/h) is shown on the x-axis and c is the y-intercept (set at 5 mL/kg/min), this can be expressed as:

$$\dot{V}O_2 = m \times \text{work rate} + 5$$

Establishing the slope (m) is the final step in describing this relationship. This is done according to the equation:

$$\text{Slope}(m) = \frac{\text{Rise}}{\text{Run}} = \frac{\Delta \dot{V}O_2}{\Delta \text{ Work rate}}$$

From the 8–10 steady state $\dot{V}O_2$'s plotted against work rate with a trendline fitted in Figure 13.5, randomly select two points that lie on or very close to the line:

Point A $\dot{V}O_2$ = _____ mL/kg/min Point A work rate = _____ W or km/h

Point B $\dot{V}O_2$ = _____ mL/kg/min Point B work rate = _____ W or km/h

Step 1: Calculate $\Delta\dot{V}O_2$

$\Delta\dot{V}O_2$ = point B $\dot{V}O_2$ − point A $\dot{V}O_2$

$\Delta\dot{V}O_2$ = _____ mL/kg/min

Step 2: Calculate Δwork rate

Δwork rate (W) = point B work rate − point A work rate

ΔW = _____ W

Step 3: Calculate m (slope)

$m = \Delta\dot{V}O_2 / \Delta$work rate

$\quad$ = _____

Step 4: Substitute the slope (m) to establish the linear regression equation

$\dot{V}O_2$ = (mL/kg/min) $m \times$ work rate + c

$\dot{V}O_2$ = _____ $\times$ work rate + 5

This is the participant's linear regression equation.

MAOD testing session 2

Determine the participant's $\dot{V}O_2$max and peak power output (see Practical 10, $\dot{V}O_2$max). Ideally, this should be performed in isolation; however, depending on the purpose of the test, this session can be combined with the MAOD testing session 1 if time is limited.

MAOD testing session 3, supramaximal test

The purpose of this session is for the participant to perform a supramaximal exercise bout to volitional exhaustion; the work rate should correspond to 110%–120% $\dot{V}O_2$max. Oxygen uptake is measured during exercise and the total amount consumed is subtracted from the predicted oxygen uptake (calculated using the regression equation generated from the series of submaximal exercise bouts in the first testing session).

Test preparation (prior to the participant's arrival)

1 Initial metabolic system set-up:

a Prior to the start of the test, switch the metabolic system/analysers/pumps on so they are given adequate time to warm up. The system's manual should be consulted to check the time required, but analysers using zirconium fuel cells should be left on all the time. Most pumps need to be switched on ≈30 min before testing.

2 Prepare solutions for post-test clean-up (see Appendix A).

3 Prepare the mouthpiece/respiratory valve.

4 Have all data collection forms ready for completion and ascertain the variables on the data-recording sheet collected via the computer during the test or manually recorded during the test.

5   Measure and enter relevant environmental data into the metabolic system software on the computer (e.g. temperature, humidity and barometric pressure).

6   Calibrate analysers and volume/flow devices according to the instructions in the manual or laboratory procedures (see Practical 1, Test accuracy, reliability and validity).

7   Ensure familiarity with test termination criteria (see Appendix F)

8   Calculate the required work rate for the supramaximal exercise bout, by substituting 110%–120% (choose a work rate closer to 120% for trained participants and closer to 110% for untrained participants; 115% will be used for this example) $\dot{V}O_2$max into the individualised regression equation and solving for the work rate:

$$\text{Work rate} = \frac{[(1.15 \times \dot{V}O_2\,\text{max}) - 5]}{\text{Slope}}$$

Pre-test (with participant present)

1   Follow the pre-exercise test procedures outlined in Appendix B.

2   Check Appendix C to ensure that there are no contraindications to exercise testing.

3   Enter the participant details into the computer (e.g. name, sport (if applicable), group (if applicable), date of birth, sex, body mass).

4   Have the participant place their water bottle and towel in close proximity to the cycle ergometer/treadmill.

5   Fit the heart rate monitor and record heart rate (see Practical 3, Cardiovascular health).

6   Measure and record blood pressure in the exercising posture (e.g. standing or sitting; see Practical 3) – the blood pressure provides a baseline measure and is used to determine whether the participant has exceeded the criteria for a contraindication to exercise (see Appendix C).

7   If using a treadmill, provide treadmill safety precautions to the participant (see Appendix D). An assessment of their ability to walk/jog safely should be conducted prior to starting the test.

8   Provide details of the test, including the protocol, hand signals the participant can use during the test, explanation of the rating of perceived exertion (RPE) (see Appendix E), test termination and safety (see Appendix F).

9   The participant should complete a 5-minute warm-up. In the interest of time this can be done while the metabolic system is being calibrated and pre-testing data are being entered. The metabolic system should be set to record every 30 seconds.

10 Record the work rate and corresponding $\dot{V}O_2$ demand on the data-recording sheet.

Test

1   Encourage the participant to push themselves to his/her maximum capacity (volitional exhaustion) for as long as possible at the set work rate for valid test results.

2   With the participant on the treadmill or cycle ergometer, fit the headpiece and mouthpiece.[b]

3   Place the nose tape (e.g. Micropore tape) and nose clip on the participant. Ask the participant to check carefully for leaks by attempting to breathe in and out of the nose with the mouth closed; reposition the nose clip if necessary.

4   Count down '3, 2, 1, GO' and commence the test (using computer-controlled software or a manual start). Most software programs require you to click 'start test' on the computer keyboard or touchscreen. The work rate should be attained as quickly as possible at the start of exercise.

---

[b] If a mask that covers the mouth and nose is being used, ensure that there are no gaps between the face and mask by blocking the valve and checking suction.

5 Your primary responsibility during the test is the safety of the participant.

6 During the test, monitor closely the power output and cadence (cycle ergometer), or speed and gradient (treadmill), and overall test time even though you may be using a programmable piece of equipment. The tester should assume a position that allows these to be observed along with viewing of the participant's performance, posture, position and facial expressions. For the treadmill protocol, the tester (or assistant) may need to move towards the rear of the treadmill and put their hand behind the participant's back and provide verbal encouragement if they are tending to move to the back of the treadmill.

7 Manually record any data that is not being automatically recorded and saved by the computer.

8 During the test, it may be necessary to prematurely stop the test (see Appendix F).

9 This is a maximal test; therefore the participant should be verbally encouraged, especially when they are close to/at volitional exhaustion to complete the full last 30-second sampling period.

10 The participant's wellbeing needs to be the main focus during the test as supramaximal effort will be stressful, particularly for non-athletes.

11 Lower the work rate when the participant reaches volitional exhaustion and indicates they can no longer continue exercising and commence a cool-down.

Post-test

1 At the completion of the test the participant's wellbeing is paramount. When exercise stops, reduce the work rate immediately to as little as 3 km/h (treadmill) with no incline, or 25–50 W (cycle ergometer), so that after terminating the test a cool-down can start as soon as possible. Monitoring the heart rate during recovery will help to determine the length of the cool-down. Keep the participant on the treadmill or cycle ergometer and encourage them to start the cool-down as soon as possible.

2 Click 'end test' (or similar) on the computer or touchscreen. Save the test.

3 Remove the headpiece and nose clip. Be careful not to spill saliva from the mouthpiece and ventilation tube. A wad of tissues placed into the mouthpiece can be a useful temporary 'plug'. A bucket should be available to place the mouthpiece and tubes in to avoid saliva spilling onto the floor.

4 Provide the participant with their water bottle and towel.

5 Ensure the participant has an adequate cool-down – heart rate should return to at least 50% of HRmax. In some situations you may wish to measure the RPE, BP and heart rate during recovery (e.g. 1 and 5 minutes post-test). It is good practice to keep observing the participant at all times. If they walk away from the treadmill or cycle ergometer, ensure that they are steady on their feet.

6 Verify gas analysers to ensure that there was minimal drift during the test (see Practical 1, Test accuracy, reliability and validity). Accept the test results if the drift is less than 0.1% (absolute) in each of the two analysers.

7 Save and record the work rate and $\dot{V}O_2$ data. Alternatively, data may be exported into data analysis software (e.g. Microsoft Excel) where the formulae can be used to develop a spreadsheet that determines MAOD.

8 Shut down the metabolic system and computer.

9 Clean and disinfect all equipment (see Appendix A), including the ergometer/treadmill, as sweat can cause corrosion of mechanical and electronic components.

Data recording

Participant's name: _____   Date: _____

Age: _____ years   Sex: _____   Body mass: _____kg

Work rate

Individual regression equation calculation:

$$= \frac{[(1.15 \times \dot{V}O_2 \text{max}) - 5]}{\text{Slope}}$$

$$= \frac{[(1.15 \times \text{_____}) - 5]}{\text{_____}}$$

$$= \frac{[\text{_____} - 5]}{\text{_____}}$$

$$= \text{_____}W(\text{or km/h})$$

$\dot{V}O_2$ demand (115% $\dot{V}O_2$max) $=$ _____ mL/kg

TIME (min:s)	$\dot{V}O_2$ (mL/kg/min)	$\dot{V}O_2$ (mL/kg/30 s)	$\dot{V}O_2$ DEMAND (mL/kg/30 s)
00:00			
00:30			
01:00			
01:30			
02:00			
02:30			
03:00			
03:30			
04:00			
04:30			
05:00			
05:30			
06:00			
06:30			
07:00			
07:30			
08:00			

Note: When the test does not finish on a whole or half minute, a pro-rata estimate of oxygen consumption should be used. The pro-rata is estimated by multiplying the final 30-second $\dot{V}O_2$ by the fraction of the 30-second time period that was completed to estimate O_2 consumed

Data analysis

Calculating MAOD is a three-step process.

1 The first step is to calculate accumulated oxygen consumption. This is the volume of oxygen consumed from the onset of exercise until volitional exhaustion. Practically, this is the sum (Σ) of the 30 s $\dot{V}O_2$ values (mL/kg) consumed over the testing period, divided by two (the sum is divided by two, because the sampling rate was twice per minute; i.e. every 30 seconds). This is expressed as:

$$\text{Accumulated } \dot{V}O_2 = \sum_{n_{start}}^{n_{finish}} \left(\frac{\dot{V}O_{2\,Measured}}{2} \right)$$

where n_{start} = the final resting $\dot{V}O_2$ sample and n_{finish} = the final $\dot{V}O_2$ sample.

2 The second step is to calculate the accumulated $\dot{V}O_2$ demand. This is the theoretical volume of oxygen required to sustain the work performed during the test. Practically, this is the sum of the predicted $\dot{V}O_2$ demand (mL/kg) for each 30-second epoch over the testing period, divided by two (the sum is divided by two because the measure is recorded per minute and the sampling rate was twice per minute; i.e. every 30 seconds). This is expressed as:

$$\text{Accumulated } \dot{V}O_{2,\,Demand} = \sum_{n_{Start}}^{n_{Finish}} \left(\frac{\dot{V}O_{2\,Demand}}{2} \right)$$

where n_{start} = the final resting $\dot{V}O_2$ and n_{finish} = the final $\dot{V}O_2$.

3 The third step calculates MAOD. This is the difference between the accumulated $\dot{V}O_2$ demand and the accumulated $\dot{V}O_2$. Given the test was performed to volitional exhaustion, this is considered the maximal accumulated oxygen deficit and reflects the capacity of the anaerobic energy systems. It can be expressed as:

$$\text{MAOD} = \text{Accumulated } \dot{V}O_2 \text{ Demand} - \text{Accumulated } \dot{V}O_2$$

or by:

$$\text{MAOD} = \sum_{n_{Start}}^{n_{Finish}} \left(\frac{\dot{V}O_{2\,Demand} - \dot{V}O_{2\,Measured}}{2} \right)$$

where n_{Start} = the final resting $\dot{V}O_2$ sample and n_{Finish} = the final $\dot{V}O_2$ sample.

Data recording

Participant's name: _____   Date: _____

Age: _____ years   Sex: _____   Body mass: _____kg

Calculate accumulated $\dot{V}O_2$:

$$\text{Accumulated } \dot{V}O_2 = \sum_{n_{Start}}^{n_{Finish}} \left(\frac{\dot{V}O_{2\,Measured}}{2} \right) = \left(\frac{}{2} + \frac{}{2} + \frac{}{2} + \frac{}{2} + \dots \right) = \text{_____}$$

Accumulated $\dot{V}O_2$ = _____ mL/kg

continued overpage

Data recording (continued)

Calculate accumulated $\dot{V}O_2$ Demand:

$$\text{Accumulated } \dot{V}O_2 \text{ Demand} = \sum_{n_{Start}}^{n_{Finish}} \left(\frac{\dot{V}O_{2\,Demand}}{2} \right) = \left(\frac{}{2} + \frac{}{2} + \frac{}{2} + \frac{}{2} + \ldots \right) = \underline{\hspace{2cm}}$$

Accumulated $\dot{V}O_2$ Demand = _____ mL/kg

Calculate accumulated $\dot{V}O_2$ Deficit:

Accumulated $\dot{V}O_2$ Deficit = Accumulated $\dot{V}O_2$ Demand − Accumulated $\dot{V}O_2$

Accumulated $\dot{V}O_2$ Deficit = _____ mL/kg

Accumulated $\dot{V}O_2$ Deficit $\times 0.9^c$ = _____ mL/kg

$$\frac{\text{Accumulated } \dot{V}O_2 \text{ deficit} \times \text{body mass}}{1000} = \frac{\underline{\hspace{1cm}} \times \underline{\hspace{1cm}}}{1000}$$

$$= \underline{\hspace{3cm}} \text{L. This is the MAOD.}$$

Interpretation

First, consider the four steps of interpretation outlined in Appendix G, and refer to Table 13.6.[9]

The MAOD test may have particular relevance for identifying strengths and weaknesses in athletic events that stress the anaerobic systems maximally (i.e. 400–1500 m running, 200–400 m swimming). Results gained from MAOD testing are concurrently valid in identifying a greater capacity for anaerobic energy release in sprint- vs endurance-trained athletes,[3] and are also sensitive enough to track the development of this capacity in response to targeted training interventions.[7] The MAOD represents the total energy yield that can be derived anaerobically from intramuscular phosphagens and anaerobic glycolysis (i.e. phosphagen and glycolytic systems); however, it does not distinguish between the two

TABLE 13.6 MAOD test normative data

	FEMALES (L)		MALES (L)	
	TRAINED	**UNTRAINED**	**TRAINED**	**UNTRAINED**
Very poor	<3.12	<2.61	<4.44	<3.75
Poor	3.12–3.23	2.61–2.70	4.44–4.70	3.75–3.87
Average	3.24–3.32	2.71–2.79	4.71–4.94	3.88–3.98
Good	3.33–3.44	2.80–2.89	4.95–5.21	3.99–4.11
Excellent	>3.44	>2.89	>5.21	>4.11

Based on data from seven male and seven female initially untrained participants (aged 23.7 ± 1.6 and 22.7 ± 2.6 years for males and females, respectively). MAOD testing was completed pre- and post-training at 82.5%–100% power output at MAOD three times per week for 8 weeks. Very poor $\leq$20th percentile; poor = 21st–40th percentile; average = 41st–60th percentile; good = 61st–80th percentile; excellent $\geq$81st percentile
Source: Weber and Schneider[8]

---

[c] Typically, this value is reduced by 9% to correct for reductions in the O_2 stores of the body.[9]

anaerobic components. Where relevant, targeted follow-up testing may be conducted in order to further distinguish between these capacities (i.e. short sprint testing for the phosphagen system). Furthermore, in place of the constant supramaximal load test to volitional exhaustion (110%–120% $\dot{V}O_2$max), a test of specific event distance or duration can be used to increase the practical relevance of the results (i.e. 2000 m rowing ergometer test or 4000 m cycling time trial). Here, the results would identify the relevant contributions of aerobic and anaerobic systems to the specific event execution, which may provide meaningful insight into pacing strategies or areas in need of further development through training. Importantly, however, this type of testing cannot be termed MAOD as the complete exhaustion of anaerobic systems cannot be guaranteed during tests of fixed duration or distance (i.e. potential influence of pacing). Rather, the accumulated oxygen deficit would allow for an assessment of how each energy system has contributed to the performance of a specific effort.

SECTION 2: TESTS OF RUNNING SPEED AND ACCELERATION

Activity 13.3 Assessing speed and acceleration over 20 metres

AIMS: to assess speed and acceleration over 20 m, interpret the results and provide feedback to a participant.

Background

Acceleration is the rate of change of velocity and is recognised as an important characteristic in many court- and field-based sports; it is particularly important in determining speed over relatively short distances. Sprint-based assessments can also predict sporting career progression, with 14- to 17-year-old academy soccer players who were subsequently drafted to play at the international youth soccer level having superior 20 m sprint performance compared with those who were not drafted.[10] Furthermore, there is moderate level evidence that slow sprint speed is associated with increased risk of musculoskeletal injury.[11]

Protocol summary

The participant sprints a distance of 20 m as fast as possible with the time to complete 5, 10 and 20 m recorded. Depending on the equipment available, speed gates (timing lights) or stopwatches may be used to calculate split times (see Box 13.1).

Protocol

Course set-up

1 In an indoor sports hall (where possible), measure and mark a start line, 5 m, 10 m and 20 m positions with masking tape for split times to be taken (Figure 13.6). Place cones on top of the masking tape to aid in visual assessment of split times using a stopwatch. Alternatively, place speed gates (timing lights) on top of the masking tape and follow the manufacturer's

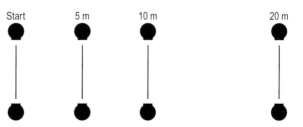

Figure 13.6 Equipment set-up for 20 m sprint test. Black markers indicate placement of cones or timing gates

instructions to establish connections to the gates, enter participant data and select a multi-gate unidirectional testing protocol.

Pre-test

1 Follow the pre-exercise test procedures outlined in Appendix B.

2 Check Appendix C to ensure that there are no contraindications to exercise testing.

3 The participant should warm up by performing light aerobic exercise followed by dynamic range of motion (ROM) exercises and short sprint efforts, building in intensity.

Test

1 Familiarise the participant with the test procedure. Explain that they are to sprint from a stationary start through the 20 m mark *before* slowing down. They are to position themselves as close as possible to the start line and remain stationary, before accelerating as fast as possible. They may commence the trial in their own time once indicated by the timer/timing light.

2 Demonstrate one repetition of the sprint, and check that the participant understands what is required.

3 If using a stopwatch, indicate that the participant may commence the trial when the tester counts down '*3, 2, 1, GO*'. If using timing gates, follow the system-specific instructions to save the data.

4 Allow a practice trial, followed by a 2–3-minute cool-down prior to starting data collection.

5 Instruct the participant that they will perform three maximal trials where they will sprint 20 m as fast as they can, with a 2–3-minute recovery in between sprints.

6 If using a stopwatch, have at least two testers with stopwatches timing the sprint and appropriately positioned to optimise accuracy. Both testers should start timing as soon as the athlete's back foot moves.

7 Measure the splits at the 5 m, 10 m and 20 m marks using the split function on the stopwatch with the average time across stopwatches recorded.

Post-test

1 Following the test, the participant completes a walk/jog cool-down.

2 If using timing gates, follow the system-specific instructions to save the data.

3 Record the data below and use the fastest splits over all trials for comparison with normative data in Table 13.7.

4 Use basic motion formulae to estimate average running speed and acceleration from the displacement and time data.

TABLE 13.7 20 M sprint normative data

| | 5 M SPRINT TIME (s) | | 10 M SPRINT TIME (s) | | 20 M SPRINT TIME (s) | | AVERAGE VELOCITY FROM 10–20 M (m/s) | | AVERAGE ACCELERATION FROM 0–5 M (m/s²) | |
	FEMALES	MALES	FEMALES	MALES	FEMALES	MALES	FEMALES	MALES	FEMALES	MALES
Very poor	>1.33	>1.18	>2.29	>1.93	>3.90	>3.29	<5.94	<7.40	<3.31	<4.37
Poor	1.28–1.33	1.12–1.18	2.17–2.29	1.86–1.93	3.80–3.90	3.18–3.29	5.94–6.25	7.40–7.60	3.31–3.61	4.37–4.77
Average	1.24–1.27	1.10–1.11	2.12–2.16	1.83–1.85	3.65–3.79	3.11–3.17	6.26–6.58	7.61–7.75	3.62–3.79	4.78–4.99
Good	1.21–1.23	1.06–1.09	2.08–2.11	1.77–1.82	3.44–3.64	3.06–3.10	6.59–6.80	7.76–7.94	3.80–3.93	5.00–5.24
Excellent	<1.21	<1.06	<2.08	<1.77	<3.44	<3.06	>6.80	>7.94	>3.93	>5.24

Based on data from 215 Australian exercise science students (females, $n = 102$) aged 18–30. Very poor $\leq$20th percentile; poor $=$ 21st–40th percentile; average $=$ 41st–60th percentile; good $=$ 61st–80th percentile; excellent $\geq$81st percentile

Data analysis

From distance and time data, velocity and acceleration can be calculated at various phases of the sprint. Note that an actual velocity at a specific distance cannot be obtained here; rather an average velocity between two distances is used. The following two equations show how to calculate average velocity and average acceleration.

$$\text{Average velocity} = \frac{\text{Distance travelled}}{\text{Elapsed time}} = \frac{(d_f - d_i)}{(t_f - t_i)}$$

where d_f = final distance, d_i = initial distance, t_f = final time, t_i = initial time.

$$\text{Average acceleration} = \frac{\text{Change in velocity}}{\text{Elapsed time}} = \frac{(v_f - v_i)}{(t_f - t_i)}$$

where v_f = final velocity, v_i = initial velocity, t_f = final time, t_i = initial time.

These equations form the basis for estimating average running velocity (between the 10 m and 20 m timing gates) and average acceleration (between the start and the 5 m timing gate).

Data recording

20 M sprint data recording sheet

Participant's name: _____   Date: _____

Age: _____ years   Sex: _____

TRIAL	5 M SPLIT	10 M SPLIT	20 M SPLIT
1			
2			
3			
Best			
Classification (according to Table 13.7)			

Estimating average running velocity

Calculate average velocity from 10 m–20 m gates.

Average velocity $= (d_f - d_i) / (t_f - t_i)$

$\qquad = (\underline{\quad} - \underline{\quad}) / (\underline{\quad} - \underline{\quad})$

$\qquad = \underline{\quad}$ m/s

Classification of average velocity from 10 m to 20 m (according to Table 13.7): _____

Estimating average acceleration

This is a two-step calculation. First, determine the velocity of the runner at the 5 m mark. This is then used to calculate acceleration from 0 to 5 m.

Calculate the velocity at the 5 m mark – that is, average velocity from 0 to 10 m.

Average velocity $= (d_f - d_i) / (t_f - t_i)$

$\qquad = (\underline{\quad} - \underline{\quad}) / (\underline{\quad} - \underline{\quad})$

$\qquad = \underline{\quad}$ m/s

continued

Data recording *(continued)*

Calculate average acceleration from 0 to 5 m.

Average acceleration $= (v_f - v_i) / (t_f - t_i)$

$$= (\underline{\hspace{2em}} - \underline{\hspace{2em}}) / (\underline{\hspace{2em}} - \underline{\hspace{2em}})$$

$$= \underline{\hspace{2em}} \text{ m/s}$$

Classification of average acceleration from 0 to 5 m (according to Table 13.7): _____

Interpretation

First, consider the four steps of interpretation outlined in Appendix G, and refer to Table 13.7.

Many sports involve sprints over relatively short distances. Indeed, research has consistently shown that, in rugby union, rugby league and soccer, the *average* distance players sprint is not more than 20 m (despite players sometimes being required to sprint >40 m). Speed over these relatively short distances is very much determined by acceleration – players rarely have the time or distance to reach the maximal speeds they would be able to achieve in, for example, a 100 m sprint. Similarly, if we were to assess a 400 m runner, maximal speed and speed maintenance are more important than acceleration because of the longer distance run and the longer overall time for the event. In this instance, a longer sprint test that allows the time to reach all three sprint phases, such as the 40 m test, is a more valid assessment of their sprint capabilities. If a player is looking to improve their 20 m and 40 m sprint times, the kind of training that will improve their performance will involve acceleration drills that focus on body position, use of arms and explosive driving of their legs. From a practical perspective, it should also be recognised that team and field players in actual competition may not always begin their sprint from a stationary position; many are already moving slowly before having to accelerate quickly. In this case, the 40 m sprint test may be modified so that the athlete does a 'flying start' (i.e. the athlete starts jogging from 20–40 m behind the first gate) and the 0 m, 10 m, 20 m and 30 m splits are timed. The variables of acceleration, maximal speed and speed maintenance can then be determined. Training drills used to develop sport-specific acceleration should try to make the circumstances as realistic as possible to competition or game situations, keeping in mind that some players may need to carry a ball, stick or racket while accelerating. Be creative in your test design!

SECTION 3 TESTS OF AGILITY AND CHANGE OF DIRECTION SPEED

Agility is the ability to rapidly change direction and position in response to a stimulus; its expression is multi-faceted, influenced by perceptual and decision-making factors as well as factors influencing change of direction speed (e.g. muscle strength and power). It is a characteristic of those who excel in evasion-type sports such as hockey, basketball and the various football codes.

A change of direction task that is pre-planned has been described as change of direction speed, which distinguishes this closed skill from agility involving a reaction.

Activity 13.4 5–0–5 Test

AIMS: to measure the time taken to complete a single, rapid change of direction over a short course, interpret the results and provide feedback to a participant.

Background

The 5–0–5 test provides a measure of the time taken to complete a single, rapid change of direction over a short course. This test is designed to minimise the influence of individual differences in running speeds whilst accentuating the effect of acceleration immediately before, during and after the change of direction. The 5–0–5 test has superior reliability compared with other change of direction speed tests in rugby league players ($r = 0.90$, typical error of measurement $= 1.9\%$).[12]

Protocol summary

The participant sprints 15 m from a stationary start, placing one foot completely over the 15 m mark, then turning and sprinting back to the start position.

Protocol

Course set-up

1 In an indoor sports hall (where possible), measure and mark a start line, 10 m and 15 m line using masking tape (Figure 13.7).

2 Position timing gates at the 10 m mark, or where a stopwatch is used, position a marker on top of the masking tape to aid in visual assessment. If using timing gates, follow the manufacturer's instructions to establish connections to the gates, enter participant data and select the '5–0–5 single gate, multidirectional' testing protocol.

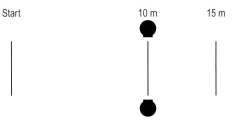

Figure 13.7 Equipment set-up for the 5–0–5 test. Black markers indicate placement of timing gates; straight lines indicate cone placement

Pre-test

1 Follow the pre-exercise test procedures outlined in Appendix B.

2 Check Appendix C to ensure that there are no contraindications to exercise testing.

3 The participant should warm up by performing light aerobic exercise followed by dynamic range of motion (ROM) exercises and short sprint efforts with changes of direction, building in intensity.

Test

1 Explain to the participant that they are to sprint as fast as they can from a stationary start through the 10 m mark, placing one foot completely over the 15 m mark, then turn and sprint as fast as they can back to the start position. They are to position themselves as close as possible to the start line and remain stationary, before accelerating as fast as possible. They may commence the trial in their own time once indicated by the timer or timing light.

2 Demonstrate one repetition of the sprint and check that the participant understands what is required.

3 Allow two practice trials (one turning on the right foot and the other turning on the left foot) prior to starting data collection.

4 Instruct the participant that they will perform three maximal trials sprinting and changing direction on each foot as fast as they can, with a 2-minute recovery in between sprints.

5 If using a stopwatch, have at least two testers with stopwatches timing the sprint and appropriately positioned to optimise accuracy. Both testers should start timing as the participant passes the 10 m mark, and stop the stopwatch as the participant returns past the 10 m mark after the $180°$ turn. The average time across stopwatches is recorded.

Post-test

1 Following the test, the participant completes a walk/jog warm down.

2 If using timing gates, follow the system-specific instructions to save the data. Record the best split times in the recording sheet.

Data recording

5–0–5 Test data recording sheet

Participant's name: _____ Date: _____

Age: _____ years   Sex: _____

TRIAL	5 m – 0 – 5 m SPLIT (s)	
	RIGHT FOOT	LEFT FOOT
1		
2		
3		
Best		

Interpretation

First, consider the four steps of interpretation outlined in Appendix G, and refer to Table 13.8.[13]

Change of direction speed is an important component of many team, field and racket sports. Indeed, rapid changes in direction are often needed in attack and defence. Acceleration and quick footwork are key determinants of change of direction speed and those athletes who are especially agile are generally explosive in their movements, take small, rapid steps when turning and stay fairly low to the ground when changing direction. Change of direction speed can be improved through specific training, where an individual sprints multiple times between cones or markers placed 5–10 m apart. Starting a sprint from a prone (lying) position and having the individual fall to the ground at each marker can encourage the necessary short, rapid footwork needed to develop acceleration following the change of direction. Making training drills sport specific should also be considered. This may involve carrying a ball, stick or racket and/or having someone point to a specific marker or cone to run to, once the sprint has begun. This will make the drill both challenging and realistic.

TABLE 13.8 5–0–5 Test normative data

SPORT	SQUAD		RIGHT FOOT (s)			LEFT FOOT (s)		
			MEAN	SD	RANGE	MEAN	SD	RANGE
Basketball	Female							
	ACT	7	2.59	0.16	2.39–2.81	2.55	0.18	2.38–2.88
	Male							
	ACT state league	13	2.20	0.04	2.06–2.34	2.21	0.11	2.03–2.37
	State league	25	2.18	0.08	2.03–2.38	2.23	0.08	2.03–3.40
Hockey	Female							
	ACT	10	2.51	0.12	2.30–2.75	2.48	0.10	2.28–2.64
	SASI[a]	20	2.57	0.10	2.36–2.78	—	—	—
	WA[a]	124	2.49	0.12	2.22–2.99	—	—	—
	Senior[a]	287	2.47	0.13	2.25–2.96	—	—	—
	Male							
	ACT	15	2.28	0.14	2.10–2.60	2.27	0.06	2.18–2.40
	WA[a]	52	2.26	0.12	2.05–2.54	—	—	—
	Senior[a]	74	2.30	0.11	2.10–2.78	—	—	—
Netball	Female							
	National senior	16	2.47	0.13	2.22–2.65	2.48	0.18	2.18–2.74
	ACT	15	2.49	0.10	2.35–2.75	2.49	0.08	2.40–2.63
	AUS/u21	12	2.40	0.10	2.33–2.54	2.44	0.10	2.36–2.60
	QAS/u19	22	2.47	0.11	2.32–2.65	2.48	0.09	2.30–3.71
	SASI/u19	9	2.57	0.05	2.48–2.67	2.57	0.08	2.43–2.72
	SASI/u17	11	2.50	0.07	2.40–2.67	2.51	0.08	2.369–2.68
Tennis	Female							
	A15/V15	12	2.38	0.08	2.21–2.46	2.42	0.05	2.31–2.58
	NSW15	3	2.54	0.04	2.52–2.59	2.53	0.06	2.49–2.58
	Male							
	A15/V15	11	2.25	0.06	2.17–2.36	2.24	0.07	2.14–2.37
	NSW15	4	2.31	0.06	2.27–2.49	2.23	0.03	2.20–2.26

[a]Tested on preferred foot only. SD = standard deviation
Source: Australian Institute of Sport[13]

SECTION 4 TESTS OF REPEATED HIGH-INTENSITY EXERCISE PERFORMANCE

Activity 13.5 Repeat Sprint Ability (RSA) Tests

AIM: to determine repeat sprint ability, interpret the results and provide feedback to a participant.

Background

Time–motion analysis has shown that team sport athletes engage in repeated bouts of high-intensity running throughout the course of play. A key feature of this type of exercise demand is that recovery between each bout is likely to be incomplete with regard to resynthesis of PCr and restoration of intramuscular pH.[14] There are several protocols that have been used to evaluate the ability of individuals to maintain speed and resist fatigue during repeated short sprints.[15] The chosen protocol should reflect the work–rest pattern and physiological demands of the individual's sport.[16] For example, the total sprint time of the 6 $\times$ 20 m sprint protocol was concurrently valid in discriminating between national- and state-level women's soccer players, and proved to be highly reproducible (intraclass correlation coefficient = 0.91; typical error of measurement = 1.5%). However, the percentage decrement was less reliable (intraclass correlation coefficient = 0.14, typical error of measurement = 19.5%). Table 13.9 shows three common repeat sprint test protocols.

TABLE 13.9 Repeat sprint ability test common testing protocols			
PROTOCOL	WORK BOUTS	RECOVERY BOUTS	ESTIMATED WORK:REST RATIO[a]
1	12 $\times$ 20 m sprints, departing every 20 seconds	Slow walk/jog	1:7
2	6 $\times$ 40 m sprints, departing every 30 seconds		1:6
3	6 $\times$ 30 m sprints, departing every 20 seconds		1:5
4	6 $\times$ 20 m sprints, departing every 15 seconds		1:4

a Estimates will vary depending on athletic ability. Deceleration time excluded

Protocol Summary

The participant performs repeated maximal sprints separated by slow walk/jog recovery bouts.

Protocol

Course Set-up

1 Mark the test area as shown in Figure 13.8 using timing gates, masking tape and/or cones. The sprint distance will vary according to the protocol selected.

2 If using timing gates, follow the manufacturer's instructions to establish connection to the gates, enter participant date and select the 'RSA multi-gate, multidirectional' testing protocol.

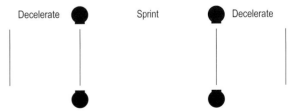

Figure 13.8 Equipment set-up for repeat sprint ability testing. Black markers indicate timing gates or masking tape and cones if using a stopwatch

Pre-test

1 Follow the pre-exercise test procedures outlined in Appendix B.

2 Check Appendix C to ensure that there are no contraindications to exercise testing.

3 The participant should warm up by performing light aerobic exercise followed by dynamic ROM exercises and short sprint efforts, building in intensity. They should be ready to sprint maximally *before* starting the test.

Test

1 Participants should be instructed to sprint as fast as they can for each sprint and avoid 'pacing' themselves.

2 During the recovery period, participants can jog slowly out to the deceleration line/marker and back before getting ready on the start line for the next sprint. Explain that you will give a 5-second countdown before each sprint.

3 Demonstrate one repetition of the sprint and recovery period to check that the participant understands what is required.

4 Allow a practice trial, followed by a 2–3-minute recovery prior to starting data recording.

5 If using a stopwatch, have at least two testers with stopwatches timing the sprint and appropriately positioned to optimise accuracy.

6 Have the participant assume the start position (i.e. staggered stance, stationary and as close to the start gate as possible). If using timing gates, have the system ready to record.

7 Explain to the participant that they are to sprint as fast as they can on the tester's call of '3, 2, 1, GO'. Both testers should start timing as soon as 'GO' is called.

8 The participant completes the sprints, departing at the nominated interval. Count down the last 5 seconds of each recovery interval by calling '5, 4, 3, 2, 1, GO' before each sprint and provide encouragement (Figure 13.9). The average time across stopwatches is recorded.

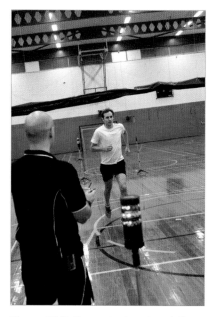

Figure 13.9 Repeated sprint ability

Used with permission from Fusion Sport

Post-test

1 Following the test, the participant completes a walk/jog warm-down.

2 If using timing lights, follow the system-specific instructions to save the data. Record the sprint times and calculate the total sprint time.

CALCULATIONS

The total sprint time (sum of all sprint times) is an index of repeat sprint ability; that is, those with poorer repeat sprint ability will have higher total time. This is attributable to the onset of fatigue in the later sprints. Another method of analysing repeat sprint ability test data is to quantify the decrement in sprint times. A theoretical decrement of zero would be optimal; in this case the participant's fastest sprint time would have been repeated for all sprints. This theoretical benchmark is calculated as:

$$\text{Best total sprint time} = \text{Best sprint time} \times \text{Number of sprints performed}$$

The ratio between total sprint time and best total sprint time reflects the actual decrement in performance. This is calculated as a percentage decrement by:

$$\text{Sprint performance decrement (\%)} = \left[1 - \left(\frac{\text{Best total sprint time}}{\text{Total sprint time}} \right) \right] \times 100$$

Data recording

Participant's name: _____ Date: _____

Age: _____ years   Sex: _____

Protocol:

Sprint	Sprint Time (s)
1	
2	
3	
4	
5	
6	
7[a]	
8[a]	
9[a]	
10[a]	
11[a]	
12[a]	
Total sprint time	

[a] If using the 12 × 20 m protocol

Best total sprint time (s) = best sprint time × number of sprints performed

$$= \rule{2cm}{0.4pt} \times \rule{2cm}{0.4pt}$$

$$= \rule{1.5cm}{0.4pt} \text{ s}$$

Calculation of sprint performance decrement

Decrement (%) = [1 − (best total sprint time/total sprint time)] × 100

$$= [1 - (\rule{2cm}{0.4pt} / \rule{2cm}{0.4pt})] \times 100$$

$$= \rule{1.5cm}{0.4pt} \%$$

Classification (according to Table 13.10): _____

Interpretation

First, consider the four steps of interpretation outlined in Appendix G, and refer to Table 13.10.[15,17] Note that the female RSA normative data are based on different protocols for males and females owing to limited available normative data.

Team and field sport players rarely have time to fully recover between sprints during a match, and many repeat sprints have to be performed in competition while a player is partially fatigued. Well-trained team and field athletes are characterised by an ability to recover quickly (though rarely

TABLE 13.10 Repeated sprint ability test normative data

PERCENTAGE DECREMENT IN SPRINT PERFORMANCE

	FEMALES 6 × 20 M RSA PROTOCOL	MALES 12 × 20 M RSA PROTOCOL
Very poor	>6.9	>8.3
Poor	6.0–6.8	6.3–8.3
Average	5.2–5.9	4.7–6.2
Good	4.3–5.1	2.7–4.6
Excellent	<4.2	<2.7

Male norms are based on data from 17 AFL players completing the 12 × 20 m RSA protocol departing every 20 seconds. Female norms are based on data from 19 elite soccer players completing the 6 × 20 m RSA protocol departing every 15 seconds.[17] Very poor ≤20th percentile; poor = 21st–40th percentile; average = 41st–60th percentile; good = 61st–80th percentile; excellent ≥81st percentile
Adapted from: Wadley and Le Rossignol[15]

completely) between sprints. This can be attributed, at least in part, to a well-developed capacity of the skeletal muscles to buffer the lactic acid accumulation and minimise the decrease in pH level, which is a contributor to fatigue. Sprint interval training elicits the necessary improvements in muscle that will be reflected in better RSA test scores. The key element or feature of repeated sprint training is that the recovery between sprints is kept deliberately brief – too brief for the complete removal of lactic acid thus preventing complete recovery – and fatigue is therefore inevitable. By keeping the recovery brief, the muscles will be deliberately 'overloaded' with lactic acid production and accumulation during a training session – this will promote the adaptation in muscle-buffering capacity that will eventually translate into improved RSA test performance.

Discussion and feedback

First, consider the three steps of feedback and discussion outlined in Appendix G. Feedback regarding high-intensity exercise performance should include more than just stating the result and relevant descriptor; it is important to consider the participant and the purpose of the test. When the test has been conducted on athletes, it is important to consider the extent to which the measure of high-intensity exercise performed is relevant to their specific sport. This should be the first consideration when selecting a test to measure high-intensity exercise performance, and the relationship of the test to sport-specific performance will need to be carefully explained to the participant following the test, as this will influence the recommendations provided. For example, if the test has been found to correlate highly with the participant's sporting performance and/or there are specific normative data available for elite athletes within their sport or from previous testing on this participant, then this should be included in the feedback. Where the participant's test result falls below expected values for their age, sex and sport, specific recommendations need to be provided to assist the athlete to improve their high-intensity exercise performance.

Case studies

Case Study 1

Setting: You are conducting a talent identification search for female cyclists for a new road cycling team, and looking to recruit cycle-trained individuals who are able to achieve high peak power and low fatigue index during a Wingate test – that is, >75th percentile relative to their age and sex

continued

Case studies *(continued)*

compared with the Maud and Schultz[3] normative data provided in this manual. You use a trial to determine whether potential clients are eligible for the team.

The first client is a female aged 20 years and weighs 61.2 kg. You calculate the required resistance setting to be 4.6 kp, using the following equation:

$$\text{Resistance (kp)} = 0.075 \times \text{body mass (kg)}$$
$$= 0.075 \times 61.2 = 4.6 \text{ kp}$$

The pedal revolutions for each 5-second interval from the test are provided in the following data-recording sheet.

Wingate test revolutions counted per 5-second period data-recording sheet

Time (s)	Revs ($n=$)
0–5	10
5–10	8
10–15	7
15–20	6
20–25	5
25–30	4
Total revs	40

Task: Calculate and interpret the results, providing feedback to the client regarding their eligibility for the study.

Case Study 2

Setting: You are conducting an exercise intervention research study comparing the MAOD of trained cyclists with those of untrained clients. One of your clients for the study is a 22-year-old untrained male with a body mass of 78 kg. He completed MAOD testing on a cycle ergometer as part of the intervention. The results of the testing sessions are outlined below.

Task: Calculate and interpret the results, providing feedback to the client.

TESTING DAY 1 RESULTS
Establishing the work rate and $\dot{V}O_2$ relationship data recording sheet

Exercise Bout	Work Rate (W for Cycle Ergometry) (km/h for Treadmill Running)	Steady-state $\dot{V}O_2$ (mL/kg/min)
Resting	0	5 *(given)*
1	35	11.23
2	70	16.42
3	105	19.38
4	140	26.02

continued overpage

Case studies (continued)

Exercise Bout	Work Rate (W for Cycle Ergometry) (km/h for Treadmill Running)	Steady-state $\dot{V}O_2$ (mL/kg/min)
5	175	31.98
6	210	34.79
7	245	39.99
8	280	45.86
9		
10		

TESTING DAY 2 RESULTS

$\dot{V}O_2$max = 44.96 mL/kg/min

TESTING DAY 3 RESULTS

Participant's 3-minute bout to volitional exhaustion

Work rate (3 min and 30 s)	329 watts
$\dot{V}O_2$ demand (115% $\dot{V}O_2$max) = 1.15 × $\dot{V}O_2$max	
$\dot{V}O_2$max = 1.15 × 44.96 = 51.7 mL/kg/min	

Time (min:s)	$\dot{V}O_2$ (mL/kg/min)	$\dot{V}O_2$ (mL/kg/30 s)	$\dot{V}O_2$ Demand (mL/kg/30 s)
00:00	5.00 (given)	2.50	2.50
00:30	11.00	5.50	51.7/2 = 25.85
01:00	23.00	11.50	25.85
01:30	33.00	16.50	25.85
02:00	39.00	19.50	25.85
02:30	42.00	21.00	25.85
03:00	44.90	22.45	25.85
03:30	44.90	22.45	25.85
04:00			
04:30			
05:00			
05:30			

continued

Case studies (continued)

Time (min:s)	$\dot{V}O_2$ (mL/kg/min)	$\dot{V}O_2$ (mL/kg/30 s)	$\dot{V}O_2$ Demand (mL/kg/30 s)
06:00			
06:30			
07:00			
07:30			
08:00			

Case Study 3

Setting: You are an athletic trainer working with the Women's U21 rugby league team. At the start of the pre-season training, all athletes must complete a battery of exercise tests to determine their sprint ability. The 20 m sprint test data for 19-year-old Kerry is included in the table below.

Task: Calculate Kerry's average velocity and acceleration, interpret the results and provide feedback.

20 M SPRINT TIMING GATE DATA FOR A 19-YEAR-OLD FEMALE CLIENT

Distance (m)	0	5	10	20
Time (s)	*0.00*	*1.19*	*2.10*	*3.82*

Case Study 4

Setting: As a musculoskeletal rehabilitation specialist, you are working with an 18-year-old male 400 m runner who is recovering from knee surgery. The coach has asked you whether he is at full recovery and able to return to competition. In order to determine the athlete's fitness and suitability to compete once again, you conduct a 6 × 40 m sprint test. The results are shown below.

REPEAT SPRINT ABILITY TEST 6 × 40 M TEST DATA
Protocol: 6 × 40 m

Sprint	Sprint Time (s)
1	*4.80*
2	*4.91*
3	*5.02*
4	*5.16*
5	*5.28*
6	*5.39*
Total sprint time	*30.56*

Task: Calculate the athlete's fatigue decrement, interpret the results and provide feedback.

References

[1] Hofman N, Orie J, Hoozemans MJM, Foster C, de Koning JJ. Wingate Test as a strong predictor of 1500-m performance in elite speed skaters. Int J Sports Physiol Perform 2017;12:1288–92.

[2] Bar-Or O. The Wingate anaerobic test. An update on methodology, reliability and validity. Sports Med 1987;4:381–94.

[3] Maud PJ, Schultz BB. Norms for the Wingate Anaerobic Test with comparison to another similar test. Res Q Exerc Sport 1989;60:146–8.

[4] Medbø JI, Mohn AC, Tabata I, Bahr R, Vaage O, Sejersted OM. Anaerobic capacity determined by maximal accumulated O_2 deficit. J Appl Physiol (1985) 1988;64:50–60.

[5] Scott CB, Roby FB, Lohman TG, Bunt JC. The maximally accumulated oxygen deficit as an indicator of anaerobic capacity. Med Sci Sports Exerc 1991;23:618–24.

[6] Whipp BJ, Wasserman K. Oxygen uptake kinetics for various intensities of constant-load work. J Appl Physiol 1972;33:351–6.

[7] Noordhof DA, de Koning JJ, Foster C. The maximal accumulated oxygen deficit method: a valid and reliable measure of anaerobic capacity? Sports Med 2010;40:285–302.

[8] Tanaka H, Monahan KD, Seals DR. Age-predicted maximal heart rate revisited. J Am Coll Cardiol 2001;37:153–6.

[9] Weber CL, Schneider DA. Increases in maximal accumulated oxygen deficit after high-intensity interval training are not gender dependent. J Appl Physiol (1985) 2002;92:1795–1801.

[10] Gonaus C, Muller E. Using physiological data to predict future career progression in 14- to 17-year-old Austrian Soccer Academy players. J Sports Sci 2012;30:1673–82.

[11] de la Motte SJ, Lisman P, Gribbin TC, Murphy K, Deuster PA. A systematic review of the association between physical fitness and musculoskeletal injury risk: part 3 – flexibility, power, speed, balance, and agility. J Strength Cond Res 2019;33(6):1723–35.

[12] Gabbett TJ, Kelly JN, Sheppard JM. Speed, change of direction speed, and reactive agility of rugby league players. J Strength Cond Res 2008;22:174–81.

[13] Australian Institute of Sport. Physiological tests for elite athletes. Champaign, IL: Human Kinetics; 2013.

[14] Spencer M, Bishop D, Dawson B, Goodman C. Physiological and metabolic responses of repeated-sprint activities: specific to field-based team sports. Sports Med 2005;35:1025–44.

[15] Wadley G, Le Rossignol P. The relationship between repeated sprint ability and the aerobic and anaerobic energy systems. J Sci Med Sport 1998;1:100–10.

[16] Meckel Y, Machnai O, Eliakim A. Relationship among repeated sprint tests, aerobic fitness, and anaerobic fitness in elite adolescent soccer players. J Strength Cond Res 2009;23:163–9.

[17] Gabbett TJ. The development of a test of repeated-sprint ability for elite women's soccer players. J Strength Cond Res 2010;24:1191–4.

PRACTICAL 14
NUTRITION

Jeff Coombes and Veronique Chachay

LEARNING OBJECTIVES

- Demonstrate an understanding of the scopes of practice of exercise and sport scientists and Accredited Exercise Physiologists with regard to nutritional analysis and providing advice
- Explain the scientific rationale, purposes, reliability, validity, assumptions and limitations of various approaches towards nutrition intake assessments
- Identify and explain the common terminology and techniques required to assess dietary intake and nutritional status
- Identify the need for guidance or further information from an appropriate health professional
- Select and conduct appropriate protocols for effective diet and nutrition assessments, including instructing participants on the correct use of common tools (e.g. diet diary)
- Record, analyse and interpret information from a dietary assessment and convey the results, including the validity and limitations of the approach, within the appropriate scope of practice, through relevant verbal and/or written communication

Equipment and other requirements

- Nutritional analysis software (e.g. FoodWorks Version 10 available at www.xyris.com.au)
- Computer/tablet
- Calculator
- Printer (optional)

Knowledge pre-requisite
- Have an understanding of the basic characteristics of macronutrients and micronutrients, including common food sources of these nutrients, and their role in energy balance, physiological function and general wellbeing

INTRODUCTION

Given the close relationship between nutrition and physical activity it is expected that practitioners in various exercise and sports science settings will have some fundamental knowledge and skills in dietary analysis. The major application of this knowledge and skills will probably involve referring individuals to a practitioner (e.g. a dietitian or sports dietitian) who has more specific and detailed expertise. Indeed, it is essential all professions recognise the need for cross-referral in order to deliver complete management appropriately. Practitioners should see cross-referrals as a way of delivering a superior standard of care and a vehicle for developing valuable collaborations with other allied health professionals.

Exercise and Sports Science Australia (ESSA) and the Dietitians Australia (DA) produced a joint position statement[1] to assist practitioners in understanding the relevant scopes of practice. The document describes a model of collaboration where Accredited Exercise Physiologists (AEPs) can provide general nutrition advice using guidelines for healthy eating.[2] Although the scope of practice was designed for AEPs, exercise and sport scientists are expected to have similar nutritional knowledge, skills and scope of practice with regards to nutrition. Indeed, in the ESSA exercise science standards,[3] nutrition is one of the 15 study areas. The guiding principle of this area is that graduates from an exercise science program will have the knowledge and confidence to provide general nutritional advice to apparently healthy participants. An important distinction in the model is that when an individual requires specific nutrition needs (e.g. as part of the management of their chronic disease or for optimising sporting performance), this needs to be provided by an Accredited Practising Dietitian (APD). It is recommended that a dietitian assist with the activities contained in this practical.

In this practical, you will be required to use various methods of nutritional assessment to evaluate your own dietary intake against the most recent Australian dietary guidelines (see Table 14.1).[4] An important consideration when implementing the guidelines is the fact they were designed to meet the nutritional requirements for the general healthy population through foods alone with respect to economic, cultural and environmental sustainability issues. Although some foods may contain more of certain nutrients, recommending their consumption over others would create an imbalance in our food supply chain or be not possible for certain socioeconomic classes. Therefore, recommendations must remain generalised to ensure that public health messages are practical and feasible.

TABLE 14.1 Australian dietary guidelines	
Guideline 1	To achieve and maintain a healthy weight, be physically active and choose amounts of nutritious food and drinks to meet your energy needs. • Children and adolescents should eat sufficient nutritious food to grow and develop normally. They should be physically active every day and their growth should be checked regularly. • Older people should eat nutritious foods and keep physically active to help maintain muscle strength and a healthy weight.
Guideline 2	Enjoy a wide variety of nutritious foods from these five groups every day: • plenty of vegetables, including different types and colours, and legumes/beans • fruit • grain (cereal) foods, mostly wholegrain and/or high-fibre cereal varieties, such as breads, cereals, rice, pasta, noodles, polenta, couscous, oats, quinoa and barley • lean meats and poultry, fish, eggs, tofu, nuts, seeds and legumes/beans • milk, yoghurt, cheese and/or their alternatives, mostly reduced fat (reduced fat milks are not suitable for children under the age of 2 years). And drink plenty of water.

Guideline 3	Limit intake of foods containing saturated fat, added salt, added sugars and alcohol.
	
	a Limit intake of foods high in saturated fat, such as many biscuits, cakes, pastries, pies, processed meats, commercial burgers, pizza, fried foods, potato chips, crisps and other savoury snacks.
	
	  • Replace high-fat foods that contain predominantly saturated fats such as butter, cream, cooking margarine, coconut and palm oil with foods that contain predominantly polyunsaturated and monounsaturated fats such as oils, spreads, nut butter/pastes and avocado.
	  • Low-fat diets are not suitable for children under the age of 2 years.
	
	b Limit intake of foods and drinks containing added salt.
	
	  • Read labels to choose lower sodium options among similar foods.
	
	Do not add salt to foods in cooking or at the table.
	
	c Limit intake of foods and drinks containing added sugars such as confectionary, sugar-sweetened soft drinks and cordials, fruit drinks, vitamin waters, energy and sports drinks.
	
	d If you choose to drink alcohol, limit your intake. For women who are pregnant, planning a pregnancy or breastfeeding, not drinking alcohol is the safest option.

Guideline 4	Encourage, support and promote breastfeeding.
Guideline 5	Care for your food; prepare and store it safely.

Source: National Health and Medical Research Council[4]

DEFINITIONS

Acceptable macronutrient distribution range (AMDR): the intake range for a macronutrient (expressed as percent contribution to EER) to maximise health.

Adequate intake (AI): the daily nutrient intake level based on observed or experimentally determined approximations. It is used when a recommended dietary intake (RDI) cannot be determined.

Basal metabolic rate (BMR): is the rate of energy expenditure needed to perform basic (basal) functions such as breathing, circulating blood and cell production. BMR should be measured under very restrictive conditions; however, as this is not always possible, resting metabolic rate (RMR) is usually assessed and the two are sometimes used synonymously.

Estimated average requirement (EAR): a daily nutrient level estimated to meet the requirements of half the healthy individuals in a particular life stage and sex group. It is determined with a biomarker of deficiency (e.g. scurvy for vitamin C). Note: this has not been determined for all micronutrients in humans because of ethical reasons.

Estimated energy requirement (EER): the average dietary energy intake in kilojoules (kJ) that is predicted to be needed to maintain energy balance in a healthy adult of defined age, sex, body mass, height and level of physical activity, consistent with good health. In children or pregnant or lactating women, the EER is adjusted to include the additional needs (growth or production of milk).

Macronutrient: any nutritional component of the diet, such as carbohydrates, fats and proteins, that is required in a relatively large amount.

Micronutrient: any nutritional component of the diet, such as a vitamin or mineral, that is essential in relatively small amounts.

Nutrient reference values (NRV): a set of recommendations for nutritional intake based on currently available scientific knowledge. The levels are considered to be adequate to meet the known nutritional needs of most healthy people for prevention of deficiency states.

Resting metabolic rate (RMR): the rate of energy expenditure at rest. RMR is usually measured after controlling for the intake of food, stimulants and physical activity in the preceding hours and having the participant in a supine position for at least 20 minutes prior to starting the measure.[5] The terms RMR and BMR are sometimes used synonymously.

Recommended dietary intake (RDI): the average daily dietary intake level that is sufficient to meet the nutrient requirements of nearly all (97%–98%) healthy individuals in a particular life stage and sex group. It is determined by increasing the dosage by two standard deviations to the right of the EAR.

Suggested dietary target (SDT): a daily average intake for certain nutrients that may help in chronic disease prevention.

Upper level of intake (UL): the highest average daily nutrient intake level likely to pose no adverse health effects to almost all individuals in the general population. As intake increases above the UL, the potential risk of adverse effects increases.

Activity 14.1 Eating for health quiz

AIM: perform an assessment of your dietary pattern using the quiz 'Are you eating for health?'

Background

Performing a quick dietary intake assessment of a participant may be all that is possible in certain situations. This activity will use a 10-question survey developed by Australia's National Health and

Medical Research Council that is available online in a document summarising the Australian dietary guidelines.[4] The quiz can be used on a participant to (1) obtain a general summary of their dietary intake and (2) supply an educational experience regarding foods that are healthy, the recommended daily intake and those that need to be limited. Incorporating these eating habits is critical to good health and the prevention of a number of diseases.

Protocol summary

Assess your diet using the 'Are you eating for health?' quiz.

Protocol

1 Figure 14.1 provides the quiz.

2 Tick each box where you believe you are meeting the statement.

QUIZ: ARE YOU EATING FOR HEALTH?

Take this quick quiz for adults to find out the answer – be honest! Give yourself one point for each box you tick if you:

- Eat at least 5 serves of vegetables every day. A serve is ½ cup cooked vegetables (hot chips don't count!) or 1 cup of salad.

- Eat at least 2 serves of fruit every day. A serve is 1 medium piece or 2 small pieces of fresh fruit, or one cup of chopped or canned fruit (no added sugar).

- Have at least 2 serves of reduced fat milk, yoghurt, cheese or alternatives every day (for example, 1 slice of reduced fat cheese, a small tub of reduced fat yoghurt (preferably no added sugar), 1 cup of milk or 1 cup of soy milk with added calcium).

- Eat mostly wholegrain cereals (such as high fibre breakfast cereal and wholemeal bread).

- Eat at least a small serve of lean meat or chicken (fat and/or skin cut off) or fish, or eggs or some nuts or legumes (for example, lentils, chickpeas, beans such as kidney beans or baked beans) every day.

- Drink plenty of water every day and limit drinks with added sugars, such as soft drinks, cordial, energy drinks and sports drinks.

- Limit takeaway foods such as pizzas, commercial burgers, hot chips or other deep fried foods to once a week or less.

- Limit store-bought cakes, muffins, pastries, pies and biscuits to once a week or less.

- Limit salty foods like processed meats (for example, salami and bacon), crisps and salty snacks to once a week or less, and avoid adding salt during cooking or at the table.

- Drink no more than 2 standard drinks containing alcohol on any one day.

How did you rate?

8–10 points Congratulations, you're already a pretty healthy eater!

6–8 points Keep going, you're nearly there!

4–6 points There's plenty of room for improvement.

Less than 4 It's time for a serious overhaul.

Use the information in this booklet for some great ideas.

Poor eating habits are sometimes hard to break. For adults, it's not too late to make changes if poor eating habits have crept up, but it's important to keep changes realistic using the practical information in this booklet should help.

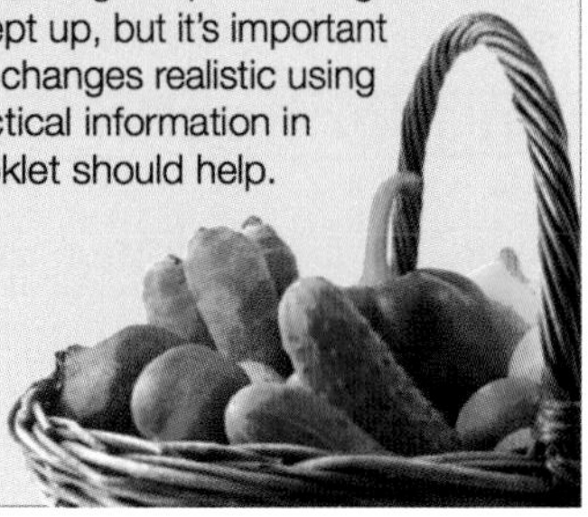

For more information go to:
www.eatforhealth.gov.au

Figure 14.1 Quiz: Are you eating for health?
Source: National Health and Medical Research Council[4]

3 Each tick is 1 point and the number out of 10 should be entered in the data-recording sheet.

4 Answer the questions below.

Data recording

Number of points: _____ / 10

How could you improve your score? _____

_____

_____

_____

_____

_____

Is your diet different during periods of high vs low stress (e.g. during exams)? Clarify what dietary changes you typically make. _____

_____

_____

_____

_____

Activity 14.2 The Australian dietary guidelines

AIM: to better understand the Australian dietary guidelines.

Background

The Australian dietary guidelines (Table 14.1) provide advice about the amounts and kinds of foods that we need to eat for health and wellbeing. The recommendations were developed by a working group from the National Health and Medical Research Council of Australia based on scientific evidence from available robust research.[4] The guidelines are supported by a number of resources available at the Australian Government's 'Eat for health' website such as the brochure 'Healthy eating for adults' (Figure 14.2).[2]

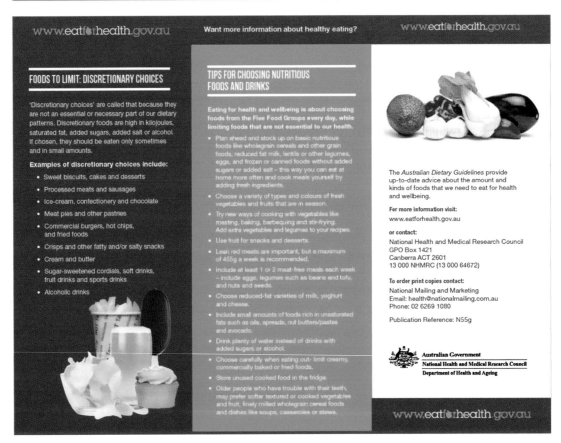

Figure 14.2 Healthy eating for adults

Source: National Health and Medical Research Council[2]

continued

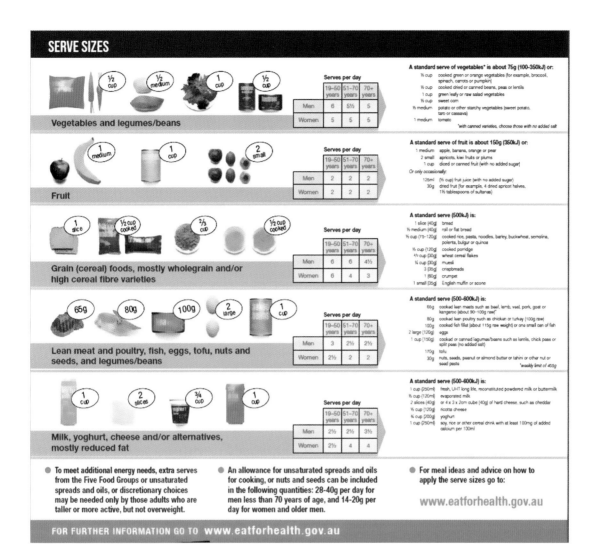

SERVE SIZES

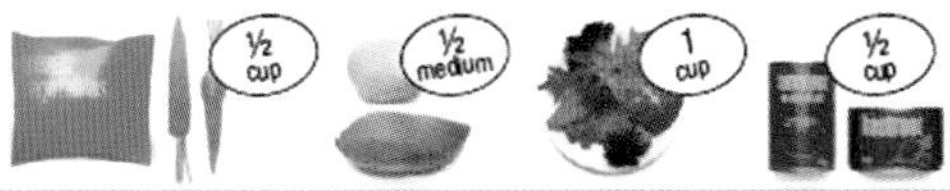

Vegetables and legumes/beans

	Serves per day		
	19–50 years	51–70 years	70+ years
Men	6	5½	5
Women	5	5	5

A standard serve of vegetables* is about 75g (100-350kJ) or:

½ cup	cooked green or orange vegetables (for example, broccoli, spinach, carrots or pumpkin)
½ cup	cooked dried or canned beans, peas or lentils
1 cup	green leafy or raw salad vegetables
½ cup	sweet corn
½ medium	potato or other starchy vegetables (sweet potato, taro or cassava)
1 medium	tomato

**with canned varieties, choose those with no added salt*

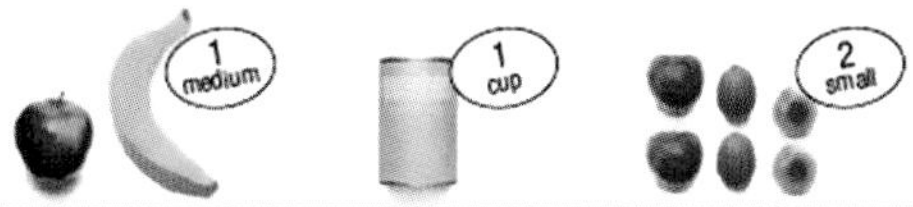

Fruit

	Serves per day		
	19–50 years	51–70 years	70+ years
Men	2	2	2
Women	2	2	2

A standard serve of fruit is about 150g (350kJ) or:

1 medium	apple, banana, orange or pear
2 small	apricots, kiwi fruits or plums
1 cup	diced or canned fruit (with no added sugar)

Or only occasionally:

125ml	(½ cup) fruit juice (with no added sugar)
30g	dried fruit (for example, 4 dried apricot halves, 1½ tablespoons of sultanas)

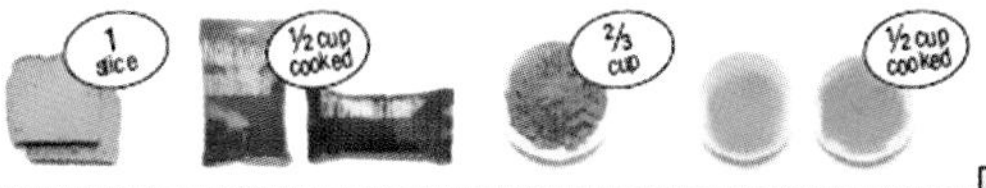

Grain (cereal) foods, mostly wholegrain and/or high cereal fibre varieties

	Serves per day		
	19–50 years	51–70 years	70+ years
Men	6	6	4½
Women	6	4	3

A standard serve (500kJ) is:

1 slice (40g)	bread
½ medium (40g)	roll or flat bread
½ cup (75–120g)	cooked rice, pasta, noodles, barley, buckwheat, semolina, polenta, bulgur or quinoa
½ cup (120g)	cooked porridge
⅔ cup (30g)	wheat cereal flakes
¼ cup (30g)	muesli
3 (35g)	crispbreads
1 (60g)	crumpet
1 small (35g)	English muffin or scone

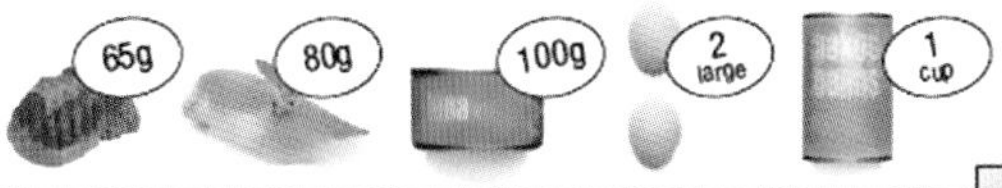

Lean meat and poultry, fish, eggs, tofu, nuts and seeds, and legumes/beans

	Serves per day		
	19–50 years	51–70 years	70+ years
Men	3	2½	2½
Women	2½	2	2

A standard serve (500-600kJ) is:

65g	cooked lean meats such as beef, lamb, veal, pork, goat or kangaroo (about 90–100g raw)*
80g	cooked lean poultry such as chicken or turkey (100g raw)
100g	cooked fish fillet (about 115g raw weight) or one small can of fish
2 large (120g)	eggs
1 cup (150g)	cooked or canned legumes/beans such as lentils, chick peas or split peas (no added salt)
170g	tofu
30g	nuts, seeds, peanut or almond butter or tahini or other nut or seed paste

**weekly limit of 455g*

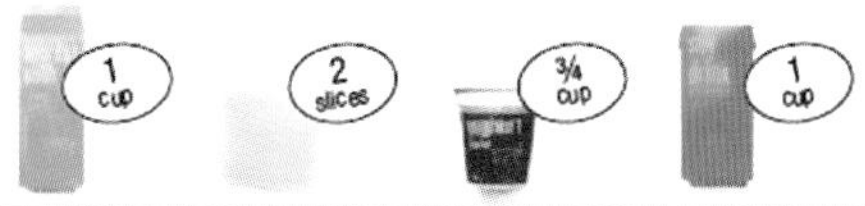

Milk, yoghurt, cheese and/or alternatives, mostly reduced fat

	Serves per day		
	19–50 years	51–70 years	70+ years
Men	2½	2½	3½
Women	2½	4	4

A standard serve (500-600kJ) is:

1 cup (250ml)	fresh, UHT long life, reconstituted powdered milk or buttermilk
½ cup (120ml)	evaporated milk
2 slices (40g)	or 4 x 3 x 2cm cube (40g) of hard cheese, such as cheddar
½ cup (120g)	ricotta cheese
¾ cup (200g)	yoghurt
1 cup (250ml)	soy, rice or other cereal drink with at least 100mg of added calcium per 100ml

- **To meet additional energy needs, extra serves from the Five Food Groups or unsaturated spreads and oils, or discretionary choices may be needed only by those adults who are taller or more active, but not overweight.**
- **An allowance for unsaturated spreads and oils for cooking, or nuts and seeds can be included in the following quantities: 28-40g per day for men less than 70 years of age, and 14-20g per day for women and older men.**
- **For meal ideas and advice on how to apply the serve sizes go to:**

www.eatforhealth.gov.au

FOR FURTHER INFORMATION GO TO www.eatforhealth.gov.au

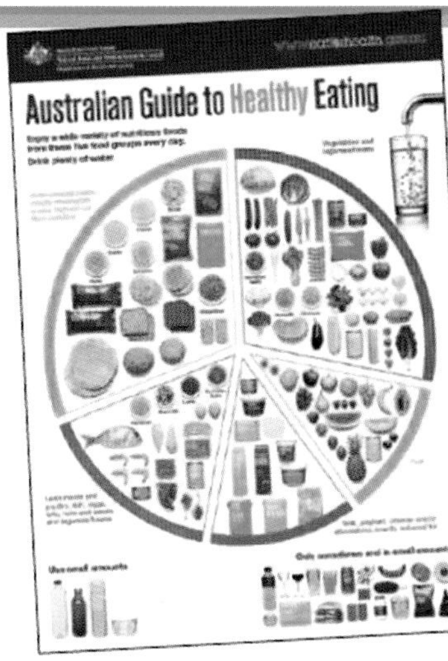

WHICH FOODS SHOULD I EAT AND HOW MUCH?

The *Australian Dietary Guidelines* provide up-to-date advice about the amount and kinds of foods and drinks that we need regularly, for health and well-being.

By eating the recommended amounts from the Five Food Groups and limiting the foods that are high in saturated fat, added sugars and added salt, you get enough of the nutrients essential for good health. You may reduce your risk of chronic diseases such as heart disease, type 2 diabetes, obesity and some cancers. You may also feel better, look better, enjoy life more and live longer!

The amount of food you will need from the Five Food Groups depends on your age, gender, height, weight and physical activity levels, and also whether you are pregnant or breastfeeding. For example, a 43-year-old man should aim for 6 serves of vegetables a day, whereas a 43-year-old woman should aim for 5 serves a day. A 61-year-old man should aim for 6 serves of grain (cereal) foods a day, and a 61-year-old woman should aim for 4 serves a day. Those who are taller or more physically active (and not overweight or obese) may be able to have additional serves of the Five Food Groups or unsaturated spreads and oils or discretionary choices.

For further information go to www.eatforhealth.gov.au.

HOW MUCH IS A SERVE?

It's helpful to get to know the recommended serving sizes and serves per day so that you eat and drink the right amount of the nutritious foods you need for health – as shown in the tables above. We've given you the serve size in grams too, so you can weigh foods to get an idea of what a serve looks like.

The 'serve size' is a set amount that doesn't change. It is used along with the 'serves per day', to work out the total amount of food required from each of the Five Food Groups. 'Portion size' is the amount you actually eat and this will depend on what your energy needs are. Some people's portion sizes are smaller than the 'serve size' and some are larger. This means some people may need to eat from the Five Food Groups more often than others.

HOW MANY SERVES A DAY?

Few people eat exactly the same way each day and it is common to have a little more on some days than others. However, on average, the total of your portion sizes should end up being similar to the number of serves you need each day.

If you eat portions that are smaller than the 'serve size' you will need to eat from the Food Groups more often. If your portion size is larger than the 'serve size', then you will need to eat from the Food Groups less often.

Figure 14.2, cont'd

Protocol summary

Answer questions regarding the Australian dietary guidelines.

Protocol

You are asked the following questions (related to the respective Australian Dietary Guideline) by a participant. Use resources such as those available at the 'Eat for health' website (https://www. eatforhealth.gov.au)[2] to provide written responses to the questions using lay language.

Guideline 1: What is a healthy body mass?

Guideline 1: How do I calculate my estimated energy need?

Guideline 2: What is a 'wide variety' of foods?

Guideline 2: What does 'nutritious' mean?

Guideline 3: What is saturated fat, and which foods contain saturated fat?

Guideline 3: Which foods have added sugars?

Guideline 3: What is a 'standard alcoholic drink' and what are some examples?

Guideline 4: What is the difference in composition between breast milk and formula milk?

Guideline 5: What is an example of proper food preparation?

Guideline 5: What is an example of proper food storage?

Activity 14.3 Nutrition information panel

AIM: understand what is stated on the nutrition information panel

Background

In Australia and New Zealand, all packaged foods are required to have a label with important information to help people make informed choices about food products. The information required varies depending on the food. Food Standards Australia New Zealand (FSANZ) is responsible for developing and maintaining the Australia New Zealand Food Standards Code, which includes standards for food labelling. Food labels help to protect public health and safety by displaying information such as use-by dates, ingredients, certain allergens, instructions for storage and preparation, and advisory and warning statements.

One component of the food label is the nutrition information panel (NIP) that provides information on the average amount of energy, protein, fat, saturated fat, carbohydrate, sugars and sodium. The amount of other selected food constituents found in the food for which a claim is made on the packaging must be indicated in the NIP. For example, if a food is claimed to be a 'good source of fibre' then the amount of fibre in the food must be stated in the NIP. The panel must be presented in a standard format that shows the average amount per manufacturer-determined serve and per 100 g (or 100 mL if liquid) of the product. Foods in small packages of less than 4 cm in length or width are not required to have an NIP. Figure 14.3 shows an NIP and explains what the different areas represent.[6]

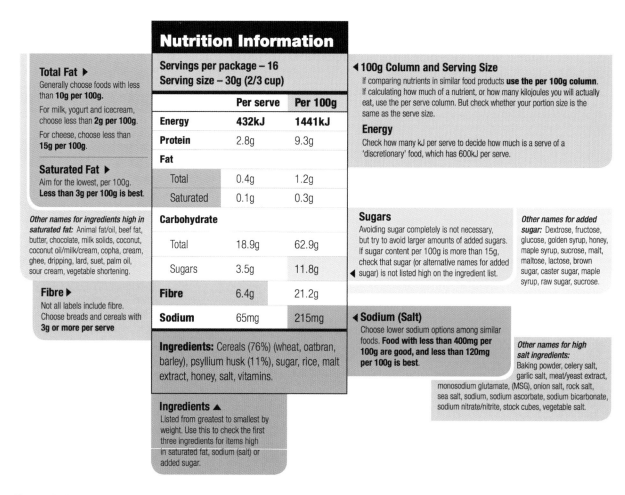

Figure 14.3 Understanding a nutrition information panel
Source: National Health and Medical Research Council[6]

Protocol summary

Answer questions about the nutrition information panel.

Protocol

1 Answer the questions below.

Question 1: When do I use the 'per serve' vs. the 'per 100 g' column?

Question 2: How do I know what a serve is?

Question 3: What does 'total fat' mean?

Question 4: What is the difference between 'carbohydrate' and 'sugar'?

Question 5: How do I know if there is added sugar in the product?

Question 6: Is the 'sugar' row about added or naturally occurring sugar?

Question 7: What is a good amount of fibre to have in a product?

Question 8: How do I know how much of each ingredient is contained in the product?

Activity 14.4 Estimated energy requirement

AIM: using the Schofield equation,[7] estimate your average daily energy requirement.

Background

A person's energy requirement from food and beverages depends on their energy expenditure. Energy expenditure is influenced by basal metabolic rate (BMR), often referred to as resting metabolic rate (RMR), physical activity levels, age, body composition, growth, the thermogenic effect of food and any special condition (e.g. pregnancy, lactation, injury, disease) that will impact metabolism. BMR can be measured by complex methodology such as direct or indirect calorimetry, or estimated. A number of equations have been developed to estimate basal energy expenditure/requirement. A factor is then applied to account for physical activity level, growth, pregnancy, lactation, etc. to determine the estimated energy requirement (EER). The following activity uses the Schofield equations[7] and will use the product of estimated BMR and physical activity level (PAL)[8] to determine EER.

$$EER = BMR \times PAL$$

Protocol summary

Calculate your estimated energy requirement.

Protocol

1 Determine your BMR from the relevant equation in Table 14.2. Note that this will give you a value in megajoules (MJ), which you will need to convert to kilojoules (kJ).

2 From Table 14.3, estimate your physical activity level (expressed as a multiple of BMR).

3 Determine your daily energy requirement by multiplying the BMR by the physical activity level.

4 Show calculations and enter your estimated daily energy requirement in kJ in the data-recording sheet on p. 397. The estimation from FoodWorks (next column) will come from Activity 14.10.

TABLE 14.2 Equations for estimating basal metabolic rate in MJ/day from body mass (kg) of adults and children over the age of 10 years

	AGE (years)	EQUATION
Males	10–18	0.074 BM + 2.754
	19–30	0.063 BM + 2.896
	31–60	0.048 BM + 3.653
	Over 60	0.049 BM + 2.459
Females	10–18	0.056 BM + 2.898
	19–30	0.062 BM + 2.036
	31–60	0.034 BM + 3.538
	Over 60	0.038 BM + 2.755

BM = body mass (kg)
Source: Schofield[7]

TABLE 14.3 Activity factors

PHYSICAL ACTIVITY LEVEL	ACTIVITY FACTOR
Bed or chair bound: no more than 2 hours out of bed/chair per day	1.2
Very sedentary: very physically inactive in both work and leisure	1.4
Sedentary: physically inactive in both work and leisure	1.5
Light: some moderate-to-vigorous exercise at least twice per week while in full-time employment that is sedentary.	1.6
Light–moderate: at least 75 min/week of moderate-intensity or 35 min/week of vigorous exercise while in full-time employment that is sedentary.	1.7
Moderate: at least 150 min/week of moderate-intensity or 75 min/week of vigorous exercise or full-time employment that is physically demanding.	1.8
Heavy: at least 250 min/week of moderate-intensity or 125 min/week of vigorous exercise or full-time employment that is physically demanding.	2.0
Very heavy: at least 350 min/week of moderate-intensity or 175 min/week of vigorous exercise or full-time employment that is very physically demanding.	2.2

Source: FoodWorks[8]

Data recording for Activities 14.4, 14.5, 14.7, 14.10–14.12

Participant's name: _____   Date: _____

Age group (circle) Male: 9–13 yrs   14–18 yrs   19–30 yrs   31–50 yrs   51–70 yrs   >70 yrs

Female[a]: 9–13 yrs   14–18 yrs   19–30 yrs   31–50 yrs   51–70 yrs   >70 yrs

Activities 14.4 and 14.10: Energy requirement and intake

	DAILY ESTIMATED ENERGY REQUIREMENT IN kJ	YOUR ACTUAL INTAKE BASED ON THE DIET DIARY ANALYSIS (kJ)
From Schofield equation (Activity 14.4)		
From FoodWorks (Activity 14.10)		

Activities 14.5 and 14.10: Nutrient reference values

MACRONUTRIENTS AND RELATED MICRONUTRIENTS	RANGE OR TARGET BASED ON AMDR OR NRVs (ACTIVITY 14.5)	EQUIVALENT IN g/mg FOR YOUR EER (USE EER FROM THE SCHOFIELD EQUATION – ACTIVITY 14.4)	YOUR INTAKE IN g/m FROM FOODWORKS (Activity 14.10)
Total fat			
Saturated fat and trans fat			
Long-chain n-3 PUFA			
Total carbohydrate			
Protein			
Dietary fibre			

VITAMINS	DAILY NRV (ADD VALUE WHERE APPLICABLE) – PROVIDE UNITS				YOUR DAILY INTAKE (PROVIDE UNITS)
	RDI	AI	SDT	UL	
Total vitamin A equivalent					
Thiamin (B1)					
Riboflavin (B2)					
Niacin equivalent (B3)				The UL for niacin is for nicotinic acid (from fortified foods or supplements)	
Vitamin B6					
Vitamin B12					
Folate, total dietary folate equivalent				The UL for folate is for folic acid (from fortified foods or supplements)	
Vitamin C					
Vitamin E					

[a] not pregnant or lactating

AI = adequate intake; AMDR = acceptable macronutrient distribution range; EER = estimated energy requirement; PUFA = polyunsaturated fatty acid; RDI = recommended dietary intake; SDT = suggested dietary target; UL = upper level of intake

continued

Data recording for Activities 14.4, 14.5, 14.7, 14.10–14.12 *(continued)*

MINERALS	DAILY NRV (ADD VALUE WHERE APPLICABLE) – PROVIDE UNITS				YOUR DAILY INTAKE (PROVIDE UNITS)
	RDI	AI	SDT	UL	
Calcium					
Iodine					
Iron					
Magnesium				The UL for magnesium is from supplements	
Potassium					
Sodium					
Zinc					

AI = adequate intake; NRV = nutrient reference values; RDI = recommended dietary intake; SDT = suggested dietary target; UL = upper level of intake

Activities 14.6 and 14.10: Food groups

FOOD GROUP	RECOMMENDED NUMBER OF SERVES (ACTIVITY 14.6)	NUMBER OF SERVES IN YOUR DIET FROM FOODWORKS ANALYSIS (ACTIVITY 14.10)
Vegetables and legumes/beans		
Fruit		
Bread /grain and cereals		
Lean meat, poultry, fish, eggs, nuts and seeds, legumes/beans		
Milk, yoghurt, cheese and/or alternatives		

Activities 14.7 and 14.10: Alcohol

	RECOMMENDATIONS TO REDUCE HARM FROM ALCOHOL CONSUMPTION' (ACTIVITIES 14.7 AND 14.8)	INTAKE FROM FOODWORKS ANALYSIS
Alcohol (grams)		

Activities 14.10 and 14.11: Diet diary validity

YOUR ENERGY INTAKE (EI) FROM FOODWORKS (ACTIVITY 14.10)	YOUR EER FROM FOODWORKS (ACTIVITY 14.10)	EI:EER BIAS CUT-OFFS	ENTER YOUR EI:EER AND STATE ANY BIAS (E.G. 'UNDER-REPORTER')
		'Under-reporters' <0.76 'Over-reporters' >1.24	

EER = estimated energy requirement

continued overpage

Data recording for Activities 14.4, 14.5, 14.7, 14.10–14.12 *(continued)*

If these were valid (prognostic) data, what would the expected outcome on your body mass be over time?

What are the reasons why your ratio is in either the over- or the under-reporting category?

Activity 14.12: Interpretation, feedback and discussion

Looking at the diet analysis, provide feedback by pointing out four positives and four points of improvement. Is there any reason to refer to a dietitian? Points to consider: the number of serves per food group, the EI: EER ratio, comparing recommended targets for macronutrients and micronutrients to actual intake.

Four positive points about the diet

Four improvements that you could make to the diet

Additional comments:

Activity 14.5 Nutrient reference values

AIMS: based on the nutrient reference values, determine your macronutrients and micronutrients targets.

Background

The Australian and New Zealand Governments established a scientific working party that, in 2006, developed nutrient reference values (NRVs) for over 40 nutrients. Depending on the available scientific evidence about the nutrient, the NRV could be presented as an estimated average requirement (EAR) and a recommended dietary intake (RDI), or an adequate intake (AI), and could indicate an upper level of intake (UL). Figure 14.4[9] shows the relationships between these various values/ranges.

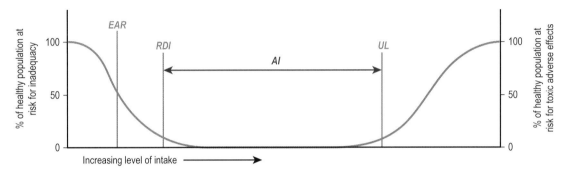

Figure 14.4 Nutrient reference values
Source: Byrd–Bredbenner (2018)[9]

To address the issue of chronic disease prevention, and healthy eating macronutrient distribution, two additional sets of reference values were developed for which sufficient evidence exists.[10] The set dealing with macronutrients is the acceptable macronutrient distribution range (AMDR) and for micronutrients it is the suggested dietary targets (SDTs). These both relate to nutrients for which there was a reasonable body of evidence of a potential chronic disease preventive effect at levels either substantially higher than the RDI or AI, or at a controlled level of intake (e.g. sodium).

Protocol summary

Determine your target reference values for selected nutrients. These may be dependent on age and sex.

Protocol

1 In the data-recording sheet, add your target reference values for the selected macro- and micronutrients.

2 For total fat, total carbohydrate and protein, find the AMDRs at https://www.nrv.gov.au/chronic-disease/summary (Table 2: Acceptable macronutrient distribution ranges for macronutrients to reduce chronic disease risk while still ensuring adequate micronutrient status). For long-chain omega-3 (n-3) polyunsaturated fatty acids (PUFA), the recommendation is that this is 0.2% of total energy intake.[10]

3   To calculate the range in grams, use the following:

- Carbohydrate $= 16.7$ kJ/g

- Proteins $= 16.7$ kJ/g

- Fats (including 'saturated fat and trans fat' and 'long-chain n-3 PUFA' $= 37.7$ kJ/g

4   To determine whether a vitamin or a mineral has an RDI or an AI and a UL go to https://www.nrv.gov.au/introduction, where there are links to pages for each nutrient.

5   To determine whether a vitamin or mineral has an SDT go to https://www.nrv.gov.au/chronic-disease/summary (Table 1. Suggested dietary targets (SDTs) to reduce chronic disease risk).

6   Your intake (in the next column) will come from the FoodWorks analysis of your diet diary (Activity 14.10).

7   Ensure that units are always provided.

Activity 14.6 Food groups

AIMS: enhance understanding of the five food groups and determine the number of serves of each food group that you require.

Background

The second Australian Dietary Guideline (ADG) states that the key to eating well is to enjoy a variety of nutritious foods from each of the five food groups. The ADGs are underpinned by the grouping of foods. Foods are grouped together according to the main nutrients they provide. The guideline goes on to say that it is not necessary to eat from each food group at every meal. Furthermore, it states that it is important to enjoy a variety of foods within each of the five food groups because different foods vary in the amount of the key nutrients that they provide. Given all this, it is important to have a good understanding of the five groups.

The brochure 'Healthy eating for adults' (see Figure 14.2) is available to complement the second ADG. The Australian guide to healthy eating is a pictorial representation of the proportion of the five food groups recommended for consumption each day. The recommended dietary pattern provides the nutrients and energy required by men and women of average height who have sedentary to moderate activity levels. The dietary pattern is based on the consumption of plant and animal foods (an omnivore diet). Other dietary patterns, including vegetarian and vegan diets, can also meet nutrient and energy requirements but are not specifically addressed in this activity. Taller or more active individuals require additional portions of the five food groups to meet their higher energy requirements. It is important to remember that these recommendations are targeted at the healthy general population. Increased requirements by an athlete would not be met by these guidelines and would require tailored recommendations.

Protocol summary

Determine the number of serves of each food group that you require.

Protocol

Using Figure 14.2 and/or www.eatforhealth.gov.au, fill in the adequate number of serves of each food group in the data-recording sheet. The number of serves in your diet (in the next column) will come from the FoodWorks analysis of your diet diary (Activity 14.10).

Activity 14.7 Alcohol

AIMS: enhance understanding of the Australian guidelines for safe alcohol drinking and the concept of the Australian standard alcoholic drink.

Background

In 2020 Australia's National Health and Medical Research Council revised the Australian guidelines to reduce health risks from consuming alcohol.[11] The guidelines provide health professionals and policy makers with evidence-based recommendations on the health effects of consuming alcohol, and help individuals make informed decisions about their alcohol consumption to keep the risk of harm as low as possible. The three new guidelines are:

1. To reduce the risk of harm from alcohol-related disease or injury, healthy men and women should drink no more than 10 standard drinks a week and no more than 4 standard drinks on any one day.

2. To reduce the risk of injury and other harms to health, children and young people under 18 years of age should not drink alcohol.

3. To prevent harm from alcohol to their unborn child, women who are pregnant or planning a pregnancy should not drink alcohol. For women who are breastfeeding, not drinking alcohol is safest for their baby.

The concept of a standard drink is widely used internationally, though the definition varies between countries. The Australian guidelines define the Australian standard drink as containing 10 g of alcohol (equivalent to 12.7 mL of pure alcohol, because the specific gravity of alcohol is 0.789). A 'serving' of an alcoholic beverage frequently differs from a standard drink depending on the beverage's alcohol concentration. For example, a *standard drink* of average red wine may correspond to just above 100 mL (for red wine at 14.5% alc/vol), whereas a typical serve may be 150 mL. In Australia all bottles, cans and casks containing alcoholic beverages are required by law to state on the label the approximate number of standard drinks they contain, and the concentration of alcohol in volume (% alc/vol) to assist the public in being aware of their consumption. Note that alcoholic drinks also yield energy. Alcohol yields 29 kJ per gram. Alcoholic drinks may also yield additional energy from other components such as sugars and starch.

Protocol summary

State the guideline for the amount of alcohol/day for you.

Protocol

1 Provide the guideline for the amount of alcohol (g)/day for you. Your intake (in the next column) will come from FoodWorks (Activity 14.10).

2 Compare your intake with recommendations and comment on how this was distributed over the 3 days.

Activity 14.8 Discretionary foods and beverages

AIMS: enhance understanding of discretionary foods/beverages and how much energy one serving contains.

Background

Some foods and beverages do not fit into the five food groups because they are too high in saturated fat, added sugars or salt, and/or low in fibre. These foods/beverages are referred to as 'discretionary'. They are often high in energy density and low in nutrient density. They often replace nutritious foods in the diet. The higher amounts of kilojoules, saturated fat, added sugars and salt that they contain are associated with increased risk of chronic disease.

For a person trying to lose weight, consuming these foods/beverages will contribute to excess energy intake with low satiation. For people in the normal weight range, consuming these foods/beverages occasionally in small amounts can add variety and enjoyment.

One serving of a discretionary food is equivalent to 600 kJ. The nutrition information panel allows people to calculate the amount of the food/beverage that would contain 600 kJ.

Protocol summary

Answer questions about discretionary foods.

Protocol

Question 1: What is one serving of discretionary foods in the ADG?

Question 2: What is one serving of a discretionary food equivalent to in a savoury food?

Question 3: What is one serving of a discretionary food equivalent to in a sweet food?

Question 4: What is one serving of a discretionary food equivalent to in a sweet drink?

Activity 14.9 Diet diary

AIM: collect a 3-day diet diary of the foods and beverages you have consumed as accurately as possible. Ideally, you have prepared this in the week before the tutorial as instructed.

Background

One approach to assess the diet of an individual is to ask them to keep a diary of the foods and beverages they have consumed over a certain period of time (e.g. 3 days). The more details it contains about the type of foods and the amount consumed, the more valid the analysis will be. Table 14.4 provides an example of a food diary with instructions.

Assumptions and limitations

- Ideally, the diary should be filled in throughout the day (each time a person eats something or takes a drink). However, this is not always possible and attempting to recall what has been consumed can easily lead to misreporting.

- It is often difficult to include full and correct information, especially with processed or restaurant food. Some nutrition information panels may be helpful and additional information may be found online to estimate composition.

- Quantities may be difficult to estimate accurately.

- A participant may not be truthful in recording what they have eaten, or they may change (improve) their behaviour over the 3 days so that they appear to be eating more healthily.

- A participant may have a very different diet across the week, so the 3 days they choose should reflect usual eating behaviour as much as possible.

TABLE 14.4 Diet diary

The more honest and accurate you are, the more useful this information will be.

Instructions:

1 Record all food and beverage intake over 2 weekdays and 1 weekend day (don't need to be consecutive).

2 To improve accuracy, try to record the details as soon after consumption as possible.

3 Record the amounts of food served in common portion sizes such as cups, slices, teaspoons, weight, or describe size (e.g. 1 large banana – 20 cm long).

4 Provide composition details (e.g. sweetened, low-fat, flavoured, wholemeal, etc.).

5 Indicate how the food was prepared (e.g. fried, steamed, baked, raw, etc.).

6 List brand names if known.

7 Record the source if known (e.g. name of the fast food chain where the food was obtained).

8 Be as specific as possible (e.g. instead of 'ham sandwich', write, 'ham sandwich with 2 slices (brand name) white bread, 2 slices of (brand name) ham, 1 tablespoon (brand name) reduced fat mayonnaise, and two 8 cm pieces of romaine lettuce'.

9 Record any added ingredients (gravies, salad dressings, sauce, sugar, salt, margarine, etc.) and indicate the amounts.

10 Include recipes for any unusual items you prepared at home.

DAY (e.g. 1 SAT.)	TIME (e.g. 7a.m.)	FOOD/FLUID (e.g. WEET-BIX)	BRAND NAME (e.g. SANITARIUM)	FOOD PREPARATION (e.g. COOKED)	AMOUNT (e.g. 100 g, ½ CUP)

continued overpage

TABLE 14.4 Diet diary *(continued)*

DAY (e.g. 1 SAT.)	TIME (e.g. 7a.m.)	FOOD/FLUID (e.g. WEET-BIX)	BRAND NAME (e.g. SANITARIUM)	FOOD PREPARATION (e.g. COOKED)	AMOUNT (e.g. 100 g, ½ CUP)

- Recording a diet diary is time-consuming compared with other dietary analysis approaches (e.g. food frequency questionnaires).

After taking these into account, an accurate diet diary can still provide important information to assist in understanding a participant's eating behaviour.

Protocol summary

Complete a 3-day diet diary.

Protocol

Following the instructions at the top of Table 14.4, write down the required details for all the foods and beverages you consumed over 3 days (2 weekdays and 1 weekend day).

Activity 14.10 Nutritional analysis software

AIM: perform an assessment of your dietary intake using the nutritional analysis software FoodWorks.

Background

The past decade has seen major improvements in the way technology is used to analyse dietary intakes. One of these approaches is nutritional analysis software that combines food composition databases with an easy-to-use interface. It provides a detailed quantitative analysis of daily energy and macro- and micronutrient intakes. One example is FoodWorks,[8] which uses Australian and New Zealand foods composition databases such as AusFoods 2017, AusBrands 2017, AUSNUT 2011–2013 and New Zealand FOODfiles 2016. The protocol in this practical is for FoodWorks version 10.

At first glance a nutritional analysis program would appear to be a powerful method of analysing dietary information. However, there are major limitations to this approach, including the need to keep detailed food records, difficulties in knowing what specific ingredients are in certain foods (e.g. stir fry) and problems locating uncommon foods in the database. Furthermore, the output needs to be contextualised against the foods that have been eaten. This will be discussed in detail in the background to Activity 14.11.

Protocol summary

Enter your 3-day food diary into FoodWorks to obtain an average daily energy, macronutrient and micronutrient composition of your diet.

Protocol

1 Open the FoodWorks application.

2 Create your new FoodWorks database (this is a repository for the work you do in FoodWorks).

3 Select an appropriate database: for Australia, AUSFOODS 2017; for New Zealand, FOODfiles.

4 Save the database using an identifiable file name (e.g. your name or student number).

5 FoodWorks then starts with your new database open.

Create a new food record

6 A new food record will open.

7 On the 'General' tab, enter your name, age, body mass, height, pregnancy and lactation status, sex and physical activity level (for help in choosing the appropriate activity level, click the (….) button). You can then see the values for BMI, EER and BMR on this tab. Add the EER from here to the data-recording sheet.

Enter the foods

8 Click the 'Foods' tab. Figure 14.5[12] shows the major elements of the FoodWorks window on the 'Foods' tab.

9 In the first row of the 'Day' column, enter the date of your first food record.

10 In the 'Meal' column, enter the meal (e.g. 'Breakfast').

11 In the 'Food' column, type the first few letters of each word of the food. Use the arrow keys to select the food from the drop-down box, then press 'Enter'.

12 In the 'Quantity' column, type the number of units for the measure that you want to use. Then use the arrow keys to select the measure, then press 'Enter'.

13 Repeat steps 11 and 12 for each food in the meal. If the exact food is not in the database, use a food that is as similar as possible.

14 Repeat from step 10 to start the next meal.

15 Repeat from step 9 to start the next day.

16 Save the food record.

17 On the FoodWorks toolbar, click 'Save'.

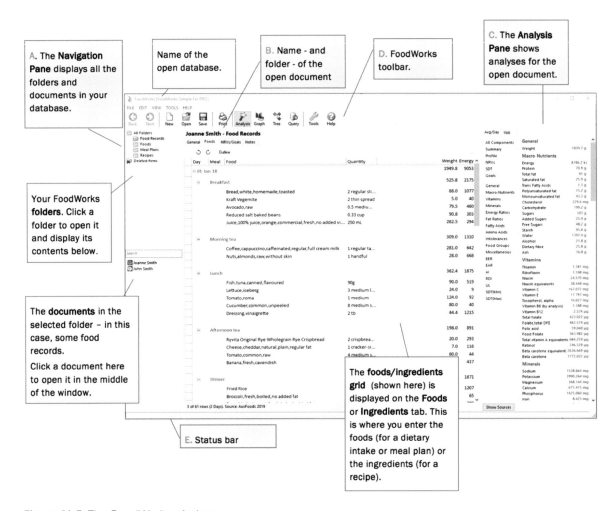

Figure 14.5 The FoodWorks window
Used with permission from Xyris software

Data analysis

1 To choose the unit of analysis for the food record, click the tabs at the top of the 'analysis pane' on the right. You can view the analyses as an 'average per day' or 'per megajoule'.

2 In the 'analysis pane', you can view nutrient reference values (NRV) analyses, as shown in Figure 14.6.[12]

3 Complete the data-recording sheet with your values.

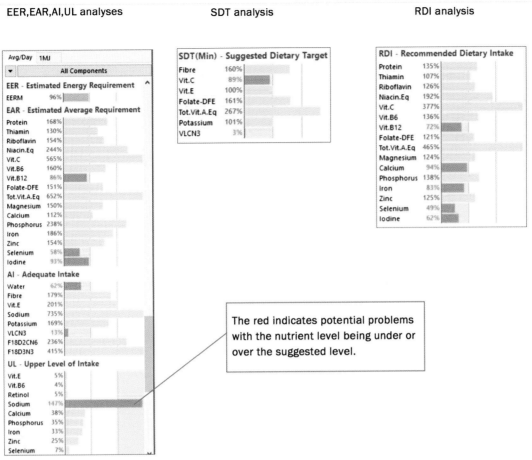

EER,EAR,AI,UL analyses　　　　SDT analysis　　　　RDI analysis

The red indicates potential problems with the nutrient level being under or over the suggested level.

Figure 14.6 The NRV analyses in FoodWorks
Used with permission from Xyris software

Activity 14.11 Diet diary validity

AIM: to determine the validity of your diet diary.

Background

As previously discussed, the collection of self-report diet information is problematic. A term that is commonly used is 'misreporting', or 'bias of self-report', which implies the participant has inaccurately completed the task on purpose. However, other factors may be occurring (e.g. they may improve their dietary behaviour because they do not wish others to see their normal dietary intake). This would result in an accurate diet diary; however, it is invalid (concurrent), with regards to representing the usual eating habits of the individual.

The usual bias is for people to under-report the foods and beverages they have consumed and this has implications for the analysis and interpretation of the dietary intake, because less or more energy intake means also less or more macro- and micronutrients. Indeed, under-reporting has been shown to be as high as 70% in particular individuals.[13] One attempt to assess the concurrent validity of the diet diary is to use the ratio of energy intake (e.g. calculated from the diet diary by FoodWorks) to the estimated energy requirement (e.g. calculated using the Schofield equations). This ratio is then compared with bias cut-offs ('Under-reporters' <0.76; 'Over-reporters' >1.24).

Protocol summary

Determine whether your diet diary has bias.

Protocol

1 Obtain your average daily energy intake calculated from FoodWorks (Activity 14.10) and add this to the data-recording sheet for this Activity.

2 Add your daily estimated energy requirement calculated from FoodWorks (Activity 14.10) and add this to the data-recording sheet for this Activity.

3 Calculate your EI:EER ratio, compare your value with the bias cut-offs provided above and state whether there is any bias.

4 Answer the question in the data-recording sheet regarding the potential impact on your body mass over time if this ratio was maintained.

Interpretation, feedback and discussion

The use of nutritional software can lead to an undue focus on the nutrients. Interpretation of a nutritional analysis requires knowledge of the following important nutritional concept:

The benefits from whole foods are greater than the sum of their individual nutrients.

For example, it is relatively easy to consume all the required macronutrients and micronutrients through processed foods complemented with supplementation. However, if there is a lack of natural whole foods in your dietary intake, you risk not receiving all of the health benefits that food can offer such as the synergy of food components and phytonutrients. Therefore, at all times during a nutritional assessment it is critical to promote the message that the majority of the nutrients should come from unprocessed plant and animal foods and these should be favoured in priority over supplementation or processed dietary products.

Interpreting the results from a nutritional assessment point of view, using the Australian dietary guidelines and/or the Guide to healthy eating is done with the knowledge that a person's optimal nutritional intake will depend on:

- meeting the relevant guidelines overall
- attaining the recommended number of serves within each food group.

Interpretation of the individual nutrient intake from the nutritional analysis software needs to be done in conjunction with an assessment of the food groups that the person is consuming, also provided by FoodWorks. The interpretation can also consider the quality of the foods consumed within each food group (e.g. whole grain bread and cereals instead of refined flour bread and cereals, which may influence the overall fibre intake).

Energy intake is usually the first value analysed. This needs to be done in the context of whether the participant is wishing to change their body mass or body composition. As discussed in Activity 14.11, the collection and analysis of food diary information using this approach has a high risk that the calculated energy intakes are less than the suggested requirements for weight maintenance. Therefore, interpretation of the energy intake values must be done with caution, especially in situations where individuals are wishing to lose body mass. The calculation of EI:EER may assist in interpreting the energy intake data. Asking whether the diet diary is representative of the usual intake may help to determine the value of the data collected.

The high probability of under-reporting will also impact on the analysis of other nutrients. For example, if a participant has reported only two-thirds of the foods they have consumed, there will be considerable errors in the analysis of the nutrients due to not including the other one-third of the foods.

The interpretation of a FoodWorks analysis is often used to identify individual dietary nutrients that may be out of a recommended range. This then needs to lead to a closer examination of the food groups that the person has consumed (or not consumed) that have caused a nutrient to be outside a recommendation. Caution should be used when interpreting results as the analysis relies on the 3-day record being representative of normal eating habits. It may, however, prompt further discussion regarding foods containing particular nutrient/s with a participant.

When deciding what feedback to provide to a participant, it is important to reflect on the scope of practice of your profession. For exercise and sport scientists and AEPs, this is to provide general nutrition advice to apparently healthy participants. If a person has a special need, a medical condition or is eating an exclusion diet (where they are attempting to exclude certain foods from their diet or are following a vegan pattern) then they should be referred to a dietitian.

It is very important to look at both qualitative and quantitative assessments of food intake to determine the overall quality of the diet. These activities should demonstrate the importance of not relying on one method (e.g. micronutrient content analysis) for assessing dietary quality. Quantitative assessments of food groups, and ensuring whole foods are being consumed within each food group (qualitative assessment), is essential not just to nutritional adequacy, but also to health maintenance and disease prevention.

Two components of the dietary intake that should be covered are alcohol intake and discretionary foods. Activities 14.7 and 14.8 provide information to assist with supplying feedback regarding these.

When you consume foods in line with the food group recommendations, you make positive changes to your overall consumption of all nutrients: amount and types of fat, fibre, vitamins and minerals.

General recommendations are a good start. Passing on food group knowledge is helpful. Some participants will need a more-personalised plan and this provides an excellent opportunity to collaborate with a dietitian.

When providing feedback, first consider the three steps of feedback and discussion outlined in Appendix G. The objective is to provide feedback that is within the scope of practice for the practitioner and that aims to have the participant understand which foods are healthier and which foods need to be limited. Participants should be encouraged to ask questions and discuss the feedback.

The following questions should be considered when giving feedback to the participant:

- Is this a usual intake, or was this intake recorded in any way different owing to circumstances during the 3 days?
- What does the EI:EER indicate about the likely effect on body mass over time? Have they lost or gained weight lately? Are they aiming to do so?
- Where could you direct your participant for more information on food composition and healthy eating tips?
- Ask whether they are using any supplements, as this may compensate for any low intakes of micronutrients. Recommending someone to take a supplement is not within the scope of an exercise and sport science professional; nor is the assessment of whether using the supplement is adequate or not.
- Is your participant likely to need a referral to a dietitian, and why?

After examining your data from Activities 14.4–14.11, provide four positive points and four points of improvement you could make regarding your diet in the data-recording sheet.

Case studies

Case Study 1

Setting: You are completing an exercise science degree and a friend has told you she is having trouble losing weight. She has been limiting her energy intake to 10,000 kJ/day but is now wondering whether this is an accurate target.

Task: Calculate her estimated energy expenditure. She is a non-pregnant, non-lactating woman aged 32 years, with a mean body mass of 60 kg and a light activity level.

Case Study 2

Setting: You are working as an Accredited Exercise Scientist delivering a corporate health program in a large company. Your main task is to improve the health of the employees and you have developed a program that aims to identify and support individuals who may benefit from a visit to an allied health professional.

An employee, Ruth, has approached you about her health. During the consultation you learn that she is a 32-year-old female with low physical activity levels. Her body mass is 72 kg and her height is 162 cm. She states she has no medical conditions. She identifies that 'she does not eat very well'.

You provide her with the 'Are you eating for health?' quiz and ask her to be honest and tick each box that applies to her current eating pattern. As Ruth completes the form, you encourage her to ask questions if any of the guidelines are not clear. Her completed sheet is provided in Figure 14.7.

Task: Determine the appropriate course of action for Ruth.

continued

Case studies *(continued)*

QUIZ: ARE YOU EATING FOR HEALTH?

Take this quick quiz for adults to find out the answer – be honest! Give yourself one point for each box you tick if you:

☐ Eat at least 5 serves of vegetables every day. A serve is ½ cup cooked vegetables (hot chips don't count!) or 1 cup of salad.

☐ Eat at least 2 serves of fruit every day. A serve is 1 medium piece or 2 small pieces of fresh fruit, or one cup of chopped or canned fruit (no added sugar).

☐ Have at least 2 serves of reduced fat milk, yoghurt, cheese or alternatives every day (for example, 1 slice of reduced fat cheese, a small tub of reduced fat yoghurt (preferably no added sugar), 1 cup of milk or 1 cup of soy milk with added calcium).

☑ Eat mostly wholegrain cereals (such as high fibre breakfast cereal and wholemeal bread).

☐ Eat at least a small serve of lean meat or chicken (fat and/or skin cut off) or fish, or eggs or some nuts or legumes (for example, lentils, chickpeas, beans such as kidney beans or baked beans) every day.

☑ Drink plenty of water every day and limit drinks with added sugars, such as soft drinks, cordial, energy drinks and sports drinks.

☐ Limit takeaway foods such as pizzas, commercial burgers, hot chips or other deep fried foods to once a week or less.

☐ Limit store-bought cakes, muffins, pastries, pies and biscuits to once a week or less.

☐ Limit salty foods like processed meats (for example, salami and bacon), crisps and salty snacks to once a week or less, and avoid adding salt during cooking or at the table.

☐ Drink no more than 2 standard drinks containing alcohol on any one day.

How did you rate?

8–10 points Congratulations, you're already a pretty healthy eater!

6–8 points Keep going, you're nearly there!

4–6 points There's plenty of room for improvement.

Less than 4 It's time for a serious overhaul.

Use the information in this booklet for some great ideas.

Poor eating habits are sometimes hard to break. For adults, it's not too late to make changes if poor eating habits have crept up, but it's important to keep changes realistic using the practical information in this booklet should help.

For more information go to:

www.eatforhealth.gov.au

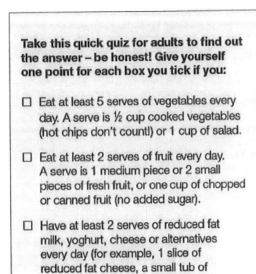

Figure 14.7 Completed quiz for Case study 2

continued overpage

Case studies *(continued)*

Case Study 3

Setting: you work as an Accredited Exercise Physiologist in your own business.

Bruce is a client requesting help to 'meet his goals'. He tells you that he has gained weight in the last few months and wants to lose it. This has coincided with starting a new job. He also states he wants to 'get my fitness back to where it was when I was younger'. During an initial assessment you determine the following:

- 29-year-old male, light physical activity levels
- body mass: 92 kg; height: 172 cm; gained 3–4 kg in last 2 months
- medical conditions: none identified.

You provide him with the 'Are you eating for health?' quiz and ask him to place a tick against those relevant to his current eating habits. He scores only 2/10. Based on this, you decide to ask him to complete a 3-day food diary including 1 weekend day. He presents the following information.

FOOD DIARY

Day 1 (Thursday)

Breakfast

4 pieces of wholemeal bread toasted with butter and raspberry jam

1 cup of tea with milk and 1 teaspoon of sugar

Morning tea

500 mL chocolate milk

1 ham and cheese toasted sandwich

Lunch

Large hot chips

2 glasses of water

Afternoon tea

2 packets of 2-minute noodles (with beef flavour sachet)

Dinner

Steak (500 g) and large hot chips

2 beers

Day 2 (Friday)

Breakfast

4 pieces of wholemeal bread toasted with butter and raspberry jam

1 cup of tea with milk and 1 teaspoon of sugar

Morning tea

500 mL chocolate milk

1 ham and cheese toasted sandwich

Lunch

4 slices of a frozen vegetarian pizza

2 glasses of water

Afternoon tea

2 packets of 2-minute noodles

Dinner

500 g of ravioli with beef bolognese sauce

2 glasses of water

Day 3 (Saturday)

Breakfast

4 pieces of wholemeal bread toasted with butter and raspberry jam

1 cup of tea with milk and 1 teaspoon of sugar

Morning tea

Sausage roll

Meat pie

Lunch

2 chicken and salad sandwiches

2 glasses of water

Afternoon tea

2 slices of a frozen vegetarian pizza

Dinner

Fish and chips

Drinks

4 beers

continued

Case studies *(continued)*

Task:

1 What is some critical information that has been omitted from Bruce's diet history that will aid your assessment of his intake? How would you reliably gather this information?

2 Should you be asking any further questions about his intake, or should you just analyse what he has written? Why?

3 What further steps would you take to analyse the data?

References

[1] Exercise and Sports Science Australia and the Dietitians Association of Australia. The collaboration of exercise physiologists and dietitians in chronic disease management. Albion, Qld: ESSA; 2014. https://www.essa.org.au/Public/Advocacy/Position_Statements/Public/Advocacy/Position_Statements.aspx.

[2] National Health and Medical Research Council. Healthy eating for adults. Canberra, ACT: NHMRC; 2013. https://www.eatforhealth.gov.au/sites/default/files/content/The%20Guidelines/n55g_adult_brochure.pdf.

[3] Exercise and Sport Science Australia. Exercise science standards. Albion, Qld: ESSA; 2013. https://www.essa.org.au/Public/Professional_Standards/The_professional_standards.aspx.

[4] National Health and Medical Research Council. Australian dietary guidelines. Canberra, ACT: NHMRC; 2013. https://www.eatforhealth.gov.au/sites/default/files/content/The%20Guidelines/n55a_australian_dietary_guidelines_summary_131014_1.pdf.

[5] Compher C, Frankenfield D, Keim N, Roth-Yousey L; Evidence Analysis Working Group. Best practice methods to apply to measurement of resting metabolic rate in adults: a systematic review. J Am Diet Assoc 2006;106:881–903.

[6] National Health and Medical Research Council. How to understand food labels. Canberra, ACT: NHMRC; 2013. https://www.eatforhealth.gov.au/sites/default/files/files/eatingwell/efh_food_label_example_130621.pdf.

[7] Schofield WN. Predicting basal metabolic rate, new standards and review of previous work. Hum Nutr Clin Nutr 1985;39(Suppl 1):5–41.

[8] Xyris. FoodWorks software. Version 10. Highgate Hill, Qld: Xyris; 2019. https://xyris.com.au/.

[9] Byrd-Bredbenner C. Wardlaw's perspectives in nutrition. New York: McGraw-Hill Higher Education; 2018.

[10] National Health and Medical Research Council. Nutrient reference values for Australia and New Zealand. Canberra, ACT: NHMRC; 2017. https://www.nhmrc.gov.au/sites/default/files/images/nutrient-refererence-dietary-intakes.pdf.

[11] National Health and Medical Research Council. Australian guidelines to reduce health risks from drinking alcohol. Canberra, ACT: NHMRC; 2020. https://www.nhmrc.gov.au/about-us/publications/australian-guidelines-reduce-health-risks-drinking-alcohol.

[12] Xyris. Introduction to dietary analysis with FoodWorks 10. Highgate Hill, Qld: Xyris; 2019. https://support.xyris.com.au/hc/en-us/articles/204538859-Introductory-Guide-FoodWorks-Professional.

[13] Macdiarmid J, Blundell J. Assessing dietary intake: who, what and why of under-reporting. Nutr Res Rev 1998;11:231–53.

PRACTICAL 15
FUNCTIONAL MEASURES

Tina Skinner and Kate Bolam

LEARNING OBJECTIVES

- Identify and explain the common terminology, processes and equipment required to conduct accurate and safe functional measures

- Identify and describe the limitations, contraindications or considerations that may require the modification of functional measures, and make appropriate adjustments for relevant populations or participants

- Explain the scientific rationale, purposes, reliability, validity, assumptions and limitations of common functional measures

- Conduct appropriate pre-assessment procedures, including explaining the test and obtaining informed consent and a focused medical history, and performing a pre-exercise risk assessment

- Identify the need for guidance or further information from an appropriate health professional, and recognise when to cease a test

- Select and conduct appropriate protocols for safe and effective assessment of functional measures, including instructing participants on the correct use of equipment

- Record, analyse and interpret information from functional measures and convey the results, including the validity and limitations of the assessments, through relevant verbal and/or written communication with the participant or involved professional

- Integrate knowledge of and skills in functional measures with other study areas of exercise science, in particular the physiology that underpins common exercise contraindications

Equipment and other requirements

- Information sheet and informed consent form
- Stopwatch
- Electronic speed gates/timing lights (optional – see Box 13.1 for a comparison between stopwatch and timing lights)
- Exercise mat (high density)
- Anthropometry tape or segmometer
- Brightly coloured marking cones
- Masking tape (normal and brightly coloured)
- Measuring tape (at least 6 m)
- Straight-backed arm chair (seat height approximately 46 cm)
- Calculator
- Cleaning and disinfecting equipment (see Appendix A)

INTRODUCTION

The life expectancy of Australian and New Zealand adults is among the highest in the world. Improvements in healthcare and medical science have meant that people are living longer. While older Australians and New Zealanders are living longer, they are not necessarily ageing 'well' and this is of severe consequence for the health system of each country, the carers and families of these people and the quality of life of these individuals. Due to the physiological changes that generally occur with the normal ageing process, older adults' functional capacity or their ability to undertake activities of daily living (ADL) often decreases. This can lead to an increased dependence on others as well as increased risk for developing chronic diseases and mortality.[1]

Researchers have typically described functional declines according to changes in functional capacity or physical performance. There are numerous different functional tests that have been developed to assess these parameters; these typically require minimum equipment and standardised instruction. Tests of functional capacity objectively evaluate specific aspects of physical performance by having the individual perform standardised tasks that reflect ADL. These tests are used to predict future disability and/or mortality in both healthy populations and individuals with chronic disease. Selection of an appropriate test/s of function for each participant requires clinical judgment to ensure that the test: (i) is sufficiently challenging to avoid a ceiling or floor effect, (ii) is safe for the participant to perform (see safety considerations section within this practical), (iii) provides an accurate and concurrently valid measure of the outcome of interest, and (iv) can be compared against normative data if the test is performed on a single occasion, or is sufficiently sensitive to detect differences across time with repeated measures.

Exercise professionals are likely to administer these tests during an initial health assessment of an older adult to determine a baseline level of functional status prior to prescribing an exercise program. These tests may also be used as a measure of the effectiveness during or following an exercise program.

A limitation of many of these tests is the absence of reference ranges for 'normal' or 'desired' values. Typically, functional capacity measures are collected pre- and post-intervention for a within-individual comparison. Where available, normative values have been included in this practical; however, they refer only to persons aged 60 years and over. A further limitation is that many older adults are apparently healthy with no or few functional limitations. As such, certain tests described within this practical may be too easy for active, healthy older adults.

If the aim of functional testing is to practise the testing procedures and involves young, healthy participants, it is recommended that role-play is involved to more closely mimic conditions when testing older adults, and to ensure that the feedback provided has some purpose. Role-play, for example '*your participant is an 89-year-old female who has had a fall and has come in today to test their balance*', will enhance the ability for a young, healthy tester to consider safety precautions, and provide and discuss meaningful feedback.

DEFINITIONS

Dynamic balance: the ability to balance whilst in motion or when switching between positions.

Fall: an event which results in a person coming to rest inadvertently on the ground or other lower level.

Frailty: a dynamic condition of increased vulnerability that limits one's social, psychological and physical functioning.

Intraclass correlation coefficient (ICC): a measure of the reliability of two or more measurements.

Odds ratio (OR): a measure of association between an exposure and an outcome. The OR represents the odds that an outcome will occur given a particular exposure, compared with the odds of the outcome occurring in the absence of that exposure.

Orthostatic hypotension: also known as postural hypotension, this occurs when an individual becomes dizzy or lightheaded owing to a sudden drop in blood pressure when sitting or standing up.

Osteoporosis: a medical condition in which the bones become brittle and fragile from loss of tissue. It is characterised by decreased bone mineral density (2.5 standard deviations or more below the mean for young adults) and altered micro-architecture, resulting in compromised bone strength and increased risk for fracture.

Relative risk (RR): a comparison of the risk of a particular illness or cause of death for a group compared with another group (e.g. a separate intervention group or control group).

SAFETY CONSIDERATIONS

Older adults and individuals with functional deficits are the target populations for most of the tests included within this practical. Therefore, the importance of appropriate risk stratification and health assessment, as well as laboratory safety and infection control (see Appendix A), is heightened in this population. Although many older adults are otherwise healthy, for those older adults who have reduced functional capacity and/or poor balance, sight and/or hearing, special consideration must be given to safety measures when conducting these tests.

Falls risk

Ensure that the testing environment is clear of trip hazards (such as objects on the floor or risen-up mats) to reduce the risk of the participant tripping or falling. Select well-lit testing areas with level, non-slip surfaces where possible.

Fatigue

Due to the physiological changes that occur to our bodies as we age, become more frail and/or less fit, the participant may report feeling fatigued more quickly and work at a lower rate than a younger, less frail and/or fitter participant. Therefore, the time needed to recover between exercises can be longer than for a younger and/or fitter person. The duration of the rest periods between exercises will need to be adapted to suit the participant. In addition, testing order is more important in this population to minimise the effect of fatigue from one test influencing the results of subsequent tests.

Hydration

Older adults are also more likely to be dehydrated than younger adults and so reminding the participant of the importance of hydration is important not only for the health of the participant but also for their performance during the testing session.

Vision/hearing/cognition

Older adults may have impaired vision, hearing and/or cognition and thought must be given to how to communicate with the participant (e.g. hearing aid device). Ensure that the instructions are explained slowly, clearly and at a volume that provides the participant with the best chance of understanding the directions and questions. Noisy teaching laboratories may make this process difficult. Provide the participant with sufficient opportunities to ask questions or clarify procedures before the test. Check the participant is both paying attention and understands the instructions. Carefully select concise and directive cueing using appropriate and respectful lay language (i.e. avoiding condescension and oversimplification). It is also advisable to clearly demonstrate each measure before the participant is asked to perform the test.

It is important to use your clinical judgment to determine which tests are appropriate to select for your participant, and how quickly to advance these tests. Some of the tests included in this practical may be too advanced for certain participants, which may compromise their safety and result in a floor effect of the test (i.e. a zero result). In contrast, some tests may be too easy for certain participants, resulting in a ceiling effect of the test (i.e. maximal result with no capacity to identify improvement following exercise training). This is especially the case with tests that have a maximum distance or time (e.g. various balance tests). Test selection should therefore consider what you specifically want to measure (and why), comorbidities and functional deficits (including observation of their gait and mobility as soon as you meet them) and the safety considerations listed above.

Above all else, the participant must feel safe when performing these measures. If the participant indicates that they do not feel capable or safe to begin performing the measure, do not try to persuade or pressure them to continue with the test. During the test it may be necessary to prematurely stop the test; follow the indications for stopping an exercise test described in Appendix F. An appropriate cool-down (e.g. slower walking for 2–3 minutes) should be administered after the test is terminated. For older, more frail and/or less fit individuals, monitoring heart rate during recovery will help to determine the length of the cool-down.

Activity 15.1 Physical performance battery

....

AIMS: conduct a physical performance battery, interpret the results and provide feedback to a participant.

Background

A battery of tests is commonly used in clinical and research settings to provide a complete and objective assessment of physical function and adverse outcomes in older adults. These tests can be used as standalone measures to assess an individual's balance, gait speed and/or lower body strength.

Several variations of these tests have been developed, including the three-stage (side-by-side, semi-tandem and tandem stand) balance test in the Short Physical Performance Battery, coordinated stability (a measure of controlled leaning balance),[2] the 3, 4, 6 and 10 m usual and maximal gait speed tests and the 30-second chair stand test from the Seniors Fitness Test.[3]

The test–retest reliability is good to excellent for the balance tests (tandem stance: percentage agreement = 52.6%; semi-tandem stance = 73.7%)[4] and usual walk speed tests (intraclass correlation coefficient (ICC) = 0.97),[5] and good-to-high for the sit to stand test (ICC = 0.81).[6]

Protocol summary

Conduct a physical performance battery that includes tests of balance, usual walk speed and functional leg strength.

Protocol

1 Follow the pre-exercise test procedures outlined in Appendix B.

2 Check Appendix C to ensure that there are no contraindications to exercise testing.

3 Instructions to the participants are shown in the text and should be delivered exactly as they are written in this script to enhance reliability of testing procedures (see Practical 1, Test accuracy, reliability and validity).

4 This functional test battery can be used as described or as single separate measures according to the needs of the situation. If you are performing all of the tests from the battery in one session, the tests should be performed in the order presented in this protocol.

1. Balance
The participant must be able to stand unassisted without the use of a cane or walker, although they may be assisted to get up out of the chair.

PERFORMING THE TEST
Deliver the following script.

'Now let's begin the evaluation. I would now like you to try to move your body in different movements. I will first describe and show each movement to you. Then I'd like you to try to do it. If you cannot do a particular movement, or if you feel it would be unsafe to try to do it, tell me and we'll move on to the next one. Let me emphasise that I do not want you to try to do any exercise that you feel might be unsafe. Do you have any questions before we begin?'

SEMI–TANDEM STAND

1 *'Now I will show you the first movement.'*

2 (Demonstrate) *'I want you to try to stand with the side of the heel of one foot touching the big toe of the other foot for 30 seconds. You can put either foot in front, whichever is more comfortable for you'* (Figure 15.1).

3 *'You may use your arms, bend your knees, or move your body to maintain your balance, but try not to move your feet. Try to hold this position until I tell you to stop.'*

4 Stand next to the participant to help them into the semi-tandem position.

5 Supply just enough support to the participant's arm to prevent loss of balance.

6 When the participant has their feet in the correct position, ask *'Are you ready?'*

7 Safely let go of the participant and begin timing after saying *'ready, begin'*.

8 Stop the stopwatch and say *'stop'* after 30 seconds, or when the participant steps out of position or grabs your arm.

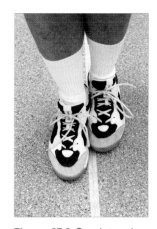

Figure 15.1 Semi-tandem stand test

9 If the participant is unable to hold the position for 30 seconds, allow the participant a second attempt at the test. If unable to hold the position for 30 seconds on the second attempt, record their best time to the nearest 0.1 of a second, stop the test and move on to the usual walk speed test.

TANDEM STAND

1 *'Now I will show you the second movement.'*

2 (Demonstrate) *'I want you to try to stand with the heel of one foot in front of and touching the toes of the other foot for 30 seconds. You may put either foot in front, whichever is more comfortable for you.'*

3 *'You may use your arms, bend your knees, or move your body to maintain your balance, but try not to move your feet. Try to hold this position until I tell you to stop.'*

4 Stand next to the participant to help them into the tandem position.

5 Supply just enough support to the participant's arm to prevent loss of balance (Figure 15.2).

6 When the participant has their feet in the correct position, ask *'Are you ready?'*

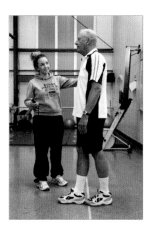

Figure 15.2 Tandem stand test

7 Safely let go of the participant and begin timing after saying, *'ready, begin'*.

8 Stop the stopwatch and say *'stop'* after 30 seconds or when the participant steps out of position or grabs your arm.

9 If the participant is unable to hold the position for 30 seconds, allow the participant a second attempt at the test.

10 If the participant is unable to hold the position for 30 seconds on the second attempt, record their best time to the nearest 0.1 of a second, stop the test and move on to the usual walk speed test.

SINGLE-LEG STAND

1 *'Now I will show you the third movement.'*

2 (Demonstrate) *'I want you to try to stand on one leg for 30 seconds. You may stand on either leg, whichever is more comfortable for you.'*

3 *'You may use your arms, bend your knees, or move your body to maintain your balance, but try not to drop your foot onto the floor or let it touch your standing leg. Try to hold this position until I tell you to stop.'*

4 Stand next to the participant to help them into the single-leg position.

5 Supply just enough support to the participant's arm to prevent loss of balance.

6 When the participant is in the correct position, ask *'Are you ready?'*

7 Safely let go of the participant and begin timing after saying, *'ready, begin'*.

8 Stop the stopwatch and say *'stop'* after 30 seconds or when the participant touches their second foot to the floor or to their standing leg, or grabs your arm.

9 If the participant if unable to hold the position for 30 seconds, allow the participant a second attempt at the test.

10 If the participant is unable to hold the position for 30 seconds on the second attempt, record their best time to the nearest 0.1 of a second, stop the test and move on to the usual walk speed test.

Data recording

Participant's name: _____   Date: _____

Age: _____ years   Sex: _____

Semi-tandem stand score:

Time held: _____._____ s

Not attempted   ☐

Tandem stand score

Time held: _____._____ s

Not attempted   ☐

Single-leg stand score

Time held: _____._____ s

Not attempted   ☐

Total balance test time: _____ (sum time from all three balance tests).

If the participant did not attempt a test mark the box that best describes why.

Participant not able to understand instructions   ☐

Participant refused   ☐

Not attempted, tester felt unsafe   ☐

Not attempted, participant felt unsafe   ☐

Other (specify): _____   ☐

2. Usual walk speed

1 Using brightly coloured masking tape, mark out a 5, 6, or 8 m distance on the ground.

> **Note:** The 8 m distance is the preferred option for this test. However, should space be limited, the 5 or 6 m course can be substituted for the 8 m course.

Then mark out clear perpendicular lines 1 m either side of the ends of coloured masking tape (i.e. if using an 8 m course, then there will be coloured masking tape at 0, 1, 7 and 8 m on the line).

> **Note:** 1 m is marked either side of the 6 m track to minimise the influence of reaction time, acceleration and deceleration.

2 If using timing lights, place the gates at the 1 m and 7 m marks (or at 0, 1, 7 and 8 m if using a four-gate system) and follow the manufacturer's instructions to establish connections to the gates, enter participant details, and select the appropriate multi-gate, single-direction testing protocol ready for testing.

3 'Now I am going to observe how you normally walk. If you use a cane or other walking aid and you feel you need it to walk a short distance, then you may use it.'

FIRST USUAL WALK SPEED TEST

1 'This is our walking course. I want you to walk to the other end of the course at your usual walking speed, just as if you were walking down the street to go to the shops.'

2 Demonstrate the walk for the participant.

3 'Walk all the way past the other end of the tape before you stop. I will walk with you. Do you feel this would be safe?'

4 Have the participant stand with both feet touching the starting line.

5 'When I want you to start, I will say ready, begin.' When the participant acknowledges this instruction say 'ready, begin'.

6 The participant walks the total distance of 8 m, but the tester times the middle 6 m (Figure 15.3). Start timing when the participant's toes first cross the 1 m mark and stop timing when one of the participant's feet is completely across the 7 m line.

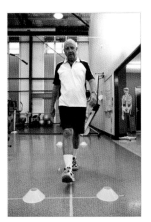

Figure 15.3 Usual walk speed test

7 If balance is an issue, walk directly behind and to the side of the participant to optimise safety.

8 Record the time taken to the nearest 0.1 of a second.

9 Allow ≥30 seconds rest.

SECOND USUAL WALK SPEED TEST

1. 'I want you to repeat the walk. Remember to walk at your usual pace, and go all the way past the other end of the course.'

2. Repeat stages 4 to 9 from the first usual walk speed test outlined above.

Data recording

Time for first usual walk speed test: _____._____ s

Time for second usual walk speed test: _____._____ s

Best usual walk speed score: _____._____ s

> **Note:** If only one walk was completed, record that time.

Usual walk speed = distance covered (m)/time taken (s)

= _____ / _____

= _____ m/s

continued

Data recording *(continued)*

Percentile (see Table 15.1): _____

For example, if the participant took 5.0 seconds to complete the 6 m course, the calculation would be $6 \div 5 = 1.2$ m/s.

If the participant did not attempt a test mark the box that best describes why.

Participant not able to understand instructions ☐

Participant refused ☐

Not attempted, tester felt unsafe ☐

Not attempted, participant felt unsafe ☐

Other (specify): _____ ☐

Walk aid used:

   None ☐

   Cane ☐

   Other (specify): _____ ☐

TABLE 15.1 Usual walk speed normative data (m/s)				
	FEMALES		**MALES**	
	70–79 years	**≥80 years**	**70–79 years**	**≥80 years**
Unable to complete (%)	3.2%	8.7%	3.3%	6.2%
10th percentile	0.3	0.2	0.4	0.3
25th percentile	0.5	0.4	0.5	0.4
50th percentile	0.6	0.5	0.7	0.6
75th percentile	0.8	0.6	0.8	0.7
90th percentile	0.9	0.8	1.0	0.8
Mean	0.5	0.4	0.6	0.5

Based on data from independent living, community-dwelling American adults aged 70–79 years (females = 2030; males = 1239) and ≥80 years (females = 1282; males = 546) of age
Adapted from: Guralnik et al[7]

3. Chair stand

This test is used to measure functional leg power and strength.

SINGLE CHAIR STAND

1 Equipment set-up: place a chair firmly against the wall to prevent it from tipping over. Check that the participant feels that it is safe to stand up from a chair without using their arms. *'Let's do the last movement test. Do you think it would be safe for you to try to stand up from a chair without using your arms?'*

2 If the participant answers no, this is the end of their test. Record the result and go to the scoring page.

3 'The next test measures the strength in your legs.'

4 Demonstrate and explain the procedure. 'First, fold your arms across your chest and sit so that your feet are flat on the floor; then stand up keeping your arms folded across your chest.'

5 Record the result.

6 If the participant cannot rise to a standing position while keeping their arms across their chest, say 'Okay, try to stand up using your arms' (Figure 15.4a–15.4c). This is the end of their test. Record the result and go to the scoring page.

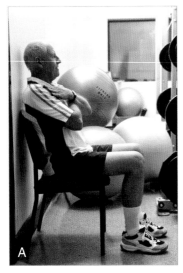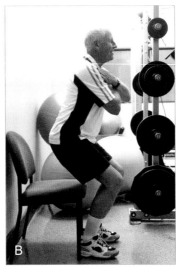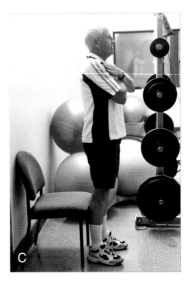

Figure 15.4 a: Start and finish position of the chair stand test. b and c: Performing the chair stand test.

7 If the participant can rise to a standing position without using their arms, continue to step 1 of the repeated chair stand test.

Data recording

Single chair stand score

Safe to stand without help	☐ Yes ☐ No
Participant stood without using arms	☐ go to repeated chair stand test
Participant used arms to stand	☐ end test
Test not completed	

REPEATED CHAIR STANDS

Note: Do not attempt the repeated chair stand test if the participant did not want to attempt the single chair stand, was not able to stand unassisted or had to use their arms in the single chair stand test.

1 First check with the participant; 'Do you think it would be safe for you to try to stand up from a chair five times without using your arms?'

2 Demonstrate and explain the procedure (Figure 15.4a–15.4c). 'Please stand up straight five times as quickly as you can, without stopping in between. After standing up each time, sit down and then stand up again. Keep your arms folded across your chest. Your back must touch the backrest every time you sit down. I'll be timing you with a stopwatch.'

3 When the participant is properly seated, say: 'ready, stand' and start the stopwatch.

4 Count out loud as the participant rises each time, up to five times.

5 Stop the test if:

   a the participant becomes short of breath during the repeated chair stands

   b the participant uses their arms to help them rise out of the chair

   c after 1 minute, if the participant has not completed the rises

   d at the tester's discretion, if concerned for the participant's safety.

6 If the participant stops and appears to be fatigued before completing the five stands, confirm this by asking, 'Can you continue?'

   a If the participant says 'yes', continue timing.

   b If the participant says 'no', stop the test.

7 When the participant has sat down with their back touching the backrest of the chair for the fifth time, stop the stopwatch.

8 Record the time taken to the nearest 0.1 of a second.

Data recording

Repeated chair stand score

1 Safe to stand five times   ☐ Yes   ☐ No

2 Time to complete five stands: _____._____ s

   a Participant unable to complete five chair stands   ☐

   b Participant fails to complete five stands in 60 s   ☐

If the participant did not attempt the test or failed to complete the test, mark the box that best explains why.

Participant not able to understand instructions   ☐

Participant refused   ☐

Not attempted, tester felt unsafe   ☐

Not attempted, participant felt unsafe   ☐

Participant could not hold the position unassisted   ☐

Participant tried but was unable to finish the test   ☐

Other (specify): _____   ☐

Interpretation

First, consider the four steps of interpretation outlined in Appendix G, and refer to Tables 15.2 and 15.3.[7,8]

The clinical implications for individuals who score poorly in these tests are that they may be at risk for falls and an inability to independently perform ADLs. The results of these standalone tests can also be used clinically to determine which physical function deficits should be targeted when prescribing exercise, as well as which safety-related precautions should be considered for the person.

Balance, usual walk speed and chair stand collectively, and independently, can predict poor outcomes in older individuals. Poorer performance on physical performance batteries, consistent with Tables 15.1–15.3, have been found to be associated with an increase in age- and sex-adjusted

TABLE 15.2 Repeated chair stand normative data (s)

	FEMALES		MALES	
	70–79 years	≥80 years	70–79 years	≥80 years
Unable to complete (%)	16.4%	35.2%	13.3%	27.6%
10th percentile	20.1	23.3	18.0	21.0
25th percentile	16.6	18.7	15.0	17.3
50th percentile	13.7	15.0	12.6	14.0
75th percentile	11.1	12.3	10.6	11.5
90th percentile	9.5	10.3	9.0	10.0
Mean	14.4	16.1	13.2	15.0

Based on data from independent living, community-dwelling American adults aged 70–79 years (females = 2033; males = 1239) and ≥80 years (females = 1287; males = 547) of age
Adapted from: Guralnik et al[7]

TABLE 15.3 Physical performance battery normative data

	BALANCE TEST (s)	USUAL WALK SPEED TEST (m/s)	CHAIR STAND TEST (s)
High risk	<53	<1.0	≥17
Not at high risk	≥53	≥1.0	<17

Based on data from 3024 well-functioning older persons aged 70–79 years (female = 52%). Risk refers to risk of persistent and severe functional limitation, future hospitalisation and premature mortality
Adapted from: Cesari et al[8]

mortality rate, with those in the 25th percentile having double the mortality rate of those in the 75th percentile.[7] Risk of all-cause mortality increases by 89% when comparing the lowest with the highest usual walking speed among older adults,[9] with improvements of as little as 0.1 m/s increasing survival across the full range of gait speeds.[10] Furthermore, usual walk speed has been shown to be an important predictor of mobility limitations, cognitive decline and institutionalisation in older adults,[11] while impaired balance and reduced lower limb muscle strength are also associated with increased falls risk[12] and mortality.

Activity 15.2 Floor rise to standing

AIMS: conduct the floor rise to standing test, interpret the results and provide feedback to a participant.

Background

The floor rise to standing test is designed to measure dynamic balance and leg strength through determining the ability to rise from a supine position to upright standing. The assessment of functional ability to rise from a supine position on the floor may provide information on an older adult's ability to regain standing posture following a fall without assistance in the home. This test has been shown to have a good test–retest reliability (ICC $=$ 0.87), excellent inter-tester reliability (ICC $=$ 0.99) in school-aged children[13] and good inter-tester reliability (ICC $=$ 0.73–1.00) for community-dwelling older adults.[14] A practical application for this test can be as a screening tool to assess readiness for independent living for adults living in the community.[14] The test may also help to identify which individuals would benefit from exercises that specifically aim to improve their ability to rise independently from the floor.

Protocol summary

The participant rises from the floor as fast as safely possible.

Protocol

This test involves a participant being willing and able to safely move from a standing to a lying position and back again. This can be a very difficult task for a frail individual, therefore carefully consider whether this test is appropriate for the participant. In addition, if the participant has low blood pressure they may experience orthostatic hypotension.

1 Follow the pre-exercise test procedures outlined in Appendix B.

2 Check Appendix C to ensure that there are no contraindications to exercise testing.

3 A high-density mat (e.g. exercise mat) should be used on a non-slip floor for this test.

4 If the participant uses a cane or walking aid to walk short distances then they may use it in this test; however, scores should not be compared with the normative data provided within this practical.

5 Position the participant (they may be assisted to assume this position if required) lying supine on the mat with their legs and feet together, arms by their side and palms face down against the mat (Figure 15.5).

6 Instruct the participant to 'Stand up as quickly as safely possible after I say 3, 2, 1, GO' (Figure 15.6).

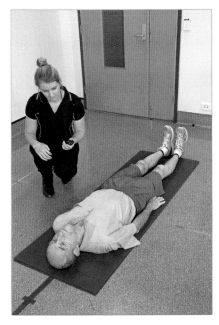

Figure 15.5 Floor to stand test start position

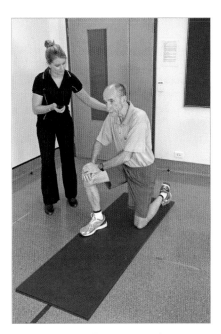

Figure 15.6 Performing the floor to stand test

7 Start the stopwatch after saying 'GO' and press stop when the participant has reached an upright standing position.

8 Complete three trials and record the time taken to the nearest 0.1 of a second.

9 Allow $\geq$30 seconds rest between trials.

10 Clean and disinfect all equipment (see Appendix A).

Data recording

Participant's name: _____ Date: _____

Age: _____ years   Sex: _____

Aid used: Yes/No   Details of aid used: _____

Participant was deemed safe to stand from the floor   ☐ Yes   ☐ No

Trial 1 time: _____._____ s   Trial 2 time: _____._____ s   Trial 3 time: _____._____ s

Best time: _____._____ s   Rating: _____

Aids used for floor to stand test:

None ☐

Wall ☐

Other (specify): _____ ☐

If participant did not attempt test or failed to complete the test, mark the box that best explains why.

Participant not able to understand instructions ☐

Participant refused ☐

Not attempted, tester felt unsafe ☐

Not attempted, participant felt unsafe ☐

Participant could not hold the position unassisted ☐

Participant tried but was unable to finish the test ☐

Other (specify): _____ ☐

Interpretation

First, consider the four steps of interpretation outlined in Appendix G, and refer to Table 15.4.

A poor performance on the floor rise to standing test may indicate insufficient muscle strength and future difficulty rising from the floor after sustaining a fall. The floor to rise test has shown to be a valid (concurrent) measure for screening physical disability, frailty and functional mobility.[14] Inability to rise independently without help during the test has shown to be able to discriminate between those with and without physical disabilities.[14] The inability to rise after a fall is one of the most common reasons emergency services are called to help people found helpless in their homes.[15] Although most of the falls associated with the inability to rise without help are not associated with serious injury, less than 50% of community-dwelling fallers are able to rise after a fall without assistance.[16]

TABLE 15.4 Floor rise to stand test normative data (s)

	FEMALES		MALES	
	60–69 years	70–80 years	60–69 years	70–80 years
Very poor	>5.1	>5.1	>3.1	>4.7
Poor	4.3–5.1	4.5–5.1	2.8–3.1	4.3–4.7
Average	3.8–4.3	4.1–4.5	2.6–2.8	3.5–4.3
Good	3.1–3.8	3.8–4.1	2.3–2.6	3.1–3.5
Excellent	<3.1	<3.8	<2.3	<3.1
Mean	4.1	4.5	2.7	4.0
Standard deviation	1.1	1.0	0.5	1.2
Minimum	2.2	3.2	1.3	2.0
Maximum	7.7	6.9	3.7	7.2

Based on data from 118 independent living, community-dwelling exercise study volunteers in Australia (females, $n = 35$). Very poor <20th percentile; poor = 21st–40th percentile; average = 41st–60th percentile; good = 61st–80th percentile; excellent >80th percentile

Activity 15.3 Functional forward reach

AIMS: conduct the functional forward reach test, interpret the results and provide feedback to a participant.

Background

The functional forward reach test is designed to measure dynamic balance[17] during voluntary movement. Functional reach is the maximal distance one can reach forwards beyond arm's length while maintaining a fixed base of support in the standing position. The functional forward reach test has high test–retest reliability, with an ICC of 0.81 and a coefficient of variation of 2.5%, measured across three different days.[18]

Protocol summary

The participant reaches as far forward as safely possible with the distance reached subtracted from the initial standing reach position.

Protocol

Equipment set-up

1 This test needs to be administered beside a wall that has a measuring tape positioned at the height of the subject's acromiale (the point on the superior aspect of the most lateral part of the acromion border) on the dominant arm.

2 Place an exercise mat in front of the participant as a safety precaution in case the participant loses balance and falls forwards.

> **Note:** Ensure the participant is not standing on the exercise mat as this will make the balance test more difficult.

Test

1 Follow the pre-exercise test procedures outlined in Appendix B.

2 Check Appendix C to ensure that there are no contraindications to exercise testing.

3 Demonstrate and explain the movement to the participant before asking them to attempt the test.

4 Instruct the participant to stand comfortably, to make a fist with their dominant arm and to raise their fist until it is parallel with the tape (Figure 15.7a).

5 Mark the position where the most distal aspect of the participant's third metacarpal is positioned along the measuring tape and record the distance to the nearest 0.1 of a cm.

6 Instruct the participant to 'Reach forward as far as safely possible without moving your feet or lifting your heels and without losing your balance. Keep your arm at the height of the tape and wrist straight as you reach forwards' (see Figure 15.7b).

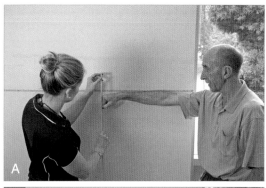

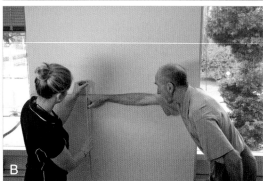

Figure 15.7 a: Forward reach test start position. b: Forward reach test finish position

7 If the participant loses their balance by raising their heels or taking a step, or if they touch the wall at any time during the manoeuvre, the test is invalid and must be repeated.

8 The participant may bend at the hips, however, their legs must remain straight at all times.

9 Provide encouragement to the participant and stand at a close distance to support the participant if they lose their balance.

10 Mark the point on the wall where the most distal aspect of the participant's third metacarpal travels to along the measuring tape.

11 The measured reach is the difference between where the third metacarpal is positioned at rest and where it is positioned at the end of the reach.

12 Complete three trials and record the measured reach to the nearest 0.1 of a cm.

13 Allow $\geq$30 seconds rest between trials.

Data recording

Participant's name: _____   Date: _____

Age: _____ years   Sex: _____

Trial 1: _____._____ cm   Trial 2: _____._____ cm   Trial 3: _____._____ cm

Best: _____._____ cm   Rating: _____

Interpretation

First, consider the four steps of interpretation outlined in Appendix G, and refer to Table 15.5.

This test provides a good indication of functional forward-reaching ability and the risk of falls in performing such tasks.[16,18] The odds ratio (OR) of falling twice for an older adult (aged 70–104 years) who is unable to reach (e.g. due to inability to stand without support) is 8.1, compared with an OR of 4.0 for an older adult who reaches 0.1–15.2 cm, and an OR of 2.0 for those who reach 15.3–25.4 cm.[19]

TABLE 15.5 Functional forward reach test normative data (cm)

	FEMALES		MALES	
	60–69 years	70–80 years	60–69 years	70–80 years
Very poor	<24.2	<26.0	<29.1	<26.2
Poor	24.2–28.6	26.0–28.2	29.1–32.4	26.2–31.5
Average	28.7–31.6	28.3–29.8	32.5–34.8	31.6–33.9
Good	31.7–33.9	29.9–32.7	34.9–38.4	34.0–36.7
Excellent	>33.9	>32.7	>38.4	>36.7
Mean	29.3	28.7	33.5	32.4
Standard deviation	5.3	4.8	5.2	5.8
Minimum	15.1	15.0	20.5	22.9
Maximum	38.2	35.9	43.8	44.4

Based on data from 118 independent living, community-dwelling exercise study volunteers in Australia (females, $n = 35$). Very poor <20th percentile; poor = 21st–40th percentile; average = 41st–60th percentile; good = 61st–80th percentile; excellent >80th percentile

Activity 15.4 Timed up and go test

AIMS: conduct the timed up and go test, interpret the results and provide feedback to a participant.

Background

The timed up and go test is designed to assess agility and dynamic balance, typically in elderly and/or frail individuals.[20] This test measures the participant's ability to rise from a chair, walk a short distance and change the direction of their walking, which are all important and common ADLs. The timed up and go test has an excellent test–retest reliability, with an ICC of 0.96 for time to complete the test in older adults.[21]

Protocol summary

The participant stands up from sitting in a chair, walks around a brightly coloured cone placed 3 m away and returns to a seated position in the chair.

Protocol

Course set-up

1 Place a chair firmly against the wall or support the chair firmly from behind to prevent it from tipping over.

2 Place a cone marker 3 m away, measured from the back of the cone to a point on the floor even with the front edge of the chair.

Test

1 Follow the pre-exercise test procedures outlined in Appendix B.

2 Check Appendix C to ensure that there are no contraindications to exercise testing.

3 Demonstrate and explain the test procedures to ensure correct form.

4 If the participant uses a cane or walking aid to walk short distances then they may use it in this test; however, scores should not be compared with the normative data provided within this practical.[22,23]

5 One practice trial is given before scoring the test.

6 Instruct the participant to sit in the middle of the chair with their:

   a back straight

   b feet flat on the floor

   c hands on their thighs

   d one foot slightly in front of the other foot

   e torso slightly leaning forwards (Figure 15.8).

7 On the signal 'GO' start the stopwatch as the participant gets up from the chair, walks around one side of the cone (Figure 15.9) and returns to sit down in the chair (Figure 15.8) as quickly and safely as possible.

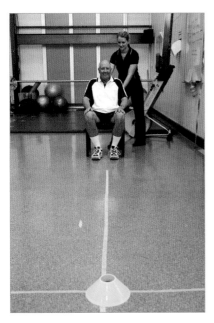

Figure 15.8 Timed up and go test start and finish position

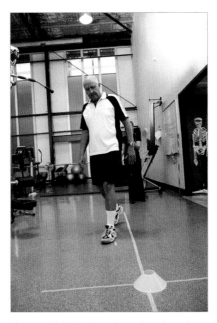

Figure 15.9 Navigating the timed up and go test course

8 Discontinue the test if the participant becomes short of breath.

9 When the participant returns and sits down on the chair, stop the stopwatch.

10 Record times to the nearest 0.1 of a second.

11 Complete two trials and record the time taken to the nearest 0.1 of a second.

12 Allow $\geq$30 seconds rest between trials.

Data recording

Participant's name: _____   Date: _____

Age: _____ years   Sex: _____

Walking aid used: Yes/No

Details of aid used: _____

Trial 1 time: _____._____ s   Trial 2 time: _____._____ s

Best: _____._____ s   Rating: _____

Interpretation

First, consider the four steps of interpretation outlined in Appendix G, and refer to Table 15.6.[24]

The clinical implications for this test are mixed. There is a significant association between the timed up and go test time and a history of falls, but the clinical relevance of this association is limited, as its ability to predict future falls is poor.[25] The limited predictive value of the timed up and go test may be explained by the fact that it is a single test which reflects a combination of power, balance and mobility. Therefore, it is recommended that the timed up and go test be used to detect differences in pre- to post-exercise testing, rather than as a risk factor for falling. Nonetheless, the transition from the sit to stand to walking is highly relevant to ADLs. Poor scores or problems performing components of this test can help to determine which exercises should be included in an exercise program for the individual.

TABLE 15.6 Timed up and go normative data (s)			
	60–69 YEARS	**70–79 YEARS**	**80–99 YEARS**
Very poor	<7.4	<8.0	<9.3
Poor	7.4–8.0	8.0–8.9	9.3–10.7
Average	8.1–8.3	9.0–9.7	10.8–11.8
Good	8.4–8.9	9.8–10.6	11.9–13.2
Excellent	>8.9	>10.6	>13.2
Mean	8.1	9.2	11.3

Based on data from 176 60–69-year-olds, 798 70–79-year-olds and 1102 80–99-year-olds across 21 studies. Very poor <20th percentile; poor = 20st–40th percentile; average = 41st–60th percentile; good = 61st–80th percentile; excellent >80th percentile
Adapted from: Bohannon[24]

Activity 15.5 Activities-specific Balance Confidence Scale (ABC-S)

AIMS: conduct the Activities-specific Balance Confidence Scale (ABC-S), interpret the results and provide feedback to a participant.

Background

The ABC-S test is designed to assess balance confidence.[26] Consistent with other standardised tests, the ABC-S is designed in such a way that the questions, conditions for administering, scoring procedures and interpretations are consistent and are administered and scored in a predetermined, standardised manner. This enables a more reliable comparison of outcomes across all questionnaire respondents. The ABC-S is a reliable measure for the assessment of balance confidence among community-dwelling older adults, with a high test-retest reliability ($r = 0.92$).[27,28]

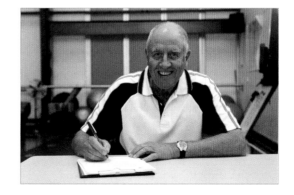

Protocol summary

The ABC-S requires respondents to self-rate their degree of confidence in their balance associated with the performance of ADLs.

Protocol

Respondents provide ratings on a 0–10 continuous scale based on the following cue question: *'How confident are you that you will not lose your balance or become unsteady when you* [list of items]' (Table 15.7).

TABLE 15.7 ABC-S test

How confident are you that you will not lose your balance or become unsteady when you …

1. walk around the house?

0	1	2	3	4	5	6	7	8	9	10
Not at all confident			Somewhat confident		Moderately confident		Quite confident		Completely confident	

2. walk up and down stairs?

0	1	2	3	4	5	6	7	8	9	10
Not at all confident			Somewhat confident		Moderately confident		Quite confident		Completely confident	

3. pick up a slipper from the floor?

0	1	2	3	4	5	6	7	8	9	10
Not at all confident			Somewhat confident		Moderately confident		Quite confident		Completely confident	

4. reach at eye level?

0	1	2	3	4	5	6	7	8	9	10
Not at all confident			Somewhat confident		Moderately confident		Quite confident		Completely confident	

5. reach while standing on your tip toes?

0	1	2	3	4	5	6	7	8	9	10
Not at all confident			Somewhat confident		Moderately confident		Quite confident		Completely confident	

6. stand on a chair to reach?

0	1	2	3	4	5	6	7	8	9	10
Not at all confident			Somewhat confident		Moderately confident		Quite confident		Completely confident	

7. sweep the floor?

0	1	2	3	4	5	6	7	8	9	10
Not at all confident			Somewhat confident		Moderately confident		Quite confident		Completely confident	

continued

TABLE 15.7 ABC–S test *(continued)*

8. walk outside to a nearby car?

0	1	2	3	4	5	6	7	8	9	10
Not at all confident			Somewhat confident		Moderately confident		Quite confident		Completely confident	

9. get in and out of a car?

0	1	2	3	4	5	6	7	8	9	10
Not at all confident			Somewhat confident		Moderately confident		Quite confident		Completely confident	

10. walk across a parking lot?

0	1	2	3	4	5	6	7	8	9	10
Not at all confident			Somewhat confident		Moderately confident		Quite confident		Completely confident	

11. walk up and down a ramp?

0	1	2	3	4	5	6	7	8	9	10
Not at all confident			Somewhat confident		Moderately confident		Quite confident		Completely confident	

12. walk in a crowded mall?

0	1	2	3	4	5	6	7	8	9	10
Not at all confident			Somewhat confident		Moderately confident		Quite confident		Completely confident	

13. walk in a crowd or get bumped?

0	1	2	3	4	5	6	7	8	9	10
Not at all confident			Somewhat confident		Moderately confident		Quite confident		Completely confident	

14. ride an escalator holding the rail?

0	1	2	3	4	5	6	7	8	9	10
Not at all confident			Somewhat confident		Moderately confident		Quite confident		Completely confident	

15. ride an escalator, while not holding the rail?

0	1	2	3	4	5	6	7	8	9	10
Not at all confident			Somewhat confident		Moderately confident		Quite confident		Completely confident	

16. walk on icy footpaths?

0	1	2	3	4	5	6	7	8	9	10
Not at all confident			Somewhat confident		Moderately confident		Quite confident		Completely confident	

Source: Powell and Myers[26]

Instructions to participants: for each of the following activities, please indicate your level of self-confidence by choosing a corresponding number from the scale of 1 (Not at all confident) to 10 (Completely confident).

Data analysis

The ABC-S is an 11-point scale and ratings should consist of whole numbers (0–10) for each item. The total rating is the sum of all 16 scores (possible range = 0–160). To calculate the ABC-S, divide the total rating by the number of scores provided (i.e. 16 if all 16 questions were answered) (Table 15.8). Item #16 may not be appropriate, depending on the location. If this item is not appropriate omit it and give the participant an ABC-S out of 150 (dividing the total rating by 15 to get their ABC-S).

TABLE 15.8 ABC-S normative data

ABC-S	LEVEL OF PHYSICAL FUNCTIONING
>8	High
5–8	Moderate
<5	Low

Source: Myers[29]

Data recording

Participant's name: _____   Date: _____

Age: _____ years   Sex: _____

Walking aid used: Yes/No   Details of aid used: _____

Total rating: _____

ABC-S rating: _____

Level of physical functioning: _____

Interpretation

First, consider the four steps of interpretation outlined in Appendix G, and refer to Table 15.8.

The ABC-S can distinguish between older adults at various levels of functional mobility.[29] ABC-S scores differentiate those at a low level of physical functioning (e.g. residents in high-care facilities) from those with moderate (e.g. residents in low-care facilities and/or with a chronic health condition) and high (e.g. physically active older adults) levels of functioning.[29] This makes the measure particularly well suited for identifying community-dwelling older adults who could benefit from a falls prevention exercise program such as those who are beginning to lose confidence in their balance and/or avoiding activity because of fear of falling.[30] If participants are classified as having a low or moderate level of functioning according to the ABC-S, then strategies to improve their balance confidence should be explored, such as balance training, exercise and rehabilitative therapies (e.g. standard physical therapy following hip or knee replacement).

Discussion and feedback

First, consider the three steps of feedback and discussion outlined in Appendix G. The main job of exercise professionals during exercise testing is to provide education and motivation before, during and after the test. This may include explaining and educating the participant on their condition and how exercise can help to prevent progression or even reverse decline of their functional capacity. A discussion should focus on what can be done to improve the participant's functional capacity. Part of this conversation should be explaining to the participant the wealth of high-quality evidence demonstrating that physical inactivity exacerbates deconditioning and physical decline with ageing, and that exercise, at any age, can improve physical function. Referral to the exercise guidelines will be helpful in this situation.

Specific feedback may vary considerably between testing sessions owing to the multitude of reasons for performing functional testing. Exercise professionals may provide participants with feedback indicating that they have an increased risk of future disability, or have very poor balance placing them at an increased risk of falls and fractures. Therefore, it is important to ensure that the discussion and feedback focus on the positives, yet remain honest. It is important to consider how the participant may handle feedback about poor test results and that the words selected to describe their results reflect this to ensure thoughtful and appropriate feedback is provided.

Case studies

Setting: You work in an exercise physiology clinic that specialises in exercise classes, one-on-one sessions and home visits for older adults. You are responsible for conducting the client's initial health assessment, which includes various functional performance measures. The results of these measures are used to prescribe an appropriate exercise program for the client's level of function. During the appointment you are expected to give feedback to the client on their results and also how those results will influence your choices as to which exercises will be prescribed for them.

Case Study 1

The client is a 76-year-old male who had right hip replacement surgery 10 months ago. He is an ex-rugby league player and reports that his hip still feels 'stiff'. He also feels that his poor balance is affecting his ability to garden and do general chores around his house. He is on blood pressure medication. You measure his resting blood pressure and heart rate and these are both normal. He lives alone and doesn't leave the house very much, other than to get the groceries. He was referred to you by his general practitioner for a muscle-strengthening program.

Task: Design an initial health assessment for this client, choosing from the battery of tests within this practical. Describe and justify the most important functional measure that you would include in this testing battery.

Within your practical session, partner with another student who will role-play the client to conduct this test. Interpret these results according to the four steps of interpretation outlined in Appendix G. Particular reference should be made to how this result will be used to design the client's exercise program.

TEST BATTERY:
Priority test

Name and describe the test:

_____

_____

_____

_____

continued overpage

Case studies *(continued)*

Justify the test, with specific reference to the case study:

Practise completing this test, including data recording and calculations as appropriate. Interpret the results and provide feedback:

How does your answer compare with the worked example provided in the Answers?

Case Study 2

The client is an 80-year-old female who is underweight and has osteoporosis. She has not done any structured exercise previously. She is worried that she sometimes loses her balance and doesn't know whether she will be able to get up if she falls down. She is currently taking calcium and vitamin D supplements. She lives with her husband, who is currently doing a resistance training program.

TASK

As part of a home visit, design a brief initial health assessment for this client, choosing from the battery of tests within this practical. Describe and justify the most important functional measure that you would include in this testing battery.

Within your practical session, partner with another student who will role play the client, to conduct this test. Interpret these results according to the four steps of interpretation outlined in Appendix G. Particular reference should be made to how this result will be used to design the client's exercise program.

TEST BATTERY:
Priority test

Name and describe the test:

continued

Case studies *(continued)*

Justify the test, with specific reference to the case study:

Practise completing this test, including data recording and calculations as appropriate. Interpret the results and provide feedback:

How does your answer compare with the worked example provided in the Answers section (p. 000)?

References

[1] Brach JS, Simonsick EM, Kritchevsky S, Yaffe K, Newman AB. The association between physical function and lifestyle activity and exercise in the health, aging and body composition study. J Am Geriatr Soc 2004;52(4):502–9.

[2] Lord SR, Ward JA, Williams P. Exercise effect on dynamic stability in older women: a randomized controlled trial. Arch Phys Med Rehabil 1996;77(3):232–6.

[3] Jones CJ, Rikli RE, Beam WC. A 30-s chair-stand test as a measure of lower body strength in community-residing older adults. Res Q Exerc Sport 1999;70(2):113–19.

[4] Ritchie C, Trost SG, Brown W, Armit C. Reliability and validity of physical fitness field tests for adults aged 55 to 70 years. J Sci Med Sport 2005;8(1):61–70.

[5] Goldberg A, Schepens S. Measurement error and minimum detectable change in 4-meter gait speed in older adults. Aging Clin Exp Res 2011;23(5-6):406–12.

[6] Bohannon RW. Test-retest reliability of the five-repetition sit-to-stand test: a systematic review of the literature involving adults. J Strength Cond Res 2011;25(11):3205–7.

[7] Guralnik JM, Simonsick EM, Ferrucci L, Glynn RJ, Berkman LF, Blazer DG, et al. A short physical performance battery assessing lower extremity function: association with self-reported disability and prediction of mortality and nursing home admission. J Gerontol 1994;49(2):M85–94.

[8] Cesari M, Kritchevsky SB, Newman AB, Simonsick EM, Harris TB, Penninx BW, et al. Added value of physical performance measures in predicting adverse health-related events: results from the Health, Aging And Body Composition Study. J Am Geriatr Soc 2009;57(2):251–9.

[9] Liu B, Hu X, Zhang Q, Fan Y, Li J, Zou R, et al. Usual walking speed and all-cause mortality risk in older people: a systematic review and meta-analysis. Gait Posture 2016;44:172–7.

[10] Studenski S, Perera S, Patel K, Rosano C, Faulkner K, Inzitari M, et al. Gait speed and survival in older adults. JAMA 2011;305(1):50–8.

[11] Abellan van Kan G, Rolland Y, Andrieu S, Bauer J, Beauchet O, Bonnefoy M, et al. Gait speed at usual pace as a predictor of adverse outcomes in community-dwelling older people an International Academy on Nutrition and Aging (IANA) Task Force. J Nutr Health Aging 2009;13(10):881–9.

[12] Lord SR, Ward JA, Williams P, Anstey KJ. Physiological factors associated with falls in older community-dwelling women. J Am Geriatr Soc 1994;42(10):1110–17.

[13] Weingarten G, Kaplan S. Reliability and validity of the timed floor to stand test-natural in school-aged children. Pediatr Phys Ther 2015;27(2):113–18.

[14] Ardali G, Brody LT, States RA, Godwin EM. Reliability and validity of the floor transfer test as a measure of readiness for independent living among older adults. J Geriatr Phys Ther 2019;42(3):136–47.

[15] Gurley RJ, Lum N, Sande M, Lo B, Katz MH. Persons found in their homes helpless or dead. N Engl J Med 1996;334(26):1710–16.

[16] Hofmeyer MR, Alexander NB, Nyquist LV, Medell JL, Koreishi A. Floor-rise strategy training in older adults. J Am Geriatr Soc 2002;50(10):1702–6.

[17] Taaffe DR, Duret C, Wheeler S, Marcus R. Once-weekly resistance exercise improves muscle strength and neuromuscular performance in older adults. J Am Geriatr Soc 1999;47(10):1208–14.

[18] Duncan PW, Weiner DK, Chandler J, Studenski S. Functional reach: a new clinical measure of balance. J Gerontol 1990;45(6):M192–7.

[19] Duncan PW, Studenski S, Chandler J, Prescott B. Functional reach: predictive validity in a sample of elderly male veterans. J Gerontol 1992;47(3):M93–8.

[20] Podsiadlo D, Richardson S. The timed "Up & Go": a test of basic functional mobility for frail elderly persons. J Am Geriatr Soc 1991;39(2):142–8.

[21] Smith E, Walsh L, Doyle J, Greene B, Blake C. The reliability of the quantitative timed up and go test (QTUG) measured over five consecutive days under single and dual-task conditions in community dwelling older adults. Gait Posture 2016;43:239–44.

[22] Galvao DA, Nosaka K, Taaffe DR, Spry N, Kristjanson LJ, McGuigan MR, et al. Resistance training and reduction of treatment side effects in prostate cancer patients. Med Sci Sports Exerc 2006;38(12):2045–52.

[23] Peiffer JJ, Galvao DA, Gibbs Z, Smith K, Turner D, Foster J, et al. Strength and functional characteristics of men and women 65 years and older. Rejuvenation Res 2010;13(1):75–82.

[24] Bohannon RW. Reference values for the timed up and go test: a descriptive meta-analysis. J Geriatr Phys Ther 2006;29(2):64–8.

[25] Barry E, Galvin R, Keogh C, Horgan F, Fahey T. Is the Timed Up and Go test a useful predictor of risk of falls in community dwelling older adults: a systematic review and meta-analysis. BMC Geriatr 2014;14:14.

[26] Powell LE, Myers AM. The Activities-specific Balance Confidence (ABC) Scale. J Gerontol A Biol Sci Med Sci 1995;50A(1):M28–34.

[27] Talley KM, Wyman JF, Gross CR. Psychometric properties of the activities-specific balance confidence scale and the survey of activities and fear of falling in older women. J Am Geriatr Soc 2008;56(2):328–33.

[28] Jorstad EC, Hauer K, Becker C, Lamb SE, ProFa NE Group. Measuring the psychological outcomes of falling: a systematic review. J Am Geriatr Soc 2005;53(3):501–10.

[29] Myers AM, Fletcher PC, Myers AH, Sherk W. Discriminative and evaluative properties of the activities-specific balance confidence (ABC) scale. J Gerontol A Biol Sci Med Sci 1998;53(4):M287–94.

[30] Myers AM, Powell LE, Maki BE, Holliday PJ, Brawley LR, Sherk W. Psychological indicators of balance confidence: relationship to actual and perceived abilities. J Gerontol A Biol Sci Med Sci 1996;51(1):M37–43.

PRACTICAL 16
EXERCISE CAPACITY

Jeff Coombes and Mia Schaumberg

LEARNING OBJECTIVES

- Understand the scientific rationale, purposes, reliability, validity, assumptions and limitations of common exercise capacity assessments
- Identify and explain the common terminology, processes and equipment required to conduct accurate and safe exercise capacity assessments
- Identify and describe contraindications or considerations that may require the modification of exercise capacity assessments, and make appropriate adjustments for relevant populations or participants
- Conduct appropriate pre-assessment procedures, including explaining the test, obtaining informed consent and a focused medical history, and performing a pre-exercise risk assessment
- Identify the need for guidance or further information from an appropriate health professional, and recognise when medical supervision is required before or during an exercise capacity assessment and when to cease a test
- Select and conduct appropriate exercise capacity assessments, including instructing clients on the correct use of equipment
- Record, analyse and interpret information from exercise capacity assessments and convey the results, including the validity and limitations, through relevant verbal and/or written communication with the participant or relevant professional

Equipment and other requirements

- Information sheet and informed consent form
- Adult Pre-exercise Screening System (APSS) form
- Measuring wheel/tape to measure up to 30 m
- 20 m multi-stage shuttle run test audio track (e.g. CD, digital track)
- Audio player (e.g. CD player, smartphone)
- Heart rate monitor set (e.g. transmitter, receiver, chest strap)
- Stopwatch
- Sphygmomanometer on stand with various size arm cuffs (with size indicators)
- Stethoscope and alcohol wipes
- Motorised programmable treadmill
- Masking tape
- A space (e.g. gymnasium) that allows participants to walk for 30 m in a straight line
- Mechanical counter and calculator

- 11 cones/markers and chairs
- Cleaning and disinfecting equipment (see Appendix A)

INTRODUCTION

Exercise capacity tests determine the aerobic endurance of an individual. They are used in clinical and sport settings as well as in schools. In rehabilitation programs they are commonly performed for assessing baseline aerobic fitness, monitoring progression through an exercise program, the response to a therapy or intervention and/or for an individual's prognosis.

Exercise capacity tests are sometimes preferred over submaximal or aerobic power ($\dot{V}O_2max$) tests because they usually require less expensive equipment, a less-skilled tester and are faster to administer. The tests generally use either. (1) self-paced activity (e.g. the 6-minute walk test, 6MWT) or (2) graded exercise, where intensity is progressively increased (e.g. the multi-stage shuttle run test, MSRT). The self-paced tests are viewed as submaximal as the participant will not usually reach their maximal heart rate. The maximal tests (i.e. graded exercise tests) are more likely to be reliable[1] and therefore a better measure of exercise capacity.

Generally, the goal of an exercise capacity test is to provide a strong aerobic physiological challenge, and walking/running induces the highest maximum metabolic rate compared with other exercise modes.[2] Exercise capacity tests are also more representative of activities of daily living (ADLs) than other tests (e.g. cardiorespiratory fitness tests). Most exercise capacity test protocols will attempt to bring the participant to the limit of exercise tolerance in around 10 minutes. This is based on recommendations from major international associations that this is an optimal time to complete a maximal test.[3]

Exercise capacity is a more powerful predictor of mortality than other established risk factors (e.g. hypertension, smoking and diabetes) for cardiovascular disease[4] and the change in exercise capacity is inversely related to all-cause mortality.[5] It is also an important factor that dictates how an individual can perform many ADLs including stair climbing, walking and participating in sport and leisure-time physical activities. When used for these purposes, exercise capacity tests may also be referred to as functional capacity tests. In some clinical situations, exercise capacity tests provide information that may be a better index of the participant's ability to perform daily activities than measures of aerobic power ($\dot{V}O_2max$); for example, the distance walked during the 6MWT is highly correlated with quality of life.[6]

It is well accepted that the protocol for an exercise capacity test should be appropriate for the participant. This practical contains four different walking/running tests; the first two have reference data for younger, fitter, more mobile individuals, whereas the final protocols are more likely to be used in clinical populations and include reference values for older adults.

DEFINITIONS

MET: or **m**etabolic **e**quivalent, is a measure of the energy cost of physical activities relative to the energy cost at rest. At rest it is convention that 1 MET of energy is expended, which is obtained by consuming 3.5 mL/kg/min of oxygen.

Cardiorespiratory fitness: ability of the circulatory and respiratory systems to supply oxygen and support the energy demands during sustained physical activity. Also known as aerobic fitness or aerobic endurance.

Exercise capacity: the maximum amount of physical exertion that a person can sustain (e.g. peak power output on a maximal cycle ergometer test or total distance covered during a treadmill graded exercise test).

Functional capacity: an individual's capacity to function in a specific situation. In an exercise test, the term functional capacity is usually synonymous with exercise capacity.

EXERCISE CAPACITY VS CARDIORESPIRATORY FITNESS/AEROBIC POWER/$\dot{V}O_2max$

In this manual we have defined exercise capacity in line with what the term implies – the physical capacity of an individual to complete an exercise task. The four activities in this practical were chosen to reflect three different ways this can be assessed: (1) the time to volitional exhaustion during a graded exercise test (e.g. multi-stage shuttle run test or BSU/Bruce treadmill test) or (2) the maximal distance travelled over a period of time (e.g. walking for 6 minutes) or (3) the quickest time to complete a set distance (walking 400 m). Therefore, an exercise capacity test will usually provide a single measure (power, time or distance). Importantly, this value reflects the integrated response of the physiological (cardiovascular, pulmonary and neuromuscular) and psychological (motivational) aspects of the participant.

The value from an exercise capacity test is commonly converted to reflect estimated cardiorespiratory fitness/aerobic power/$\dot{V}O_2$max using metabolic equations. However, students should understand that a cardiorespiratory fitness/aerobic power/$\dot{V}O_2$max test is primarily assessing the maximal cardiovascular and pulmonary responses and therefore, strictly speaking, the terms/tests should not be used interchangeably with exercise capacity. However, many older key publications in the field of exercise science still swap between the terms (cardiorespiratory fitness/aerobic power/$\dot{V}O_2$max/exercise capacity) when describing the process of conducting an exercise capacity test and then using the time/distance/work rate to calculate an estimated $\dot{V}O_2$max.[7,8]

The use of an exercise capacity value to estimate $\dot{V}O_2$max has previously occurred in large epidemiological studies, where the direct assessment of aerobic power/cardiorespiratory fitness may have been problematic owing to a lack of resources. Indeed, our early knowledge of the strong positive association between cardiorespiratory fitness and health outcomes gained during the 1970s–1990s was from an estimate of $\dot{V}O_2$max from an exercise capacity test (time to volitional exhaustion during a graded exercise test).[9] This is likely to be one of the reasons why the terms exercise capacity and cardiorespiratory fitness continue to be readily interchanged. It is recommended that more care be taken with the use of these terms so they reflect the type of test used.

METABOLIC EQUIVALENT (MET)

The ongoing use of exercise capacity data to estimate cardiorespiratory fitness/aerobic power/$\dot{V}O_2$max is facilitated by the use of the term/unit 'MET'. The 'MET' was developed to more easily understand measures of cardiorespiratory fitness/aerobic power/$\dot{V}O_2$max (e.g. 7 METs is easier to understand than 24.5 mL/kg/min). The common approach to calculate a MET value for an individual is to have them complete an exercise capacity test (e.g. BSU/Bruce treadmill test) and convert the work rate achieved at test completion (i.e. grade and speed) into a $\dot{V}O_2$ value by using a metabolic equation specific to the exercise mode and the individual. This is then converted to METs by dividing by 3.5 (e.g. 17.5 mL/kg/min = 5 METs). This approach has a number of limitations including the assumptions that the metabolic equations are valid for each individual and that a participant has a resting metabolic rate of 3.5 mL/kg/min.

ASSUMPTIONS AND LIMITATIONS

The assumptions and limitations for exercise capacity tests vary depending on whether they are self-paced (e.g. 6MWT) or use a graded exercise test to volitional exhaustion (e.g. MSRT). For self-paced tests a major assumption is that participants have paced themselves such that they are able to complete the maximal distance possible, which requires skill. It has been found that the repeatability of time-trial tests is lower than that of time-to-volitional exhaustion tests.[10] This indicates that factors such as lack of motivation may be more dramatic and influential on performance during a time-to-volitional exhaustion protocol compared with a time-trial test. For a graded exercise test it is assumed that the participant is exhausted at the end of the test and is unable to complete any further work, which requires significant psychological motivation. To overcome these potential limitations, it has been suggested that testers conduct two tests (separated by a suitable recovery period to ensure that fatigue is not a performance-limiting factor) and use the first test as a familiarisation trial.[11] However, this will often be too resource intensive for the testing site and too onerous for the participant.

An exercise capacity test does not provide specific information on the function or contribution of the physiological systems, as can be obtained from an exercise stress test or a $\dot{V}O_2$max test. For this reason, in most clinical situations, information from exercise capacity tests should be seen as complementary to more physiologically investigative assessments.

A limitation of some exercise capacity tests (e.g. 6MWT) is that they have a low test ceiling (i.e. distances vary little in those with normal or high fitness).[12]

VALIDITY AND RELIABILITY

Validity (concurrent) refers to the ability of the exercise capacity test to measure the maximal distance/duration a participant is able to complete during an endurance exercise task. Validity relies on consistent test and pre-test procedures (e.g. standardised instructions in relation to prior physical activity, caffeine and food intake, and behaviour during the test; see Practical 1, Test accuracy, reliability and validity). As an example, during a treadmill test to volitional exhaustion to determine 'time on test', if the participant is allowed to hold onto the handrails this will probably increase the time on test as their upper body strength will then be an influencing factor and stronger individuals may be able to support some of their body mass for longer than weaker individuals. Appendix B provides pre-test procedures, including instructions to the participant, that should be adhered to for all tests. Strong standardised verbal encouragement (e.g. set script) towards the end of the test will also improve the validity of tests where the participant is attempting to exercise to volitional exhaustion (e.g. MSRT, BSU/Bruce treadmill test). Accuracy will be improved if two tests are conducted (separated by a suitable recovery period to minimise the effect of fatigue on performance) and the first test used as a familiarisation trial.[11] However, as mentioned earlier, this is usually not feasible.

Given that many exercise capacity tests are used to estimate cardiorespiratory fitness/aerobic power/$\dot{V}O_2$max, it is common to see this comparison made when assessing concurrent validity. As mentioned above, these should be acknowledged as different, albeit related, measures, with $\dot{V}O_2$max representing a physiological measure (when a plateau in oxygen consumption is obtained) and exercise capacity representing an integrated response of physiological and psychological inputs. However, the comparison between the two provides useful data regarding the ability of an exercise test to estimate an established marker of health and aerobic performance. A discussion of the studies that have compared the different exercise capacity tests in the following activities with measured $\dot{V}O_2$max are provided in each activity.

The reliability of exercise capacity tests is usually assessed by participants completing the same test on two or more separate occasions. As discussed earlier, the reliability of exercise tests is complicated because most exercise capacity tests will be affected by a previous attempt that has familiarised the participant (e.g. to pacing). Some of the factors that affect the concurrent validity will also impact on the reliability of an exercise capacity test such as participant preparation, test specificity and behaviour during the test. Other factors that fall into this category include tester-related variability. This is affected by attention to detail replicating the test protocol, including timing of measures and uniformity of the instructions and/or encouragement provided to the participant. Specific data on the reliability of the selected tests is provided in their respective backgrounds.

Activity 16.1 Multi-stage shuttle run test (MSRT)

AIMS: conduct the MSRT, interpret the results and provide feedback to a participant.

Background

The MSRT, also known as the beep test, is a graded exercise test (GXT) to volitional exhaustion that requires well-motivated participants with some knowledge of pacing strategies. It is a popular and simple test for the simultaneous measurement of exercise capacity in a large group of participants. The MSRT can be administered in a relatively small space indoors or outdoors and is therefore practical for schools or sporting teams without extensive facilities or resources. It was first described in 1988 as a method of estimating $\dot{V}O_2$max using a regression equation.[13]

Accuracy
The accuracy of the MSRT will depend on:

- consistent test and pre-test procedures
- accurately measuring the 20 m course
- verifying the audio recording speed (likely that you will not be able to calibrate/adjust), although the use of digital and modern electronic devices has improved timing accuracy
- stopping a participant after they have failed to reach the line in two successive shuttle attempts.

Reliability
The reliability of the MSRT has been widely investigated in children, adolescents and young adults; however, there is little investigation into MSRT reliability in adults over the age of 30 years.[14] The MSRT has good reliability; in 42 trained male military personnel the test–retest correlation was strong

$(r = 0.95-0.96)$,[14] which is similar to previously published studies in adults. In another study, 35 active young men and women completed 3 MSRT trials.[15] The mean difference in estimated $\dot{V}O_2$max between trial 1 and 2 was -1.1 ± 4.7 mL/kg/min; however, the mean difference between trial 2 and 3 was 0.0 ± 5.0 mL/kg/min. There was an increase in performance from trial 1 to 2, but no mean difference between trials 2 and 3, reflecting the effect of familiarisation on the reliability of MSRT performance.

MSRT to estimate $\dot{V}O_2$max

Numerous equations have been developed to estimate $\dot{V}O_2$max from MSRT performance, all with strengths and limitations. Most studies report a moderate-to-high correlation between MSRT performance and $\dot{V}O_2$max[16] and good reliability.[17] Most notably, prediction equations have been determined from specific populations and therefore may not be applicable to varied population groups. Additionally, whether true maximal capacity during testing was attained is often poorly recorded within studies, limiting the concurrent validity of equations.[14] Therefore, to maximise validity of estimated $\dot{V}O_2$ max from the MSRT, it is important to choose an equation derived from a similar population to that being tested.

Protocol summary

The test involves continuously moving between two lines 20 m apart.

Protocol

The test should ideally be conducted indoors (to avoid environmental influences) on a flat, even, non-slip surface.

1 Follow the pre-exercise test procedures outlined in Appendix B.

2 Check Appendix C to ensure that there are no contraindications to exercise testing.

3 Fit a heart rate monitor (see Practical 3, Cardiovascular health).

4 Obtain a baseline heart rate and blood pressure immediately before exercise (see Practical 3). The baseline blood pressure is used to determine whether the participant has exceeded the criteria for a contraindication to exercise (see Appendix C).

5 Measure a 20 m runway and mark clearly with cones. The test area should be at least 22 m long to provide a safe turning zone at each end of the shuttle. If testing multiple participants, ensure there is at least 1 m between participants on the starting line.

6 Have the participant(s) complete an appropriate warm-up prior to the test. This will depend on the age, experience and fitness of the individual.

7 When ready, instruct the participant(s) to stand behind the line.

8 During the test the participant(s) should be encouraged not to talk as this may influence the test result; however, for safety purposes, it may be appropriate to check how the participant is feeling using 'yes/no' questioning.

9 Start the audio track and have the participant(s) listen to the instructions.

10 When instructed by the audio track commentator, the participant(s) should start slowly jogging towards the line 20 m away.

11 When instructed by the audio track recorded 'beep' the participant(s) should turn efficiently and jog back to the start line.

12 Participant(s) should continue jogging/running between the two lines, turning when instructed by the audio signals (beeps). At least one foot must be placed over the line to complete the shuttle.

13 If the line is reached before the beep sounds, ensure participant(s) wait until the sound is heard before moving back in the other direction, but emphasise to participant(s) that they should attempt to pace themselves so that arrival at the other end coincides with each beep.

14 Every minute, three distinct beeps sound, indicating completion of that level and subsequent increase in frequency of beeps for the next minute of shuttles, and therefore the running/jogging speed required. The first running/jogging speed is known as 'level 1', the second as 'level 2' and so on. The test can go to a maximum of 'level 23'.

15 If the line is not reached in time for the beep, a participant must continue to run to the line (i.e. not turn early), change direction and try to catch up with the pace before the next beep.

16 The test is terminated when a participant fails to reach the line in the time allotted (by the beep) in two consecutive shuttle attempts.

17 During the test it may be necessary to prematurely stop the test – see Appendix F for more detail and criteria.

18 Obtain the maximal heart rate immediately on completion of the test.

19 The values for the last successfully completed level and number of shuttles are recorded (e.g. level 8 shuttle 5, or 8/5).

20 Ensure that participants complete an appropriate cool-down (e.g. slower walking or jogging).

21 Add the category from Table 16.1 to the data-recording sheet.

22 Clean and disinfect all equipment (see Appendix A).

TABLE 16.1 MSRT reference data		
	FEMALES (LEVEL/SHUTTLE)	**MALES (LEVEL/SHUTTLE)**
Very poor	$<5/6$	$<7/5$
Poor	$5/6-6/8$	$7/5-8/7$
Average	$6/9-7/9$	$8/8-9/8$
Good	$7/10-9/2$	$9/9-11/3$
Excellent	$>9/2$	$>11/3$

Suitable for participants aged 20–29 years
Very poor $<$20th percentile; poor = 21st–40th percentile; average = 41st–60th percentile; good = 61st–80th percentile; excellent $>$80th percentile
Source: based on calculated estimates of $\dot{V}O_2$max from the test[13] and the American College of Sports Medicine guidelines[7]

Data recording

Participant's name: _____ Date: _____

Age: _____ years   Sex: _____

Baseline HR: _____ bpm   Baseline BP: _____ mmHg

Last successfully completed level/shuttle: _____ / _____   Category: _____

Maximal HR: _____ bpm

Interpretation

First, consider the four steps of interpretation outlined in Appendix G. Table 16.1 provides reference values for the MSRT. There is controversy regarding the highest ever score on the MSRT with reports that individuals have completed all 23 stages, likely due to errors in marking the correct distance. The Australian Football League (AFL) used to test all future hopeful players on the MSRT as part of their fitness testing prior to the draft. In 2013, Billy Hartung set a new record of 16/6 that remained until the test was replaced with the yo-yo test in 2017.

Interpreting the MSRT value requires considering the purpose of the test. For example, if the aim was to determine the aerobic capacity of an athlete involved in a sport that required high levels of endurance and the participant did not score highly, this would lead to a discussion about implementing a training program to improve the value.

Activity 16.2 BSU/Bruce treadmill test

AIMS: conduct the Ball State University (BSU)/Bruce treadmill test, interpret the results and provide feedback to a participant.

Background

For graded (incremental) exercise testing it is important to have linear increases in work rate during the protocol.[18] The BSU/Bruce treadmill test[19] (Table 16.2) was developed at Ball State University (BSU) from the Bruce protocol[20] (see Practical 10, $\dot{V}O_2$max) to overcome the relatively large and uneven increments in work rate of the Bruce protocol. The speed and grade settings for the last 20 seconds of each 3-minute segment of the BSU/Bruce protocol are identical to those of the Bruce protocol (e.g. at 3 minutes, 2.7 kph with a 10% grade). When using a treadmill protocol such as the BSU/Bruce as an exercise capacity test, either the time on the test or the highest estimated MET value achieved during the test is the main outcome measure. The estimated MET value may be calculated by using an equation[21] and is often used for its convenience and wide use in cardiology.

TABLE 16.2 BSU/Bruce treadmill protocol							
INCREMENT	TIME (min)	SPEED (km/h)	GRADE (%)	INCREMENT	TIME (min)	SPEED (km/h)	GRADE (%)
1	0:00	1.7	0.0	33	10:40	4.0	15.2
2	0:20	1.7	1.3	34	11:00	4.1	15.4
3	0:40	1.7	2.5	35	11:20	4.2	15.6
4	1:00	1.7	3.7	36[a]	11:40	4.2	16.0
5	1:20	1.7	5.0	37	12:00	4.3	16.2
6	1:40	1.7	6.2	38	12:20	4.4	16.4
7	2:00	1.7	7.5	39	12:40	4.5	16.6
8	2:20	1.7	8.7	40	13:00	4.6	16.8
9[a]	2:40	1.7	10.0	41	13:20	4.7	17.0
10	3:00	1.8	10.2	42	13:40	4.8	17.2

continued overpage

TABLE 16.2 BSU/Bruce treadmill protocol *(continued)*

INCREMENT	TIME (min)	SPEED (km/h)	GRADE (%)	INCREMENT	TIME (min)	SPEED (km/h)	GRADE (%)
11	3:20	1.9	10.2	43	14:00	4.9	17.4
12	3:40	2.0	10.5	44	14:20	5.0	17.6
13	4:00	2.1	10.7	45[a]	14:40	5.0	18.0
14	4:20	2.2	10.9	46	15:00	5.1	18.0
15	4:40	2.3	11.2	47	15:20	5.1	18.5
16	5:00	2.4	11.2	48	15:40	5.2	18.5
17	5:20	2.5	11.6	49	16:00	5.2	19.0
18[a]	5:40	2.5	12.0	50	16:20	5.3	19.0
19	6:00	2.6	12.2	51	16:40	5.3	19.5
20	6:20	2.7	12.4	52	17:00	5.4	19.5
21	6:40	2.8	12.7	53	17:20	5.4	20.0
22	7:00	2.9	12.9	54[a]	17:40	5.5	20.0
23	7:20	3.0	13.1	55	18:00	5.6	20.0
24	7:40	3.1	13.4	56	18:20	5.6	20.5
25	8:00	3.2	13.6	57	18:40	5.7	20.5
26	8:20	3.3	13.8	58	19:00	5.7	21.0
27[a]	8:40	3.4	14.0	59	19:20	5.8	21.0
28	9:00	3.5	14.2	60	19:40	5.8	21.5
29	9:20	3.6	14.4	61	20:00	5.9	21.5
30	9:40	3.7	14.6	62	20:20	5.9	22.0
31	10:00	3.8	14.8	63[a]	20:40	6.0	22.0
32	10:20	3.9	15.0				

[a] At these time points the time, speed and grade are the same as the standard Bruce protocol[20]

Accuracy

The accuracy of the test will depend on (1) accurately measuring the time on test and then (2) estimating METs from this value. The accuracy will be primarily affected by whether the participant has followed the pre-test directions and follows instructions during the test (e.g. no continuous holding the hand rails). Strong verbal encouragement towards the end of the test will also improve the accuracy of this aspect of the test.

The validity of the test to estimate METs will depend on the metabolic equations used to convert the time on test to a MET value. This activity will use equations recently developed from the FRIEND registry that have been shown to be more valid than the commonly used ACSM equations.[21]

Reliability

It appears that the reliability of the BSU/Bruce test has not been assessed. Other treadmill graded exercise tests have been evaluated by participants completing two separate attempts. The coefficient of variation for the Harvard Fitness Test protocol has been shown to be very high ($r = 0.95$), with a standard error of the measurement of 2.4% of the overall mean, indicating very good reliability.[1]

BSU/Bruce treadmill test to estimate $\dot{V}O_2$max

In the study that developed the BSU/Bruce treadmill test, the estimated $\dot{V}O_2$max had a standard error of the estimate of 3.4 mL/kg/min compared with directly measured $\dot{V}O_2$max.[19]

Protocol summary

The protocol begins with an intensity of around 2 METs and then increases in speed and/or grade (around 0.3 METs) every 20 seconds.

Protocol

1. Follow the pre-exercise test procedures outlined in Appendix B.

2. Check Appendix C to ensure that there are no contraindications to exercise testing.

3. Fit a heart rate monitor (see Practical 3, Cardiovascular health).

4. Program the treadmill with the BSU/Bruce protocol.

5. A warm-up is not generally used for this test.

6. Obtain a baseline heart rate and blood pressure immediately before exercise (see Practical 3). The baseline blood pressure is used to determine whether the participant has exceeded the criteria for a contraindication to exercise (see Appendix C).

7. Provide treadmill safety precautions to the participant (see Appendix D). An assessment of their ability to walk/jog safely should be conducted prior to starting the test.

8. Provide details of the test, including the protocol, hand signals the participant can use during the test, explanation of the rating of perceived exertion (RPE) (see Appendix E), test termination and safety (see Appendix F).

9. Start a stopwatch when the participant reaches the speed of increment 1.

10. During the test, provide strong verbal encouragement to exercise to volitional exhaustion.

11. When the participant indicates they are close to stopping, they should be encouraged to complete the interval they are currently on. If they are just about to finish an interval then they should be encouraged to complete another (20 seconds).

12. Continuous handrail support is not allowed during the protocol, but permitted for a few seconds if balance is compromised. It is encouraged when they start and stop the test.

13. During the test it may be necessary to prematurely stop the test (see Appendix F).

14. Record the time of the protocol to the nearest second (e.g. 9 minutes 22 seconds).

15. Obtain the maximal heart rate immediately on completion of the test.

16. Record whether the person was walking or running at the end of the test on the data-recording sheet. This will be useful for follow-up testing of the same participant.

17. Slow the treadmill and lower the grade and ensure that the participant completes an appropriate cool-down (e.g. slower walking or jogging) after the test. For older/less fit individuals, monitoring heart rate recovery will help to determine the length of the cool-down.

18. From the time on test, add the category from Table 16.3.

19. Clean and disinfect all equipment (see Appendix A).

TABLE 16.3 Categories based on time (minutes) on the BSU/Bruce treadmill test

	FEMALES	MALES
Very poor	<9.4	<11.6
Poor	9.4–10.9	11.6–12.5
Average	11.0–12.2	12.6–13.2
Good	12.3–13.4	13.3–14.7
Excellent	>13.4	>14.7

Suitable for participants aged 20–29 years. Very poor $<$20th percentile; poor = 21st–40th percentile; average = 41st–60th percentile; good = 61st–80th percentile; excellent $>$80th percentile
Note: 30 seconds = 0.5
Source: based on data from Kaminsky et al 1998[19] and the American College of Sports Medicine guidelines[7]

Data analysis

Calculate the estimated MET value from the grade and speed of the last completed increment using the following equation.[21]

$$\dot{V}O_2max\ (mL/kg/min) = speed \times (0.17 + fractional\ grade \times 0.79) + 3.5$$

speed in m/min where 1 km/h = 16.7 m/min

grade in % expressed as a decimal

Data recording

Participant's name: _____   Date: _____

Age: _____ years   Sex: _____   Body mass: _____kg

Baseline HR: _____bpm   Baseline BP: _____mmHg

Time on test: _____ minutes _____ seconds   Category: _____

Last full stage completed: Speed _____km/h

Maximal HR: _____bpm   Circle: Walking/running

Estimated METs achieved: _____METs

Interpretation

First, consider the four steps of interpretation outlined in Appendix G. Feedback should be provided on both the time on test category and the estimated METs. A value of $\leq$5 METs has been used as a cut-off value for categorising 'low' fitness. There is strong evidence that values in this range are highly associated with an increased risk of poor health outcomes.[4] Indeed, the relative risk of death from any cause is 4.5 times greater for those with an exercise capacity of $<$5 METs compared with those $>$8 METs.[4]

Activity 16.3 6-minute walk test (6MWT)

AIMS: conduct the 6MWT, interpret the results and provide feedback to a participant.

Background

The 6MWT is one of the most common clinical exercise tests. It is widely used in cardiac, pulmonary and musculoskeletal rehabilitation settings as it is relatively safe, well tolerated and easy to administer and interpret.[22] The test measures the distance an individual can quickly walk in 6 minutes (6MWD), while self-pacing. As most participants will not achieve a maximal heart rate during the 6MWT the test is considered submaximal. Because the majority of ADLs are performed at submaximal levels of exertion, the 6MWD may better reflect an exercise capacity for daily physical activities. More than one person can be tested at a time by staggering the starting time (e.g. by 10 seconds) and encouraging participants to walk at their own pace and not in clusters. Electrocardiography (ECG) monitoring is not routinely done with this test, which limits its prognostic validity. The protocol below is from the American Thoracic Society.[23]

Accuracy

The accuracy of the 6MWT will depend on:

- consistent test and pre-test procedures
- accurately measuring the distance covered
- the level of encouragement provided (as the 6MWT is self-paced, motivational factors will impact the distance covered).[24]

Using the average-of-two or best-of-two walk distances increases the precision of the measure and makes it more comparable with $\dot{V}O_2max$ values.[25]

Reliability

As mentioned previously, assessing the reliability of submaximal exercise capacity tests is complicated by the impact of a previous attempt that gives the participant experience in pacing. However, studies investigating the reliability of the 6MWT have generally found it to be reliable when performed twice on subsequent days (intra-class correlations of around 0.90).[26,27] However, a second 6MWT will usually have the participant walk on average 5%–10% further. Indeed, one study that conducted two 6MWT on 337 participants with chronic heart failure found that 40% of them walked around 40 m (10%) further during the second test on a subsequent day.[26] This is considered to be a clinically significant improvement and highlights how conducting a single 6MWT may affect accurate clinical decision making. Interestingly, substantial agreement was found between the two 6MWTs for the proportion of patients with a poor 6MWD (<300 m).[26] This suggests that, if the aim is to identify patients with a poor 6MWD, one test may be enough.

6MWT to estimate $\dot{V}O_2max$

The correlation between the 6MWD and $\dot{V}O_2max$ has been reported to be between 0.5 and -0.6.[28,29] Although an equation has been developed to predict $\dot{V}O_2max$ from the 6MWT, the study authors state that it has limited usefulness for individual patients.[30] This is because of random, inherent, within-participant measurement errors associated with both tests. Instead, the equation should be used to estimate mean $\dot{V}O_2max$ among groups of patients. It will not be used in the following activity.

Protocol summary

The test involves walking continuously (up and back) around a 60 m circuit on a flat, even, non-slip surface with the aim to cover as much ground as safely possible in 6 minutes.

Protocol

As it is likely the participant will not be an older individual in a learning environment, role-playing feedback between students during practice is suggested.

Course set-up

1 The walking course should be 30 m in length so that one lap (out and back) is 60 m (Figure 16.1).

2 Using masking tape, mark the starting line and turning point, 30 m apart.

3 Coloured cones ($n = 11$) should then be placed on these marks and at 3 m intervals.

4 Position chairs at several points along the outside of the walking area in case the participant needs to rest during the test.

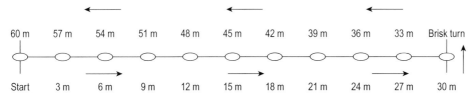

Figure 16.1 6-minute walk test course diagram

Test

1 Follow the pre-exercise test procedures outlined in Appendix B.

2 Check Appendix C to ensure that there are no contraindications to exercise testing.

3 Fit a heart rate monitor (see Practical 3, Cardiovascular health).

4 Obtain baseline heart rate and blood pressure immediately before exercise (see Practical 3). The baseline blood pressure is used to determine whether the participant has exceeded the criteria for a contraindication to exercise (see Appendix C).

5 A warm-up is not generally used for this test.

6 Older and/or less fit individuals should rest seated in a chair located near the starting position for at least 10 minutes before the test starts.

7 During the test the participant should be encouraged not to talk as this may influence the test result; however, for safety purposes, it may be appropriate to check how the participant is feeling using 'yes/no' questioning.

8 A script similar to the following text is advised to be used to ensure test accuracy:

   'The objective of this test is to walk as far as possible for 6 minutes. You will walk back and forth in this hallway/space. Six minutes is a long time to walk, so you will be exerting yourself. You will probably get out of breath or become exhausted. You are permitted to slow down, to stop and to rest as necessary. You may lean against the wall/chair while resting, but resume walking as soon as you are able. You will be walking back and forth around the furthest cones. You should pivot briskly around the cones and continue back the other way without hesitation. Now I'm going to show you. Please watch the way I turn without hesitation.'[23]

9 Demonstrate by walking one lap yourself.

10 Explain and demonstrate to the participant to always walk completely around the turning cones (at each end). When doing this, position the participant close to a turning cone and demonstrate the turn by quickly walking around the cone. Reinforce that they are to avoid walking over the cones and should continue walking in a non-stop fashion at each end.

11 When you have finished instructions and demonstrating use a script similar to the following:

'Are you ready to do that? I am going to use a counter to keep track of the number of laps you complete. I will click it each time you turn around at this starting line. Remember that the objective is to walk AS FAR AS POSSIBLE for 6 minutes, but don't run or jog. Start when I say go.'

12 Ask the participant to stand behind the start marker with a foot close to the start line and ask them if they have any questions.

13 Say *'GO'* and start the stopwatch when the participant begins walking.

14 To keep track of the distance walked, use a mechanical lap counter, or mark the counter on the data-recording sheet each time a lap is completed.

15 If the participant stops and/or rests, the stopwatch keeps running.

16 The tester should encourage participants by using the following standardised statements.

1st minute: 'You are doing well. You have 5 minutes to go.'

2nd minute: 'Keep up the good work. You have 4 minutes to go.'

3rd minute: 'You are doing well. You are halfway done.'

4th minute: 'Keep up the good work. You have only 2 minutes left.'

5th minute: 'You are doing well. You have only 1 minute to go.'

17 Do not use other words of encouragement (or body language) during the test.

18 During the test it may be necessary to prematurely stop the test – see Appendix F for more detail and criteria.

19 When the 6 minutes have elapsed, note the exact point on the floor where the participant finished, and inform them that the test is complete.

20 Obtain the peak[a] heart rate at the end of the test.

21 Ensure that the participant completes an appropriate cool-down (e.g. slower walking) after the test. For older/less fit individuals, monitoring heart rate recovery will help to determine the length of the cool-down.

22 Record the distance walked (each lap walked represents 60 m), using the cones and tape measure or measuring wheel to measure the exact distance from where the participant completed the test.

23 Complete the data analysis by adding the category from Table 16.4.[31]

TABLE 16.4 Reference data (6MWD in metres) for the 6MWT

	FEMALES				MALES			
	40–49 YEARS	50–59 YEARS	60–69 YEARS	70–80 YEARS	40–49 YEARS	50–59 YEARS	60–69 YEARS	70–80 YEARS
Very poor	<494	<474	<468	<424	<515	<482	<444	<405
Poor	494–544	474–512	468–508	424–463	515–571	482–532	444–522	405–457
Below average	545–632	513–590	509–562	464–519	572–638	533–613	523–575	458–513
Above average	633–697	591–665	563–627	520–581	639–699	614–682	576–626	514–571
Excellent	>697	>665	>627	>581	>699	>682	>626	>571

Very poor <20th percentile; poor = 21st–40th percentile; average = 41st–60th percentile; good = 61st–80th percentile; excellent >80th percentile
6MWD = 6-minute walk distance; 6MWT = 6-minute walk test
Source: based on data from independent living, community-dwelling men ($n = 238$) and women ($n = 207$) from seven countries in three continents.[31] They were healthy with no history of chronic disease that could influence their exercise capacity and were active but not involved in any competitive sport

---

[a] As this is recognised as a submaximal test, 'peak' heart rate is used instead of 'maximal' heart rate.

24 Ensure that all equipment (e.g. heart rate monitor, stethoscope earpieces) is cleaned and disinfected (see section on 'Laboratory safety, cleaning and disinfection' at the beginning of this manual).

Data recording

Participant's name: _____   Date: _____

Age: _____ years   Sex: _____

Baseline HR: _____ bpm   Baseline BP: _____ mmHg

Lap counter:

1	2	3	4	5	6	7	8	9	10	11	12	13	14
15	16	17	18	19	20	21	22	23	24	25	26	27	28

6MWD: _____ metres   Peak heart rate: _____ bpm

Interpretation

First, consider the four steps of interpretation outlined in Appendix G. A distance walked of less than 350 m is associated with increased mortality in patients with chronic obstructive pulmonary disease, chronic heart failure and pulmonary arterial hypertension.[32] Table 16.4 contains reference data for individuals aged 40–80 years.

Activity 16.4 Long-distance corridor walk (LDCW)

AIMS: conduct the long-distance corridor walk, interpret the results and provide feedback to a participant.

Background

The LDCW was designed to overcome potential limitations of the self-paced 6MWT (low test ceiling, strong influence of participant motivation, and steep learning effects).[33,34] The test aims to increase total work rate, allow for practice and provide a reference pace from which participants can increase their performance by adding a warm-up walk and using a target distance (400 m) rather than time.[33] Because distance can be visualised, it is seen to be more motivating than time and, unlike time-based tests, the faster a person walks the sooner they are finished.[33] The developers of the test found that using a distance goal encouraged older persons to work closer to their maximum effort compared with having them walk for 6 minutes over the same course.[33]

Accuracy

The accuracy of the LDCW will depend on:

- consistent test and pre-test procedures
- accurate measurement of the course distance
- the delivery of the LDCW, including following the test script and ensuring that the participant follows instructions with regards to starting and stopping at appropriate times.

Reliability

The LDCW was found to have excellent reliability when it was assessed in 66 healthy middle-aged women. From two visits, participants completed the walk in 248 and 245 seconds, respectively (intraclass correlation coefficient (ICC) = 0.95).[35]

LDCW to estimate $\dot{V}O_2$max

Performance on extended walking tests of varying times and distances has been shown to be strongly related to directly measured oxygen consumption.[30] The correlation between the 400 m time and the measured $\dot{V}O_2$max of -0.8[33] is higher than that found for 6MWD (around -0.5 to -0.6).[28,29] An estimating equation that includes the 400 m time, whether the participant has a long or short stride and their systolic blood pressure at the end of the test improved the correlation to -0.87, explaining 76% of the variance in $\dot{V}O_2$max.[33] This equation will not be used in the following activity.

Protocol summary

This is a two-stage self-paced walking test. Stage 1 is a 2-minute walk; stage 2 is a 400 m walk.

Protocol

Course set-up

1 Measure out a 20 m course and place 2 coloured cones at the beginning and end of the course.

   a Using masking tape, mark the starting line and turning point, 20 m apart.

   b Coloured cones ($n = 11$) should then be placed at 2 m intervals.

   c Position chairs at several points along the outside of the walking area in case the participant needs to rest during the test.

Test

1 Follow the pre-exercise test procedures outlined in Appendix B.

2 Check Appendix C to ensure that there are no contraindications to exercise testing.

3 Fit a heart rate monitor (see Practical 3, Cardiovascular health).

4 Obtain resting heart rate and blood pressure immediately before exercise (see Practical 3). The resting blood pressure is used to determine whether the participant has exceeded the criteria for a contraindication to exercise (see Appendix C).

5 A warm-up is not generally used for this test.

6 Older and/or less fit individuals should rest seated in a chair located near the starting position for at least 10 minutes before the test starts.

7 During the test the participant should be encouraged not to talk as this may influence the test result; however, for safety purposes, it may be appropriate to check how the participant is feeling using 'yes/no' questioning.

8 Demonstrate by walking one lap yourself.

9 Explain and demonstrate to the participant to always walk completely around the turning cones (at each end). When doing this, position the participant close to a turning cone and demonstrate the turn by quickly walking around the cone. Reinforce that they are to avoid walking over the cones and should continue walking in a non-stop fashion at each end.

Stage 1

1 The first stage of this test is a 2-minute walk in which the participant is instructed to walk to the first marker, around and back, in a continuous loop, covering as much ground as possible at a pace they can maintain for 2 minutes.

2 Ask the participant to stand behind the start marker with a foot close to the start line.

3 Ask whether the participant has any questions.

4 Say *'go'* and start the stopwatch when the participant begins walking.

5 To keep note of the distance walked, use a mechanical lap counter or mark the counter on the data-recording sheet each time a lap is completed.

6 The tester should encourage participants by using the following standardised statements:

'You have 30 seconds to go.'

'10 seconds to go.'

7 If it is necessary to prematurely stop the test, see Appendix F for more detail and criteria.

8 At the end of the 2 minutes instruct the participant to *'stop and stay where you are'*.

9 Record their heart rate and the distance covered (each lap walked is 40 m) on the data-recording sheet. Use the tape measure or measuring wheel to get the exact distance from the last marker to where the participant stopped.

10 Within 30 seconds of test completion bring the participant back to the starting marker for stage 2.

Stage 2

1 Explain to the participant that the 400 m walk is a timed test and that they should try to complete the distance in the shortest possible time at a pace they feel that they can safely sustain for the 10 laps.

2 Participants should be instructed to walk (not run) 10 laps of the course, explaining that a lap is recorded when the participant walks from the initial marker, completely around the second marker, and back to the initial marker (40 m).

3 Inform the participant that you will count out loud as they complete the laps.

4 Ask the participant to stand behind the start marker with a foot close to the start line.

5 Ask if the participant has any questions.

6 During the test the participant should be encouraged not to talk as this may influence the test result; however, for safety purposes, it may be appropriate to check how the participant is feeling using 'yes/no' questioning.

7 Exactly 1 minute following stage 1, say *'GO'* and start the stopwatch.

8 The tester should encourage participants by using the following standardised statements.

2 laps completed: *'You are doing well. You have 8 laps to go.'*

4 laps completed: *'Keep up the good work. You have 6 laps to go.'*

6 laps completed: *'You are doing well. You have 4 laps to go.'*

8 laps completed: *'Keep up the good work. You only have 2 laps to go.'*

9 If it is necessary to prematurely stop the test, see Appendix F for more detail and criteria.

10 Stop the stopwatch at the end of the 10th lap and record the time in seconds along with their peak heart rate.

11 Ensure the participant completes an appropriate cool-down (e.g. slower walking) after the test. For older/less fit individuals monitoring heart rate recovery will help to determine the length of the cool-down.

12 Complete the data analysis by adding the category from Table 16.5.[36,37]

13 Ensure that all equipment (e.g. heart rate monitor, stethoscope ear pieces) is cleaned and disinfected (see section on 'Laboratory safety, cleaning and disinfection' at the beginning of this manual).

TABLE 16.5 Reference data for the time (seconds) to complete the 400 m long-distance corridor walk

	FEMALES		MALES	
	60–69 years	70–80 years	60–69 years	70–80 years
Very poor	>282.9	>285.1	>234.7	>267.7
Poor	258.9–282.9	277.7–285.1	226.8–234.7	243.1–267.7
Average	250.0–258.8	255.3–277.6	216.2–226.7	233.7–243.0
Good	236.6–249.9	243.9–255.2	206.1–216.1	214.0–233.6
Excellent	<236.6	<243.9	<206.1	<214.0
Mean	258.4	265.3	224.7	241.4
Standard deviation	26.1	20.6	26.6	26.2
Minimum	206.1	231.9	178.9	205.0
Maximum	327.2	302.7	313.8	288.5

Very poor <20th percentile; poor = 21st–40th percentile; average = 41st–60th percentile; good = 61st–80th percentile; excellent >80th percentile
Source: Based on data from 118 independent living, community-dwelling exercise study volunteers in Australia (females, n = 35)[36,37]

Data recording

Participant's name: _____ Date: _____

Age: _____ years   Sex: _____

Baseline HR: _____bpm   Baseline BP: _____mmHg

Stage 1:

Lap counter:

1   2   3   4   5   6   7   8   9   10   11   12   13   14

Distance: _____ metres   HR at stage completion: _____bpm

Stage 2:

Time: _____ s   HR at stage completion: _____bpm

Category: _____

Interpretation

First, consider the four steps of interpretation outlined in Appendix G. In a large cohort of well-functioning community-based older adults, an inability to walk 400 m was associated with a higher risk of mortality and cardiovascular disease.[38] Among those able to complete 400 m, each extra minute to complete the test was associated with a 29% higher rate of mortality and a 20% higher rate of cardiovascular disease.[38] Table 16.5 contains reference data for individuals aged 60–80 years.

Feedback and discussion

First, consider the three steps of feedback and discussion outlined in Appendix G. Feedback regarding exercise capacity tests should include more than just stating the result and relevant descriptor or population norm. If a participant has a value that is below average, you should inform them of the important relationship between low exercise capacity and increased risk of poor health and premature death.[39] A discussion should focus on what can be done to improve the participant's exercise capacity, as feedback should always be constructive. Referring to exercise guidelines will be helpful in this situation. Similarly, if a participant has a good or high value, they should be encouraged to maintain what they are doing, and the relationship between good exercise capacity and health- and mortality-related outcomes should be reiterated.

When constructing feedback, it is important to consider *why* the exercise capacity test was performed, and tailor the feedback to address this reason. It is also important to consider what exercise capacity means to the participant in relation to their specific goals and why exercise capacity is important for achieving these goals. An example of this could be providing feedback to a sports team on their exercise capacity, and relating results to their sporting performance, their training level and their season goals. Information regarding mortality and morbidity is highly unlikely to be relevant to their health status, goals or the reason they are completing the test. In contrast, a patient with heart failure completing the LDCW to determine their exercise capacity following a cardiac rehabilitation program will probably be most interested in information about how their result relates to their long-term health outcomes.

In the case of clinical populations, it may be necessary to provide feedback on exercise capacity test results to both the patient and their medical practitioner. Consider what information is relevant to each party, but ensure both the client and the practitioner receive the same message regarding your interpretation of the test results, to minimise confusion. Consider, within the provision of feedback, whether this has been a re-test and, if so, compare the result with the participant's previous assessment. If this is an initial test, consider how much change is realistic within an allotted time frame, and suggest options for completing a re-test to assess change over time.

A practical implication of an exercise capacity test is that the prescription of aerobic exercise intensity can be based on data from the test. For example, if a person has a maximal heart rate of 170 bpm during the test and you wish them to be prescribed moderate-intensity aerobic exercise (64%–76% HRmax) then the target heart rate zone would be between 109 and 129 bpm.

Case studies

Case Study 1

Setting: You work as a sports scientist for a female AFL football team and one of your tasks is to monitor the fitness of the players. You use the multi-stage run test (MSRT) as a measure of the players' exercise capacity. At the start of pre-season training a new player to the club scores a level/shuttle of 8/2.

Task: What questions would you ask the player and what feedback would you provide?

Case Study 2

Setting: You work as an Accredited Exercise Scientist in a health and fitness centre. People joining the centre have the option of performing a fitness test that includes the BSU/Bruce treadmill exercise capacity test. You are responsible for administering the test and providing feedback to the clients.

continued

Case studies *(continued)*

The following data are collected during a test.

Participant: *Tamara*   Age: *21* yrs.   Sex: *Female*

Resting HR: *72* bpm   Resting BP: *114/76* mmHg

Time on test: *11* minutes *20* seconds   Category: _____

Last full stage completed: Speed *4.1* km/h   Grade: *15.4* %

Maximal HR: *194* bpm   Walking/Running

Estimated METs achieved: _____ METs

Task: Provide the category and calculate the estimated METs and the feedback you would give.

Case Study 3

Setting: You work as an Accredited Exercise Physiologist in a cardiac rehabilitation clinic. You use the 6MWT as a measure of the exercise capacity in the clinic's clients. A 65-year-old female client with heart failure walks for 520 m during the 6MWT.

Task: Provide the category and the feedback you would give.

Case Study 4

Setting: You work as an Accredited Exercise Physiologist in a residential aged care facility. You use the LDCW as a measure of the exercise capacity of the facility's clients. A 75-year-old male client completes the 400 m walk in 3 minutes and 40 seconds.

Task: Provide the category and the feedback you would give.

References

[1] Taylor HL, Buskirk E, Henschel A. Maximal oxygen intake as an objective measure of cardio-respiratory performance. J Appl Physiol 1955;8:73–80.

[2] Balke B, Ware RW. An experimental study of physical fitness of air force personnel. US Armed Forces Med J 1959;10:675–88.

[3] Gibbons RJ, Balady GJ, Bricker JT, Chaitman BR, Fletcher GF, Froelicher VF, et al; American College of Cardiology/American Heart Association Task Force on Practice Guidelines. Committee to Update the Exercise Testing G. ACC/AHA 2002 guideline update for exercise testing: summary article. A report of the American College of Cardiology/American Heart Association task force on practice guidelines (committee to update the 1997 exercise testing guidelines). J Am Coll Cardiol 2002;40:1531–40.

[4] Myers J, Prakash M, Froelicher V, Do D, Partington S, Atwood JE. Exercise capacity and mortality among men referred for exercise testing. N Engl J Med 2002;346:793–801.

[5] Brawner CA, Al-Mallah MH, Ehrman JK, Qureshi WT, Blaha MJ, Keteyian SJ. Change in maximal exercise capacity is associated with survival in men and women. Mayo Clin Proc 2017;92:383–90.

[6] Guyatt GH, Townsend M, Keller J, Singer J, Nogradi S. Measuring functional status in chronic lung disease: conclusions from a randomized control trial. Respir Med 1991;85 (Suppl B):17–21.

[7] American College of Sports Medicine. ACSM's guidelines for exercise testing and prescription, 10th ed. Baltimore, MD: Lippincott, Williams and Wilkins; 2018.

[8] Ross R, Blair SN, Arena R, Church TS, Despres JP, Franklin BA, et al; American Heart Association Physical Activity Committee of the Council on L, Cardiometabolic H, Council on Clinical C, Council on E, Prevention, Council on C, Stroke N, Council on Functional G, Translational B, Stroke C. Importance of assessing cardiorespiratory fitness in clinical practice: a case for fitness as a clinical vital sign: a scientific statement from the American Heart Association. Circulation 2016;134:e653–99.

[9] Wei M, Kampert JB, Barlow CE, Nichaman MZ, Gibbons LW, Paffenbarger RS Jr, et al. Relationship between low cardiorespiratory fitness and mortality in normal-weight, overweight, and obese men. JAMA 1999;282:1547–53.

[10] Laursen PB, Francis GT, Abbiss CR, Newton MJ, Nosaka K. Reliability of time-to-exhaustion versus time-trial running tests in runners. Med Sci Sports Exerc 2007;39:1374–9.

[11] Fletcher GF, Balady GJ, Amsterdam EA, Chaitman B, Eckel R, Fleg J, et al. Exercise standards for testing and training: A statement for healthcare professionals from the American Heart Association. Circulation 2001;104:1694–1740.

[12] Lipkin DP, Scriven AJ, Crake T, Poole-Wilson PA. Six minute walking test for assessing exercise capacity in chronic heart failure. Br Med J 1986;292:653–5.

[13] Leger LA, Mercier D, Gadoury C, Lambert J. The multistage 20 metre shuttle run test for aerobic fitness. J Sports Sc. 1988;6:93–101.

[14] Aandstad A, Holme I, Berntsen S, Anderssen SA. Validity and reliability of the 20 meter shuttle run test in military personnel. Mil Med 2011;176:513–18.

[15] Lamb KL, Rogers L. A re-appraisal of the reliability of the 20 m multi-stage shuttle run test. Eur J Appl Physiol 2007;100:287–92.

[16] Mayorga-Vega D, Aguilar-Soto P, Viciana J. Criterion-related validity of the 20-m shuttle run test for estimating cardiorespiratory fitness: a meta-analysis. J Sports Sci Med 2015;14:536–47.

[17] Artero EG, Espana-Romero V, Castro-Pinero J, Ortega FB, Suni J, Castillo-Garzon MJ, et al. Reliability of field-based fitness tests in youth. Int J Sports Med 2011;32:159–69.

[18] Hansen JE, Sue DY, Oren A, Wasserman K. Relation of oxygen uptake to work rate in normal men and men with circulatory disorders. Am J Cardiol 1987;59:669–74.

[19] Kaminsky LA, Whaley MH. Evaluation of a new standardized ramp protocol: the BSU/Bruce ramp protocol. J Cardiopulm Rehabil 1998;18:438–44.

[20] Bruce RA, Kusumi F, Hosmer D. Maximal oxygen intake and nomographic assessment of functional aerobic impairment in cardiovascular disease. Am Heart J 1973;85:546–62.

[21] Kokkinos P, Kaminsky LA, Arena R, Zhang J, Myers J. New generalized equation for predicting maximal oxygen uptake (from the fitness registry and the importance of exercise national database). Am J Cardiol 2017;120:688–92.

[22] Solway S, Brooks D, Lacasse Y, Thomas S. A qualitative systematic overview of the measurement properties of functional walk tests used in the cardiorespiratory domain. Chest 2001;119:256–70.

[23] American Thoracic Society Committee on Proficiency Standards for Clinical Pulmonary Function Laboratories. ATS statement: guidelines for the six-minute walk test. Am J Respir Crit Care Med 2002;166:111–17.

[24] Harada ND, Chiu V, Stewart AL. Mobility-related function in older adults: Assessment with a 6-minute walk test. Arch Phys Med Rehabil 1999;80:837–41.

[25] Chandra D, Wise RA, Kulkarni HS, Benzo RP, Criner G, Make B, et al. Optimizing the 6-min walk test as a measure of exercise capacity in COPD. Chest 2012;142:1545–52.

[26] Uszko-Lencer N, Mesquita R, Janssen E, Werter C, Brunner-La Rocca HP, et al. Reliability, construct validity and determinants of 6-minute walk test performance in patients with chronic heart failure. Int J Cardiol 2017;240:285–90.

[27] Cahalin L, Pappagianopoulos P, Prevost S, Wain J, Ginns L. The relationship of the 6-min walk test to maximal oxygen consumption in transplant candidates with end-stage lung disease. Chest 1995;108:452–9.

[28] Peeters P, Mets T. The 6-minute walk as an appropriate exercise test in elderly patients with chronic heart failure. J Gerontol A Biol Sci Med Sci 1996;51:M147–51.

[29] Alexander NB, Dengel DR, Olson RJ, Krajewski KM. Oxygen-uptake ($\dot{V}O_2$) kinetics and functional mobility performance in impaired older adults. J Gerontol A Biol Sci Med Sci 2003;58:734–9.

[30] Ross RM, Murthy JN, Wollak ID, Jackson AS. The six minute walk test accurately estimates mean peak oxygen uptake. BMC Pulm Med 2010;10:31.

[31] Casanova C, Celli BR, Barria P, Casas A, Cote C, de Torres JP, et al; Six Minute Walk Distance P. The 6-min walk distance in healthy subjects: reference standards from seven countries. Eur Respir J 2011;37:150–6.

[32] Rasekaba T, Lee AL, Naughton MT, Williams TJ, Holland AE. The six-minute walk test: A useful metric for the cardiopulmonary patient. Intern Med J 2009;39:495–501.

[33] Simonsick EM, Montgomery PS, Newman AB, Bauer DC, Harris T. Measuring fitness in healthy older adults: The health ABC long distance corridor walk. J Am Geriatr Soc 2001;49:1544–8.

[34] Swinburn CR, Wakefield JM, Jones PW. Performance, ventilation, and oxygen consumption in three different types of exercise test in patients with chronic obstructive lung disease. Thorax 1985;40:581–6.

[35] Pettee Gabriel KK, Rankin RL, Lee C, Charlton ME, Swan PD, Ainsworth BE. Test-retest reliability and validity of the 400-meter walk test in healthy, middle-aged women. J Phys Act Health 2010;7:649–57.

[36] Galvao DA, Taaffe DR. Resistance exercise dosage in older adults: Single- versus multiset effects on physical performance and body composition. J Am Geriatr Soc 2005;53:2090–7.

[37] Henwood TR, Taaffe DR. Short-term resistance training and the older adult: The effect of varied programmes for the enhancement of muscle strength and functional performance. Clin Physiol Funct Imaging 2006;26:305–13.

[38] Newman AB, Simonsick EM, Naydeck BL, Boudreau RM, Kritchevsky SB, Nevitt MC, et al. Association of long-distance corridor walk performance with mortality, cardiovascular disease, mobility limitation, and disability. JAMA 2006;295:2018–26.

[39] Blair SN, Kampert JB, Kohl HW 3rd, Barlow CE, Macera CA, Paffenbarger RS Jr, et al. Influences of cardiorespiratory fitness and other precursors on cardiovascular disease and all-cause mortality in men and women. JAMA 1996;276:205–10.

PRACTICAL 17
PULMONARY FUNCTION

Troy J Cross, Norm Morris, Surendran Sabapathy, Jeff Coombes and Tina Skinner

LEARNING OBJECTIVES

- Explain the scientific rationale, purposes, reliability, validity, assumptions and limitations of spirometry testing
- Identify and explain the common terminology, processes and equipment required to conduct accurate and safe spirometry tests
- Identify and describe considerations that may require the modification of spirometry tests, and make appropriate adjustments for relevant populations or participants
- Describe the principles and rationale for the calibration of equipment commonly used for spirometry testing
- Conduct appropriate pre-assessment procedures, including explaining the test
- Identify the need for guidance or further information from an appropriate health professional
- Perform forced vital capacity manoeuvre and peak expiratory flow rate tests using an electronic spirometer and peak flow meter
- Perform maximal inspiratory and expiratory pressure tests
- Identify the patterns of change in spirometry for obstructive, restrictive and mixed obstructive-restrictive disorders
- Become familiar with the hallmark changes in pulmonary function associated with three types of upper airways obstruction
- Record, analyse and interpret information from spirometry tests and convey the results, including the validity and limitations of the assessments, through relevant verbal and/or written communication to a participant

Equipment and other requirements

- Information sheet and informed consent form
- Electronic spirometer
- Disposable mouth pieces (**Note**: given the difficulty that some participants may experience with sealing their lips around a straight rubber hose section, the flanged mouthpiece is almost always preferred)
- Peak flow meter
- Hand-held respiratory pressure meter
- Cleaning and disinfecting equipment (see Appendix A)

461

INTRODUCTION

Spirometry is the most commonly performed component of pulmonary or lung function testing. Spirometric tests assess the capacity and effectiveness of an individual's ability to move air in and out of the lungs. Airflow and volume are the two key spirometry indices. Spirometry provides important information that can aid in the identification and management of respiratory diseases (as well as other diseases that may impact upon lung function and pulmonary gas exchange). This practical provides an applied guide to the measurement and interpretation of lung function, with a specific focus on spirometry.

PARAMETERS OF LUNG FUNCTION

Lung volumes and capacities

Lung function is typically assessed in terms of *static* and *dynamic* volumes. *Static* measurements are largely unaffected by the degree of participant effort, and do not change appreciably over short periods of time in the absence of respiratory disease. In contrast, indices of *dynamic* lung function are heavily dependent on correct participant technique and appropriate effort. These parameters describe how lung volume changes over a given period of time (i.e. motion of the lungs or respiratory airflow). Static and dynamic lung volumes are typically reported in litres (L), and changes in lung volume with respect to time reported in litres per second (L/s). Figure 17.1 displays a volume–time plot of a healthy individual during quiet breathing at rest, followed by a complete inspiration and maximal expiration.

The change in volume occurring between the beginning and end of inspiration (or expiration) is the tidal volume (V_T). This volume is noted in Figure 17.1 as the peak-to-peak amplitude while breathing at rest. The volume of air remaining in the lungs at the end of a normal tidal expiration represents an individual's functional residual capacity (FRC).

When an individual voluntarily inflates their lungs to the greatest volume achievable (i.e. until 'no more air can get in'), the volume recorded at the end of this effort represents total lung capacity (TLC; $@t = 10$ s in Figure 17.1). Conversely, when an individual exhales until 'no more air can get out' ($@t = 10-16$ s), a residual component of air remains inside the airspaces of the lungs: the residual volume (RV). The change in exhaled volume between TLC and RV represents the individual's vital capacity (VC). These lung volumes (TLC, FRC and RV) are often considered *static* because they are not determined by how 'fast' or 'slow' an individual breathes. Abnormal static lung volumes are indicative of alterations in the elastic properties of the lung and chest wall, typically occurring

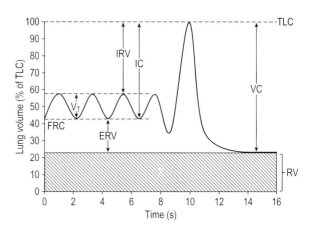

Figure 17.1 Volume–time tracing of an individual breathing at rest, followed by a complete inspiration and maximal expiration.
ERV = expiratory reserve volume; FRC = functional residual capacity; IC = inspiratory capacity; IRV = inspiratory reserve volume; RV = residual volume; TLC = total lung capacity; VC = vital capacity; V_T = tidal volume

Source: Troy J Cross, Menzies Health Institute Queensland, Griffith University

over relatively long periods of time (e.g. due to ageing and/or the progression of respiratory disease).

There are significant 'reserves' available for increasing or decreasing lung volume when breathing quietly at rest. The air inhaled from the end of a tidal inspiration to TLC is the inspiratory reserve volume (IRV). Conversely, the air exhaled from the end of tidal expiration (i.e. FRC) to RV is the expiratory reserve volume (ERV). The difference in lung volume between FRC and TLC represents the inspiratory capacity (IC) – that is, the capacity to *maximally* inflate the lungs at the beginning of inspiration. The lung volumes V_T, ERV, IRV and IC are considered *dynamic* because they are determined by tidal airflows and the magnitude of respiratory muscle effort. It is also worth noting that 'capacity' is used here to describe the sum of smaller, more 'basic' lung volumes. For example, Figure 17.1 demonstrates that TLC may be determined by the following combinations:

$$TLC = VC + RV = FRC + IC = [RV + ERV] + [V_T + IRV]$$

Hence, when a 'capacity' is classed as being abnormal or is affected by external stimuli (e.g. bronchodilators), it is important to identify the changes in the smaller 'basic' lung volumes which may have occurred.

The relationship between flow and volume

It can be argued that abnormalities in lung volumes (particularly *static* volumes) provide insight into the longer-term, structural changes that occur with respiratory disease. However, these measurements only provide *part* of the picture of lung (dys)function. For many conditions such as asthma, it is just as important to determine the speed at which an individual can move air into and out of their lungs (i.e. flow).

The most commonly used test of pulmonary function is the *forced vital capacity (FVC)* manoeuvre. This test not only provides a robust measure of an individual's vital capacity, but can also reveal the degree of dynamic airways (dys)function. Figure 17.2 demonstrates an FVC manoeuvre performed by a young, healthy male. The left panel of Figure 17.2 depicts the volume of air exhaled during a maximal expiratory effort. The participant's exhaled volume increases abruptly at the start of the forced expiratory manoeuvre, beginning to 'slow down' as the volume–time tracing approaches a final value by 6 seconds. The forced expiratory volume in 1 second (FEV_1) indicates flow through the airways and is identified by locating 1 second on the x-axis and finding the corresponding value on the y-axis. The total volume expired after 6 seconds represents the FVC. The ratio of FEV_1 to FVC is perhaps the most common, and clinically useful, parameter to obtain from the volume–time plot – a reduced FEV_1/FVC is strongly predictive of airflow limitation and may aid in the differential diagnosis between obstructive and restrictive disorders.

The flow–volume relationship of an FVC effort is displayed in the right panel of Figure 17.2. The first part of the test is exactly the same as for the previously described FVC measurement – that is, the participant takes a maximal breath in (reaching TLC as the starting point on the left side of the graph where the volume is maximal) before breathing out as hard and as fast as they can. The airflow (y-axis) rapidly increases to reach a peak expiratory flow rate (PEFR) before slowing down linearly until the only volume (x-axis) of air left in the lungs is the RV (the far right point on the curve). Instead of stopping here as for the FVC test, the participant now takes a maximal breath in (also as hard and as fast as they

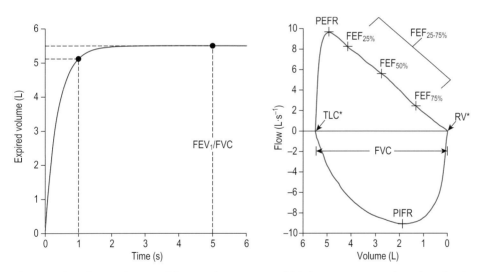

Figure 17.2 Volume–time and flow–volume curves. This is a representative plot of volume–time (left panel) and flow–volume (right panel) curves obtained from a young, healthy male during a forced vital capacity (FVC) manoeuvre. The solid red line represents the individual's maximal respiratory effort.
Note: only the individual's maximal expiratory effort is depicted on the volume–time tracing (left panel), whereas both the maximal inspiratory and expiratory efforts are displayed in the flow–volume curve (right panel). TLC and RV are displayed only for a point of reference – total lung capacity and residual volume cannot be determined via the FVC manoeuvre.
$FEF_{25\%}$, $FEF_{50\%}$ and $FEF_{75\%}$ = forced expiratory flow corresponding to 25, 50 and 75% of forced expired volume, respectively; $FEF_{25-75\%}$ = mid-expiratory flow rate; FEV_1 = forced expired volume in 1 s; PEFR = peak expiratory flow rate; PIFR = peak inspiratory flow rate.
Source: Troy J Cross, Menzies Health Institute Queensland, Griffith University

can), which is represented by the bottom part of the curve. After the peak inspiratory flow rate (PIFR) is achieved, flow progressively declines as volume increases, until the individual again reaches their TLC. Flow during inspiration is negative because it is in the opposite direction to expiration. Thus, in its entirety, the maximal flow–volume curve obtained during an FVC manoeuvre illustrates the dynamic properties of the airways over the vital capacity range (presuming that respiratory effort is maximal and the proper technique is used).

Respiratory muscle strength

It may also be useful to assess the maximal strength of the respiratory muscles. For example, global inspiratory muscle weakness is a hallmark of several clinical conditions (e.g. heart failure, chronic obstructive pulmonary disorder and the muscular dystrophies). Furthermore, there is mounting evidence demonstrating that targeted strength training of the respiratory muscles may be an effective therapeutic intervention in both the clinical and the sports performance environments.[1,2] Therefore, the ability to assess and monitor changes in respiratory muscle strength would prove advantageous to exercise professionals.

It must not be forgotten that respiratory muscles are *skeletal* muscles, whereby their maximal static (isometric) force is dictated by the 'length–tension' relationship (see Figure 7.1). Briefly, this relationship dictates that the maximal static tension occurs at the resting (optimal) length of a given skeletal muscle fibre. Furthermore, maximal static force decreases as the muscle fibre is either lengthened or shortened relative to this resting length. With specific regard to the respiratory muscles, muscle length is roughly proportional to the cubic root of lung *volume*, and muscle force is ultimately transmitted as a *pressure* to the pleural surface of the lungs. It is therefore more convenient for us to think of the 'length–tension' concept in terms of a 'volume–pressure' relationship when concerning the respiratory muscles. It is also important to make the distinction that increasing lung volume causes inspiratory muscles (e.g. the diaphragm) to shorten while the expiratory (e.g. the abdominal) muscles lengthen. Accordingly, we observe that maximal static *inspiratory* pressure (MIP) occurs at lung volumes between RV and FRC, whereas maximal static *expiratory* pressure (MEP) is observed at TLC.

Static respiratory contractions may be enforced by having a participant generate inspiratory or expiratory efforts against an occluded mouthpiece. If one neglects small contributions from gas expansion/compression (i.e. Boyle's law), respiratory efforts performed against the occluded mouthpiece do not translate into a change in lung volume. Maximal static respiratory pressures are then quantified by recording a stable mouth pressure during such manoeuvres. Figure 17.3 illustrates a typical mouth pressure–time tracing during a manoeuvre designed to measure MIP. Here, the participant has actively exhaled to RV, after which time they generated a maximal inspiratory effort against an occluded mouthpiece. The highest average mouth pressure sustained for 1 s is then reported as the participant's MIP. The MEP is assessed in a similar fashion during a maximal static expiratory effort at TLC. Detailed instructions for the MIP/MEP tests are covered in Activity 17.3. While the MIP/MEP tests are considered the standard method of estimating respiratory muscle strength, it cannot be denied that these manoeuvres are quite unfamiliar tasks to perform. As such, participants may require a number of practice attempts to achieve an acceptable level of test–retest reliability (see Practical 1, Test accuracy, reliability and validity). It should be noted that there are other methods of estimating respiratory muscle strength during more-familiar 'respiratory' tasks, such as during a sniff (inspiratory strength), or a 'reverse' sniff, a cough or even a whistle blow (expiratory strength). These alternative methods may be particularly effective when assessing paediatric participants.

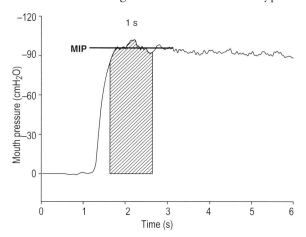

Figure 17.3 Mouth pressure–time curve. This is a representation of the mouth pressure–time curve during a maximal inspiratory effort performed at residual volume against an occluded mouthpiece. The hatched area represents the time interval over which maximal inspiratory pressure (MIP) was calculated: i.e. the highest 1-second moving average of mouth pressure observed during the manoeuvre

Source: Troy J Cross, Menzies Health Institute Queensland, Griffith University

DEFINITIONS

Dynamic lung function: spirometry tests that measure the change in volume of gas in the lungs over time (i.e. time-based tests).

Expiratory reserve volume (ERV): maximum volume of air that can be exhaled at the end of a tidal expiration to FRC.

Forced expiratory volume in 1 second (FEV$_1$): volume of air that has been exhaled at the end of the first second from a maximally forced expiratory effort.

Forced vital capacity (FVC): determination of the vital capacity from a maximally forced expiratory effort.

Functional residual capacity (FRC): the volume of air remaining in the lungs at the end of vital capacity.

Inspiratory capacity (IC): the difference in lung volume between functional residual capacity (FRC) and total lung capacity (TLC).

Inspiratory reserve volume (IRV): volume of air able to be inhaled at the end of a tidal inspiration to total lung capacity (TLC).

Maximal expiratory pressure (MEP): the maximal mouth pressure sustained over 1 s during a maximal expiratory effort performed at TLC against an occluded mouthpiece.

Maximal inspiratory pressure (MIP): the maximal mouth pressure sustained over 1 s during a maximal expiratory effort performed at RV against an occluded mouthpiece.

Mixed disorders: category of respiratory disease characterised by both obstructive and restrictive lung disease.

Obstructive disorders: category of respiratory disease characterised by airway obstruction. Types of obstructive lung disease include: asthma, bronchiectasis, bronchitis and chronic obstructive pulmonary disease (COPD).

Residual volume (RV): residual component of air remaining in the airspaces of the lungs following maximal expiration.

Restrictive disorders: category of extrapulmonary, pleural or parenchymal respiratory diseases that restrict lung expansion, resulting in a decreased lung volume, an increased work of breathing, and inadequate ventilation and/or oxygenation. Restrictive lung diseases may be intrinsic (e.g. pulmonary fibrosis) or extrinsic (e.g. neuromuscular diseases) to the parenchyma of the lung.

Static lung function: spirometry tests that measure the change in volume of gas in the lungs (i.e. purely volume-based tests).

Tidal volume (V_T): the change in volume between the beginning and end of inspiration or expiration during quiet, non-forced breathing.

Total lung capacity (TLC): maximal voluntary inflation of the lungs.

Vital capacity (VC): the change in exhaled volume between total lung capacity (TLC) and residual volume (RV).

INDICATIONS FOR SPIROMETRY

For the exercise professional, spirometric assessment of an individual may be indicated for the following reasons:
1 to evaluate general respiratory health
2 to determine the presence and severity of a lung defect or dysfunction and/or track its progress over time
3 to evaluate symptoms, including those related to physical activity or exercise intolerance
4 to assess the efficacy of interventions on parameters of lung function
5 for research purposes.

CONTRAINDICATIONS FOR SPIROMETRY

Tests of pulmonary function are generally safe for most individuals to perform. However, forced expiration and inspiration can generate relatively high intrathoracic pressures and also transiently raise blood pressure. Such pressure swings can pose a risk to some individuals, particularly those with unstable cardiovascular disease and those at risk of suffering from, or aggravation of, a thoracic or abdominal injury. In some circumstances, the exercise professional must consider whether spirometry is indicated for an individual whose test results are likely to be suboptimal (e.g. where the test may induce facial, chest or abdominal pain, or in the presence of an altered mental state). There are several contraindications for spirometric assessment (Box 17.1).[3] Most of these contraindications for lung function testing may be considered relative if the benefits of testing outweigh the perceived risks. A decision regarding whether to waive the risks should be made in consultation with the treating medical practitioner.

Box 17.1 Relative contraindications for spirometric assessment

- Thoracic/abdominal surgery
- Brain, eye, ear, nose, throat surgery
- Pneumothorax
- Recent myocardial infarction
- Ascending aortic aneurysm
- Haemoptysis (coughing up blood)
- Pulmonary embolism
- Unstable angina
- Severe hypertension (systolic >200 mmHg, diastolic >120 mmHg)
- Confused participants or people with dementia
- Participant discomfort
- Infection control issue (e.g. contagious infections).

Adapted from: Cooper[3]

In clinical practice, spirometry is typically completed twice (i.e. two series of three trials) when conducted to assess airway responsiveness. The first test provides a baseline value to assess the participant's airway function. The participants are then given a dose of a bronchodilator (usually a short-acting β_2-agonist such as salbutamol (Ventolin)) and the spirometry testing is repeated. The differences (or lack of differences) in values pre- and post-bronchodilator give just as much clinical information as the absolute values recorded. An improvement of greater than 12% in FEV_1 following administration of a bronchodilator is supportive of the diagnosis of a reversible airflow limitation, such as asthma.[4] However, for the purpose of this practical, as it may not be appropriate to provide medications to participants, the test will be completed for only one series of three trials.

DOES THE PARTICIPANT NEED TO WEAR A NOSE CLIP OR PINCH THEIR NOSE?

It is highly important that no airflow occurs through the nose of the participant during spirometric testing. A bypassing of flow through the nose will underestimate the key variables of interest, such as FEV_1, FVC and PEFR. The principal way of avoiding nasal airflow is to have the participant wear a nose clip or pinch the nose during tests; however, some participants may find wearing a nose clip to be uncomfortable or cumbersome. It is possible to breathe freely through the mouth while preventing airflow through the nose without use of a nose clip (e.g. while snorkelling) – this action is provided by cephalad movement of the soft palate. So, with adequate practice and feedback, little difference is observed in key spirometric variables whether a participant wears or does not wear a nose clip or pinches the nose.[5] Further, the highly negative pressure swings generated during the MIP test may create a small degree of middle-ear pain if a nose clip is worn. In this case, the participant's maximal inspiratory efforts may be curtailed by the presence of this discomfort. So, although a nose clip is the preferable way to avoid nasal airflow, any pain/discomfort caused by wearing it may threaten the concurrent validity and reliability of the participant's results. The tester is urged to use their judgment, and to make note of whether or not a nose clip was worn during manoeuvres – this will help to standardise future testing of the same participant.

Activity 17.1 The forced vital capacity manoeuvre

AIMS: measure the forced vital capacity and forced expiratory volume over 1 second, interpret the results and provide feedback to a participant.

Background

The most clinically useful indices derived from this test are the FVC, FEV_1, FEV_1/FVC and PEFR. The concurrent validity of these parameters is highly dependent on whether a maximal respiratory muscle effort is produced during the test; this point should be strongly emphasised to the participant.

Box 17.2 General methods for dynamic lung function testing

1. When performing lung function tests, particular care must be taken to ensure that:
   a. instructions are communicated clearly to the participant
   b. the correct posture is adopted during the test
   c. the requisite amount of 'effort' is performed by the individual
   d. recovery between tests is adequate to avoid significant fatigue
   e. acceptability/reliability criteria are met.

2. It is the tester's responsibility to ensure that the participant is comfortable and able to perform the FVC/PEFR manoeuvres successfully. Some participants may report chest or abdominal pain, fear of incontinence or emesis (vomiting), lack of confidence, tiredness, etc. Some of these concerns may be addressed by following the pre-test requirements described in Appendix B, demonstrating the test procedure to the individual and providing verbal encouragement throughout each manoeuvre.

3. Feedback from the participant should be obtained between manoeuvres (i.e. some participants may feel 'dizzy' after a manoeuvre, which may progress to fainting if not identified). Testing should be stopped if the tester thinks the participant will harm themself during the testing process.

Protocol summary

The participant completes a maximal breath in, pinches their nose (or wears a nose clip), places their lips entirely around the mouthpiece and exhales maximally and forcefully for ≥6 seconds.

Protocol

1 Follow the pre-exercise test procedures outlined in Appendix B and the general methods for dynamic lung function testing described in Box 17.2.

2 Check Box 17.1 to ensure that there are no contraindications to spirometric assessment. Check Appendix C to ensure that there are no contraindications to exercise testing.

3 Explain and demonstrate the procedure and correct technique to the participant.

4 Attach the participant's disposable mouthpiece, ensuring the tester's fingers do not come in contact with the mouthpiece. This can be done by either wearing gloves or asking the participant to attach the mouthpiece.

5 The participant should be given as many practice trials as necessary to ensure that they have mastered the correct technique, with a rest period of ≥ 1 minute between efforts.

6 Ask the participant to sit comfortably in an upright position with their head tilted slightly upwards.

7 Ensure the participant places their lips entirely around the mouthpiece so that an airtight seal is created, and pinch their nose with their fingers or wear a nose clip (Figure 17.4).

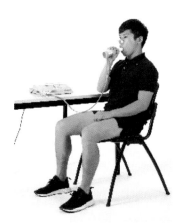

Figure 17.4 Participant positioning for the forced vital capacity manoeuvre
Used with permission from Vitalograph

> **Note:** occluding the nostrils is not mandatory, but considered best practice as it will prevent air leakage if participants partially expire through their nose despite the instruction to breathe only through their mouth.

8 Instruct the participant to inhale completely and rapidly through the mouth (not the nose), with minimal pause at TLC (<1 s) by providing the following instruction: *'breathe in all the way, completely fill up your lungs'*.

9 Instruct the participant to exhale maximally and forcefully, until absolutely no more air can be expelled. Expiratory effort must continue until the participant is indicated to stop when the entire VC has been expelled. This must be a minimum of 6 seconds, although it may be as long as 15 seconds in individuals with obstructive diseases. The participant must maintain the correct posture throughout the manoeuvre. If correct posture is compromised (e.g. the participant leans forwards), the trial is deemed invalid. Provide the following instructions: *'blast all the air out! … keep squeezing … keep going until I tell you to stop … stop!'*

10 Where the instrument allows for assessment of inspiratory volumes, instruct the participant at the end of maximal expiration to inhale rapidly and completely to TLC again to obtain maximal inspiratory flows across the vital capacity range. Provide the participant with the following instructions: *'breathe in quickly again! … all the way to the top of your lungs!'*

11 The manoeuvre should be repeated at least three times with a rest period of ≥ 1 minute between efforts.

12 End testing when the participant has met the test acceptability/reliability criteria (e.g. based on a minimum of three valid trials) and none of the common problems with dynamic lung function testing have occurred (see Box 17.3).[6]

13 Record the FVC and FEV_1 from the three completed trials on the spirometry data-recording sheet.

14 Clean and disinfect all equipment (see Appendix A).

Box 17.3 Common problems with dynamic lung function testing

- Air leak due to lips not being sealed around the mouthpiece
- Poor/submaximal/variable effort
- Not at TLC before expiration
- Long pause at TLC before expiration
- Poor start (slow 'take-off')
- Cough
- Glottic closure
- Premature termination of expiratory effort (incomplete expiration)
- Obstruction of mouthpiece by the tongue or clenching of teeth
- Vocalisation (excessive vocal 'sound' during the effort)
- Incorrect posture during the manoeuvre
- Laryngospasm
- Aspiration of sputum into flow-sensing device
- Emesis (vomiting)

TLC = total lung capacity
Adapted from: Johns and Pierce[6]

Data recording: spirometry

Participant's name: _____   Date: _____

Age: _____ years   Sex: _____   Stature: _____ cm

	TRIAL 1	TRIAL 2	TRIAL 3	BEST TRIAL
FVC (L)				
FEV_1 (L)				
FEV_1/FVC (%)				

FEV_1 = forced expired volume in 1 s; FVC = forced vital capacity.

Data analysis

To compare the participant's FVC and FEV_1 results with their predicted values according to sex, height and age, use the appropriate equations in Table 17.1.[7,8] For example, using the parameters from Table 17.1, the predicted FEV_1 for a 25-year-old, 165 cm female would be calculated as:

$$\text{Predicted FEV}_1 \text{ (L)} = [0.0342 \times \text{height(cm)}] + [-0.0255 \times \text{age(years)}] - 1.578$$
$$= [0.0342 \times 165] + [-0.0255 \times 25] - 1.578$$
$$= 3.43 \text{ L}$$

The 'Interpreting and classifying abnormal values' section later in the Practical provides guidance for the selection of arrows up/down and Table 17.2[6] for overall classification. There are no specific cut-off values for the selection of arrows, as additional clinical information would be needed to make an informed decision.

TABLE 17.1 Adult prediction equations for determining normal spirometry values

INDEX	SEX	HEIGHT (cm)	AGE (YEARS)	CONSTANT
FVC (L)	♀	$0.0491 \times$ height	$-0.0216 \times$ age	-3.590
	♂	$0.0600 \times$ height	$-0.0214 \times$ age	-4.650
FEV_1 (L)	♀	$0.0342 \times$ height	$-0.0255 \times$ age	-1.578
	♂	$0.0414 \times$ height	$-0.0244 \times$ age	-2.190

Add the columns together to obtain the normal value.
Spirometry prediction equations for adults; all lung volumes are in body temperature and pressure saturated (BTPS) (see Practical 10: VO_2max for an explanation of the differences in gas volumes). Expiratory flow rate 25%–75% of FVC; FEV_1 = forced expiratory volume in 1 second; FVC = forced vital capacity; ♀ = female participants, ♂ = male participants
Adapted from: Crapo et al[7,8]

TABLE 17.2 Classification of abnormal spirometric values

	ABSOLUTE VALUES			FEV_1/FVC	% PREDICTED	
Disorder	FEV_1(L)	FVC(L)	TLC(L)	%	FEV_1	FVC
Obstructive	↓↓	↓	↑	↓	↓↓	↓
Restrictive	↓	↓	↓	↑ or ↔	↓	↓
Mixed	↓↓	↓	↓	↓	↓	↓

FEV_1 = forced expiratory volume in 1 second; FVC = forced vital capacity; TLC = total lung capacity
Adapted from: Johns and Pierce[6]

Data recording: predicted FVC and FEV_1

FVC

Participant's best FVC result = _____ L

Predicted FVC (L)[a] = (height constant $\times$ height) + (age constant $\times$ age) + constant

= (_____ $\times$ ____) + (_____ $\times$ ___) + _____

= _____ L

Difference between participant's best FVC result vs predicted FVC (e.g. '100 mL lower than predicted'): _____

Comparison of participant's best FVC result (absolute values) vs predicted FVC (please circle) – refer to the 'Interpreting and classifying abnormal values' section for guidance:

↓↓   ↓   ↔   ↑   ↑↑

Percent (%) predicted FVC $= \dfrac{\text{Best FVC result} \times 100}{\text{Predicted FVC result}} =$ _____

= _____ %

continued

Data recording: predicted FVC and FEV$_1$ *(continued)*

Comparison of participant's best FVC result (relative values) vs predicted FVC (please circle) – refer to the 'Interpreting and classifying abnormal values' section for guidance:

$$\downarrow\downarrow \qquad \downarrow \qquad \leftrightarrow \qquad \uparrow \qquad \uparrow\uparrow$$

FEV$_1$

Participant's best FEV$_1$ result = _____ L

Predicted FEV$_1$ (L)^a = (height constant $\times$ height) + (age constant $\times$ age) + constant

$$= (\underline{\hspace{2cm}} \times \underline{\hspace{1cm}}) + (\underline{\hspace{2cm}} \times \underline{\hspace{1cm}}) + \underline{\hspace{1.5cm}}$$

$$= (\underline{\hspace{1cm}}) + (\underline{\hspace{1cm}}) \quad + \underline{\hspace{1.5cm}}$$

$$= \underline{\hspace{2cm}} L$$

Difference between participant's best FEV$_1$ result vs predicted FEV$_1$ (e.g. '100 mL lower than predicted'): _____

Comparison of participant's best FEV$_1$ result (absolute values) vs predicted FEV$_1$ (please circle) – refer to the 'Interpreting and classifying abnormal values' section for guidance:

$$\downarrow\downarrow \qquad \downarrow \qquad \leftrightarrow \qquad \uparrow \qquad \uparrow\uparrow$$

$$\text{Percent (\%) predicted FEV}_1 = \frac{\text{Best FEV}_1 \text{ result} \times 100}{\text{Predicted FEV}_1 \text{ result}} = \underline{\hspace{1.5cm}}$$

$$= \underline{\hspace{1.5cm}} \%$$

Comparison of participant's best FEV$_1$ result (relative values) vs predicted FEV$_1$ (please circle) – refer to the 'Interpreting and classifying abnormal values' section for guidance:

$$\downarrow\downarrow \qquad \downarrow \qquad \leftrightarrow \qquad \uparrow \qquad \uparrow\uparrow$$

FEV$_1$/FVC

Participant's best FEV$_1$/FVC trial = _____ %

$$\text{Predicted FEV}_1/\text{FVC} = \frac{\text{Predicted FEV}_1^a}{\text{Predicted FVC}^a}$$

$$= \underline{\hspace{1.5cm}}$$

$$= \underline{\hspace{1.5cm}} \%$$

Difference between participant's best FEV$_1$/FVC trial vs predicted FEV$_1$/FVC (e.g. '5% lower than predicted'): _____

Comparison of participant's best FEV$_1$/FVC trial vs predicted FEV$_1$/FVC (please circle) – refer to the 'Interpreting and classifying abnormal values' section for guidance:

$$\downarrow\downarrow \qquad \downarrow \qquad \leftrightarrow \qquad \uparrow \qquad \uparrow\uparrow$$

Classification of spirometric values (according to Table 17.2)

☐ 'Normal'

☐ Obstructive disorder

☐ Restrictive disorder

☐ Mixed disorder

^{a} From Table 17.1^{7,8}

Activity 17.2 Peak expiratory flow rate test

AIMS: measure PEFR, interpret the results and provide feedback to a participant.

Background

Although PEFR can be determined from the spirometry procedure demonstrated in Activity 17.1, it is often performed as a standalone test using a small portable peak flow meter (Figure 17.5). The main applications of this measurement are to monitor airway function over time in individuals with known pulmonary disease.

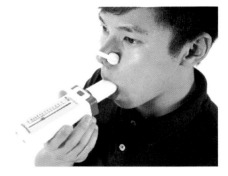

Protocol summary

Figure 17.5 Peak expiratory flow rate test
Used with permission from Vitalograph

The participant inhales completely and rapidly through the mouth, places their lips entirely around the mouthpiece and exhales as fast and forcefully as possible in a rapid 'huff'.

Protocol

1 Follow the pre-exercise test procedures outlined in Appendix B and the general methods for dynamic lung function testing described in Box 17.2.

2 Check Box 17.1 to ensure that there are no contraindications to spirometric assessment.

3 Explain and demonstrate the procedure and correct technique to the participant.

4 Attach the disposable mouthpiece, ensuring the tester's fingers do not come in contact with the mouthpiece. This can be done by either wearing gloves or asking the participant to attach the mouthpiece.

5 The participant should be given as many practice trials as necessary to ensure that they have mastered the correct technique with $\geq$30 seconds rest between efforts.

6 Ask the participant to sit comfortably in an upright position with their head tilted slightly upwards.

7 Check that the dial on the meter is reset to zero.

8 Ensure the participant places their lips entirely around the mouthpiece so that an airtight seal is created, and pinch their nose with their fingers or wear a nose clip (see Figure 17.5).

> **Note:** occluding the nostrils is not mandatory, but considered best practice as it will prevent air leakage if participants partially expire through their nose despite the instruction to breathe only through their mouth.

9 Instruct the participant to inhale completely and rapidly through the mouth (not the nose), with minimal pause at TLC ($<$1 s).

10 Instruct the participant to exhale as fast and forcefully as possible in a rapid 'huff' (as though trying to blow out the candles on a cake).

> **Note:** expiration does not need to be maintained for 6 seconds for this procedure. It is the peak speed of expiration that is being recorded.

11 The manoeuvre should be repeated at least three times with a rest period of $\geq$1 minute between efforts.

12 End testing when the participant has met the test acceptability/reliability criteria (e.g. based on a minimum of three valid trials) and none of the common problems with dynamic lung function testing (described in Box 17.3)[6] have occurred.

13 Record the results on the peak expiratory flow rate test data-recording sheet

14 Clean and disinfect all equipment (see Appendix A).

Data recording: PEFR

Participant's name: _____   Date: _____

Age: _____ years   Sex: _____   Stature: _____ cm

	TRIAL 1	TRIAL 2	TRIAL 3	BEST TRIAL	PREDICTED VALUE[a]	% OF PREDICTED VALUE
PEFR (L/min)						

PEFR = peak expiratory flow rate.
[a] L/min from Figure 17.6.

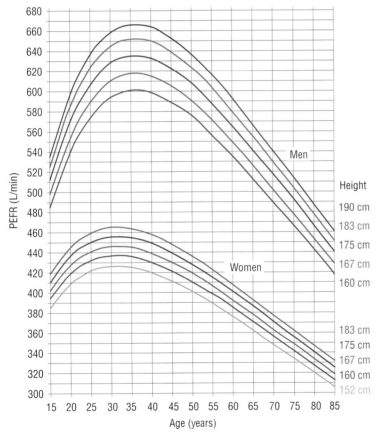

Figure 17.6 Peak expiratory flow reference data
Source: Nunn and Gregg[9]

Data analysis

Determine the predicted PEFR value by referring to Figure 17.6.

Calculate the percentage of predicted value:

$$\% \text{ predicted PEFR} = \frac{(\text{Best trial} \times 100)}{\text{Predicted value}}$$

Activity 17.3 Maximal inspiratory and expiratory pressure tests

AIMS: measure MIP and MEP, interpret the results and provide feedback to a participant.

Background

MIP and MEP are often used as estimates of global respiratory muscle strength. These values may be used to:

1 identify respiratory muscle weakness of a participant

2 evaluate the presence of globalised respiratory muscle fatigue during a dynamic breathing task (e.g. exercise)

3 monitor the progress of an individual engaged in a respiratory muscle training program.

A participant's MIP and MEP may be recorded using a commercially available handheld device. However, if these devices are not available in your laboratory, a simple testing device may be fashioned from hardware materials at low cost (see Figure 17.7 for instructions). Given that mouth pressure is the key variable being recorded during the MIP/MEP test, the instructor must encourage the participant to perform each manoeuvre with an open glottis, otherwise you may not observe a truly maximal respiratory effort (or any effort at all!).

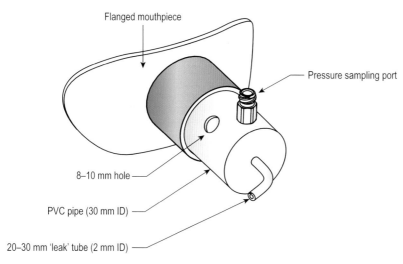

Figure 17.7 Simplified design of a device to measure maximal inspiratory pressure (MIP) and maximal expiratory pressure (MEP).
This device can be fabricated using parts available in most laboratories and hardware stores. A flexible rubber (preferably) flanged mouthpiece is affixed to a short section of PVC pipe (internal diameter (ID) = 30 mm). At the onset of the MIP/MEP manoeuvre, the participant occludes the 8–10 mm opening with their finger or thumb. A pressure 'leak' is provided by the 20–30 mm long section of tubing (ID = 2 mm) attached to the PVC pipe. This leak helps avoid glottic closure during the MIP test, and prevents excessively high mouth pressures due to buccal contraction during the MEP test. Mouth pressure is sampled by a lateral port connected to a pressure measurement device (not depicted)

Source: Troy J Cross, Menzies Health Institute Queensland, Griffith University

Protocol summary

The participant attempts to exhale (MEP) or inhale (MIP) with maximum effort against an occluded mouthpiece for at least 1.5 seconds at TLC (for the MEP) or RV (for the MIP).

Protocol

1 Follow the pre-exercise test procedures outlined in Appendix B and the general methods for dynamic lung function testing described in Box 17.2.

2   Check Box 17.1 to ensure that there are no contraindications to spirometric assessment.

3   Explain and demonstrate the procedure and correct technique to the participant.

4   Attach the participant's disposable mouthpiece, ensuring the tester's fingers do not come in contact with the mouthpiece. This can be done by either wearing gloves or asking the participant to attach the mouthpiece.

5   The participant should be given as many practice trials as necessary to ensure that they have mastered the correct technique with a rest period of ≥ 1 minute between efforts.

6   Check that your pressure measurement device is calibrated and zeroed.

7   Ask the participant to sit comfortably in an upright position with their head tilted slightly upwards.

8   Visual feedback of the mouth pressure signal should be in plain sight of the participant.

9   Ensure the participant places their lips entirely around the mouthpiece so that an airtight seal is created, but keep their lips loose so that they may continue to breathe freely despite the obstruction of the mouthpiece.

10   Instruct the participant to pinch their nose with their fingers or wear a nose clip (see Figure 17.5).

> **Note:** occluding the nostrils is not mandatory, but considered best practice as it will prevent air leakage if participants partially expire through their nose despite the instruction to breathe only through their mouth.

11a **MEP test:** allow the participant to continue tidal breathing for 4–5 breaths, and then instruct them to inhale maximally to TLC and, without delay, create an airtight seal around the mouthpiece. Instruct them to attempt to *'exhale without ballooning the cheeks against the mouthpiece with as much effort as you can generate for at least 1.5 s.'*

> **Note:** if the participant's cheeks noticeably 'balloon' outwards, the tester (or participant) may support the participant's cheeks with their hands.

11b **MIP test:** beginning again from step 6, allow the participant to continue tidal breathing for 4–5 breaths. Then, instruct them to exhale to RV and, once exhalation is complete, form an airtight seal around the mouthpiece. Instruct them to *'inhale against the mouthpiece with as much effort as you can generate for at least 1.5 s'.*

12   The participant may remove the mouthpiece once the effort is complete.

13   Each manoeuvre should be repeated at least 3 times with a rest period of ≥ 1 minute between efforts.

> **Note:** because the MIP and MEP tests are quite unfamiliar tasks to complete, the participant may require a number of practice attempts until they demonstrate the proper technique and produce consistent results. The length of this learning period varies between participants, and up to 10–18 repeated efforts may be necessary.[10,11] While completing this number of efforts may appear tedious, it is highly important to minimise any learning effects if the aim is to have a valid (concurrent) and reproducible estimate of the participant's maximal respiratory muscle strength.

14   End testing when the participant has met the test acceptability/reliability criteria (e.g. based on a minimum of three valid trials) and none of the common problems with dynamic lung function testing have occurred (described in Box 17.3).[6]

15   Record the largest/highest MIP/MEP values of all technically acceptable efforts that vary by less than 20% from other attempts on the MIP and MEP test data-recording sheet.

16   Clean and disinfect all equipment (see Appendix A).

Data recording: MIP and MEP

Participant's name: _____   Date: _____

Age: _____ years   Sex: _____   Stature: _____ cm

	TRIAL 1	TRIAL 2	TRIAL 3	BEST TRIAL
MIP (cmH$_2$O)				
MEP (cmH$_2$O)				

MEP = maximal expiratory pressure; MIP = maximal inspiratory pressure.

Data analysis

To compare the participant's MIP and MEP results with their predicted values according to sex and age, use the appropriate equations in Table 17.3.[12] The 'Interpreting and classifying abnormal values' section provides guidance for the selection of arrows up/down. There are no specific cut-off values for the selection of arrows, as additional clinical information would be needed to make an informed decision.

TABLE 17.3 Adult prediction equations for determining normal values for maximal inspiratory and expiratory pressures

	INDEX	SEX	AGE (YEARS)	CONSTANT
MIP (cmH$_2$O)	Normal	♀	$-0.61 \times$ age	108
		♂	$-0.41 \times$ age	120
	LLN	♀	$-0.50 \times$ age	62
		♂	$-0.15 \times$ age	117
MEP (cmH$_2$O)	Normal	♀	$-0.86 \times$ age	131
		♂	$-0.83 \times$ age	174
	LLN	♀	$-0.57 \times$ age	95
		♂	$-0.83 \times$ age	117

Add the columns together to obtain the normal value.
LLN = lower limit of normal; MEP = maximal expiratory pressure; MIP = maximal inspiratory pressure; ♀ = female participants; ♂ = male participants
Adapted from: Evans and Whitelaw[12]

Data recording: predicted MIP and MEP

MIP

Participant's best MIP result = _____ cmH$_2$O

Predicted MIP (cmH$_2$O)^a = (age constant $\times$ age) + constant

$$= (\rule{2cm}{0.4pt} \times \rule{1cm}{0.4pt}) + \rule{1.5cm}{0.4pt}$$

$$= (\rule{2cm}{0.4pt}) + \rule{2cm}{0.4pt}$$

$$= \rule{2cm}{0.4pt} \text{ cmH}_2\text{O}$$

continued

Data recording: predicted MIP and MEP *(continued)*

Difference between participant's best MIP vs predicted MIP (e.g. '10 cmH$_2$O lower than predicted'):

_____

Comparison of participant's best MIP result (absolute values) vs predicted MIP (please circle):

$\downarrow\downarrow$ $\quad$ $\downarrow$ $\quad$ $\leftrightarrow$ $\quad$ $\uparrow$ $\quad$ $\uparrow\uparrow$

Percent (%) predicted MIP $= \dfrac{\text{Best MIP result} \times 100}{\text{Predicted MIP result}}$

$\qquad = \underline{\hspace{2cm}}$ %

Comparison of participant's best MIP result (relative values) vs predicted MIP (please circle):

$\downarrow\downarrow$ $\quad$ $\downarrow$ $\quad$ $\leftrightarrow$ $\quad$ $\uparrow$ $\quad$ $\uparrow\uparrow$

LLN MIP (cmH$_2$O)^a = (age constant $\times$ age) + constant

$\qquad = (\underline{\hspace{2.5cm}} \times \underline{\hspace{1cm}}) + \underline{\hspace{1.5cm}}$

$\qquad = (\underline{\hspace{2cm}}) + \underline{\hspace{2cm}}$

$\qquad = \underline{\hspace{2cm}}$ cmH$_2$O

Difference between participant's best MIP vs LLN MIP (e.g. '5 cmH$_2$O above lower limit of normal'):

_____

Comparison of participant's best MIP result (relative values) vs LLN MIP (please circle):

$\downarrow\downarrow$ $\quad$ $\downarrow$ $\quad$ $\leftrightarrow$ $\quad$ $\uparrow$ $\quad$ $\uparrow\uparrow$

Classification of inspiratory muscle strength – refer to the 'Interpretation' section for guidance:

☐ 'Normal'

☐ Above average strength

☐ Below average strength

☐ Below LLN (suspect inspiratory muscle weakness)

MEP

Participant's best MEP result = _____ cmH$_2$O

Predicted MEP (cmH$_2$O)^a = (age constant $\times$ age) + constant

$\qquad = (\underline{\hspace{2.5cm}} \times \underline{\hspace{1cm}}) + \underline{\hspace{1.5cm}}$

$\qquad = (\underline{\hspace{2cm}}) + \underline{\hspace{2cm}}$

$\qquad = \underline{\hspace{2cm}}$ cmH$_2$O

Difference between participant's best MEP vs predicted MEP (e.g. '10 cmH$_2$O lower than predicted'):

_____

Comparison of participant's best MEP result (absolute values) vs predicted MEP (please circle):

$\downarrow\downarrow$ $\quad$ $\downarrow$ $\quad$ $\leftrightarrow$ $\quad$ $\uparrow$ $\quad$ $\uparrow\uparrow$

Percent (%) predicted MEP $= \dfrac{\text{Best MEP result} \times 100}{\text{Predicted MEP result}}$

$\qquad = \underline{\hspace{2cm}}$ %

continued overpage

Data recording: predicted MIP and MEP *(continued)*

Comparison of participant's best MEP result (relative values) vs predicted MEP (please circle):

$$\downarrow\downarrow \qquad \downarrow \qquad \leftrightarrow \qquad \uparrow \qquad \uparrow\uparrow$$

LLN MEP (cmH$_2$O) [a] = (age constant $\times$ age) + constant

$$= (\underline{\hspace{2cm}} \times \underline{\hspace{1cm}}) + \underline{\hspace{1.5cm}}$$

$$= (\underline{\hspace{2cm}}) + \underline{\hspace{2cm}}$$

$$= \underline{\hspace{2cm}} \ cmH_2O$$

Difference between participant's best MIP vs LLN MIP (e.g. '5 cmH$_2$O above lower limit of normal'):

_____

Comparison of participant's best MEP result (relative values) vs LLN MEP (please circle):

$$\downarrow\downarrow \qquad \downarrow \qquad \leftrightarrow \qquad \uparrow \qquad \uparrow\uparrow$$

Classification of expiratory muscle strength – refer to the 'Interpretation' section for guidance:

☐ 'Normal'

☐ Above average strength

☐ Below average strength

☐ Below LLN (suspect expiratory muscle weakness)

[a] From Table 17.3
LLN = lower limit of normal

Common participant-related problems with dynamic lung function testing

There are a number of participant-related problems one may encounter when trying to obtain acceptable breathing manoeuvres during lung function testing. These problems are outlined in Box 17.3 and Figure 17.8.[6] It is important to note that these issues may not necessarily produce 'abnormal' values.

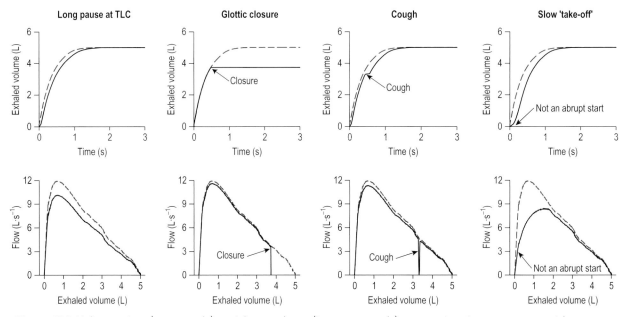

Figure 17.8 Volume–time (top panels) and flow–volume (bottom panels) curves showing common problems associated with performing forced vital capacity (FVC) manoeuvres. The dashed red lines represent the volume–time and flow–volume curves obtained from an 'ideal' FVC manoeuvre. The solid lines illustrate the flow–volume and volume–time curves obtained from 'problematic' FVC manoeuvres.

TLC = total lung capacity Adapted from: Johns and Pierce[6]

For example, if a participant coughs 3 seconds into a forced expiratory effort, or terminates the manoeuvre prematurely during an FVC test, the calculation of PEFR or FEV_1 may remain largely unaffected. Although it is recommended that *all* unacceptable efforts be rejected, there may be situations where only suboptimal manoeuvres are recorded (e.g. non-compliant participants, individuals with cognitive impairment). In such cases, the tester must use their judgment and select the parameters that are believed to still be clinically 'useful' (such as PEFR and FEV_1 in the example above). Any parameters that are recorded, but are not *technically* acceptable, should be duly noted in the data-recording sheet.

Back-extrapolated volume

An instantaneously 'maximal' expiratory effort from TLC is often difficult to achieve. On the occasion that expiration does not begin abruptly during an FVC manoeuvre (slow 'take-off'), the back-extrapolation method may be used to determine an adjusted 'zero time' to be used in the calculation of FEV_1. Figure 17.9[13] displays a volume–time tracing of an FVC effort with a relatively slow 'take-off'. The adjusted 'zero time' is found by back-extrapolating a linear segment from the steepest portion of the volume-time curve to the *x*-axis to become the new time $= 0$ (t_0). The volume corresponding to the adjusted t_0 is the volume used in the determination of FEV_1 test acceptability (Box 17.4).[14]

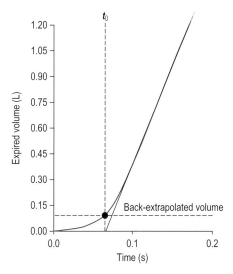

Figure 17.9 Back-extrapolation method used to determine adjusted 'zero time' (t_0) on the volume–time tracing. The red line represents the volume-time tracing from a forced vital capacity manoeuvre with a relatively slow 'take-off'. The solid line represents the linear extrapolation of the steepest portion on the volume–time curve. The dashed lines reveal the adjusted 'zero time' and the back-extrapolated volume

Adapted from: Miller et al[13]

Box 17.4 Criteria for acceptability and reliability of dynamic lung function testing

The American Thoracic Society (ATS) provides strict criteria for the acceptability and reliability of dynamic lung function testing. These guidelines are only briefly summarised here. The reader is directed to https://www.thoracic.org/statements/pulmonary-function.php for the complete list of ATS recommendations.

FVC

- Minimum of three technically acceptable efforts free from artefacts (e.g. coughing, glottic closure, leak, early termination of test, etc.).
- Expiration must start abruptly.
- Expiratory duration of at least 6 seconds.
- Consistent posture between tests (i.e. sitting).

continued overpage

> **Box 17.4 Criteria for acceptability and reliability of dynamic lung function testing *(continued)***
>
> - Reliability is achieved when the two highest FVC values differ by <0.2 L.
> - The largest FVC of all technically acceptable efforts is reported.
>
> **FEV_1**
> - Minimum of three technically acceptable efforts free from artefacts (e.g. coughing, glottic closure, leak).
> - Expiration must start abruptly.
> - Consistent posture between tests (i.e. sitting).
> - FEV_1 is reproducible when the two highest values differ by <0.2 L.
> - The largest FEV_1 of all technically acceptable efforts is reported.
>
> **PEFR**
> - Minimum of three technically acceptable efforts free from artefacts (e.g. coughing, glottic closure, leak).
> - Keep posture consistent between tests (standing is preferred).
> - Maximal expiratory duration of only $1-2$ seconds is required.
> - The largest PEFR of all technically acceptable efforts is reported.
>
> **MIP/MEP**
> - Minimum of three technically acceptable efforts free from artefacts (i.e. coughing, glottic closure, leak).
> - Keep posture consistent between tests.
> - Maximal inspiratory/expiratory effort duration must be at least $1-1.5$ seconds.

Adapted from American Thoracic Society[14]

Interpretation

First, consider the four steps of interpretation outlined in Appendix G.

Normal and predicted values — FVC and FEV_1

The interpretation of a pulmonary function test is based on a comparison with normal or predicted values obtained from a reference group of healthy participants. Factors known to influence spirometry are anthropometry (i.e. height), age, sex (see Table 17.4)[6] and ethnicity. An increase in stature results in an increase in all spirometry values except for FEV_1/FVC. Up to approximately 20 years of age for females and approximately 25 years of age for males, there is an increase in all spirometry values. The only exception is FEV_1/FVC, which decreases, suggesting that up to this age the rate of increase in FVC

TABLE 17.4 General influence of height, age and sex on spirometry					
		FEV_1	FVC	FEV_1/FVC	PEFR
Height:	↑ in standing height	↑	↑	—	↑
Age:	$<20/25$ in females/males	↑	↑	↓	↑
	$>20/25$ in females/males	↓	↓	↓	↓
Sex:	(♂ vs ♀)	♂ $>$ ♀	♂ $>$ ♀	♂sl $<$ ♀	♂ $>$ ♀

FEV_1 = forced expiratory volume in 1 second; FVC = forced vital capacity; PEFR = peak expiratory flow rate; sl = slightly; ♀ = female participants; ♂ = male participants

[A]dapted from: Johns and Pierce[6]

is greater than the increase in FEV_1. Males, as a general rule, have greater volumes than females, again except for FEV_1/FVC, which is slightly less in males compared with females.

Variations in FVC and FEV_1 occur with different ethnic groups.[15] For healthy individuals of the same age, height and sex, Caucasians tend to have the largest FVC and FEV_1, and Polynesians tend to have the lowest. Reference values for a variety of populations have been published in the literature and many electronic spirometers come pre-loaded with reference data for different ethnic populations.

Normal and predicted values — PEFR

Results for PEFR are somewhat dependent on the device being used. Therefore, peak flow meters usually come with a 'reference value chart' specific to that device. Some caution should therefore be taken when comparing results from different meters. PEFR is affected by sex, height and age, which are taken into account in the reference value charts (see Figure 17.6).[9] In contrast to FVC and FEV_1, there does not appear to be ethnic variation in PEFR.[15]

Normal and predicted values — MIP/MEP

Similar to the PEFR test, the recorded MIP and MEP values are dependent on the type of device being used; maximal pressures tend to be larger when obtained from a straight rubber mouthpiece versus a flanged mouthpiece. MIP and MEP tend to decrease with increasing age, and are systematically higher in men compared with women. Prediction equations for reference values and the lower limit of normal (LLN) for MIP and MEP are shown in Table 17.3. An MIP/MEP less than the corresponding LLN may raise suspicion of respiratory muscle weakness.

Interpreting and classifying abnormal values

Clinicians are able to determine whether a participant has abnormal pulmonary function by identifying whether FEV_1, FVC, FEV_1/FVC and PEFR are outside the 'normal' range according to predicted values. Typically, ventilatory disorders are classified into one of three types: obstructive, restrictive and mixed. The changes in FEV_1/FVC, FVC (absolute and % predicted) and FEV_1 (absolute and % predicted) for the three ventilatory conditions are outlined in Table 17.2. The volume–time curves for obstructive, restrictive and mixed disorders are shown in Figure 17.10. It should be noted that, although MIP and MEP values may aid in the assessment of respiratory muscle strength, these parameters are not typically used in the differential diagnosis of obstructive, restrictive and mixed disorders.

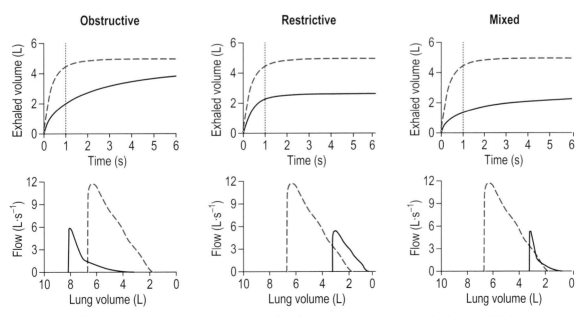

Figure 17.10 Volume–time and flow–volume curve for obstructive, restrictive and mixed ventilatory disorders. Dashed red curves are for a 'normal' individual (i.e. a healthy age-, height-, sex- and ethnicity-matched individual)

Adapted from: Johns and Pierce[6]

OBSTRUCTIVE DISORDERS

Obstructive disorders are characterised by a proportionally greater reduction in the maximal airflow from the lung relative to the maximal expired volume (FVC). Typically, obstructive disorders result in a decrease in both the absolute FVC and the FEV_1 (shown in the volume–time curve of Figure 17.10). The key features of a purely obstructive disorder are a proportionally greater reduction in FEV_1 relative to FVC, resulting in the FEV_1/FVC ratio being lower than normal (i.e. $<$70%) *and* an increase in TLC (shown in the flow–volume curve of Figure 17.10).

Obstructive disorders also result in a reduction in the PEFR compared with normal, and the slowing of the expiratory flow is shown by the concave shape of the flow–volume curve. The Global Initiative for Chronic Obstructive Pulmonary Disease (GOLD) classification system is used to define the severity of airflow limitation in chronic obstructive pulmonary disease (COPD), and is based on the reduction in the % predicted FEV1. There are four GOLD stages: GOLD I % predicted FEV1 80% (mild); GOLD II 79%–50% (moderate); GOLD III 49%–30% (severe); and GOLD IV = $<$30% with chronic respiratory failure.[16]

RESTRICTIVE DISORDERS

A restrictive disorder is characterised by a reduction in TLC, and generally also in FEV_1 and FVC (shown in the volume–time curve of Figure 17.10). However, the FEV_1/FVC ratio remains normal or slightly higher (FEV_1/FVC $>$85%), as the decreases in FVC and FEV_1 are in proportion. There is also a reduction in the PEFR compared with normal; however, the shape of the expiratory curve is normal.

MIXED DISORDERS

Mixed disorders show both obstructive and restrictive characteristics. There is a decrease in the FEV_1 and FVC in absolute terms (shown in the volume–time curve of Figure 17.10). However, *unlike* an obstructive disorder, the TLC is decreased, reflecting the restrictive component of this disease (shown in the flow–volume curve of Figure 17.10). On the other hand, *unlike* a restrictive disorder, FEV_1/FVC is decreased, indicating a proportionally greater decrease in FEV_1 relative to FVC (reflecting obstruction). Compared with 'normal', PEFR is reduced and the slowing of the expiratory flow is shown by the concave shape of the flow volume curve (reflecting the obstructive nature of the disorder).

UPPER AIRWAYS OBSTRUCTION

Airflow obstruction may also occur in the more central or upper airways of the tracheobronchial tree, referred to here as upper airways obstruction (UAO). The location of an UAO may be either extrathoracic (i.e. pharynx, larynx and extrathoracic trachea) or intrathoracic (i.e. intrathoracic trachea or primary bronchi), and termed either 'fixed' (e.g. tumour or goitre) or 'variable' (e.g. vocal cord paralysis) by nature. Figure 17.11 illustrates three different types of UAO that may be encountered during spirometric

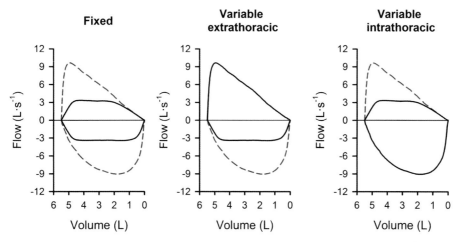

Figure 17.11 Maximal inspiratory and expiratory flow–volume curves for fixed (left panel), variable extrathoracic (middle panel) and variable intrathoracic (right panel) upper airways obstructions. Dashed red curves are for a 'normal' individual (i.e. a healthy age-, height-, sex- and ethnicity-matched individual)

Source: Troy J Cross, Menzies Health Institute Queensland, Griffith University

testing. FVC and FEV_1 are not typically affected by an UAO, whereas PEFR is almost always reduced. Accordingly, it has been suggested that an FEV_1/PEFR ratio >8 may suggest an UAO, warranting the collection of a maximal *inspiratory* flow–volume curve.[16] If the UAO is 'fixed' by nature, the resistance to airflow is present during expiration *and* inspiration, and so maximal inspiratory and expiratory flows are both reduced (Figure 17.11 left panel). Extrathoracic 'variable' obstructions are typified by a notable reduction in maximal inspiratory flows, while the maximal expiratory flow–volume curve is relatively normal (Figure 17.11 middle panel). On the other hand, intrathoracic 'variable' obstructions (e.g. functional lesion of lower trachea) decrease maximal expiratory flows, yet the maximal inspiratory flow–volume curve remains largely unaffected (Figure 17.11 right panel). It should be noted that these characteristic changes in the maximal flow–volume curve should be used only to raise the suspicion of an UAO. Radiological or endoscopic tests are required to confirm the presence (or absence) of a central/ upper airways obstruction.

Discussion and feedback

First, consider the three steps of feedback and discussion outlined in Appendix G. Before providing feedback to the participant, refer back to the initial medical history notes regarding whether the participant has any medical condition/s or is taking any medication/s that may have influenced the results. If the participant has previously performed pulmonary function testing, it would also be beneficial to obtain the past results as this may influence the details provided to ensure that the participant understands the feedback. This would also allow comparisons between the results to determine whether there have been changes over time rather than only the cross-sectional comparison with predicted data.

When providing feedback to the participant it is important to highlight that the '*diagnosis of lung disorder is given by a medically trained individual*' and is usually based on multiple measurements performed on separate occasions. Taking this into account, Table 17.2 can be used to classify (but not diagnose) lung disorders. For example, if the participant's results indicate an obstructive, restrictive or mixed lung disorder, ensure that the feedback provided highlights that this is based on categorising this single measure of lung function, and not diagnosing the disease.

Depending on the degree of severity of the obstructive, restrictive or mixed lung disorder classification, recommend to the participant that, if possible, they return for repeat spirometry testing on a separate occasion. If the participant has had their lung function measured and categorised as outside the normal range on two separate occasions, they should be referred to their medical practitioner.

Case studies

Setting: You work as an Accredited Exercise Physiologist in a large health centre. Part of your job is to supervise rehabilitation clinics for clients with a range of comorbidities.

Case Study 1

A 34-year-old female client has been complaining of shortness of breath when she exercises in the cold over the past few months. She is 167 cm tall and weighs 72 kg. She tells you she had asthma as a kid but 'doesn't take her puffers any more'. You think she may need to be referred to a GP to have the shortness of breath investigated before she commences strenuous exercise sessions.

continued overpage

Case studies *(continued)*

What additional questions would you ask the client?

_____

_____

_____

_____

You decide to test her pulmonary function so you can include the results in the letter you send with the client to her GP. You measure her FEV_1 as 2.47 L and her FVC as 3.78 L.

What are her predicted FVC, FEV_1 and FEV_1/FVC values?

FVC

Participant's best FVC result $= 3.78$ L

Predicted FVC $(L)^a =$ (height constant $\times$ height) + (age constant $\times$ age) + constant

$\qquad = ($ _____ $\times$ ____$) + ($ _____ $\times$ __$) +$ _____

$\qquad =$ _____ L

Difference between participant's best FVC result vs predicted FVC (e.g. '100 mL lower than predicted'): _____

Comparison of participant's best FVC result (absolute values) vs predicted FVC (please circle) – refer to the 'Interpreting and classifying abnormal values' section for guidance:

$$\downarrow\downarrow \qquad \downarrow \qquad \leftrightarrow \qquad \uparrow \qquad \uparrow\uparrow$$

Percent (%) predicted FVC $= \dfrac{\text{Best FVC result} \times 100}{\text{Predicted FVC result}}$

$\qquad =$ _____ %

Comparison of participant's best FVC result (relative values) vs predicted FVC (please circle) – refer to the 'Interpreting and classifying abnormal values' section for guidance:

$$\downarrow\downarrow \qquad \downarrow \qquad \leftrightarrow \qquad \uparrow \qquad \uparrow\uparrow$$

FEV_1

Participant's best FEV_1 result $= 2.47$ L

Predicted FEV_1 $(L)^a =$ (height constant $\times$ height) + (age constant $\times$ age) + constant

$\qquad = ($ _____ $\times$ ____$) + ($ _____ $\times$ __$) +$ _____

$\qquad = ($ _____ $\times$ ____$) +$ _____

$\qquad =$ _____ L

Difference between participant's best FEV_1 result vs predicted FEV_1 (e.g. '100 mL lower than predicted'): _____

continued

Case studies *(continued)*

Comparison of participant's best FEV_1 result (absolute values) vs predicted FEV_1 (please circle) — refer to the 'Interpreting and classifying abnormal values' section for guidance:

$$\downarrow\downarrow \qquad \downarrow \qquad \leftrightarrow \qquad \uparrow \qquad \uparrow\uparrow$$

Percent (%) predicted $FEV_1 = \dfrac{\text{Best FEV}_1 \text{ result} \times 100}{\text{Predicted FEV}_1 \text{ result}} = \underline{\hspace{4cm}}$

$= \underline{\hspace{2cm}}\%$

Comparison of participant's best FEV_1 result (relative values) vs predicted FEV_1 (please circle) — refer to the 'Interpreting and classifying abnormal values' section for guidance:

$$\downarrow\downarrow \qquad \downarrow \qquad \leftrightarrow \qquad \uparrow \qquad \uparrow\uparrow$$

FEV_1/FVC

Participant's best FEV_1/FVC result $= \underline{\hspace{3cm}}\%$

Predicted $FEV_1/FVC = \dfrac{\text{Predicted FEV}_1^a}{\text{Predicted FVC}^a}$

$= \underline{\hspace{2cm}}$

$= \underline{\hspace{2cm}}\%$

Difference between participant's best FEV_1/FVC result vs predicted FEV_1/FVC (e.g. '5% lower than predicted'): $\underline{\hspace{6cm}}$

Comparison of participant's best FEV_1 result (relative values) vs predicted FEV_1 (please circle) — refer to the 'Interpreting and classifying abnormal values' section for guidance:

$$\downarrow\downarrow \qquad \downarrow \qquad \leftrightarrow \qquad \uparrow \qquad \uparrow\uparrow$$

Classification of spirometric values (according to Table 17.2)

☐ 'Normal'

☐ Obstructive disorder

☐ Restrictive disorder

☐ Mixed disorder

^a From Table 17.1[7,8]

What feedback would you provide to the client?

$\underline{\hspace{14cm}}$

$\underline{\hspace{14cm}}$

$\underline{\hspace{14cm}}$

$\underline{\hspace{14cm}}$

Case Study 2

A 51-year-old male has been referred to you for cardiac rehabilitation after recently having a heart attack. He is 183 cm tall and weighs 97 kg. He tells you that his recovery has been a bit slower than he expected because he had some issues with his lungs after surgery, but he is unable to elaborate further. He has recently noticed that he is getting quite short of breath with exertion.

continued overpage

Case studies *(continued)*

What additional factors would you consider in trying to decide how to manage this patient?

_____

_____

_____

_____

After further questioning, the client tells you that his surgery was several months ago and that his surgical wounds have fully healed. He had already started rehabilitation and was exercising regularly up until a month ago, but had stopped because he rolled his ankle. He is now pain free and is keen to 'get back in to it'. He has a letter from his cardiologist stating that he is cleared to participate in rehabilitation. He has been getting breathless with exercise for several years and had some pulmonary function tests done a while ago, but can't remember the results. You decide to repeat the spirometry tests. The results show an FEV_1 of 3.02 L and his FVC of 3.17 L.

What are his predicted FEV_1 and FVC values?

FVC

Participant's best FVC result = 3.17 L

Predicted FVC_1 $(L)^a$ = (height constant × height) + (age constant × age) + constant

$\quad\quad\quad$ = (_____ × ____) + (_____ × ___) + _____

$\quad\quad\quad$ = _____ L

Difference between participant's best FVC result vs predicted FVC (e.g. '100 mL lower than predicted'): _____

Comparison of participant's best FVC result (absolute values) vs predicted FVC (please circle) – refer to the 'Interpreting and classifying abnormal values' section for guidance:

$$\downarrow\downarrow \quad\quad \downarrow \quad\quad \leftrightarrow \quad\quad \uparrow \quad\quad \uparrow\uparrow$$

Percent (%) predicted FVC $= \dfrac{\text{Best FVC result} \times 100}{\text{Predicted FVC result}} =$ _____

$\quad\quad\quad\quad\quad\quad\quad$ = _____ %

Comparison of participant's best FVC result (relative values) vs predicted FVC (please circle) – refer to the 'Interpreting and classifying abnormal values' section for guidance:

$$\downarrow\downarrow \quad\quad \downarrow \quad\quad \leftrightarrow \quad\quad \uparrow \quad\quad \uparrow\uparrow$$

FEV_1

Participant's best FEV_1 result = 3.02 L

Predicted FEV_1 $(L)^a$ = (height constant × height) + (age constant × age) + constant

$\quad\quad\quad$ = (_____ × ____) + (_____ × ___) + _____

$\quad\quad\quad$ = (_____ × ____) + _____

$\quad\quad\quad$ = _____ L

Difference between participant's best FEV_1 result vs predicted FEV_1 (e.g. '100 mL lower than predicted'): _____

continued

Case studies *(continued)*

Comparison of participant's best FEV_1 result (absolute values) vs predicted FEV_1 (please circle) — refer to the 'Interpreting and classifying abnormal values' section for guidance:

$$\downarrow\downarrow \qquad \downarrow \qquad \leftrightarrow \qquad \uparrow \qquad \uparrow\uparrow$$

$$\text{Percent (\%) predicted } FEV_1 = \frac{\text{Best } FEV_1 \text{ result} \times 100}{\text{Predicted } FEV_1 \text{ result}} = \underline{\hspace{2cm}}$$

$$= \underline{\hspace{2cm}} \%$$

Comparison of participant's best FEV_1 result (relative values) vs predicted FEV_1 (please circle) — refer to the 'Interpreting and classifying abnormal values' section for guidance:

$$\downarrow\downarrow \qquad \downarrow \qquad \leftrightarrow \qquad \uparrow \qquad \uparrow\uparrow$$

FEV_1/FVC

Participant's best FEV_1/FVC result $= \underline{\hspace{2cm}} \%$

$$\text{Predicted } FEV_1/FVC = \frac{\text{Predicted } FEV_1^a}{\text{Predicted } FVC^a}$$

$$= \underline{\hspace{2cm}}$$

$$= \underline{\hspace{2cm}} \%$$

Difference between participant's best FEV_1/FVC result vs predicted FEV_1/FVC (e.g. '5% lower than predicted'): _____

Comparison of participant's best FEV_1/FVC result (relative values) vs predicted FEV_1/FVC (please circle) — refer to the 'Interpreting and classifying abnormal values' section for guidance:

$$\downarrow\downarrow \qquad \downarrow \qquad \leftrightarrow \qquad \uparrow \qquad \uparrow\uparrow$$

Classification of spirometric values (according to Table 17.2)

☐ 'Normal'

☐ Obstructive disorder

☐ Restrictive disorder

☐ Mixed disorder

---

[a] From Table 17.1[7,8]

What feedback would you provide to the client?

_____

_____

_____

_____

Case Study 3

Jane, a 28-year old enthusiastic road cyclist, has been treated by her physician for exercise-induced asthma since she began cycling six years ago. Her symptoms include wheezing during exercise, accompanied by a sensation of tightening of the throat. These symptoms appear during higher-intensity exercise, resolve quickly when she stops exercising, and occur sporadically. Jane

continued overpage

Case studies *(continued)*

decides to undergo a battery of exercise tests to assist with her training but, because of her reported symptoms, is also advised to undergo a standard exercise and spirometry challenge to assess for exercise-induced bronchospasm. Baseline spirometry during pre-participation screening revealed normal lung function. Post-exercise spirometry tests, performed between 5 and 30 min after a high-intensity constant-load cycling bout while breathing cold dry air, elicited a 7% reduction in FVC but no clinically significant change in FEV_1 from baseline. During exercise, Jane experienced respiratory symptoms similar to that described in her history: wheezing was evident, especially during inspiration, with onset occurring early during the exercise bout. The maximal inspiratory flow-volume curves measured during the spirometric testing displayed signs of an extrathoracic 'variable' upper airways obstruction.

What feedback would you provide?

References

[1] Sales AT, Fregonezi GA, Ramsook AH, Guenette JA, Lima INDF, Reid WD. Respiratory muscle endurance after training in athletes and non-athletes: a systematic review and meta-analysis. Phys Ther Sport 2016;17:76–86.

[2] Beaumont M, Forget P, Couturaud F, Reychler G. Effects of inspiratory muscle training in COPD patients: a systematic review and meta-analysis. Clin Respir J 2018;12:2178–88.

[3] Cooper BG. An update on contraindications for lung function testing. Thorax 2011;66:714–23.

[4] [No authors listed] Lung function testing: selection of reference values and interpretative strategies. American Thoracic Society. Am Rev Respir Dis 1991;144:1202–18.

[5] [No authors listed] Standardization of spirometry, 1994 Update. American Thoracic Society. Am J Respir Crit Care Med 1995;152:1107–36.

[6] Johns DP, Pierce R. Pocket guide to spirometry. Sydney, NSW: McGraw-Hill; 2007.

[7] Crapo RO, Morris AH, Gardner RM. Reference spirometric values using techniques and equipment that meet ATS recommendations. Am Rev Respir Dis 1981;123:659–64.

[8] Crapo RO, Morris AH, Clayton PD, Nixon CR. Lung volumes in healthy nonsmoking adults. Bull Eur Physiopathol Respir 1982;18:419–25.

[9] Nunn AJ, Gregg I. New regression equations for predicting peak expiratory flow in adults. BMJ 1989;298:1068–70.

[10] Volianitis S, McConnell AK, Jones DA. Assessment of maximum inspiratory pressure. Prior submaximal respiratory muscle activity ('warm-up') enhances maximum inspiratory activity and attenuates the learning effect of repeated measurement. Respiration 2001;68:22–7.

[11] Fiz JA, Montserrat JM, Picado C, Plaza V, Agusti-Vidal A. How many manoeuvres should be done to measure maximal inspiratory mouth pressure in patients with chronic airflow obstruction? Thorax 1989;44:419–21.

[12] Evans JA, Whitelaw WA. The assessment of maximal respiratory mouth pressures in adults. Respir Care 2009;54:1348–59.

[13] Miller MR, Hankinson J, Brusasco V, Burgos F, Casaburi R, Coates A, et al. Standardisation of spirometry. Eur Respir J 2005;26:319–38.

[14] American Thoracic Society. 2005. Pulmonary function testing. https://www.thoracic.org/statements/pulmonary-function.php.

[15] Hankinson JL, Odencrantz JR, Fedan KB. Spirometric reference values from a sample of the general U.S. population. Am J Respir Crit Care Med 1999;159:179–87.

[16] Global Initiative for Chronic Obstructive Lung Disease (GOLD). Global strategy for the diagnosis, management, and prevention of chronic obstructive pulmonary disease. GOLD, 2021. https://www.goldcopd.org.

[17] Pellegrino R, Viegi G, Brusasco V, Crapo RO, Burgos F, Casaburi R, et al. Interpretative strategies for lung function tests. Eur Respir J 2005;26:948–68.

PRACTICAL 18
RESTING AND EXERCISE ELECTROCARDIOGRAPHY (ECG)

Steve Selig and Julian Sacre

LEARNING OBJECTIVES

- Explain the scientific rationale, purposes, accuracy, reliability and limitations of ECG assessments
- Identify and explain the common terminology, processes and equipment required to conduct accurate and safe ECG assessments
- Identify and describe the contraindications or considerations that may require the modification of ECG assessments, and make appropriate adjustments for relevant populations or participants
- Conduct appropriate pre-assessment procedures, including explaining the test, obtaining informed consent and a focused medical history, and performing a pre-exercise risk assessment
- Describe the principles and rationale for the calibration of the trace and adjust when necessary
- Identify the need for guidance or further information from an appropriate health professional, and recognise when medical supervision is required before or during an assessment and when to cease a test
- Conduct an appropriate protocol for safe and effective resting and exercise ECG assessments, including client instruction
- Perform basic interpretation of the resting and exercise ECG traces and demonstrate an understanding of common ECG abnormalities
- Integrate knowledge of and skills in health, exercise and sport assessment with other study areas of exercise science, in particular the cardiovascular physiology that underpins common exercise contraindications
- Record, analyse and interpret information from an ECG assessment and convey the results through relevant verbal and/or written communication with the participant or involved professional (e.g. medical practitioner)

Equipment and other requirements

- Information sheet and informed consent form
- Adult Pre-exercise Screening System (APSS) form
- Rating of perceived exertion (RPE) chart (see Appendix E)
- Bed or massage table with pillow
- Skin preparation
- Shaver

- Alcohol wipes
- Abrasive pad or sandpaper
- Programmable motorised treadmill
- Electrodes
- ECG monitor
- Sphygmomanometer on stand with various size arm cuffs (with size and position indicators)
- Stethoscope
- Pulse oximeter
- Cleaning and disinfecting equipment (see Appendix A)

INTRODUCTION

The prevalence of cardiovascular disease and increased availability of exercise stress testing in hospitals and clinics has led many exercise science graduates to gain employment as cardiac technicians. Knowledge of the key discipline areas of exercise science along with high-level communication skills and the technical competency to conduct the tests make exercise science graduates attractive employees in this field. The skills needed to conduct and interpret clinical exercise tests are also required in non-clinical environments when additional cardiovascular health monitoring is indicated or requested. For example, a Masters athlete may need an electrocardiogram (ECG) stress or exercise test before undertaking a high-intensity exercise program or competition.

DEFINITIONS

Acute myocardial infarction (AMI): also known as a heart attack, this refers to an interruption of blood flow to part of the heart muscle causing cells to die. It is commonly caused by coronary artery disease (CAD).

Angina: chest pain caused by decreased blood flow to part of the heart muscle usually caused by coronary artery disease. Angina may occur at rest or it may manifest only during exercise or other stress when there is a greater demand for coronary blood flow.

Atherosclerosis: plaque (fatty deposits) in the arteries, causing the vessel wall to thicken and the channel through which blood flows to narrow.

Cardiorespiratory fitness: ability to supply oxygen and support the energy demands during sustained physical activity. Also known as aerobic fitness or aerobic endurance.

Cardiovascular disease (CVD): an umbrella term that refers to any disease that affects the heart or blood vessels. This includes coronary heart disease (CHD), heart failure, hypertension, peripheral vascular disease and stroke (cerebrovascular accident).

Chronotropic competence: ability of the heart to increase its rate when there is demand for increased cardiac output (e.g. with exercise).

Coronary artery disease (CAD): also known as coronary heart disease (CHD) or ischaemic heart disease (IHD), this is a narrowing or blockage of the coronary arteries of the heart, usually caused by atherosclerosis. It can lead to chest pain (angina) or a heart attack (myocardial infarction) and damage to the heart muscle.

Diastole: period of the cardiac cycle during which the heart muscle relaxes and refills with blood.

ECG electrodes: the devices with conductive material attached to the participant's skin.

ECG leads: the recordings of electrical activity based on voltage differences between two electrodes (bipolar leads) or voltage differences between an electrode and a reference potential (unipolar leads).

Ectopic beats: beats that are initiated from a region in the heart outside the sinoatrial node.

Heart rate reserve: peak heart rate during maximal exercise test minus resting heart rate.

Intermittent claudication: ischaemic pain usually in the lower legs during walking that is relieved by rest. It usually manifests from peripheral artery disease.

Ischaemia: reduced blood flow to tissues (e.g. part of the heart muscle) caused by shortfall in oxygen delivery relative to demand. Ischaemia may cause symptoms (e.g. angina) or may be asymptomatic ('silent ischaemia').

J point: junction between the termination of the QRS complex and the beginning of the ST segment.

Negative test: no indication of disease, although it does not necessarily exclude the possibility.

Positive test: indication that disease is present, but this may require further clinical or diagnostic confirmation.

Sinus rhythm: normal rhythm of the heart (i.e. the heart's electrical activity is initiated by the sinoatrial (SA) node).

ST segment: represents the time between the end of ventricular depolarisation and the beginning of repolarisation.

ST segment depression: a finding on the ECG that may indicate the presence of ischaemia – defined as translation of the J point ≥ 1.0 mm below the isoelectric line and extending for 60–80 ms.[1]

Systole: period of the cardiac cycle during which the heart muscle contracts and ejects blood.

Test sensitivity: proportion of participants with disease who have a positive test.

Test specificity: proportion of participants without disease who have a negative test.

Vasospasm: when an arterial spasm leads to vasoconstriction. This can lead to tissue ischaemia and tissue death (necrosis).

Vasovagal response: when heart rate and blood pressure (BP) drop to a point that a decreased blood flow to the brain causes a range of symptoms including dizziness or fainting.

PURPOSES

It is important to appreciate why ECG monitoring is performed as part of a graded exercise test. One of the main purposes of exercise ECG monitoring is for the early detection of coronary artery disease (CAD). Because blood flow to the heart muscle (myocardium) at rest is relatively low, ECG abnormalities may not appear at rest unless the condition is advanced. In contrast, exercise at progressively higher intensities (work rates) – with consequent increases in myocardial oxygen requirements – may 'unmask' conditions, such as a limitation in coronary blood flow in people with less-advanced disease. This can lead to earlier diagnosis of the condition, resulting in earlier treatment. ECG abnormalities indicative of CAD may be observed at submaximal or maximal exercise intensities, and/or during the post-exercise recovery period. Thus, we can exploit the additional 'stress' imposed by exercise on the heart to increase the sensitivity of ECG monitoring to detect CAD. Additional purposes of ECG monitoring during exercise are to identify other cardiovascular abnormalities such as conduction defects and arrhythmias that may contraindicate exercise and need medical follow-up.

Aside from CAD detection, clinical exercise testing, including ECG, may serve important additional purposes, as outlined below.[2]

Diagnostic
- Detect and record previously undiagnosed rhythm or conduction disturbances that may indicate the need for medical interventions. These may indicate ischaemic or other (e.g. congenital) heart disease, or be benign (i.e. not needing medical treatment at this time). Some arrhythmias and conduction defects not observed at rest may be unmasked during exercise and/or recovery.

Prognostic
- Determine exercise capacity – based on maximal work rate achieved (e.g. estimated metabolic equivalents, METs). This measure, and/or maximal aerobic power ($\dot{V}O_2max$), is strongly linked to morbidity and mortality outcomes.[3,4] This includes patients with cardiovascular disease.[5]

- Determine cardiorespiratory fitness (e.g. expired gas analysis for maximal/peak aerobic power; $\dot{V}O_2$max).
- Determine the heart rate response to exercise (chronotropic competence) and post-exercise heart rate recovery – both are indications of autonomic nervous system function.
- Determine the heart rate responses to exercise and post-exercise heart rate recovery for arrhythmias (e.g. atrial fibrillation, tachyarrhythmias), tachycardias, bradycardias, conduction defects (e.g. AV blocks, re-entrant circuits), implantable pacemakers and automated implantable cardioverter defibrillators.
- Determine the blood pressure response to exercise and recovery from exercise; the latter enables screening for post-exercise hypotension and a vasovagal response.

Therapeutic

- Determine safe and effective exercise levels (submaximal) and limits (maximal) – particularly exercise intensity – for the purpose of designing appropriate exercise and physical activity interventions.
- Identify work rates associated with the onset of ischaemic symptoms (e.g. thresholds of angina or vascular claudication).
- Evaluate the effectiveness of a cardiac rehabilitation program or an exercise program.
- Evaluate the effectiveness of a medical, surgical, lifestyle or pharmacological treatment.
- Screen for safety to undergo surgery (e.g. anaerobic threshold before surgery) and/or to use exercise to improve fitness prior to surgery ('prehab').
- Motivate participants with cardiovascular disease to exercise and develop healthier lifestyles.
- Assist in maintaining the effect of an exercise intervention.

Limitations

The exercise ECG is not in itself diagnostic. Sometimes ECGs falsely indicate heart disease when it doesn't exist ('false positive') and, conversely, sometimes ECGs fail to identify heart disease when it is present ('false negative').

The most common approach to exercise ECG is the 12-lead ECG. This provides a means of obtaining an 'electrical picture' of the heart in three dimensions or two planes (frontal and transverse). Similar to cameras positioned around a sporting stadium having different views of the action on the field, the various ECG leads provide their own unique view of the electrical activity occurring in the heart. Consequently, clinically significant abnormalities may be identified in some leads, but not in others.

VALIDITY

The concurrent and prognostic validity of exercise ECG is usually expressed in terms of sensitivity and specificity. In contrast to a 'perfect' test, which would have a sensitivity of 100% (all people with disease have a positive result) and specificity of 100% (all people without disease have a negative result), the exercise ECG has been found to have around 70% sensitivity and 80% specificity for detection of CAD.[2] This will vary depending on the characteristics of people undergoing the test and the expertise of the investigators. In any case, the incidence of false positives and false negatives means that exercise ECG is an important first step in a diagnostic regimen ('gatekeeper') that may subsequently include echocardiography and other imaging and diagnostic techniques (e.g. calcium scans, radionuclide perfusion scans, angiography, cardiac computerised tomography (CT) scans and magnetic resonance imaging (MRI)). These are more sensitive and specific than ECG alone,[6] but require additional expertise, expense and time and/or are inconvenient or uncomfortable for the patient. For example, angiography is an invasive procedure involving coronary artery catheterisation to confirm CAD diagnosis. Subsequent treatment in cases of confirmed CAD may include lifestyle modifications (e.g. exercise and nutritional interventions), drug therapies or medical interventions (e.g. angioplasty, stenting or coronary artery bypass surgery).

Pulse oximetry

During an exercise ECG test in a clinical setting, it is also usual to monitor the oxygen saturation in the blood, which is the fraction of oxygen-saturated haemoglobin relative to total haemoglobin (i.e. unsaturated + saturated). This can be done non-invasively using pulse oximetry. This technique uses the light-absorptive characteristics of haemoglobin and the pulsating nature of blood flow in the arteries to determine the oxygen saturation of the blood. It is considered to be a good indicator of oxygen delivery to the peripheral tissues, and is used as a general indicator of exercise tolerance and to evaluate the need for supplemental oxygen. Normal pulse oximeter readings usually range from 95% to 100%, with values under 90% considered low. Low oxygen saturation is a manifestation of various cardiac or pulmonary disorders, but care needs to be taken in the interpretation of this measure. For example, oxygen saturation may be normal with anaemias and uncomplicated coronary artery disease, but low in some forms of heart failure and obstructive airways conditions such as asthma and chronic obstructive pulmonary disease (COPD).

SCIENTIFIC RATIONALE

To interpret changes that may occur during a resting or exercise ECG, it is essential to appreciate the physiology and electrical activities that underpin each specific characteristic of the ECG waveform.

Although all cardiac cells are capable of conducting action potentials, specific pathways in the heart enable a rapid and coordinated transmission of electrical signals throughout the heart's chambers (atria and ventricles). This signal (the action potential) is initiated at the sinoatrial node (SA node) (Figure 18.1).[7] Depolarisation of the SA node spreads in a wave-like fashion throughout the atria via the internodal tracks before reaching the atrioventricular node (AV node). It then continues to the common bundle of His before branching into the bundles (left and right bundle branches), Purkinje fibres and eventually into the myocardial cells. The depolarisation causes contraction of the heart muscle (systole). The subsequent repolarisation occurs during relaxation of the heart muscle (diastole). These events are captured by the surface ECG.

The electrical patterns and timings are tightly coupled with the mechanical/contractile function of the heart (Figure 18.2). Although most filling of the ventricles occurs during the early part of diastole and is passive, the initial conduction pathway (SA → AV node) enables contraction of the atrial chambers to 'top up' the blood volume in the ventricles (referred to as atrial 'kick'). A subsequent slowing of conduction at the AV node further facilitates this by delaying arrival of the signal at the bundle branches/Purkinje fibres and thus enabling optimal filling of the ventricles *before* they start contracting. In this way, the greatest volume of blood can be ejected to the lungs (from the right ventricle) and the rest of the body (from the left ventricle).

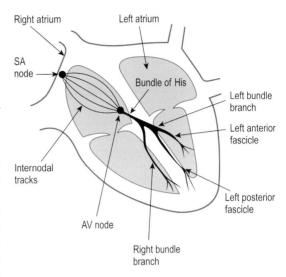

Figure 18.1 Location of SA and AV nodes and conduction pathways. Activation of the Purkinje fibres (not shown) after the bundle branches/fascicles represents the end point of the conduction pathway

Source: Jayasinghe, Figure 1.2, p 4[7]

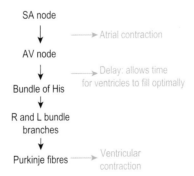

Figure 18.2 Timing of electrical activity and the contractile function of the heart

ECG LEADS AND ELECTRODES

The terms *electrode* and *lead* are not interchangeable. The standard 12-lead ECG consists of 10 separate electrodes, comprising four limb electrodes and six chest electrodes. These enable an almost 360° view of the heart. Figure 18.3 displays the torso locations for the ECG electrodes and Box 18.1[2] provides the locations for an exercise test.

Note: The electrode positioning for an exercise ECG test is different to that for a resting ECG (not followed by an exercise ECG), in which the limb electrodes (left arm (LA), right arm (RA), left leg (LL), right leg (RL)) may be placed on the wrists and ankles.

Of the four limb electrodes, the RL electrode provides a 'ground' signal while the remaining three are used to project six leads: three bipolar leads (I, II and III; forming a triangle) and three unipolar leads (aVR, aVF, aVL). These are shown in Figure 18.4. The six chest electrodes are used for the six unipolar leads (V1–V6, Figure 18.5) giving an overall total of *10 electrodes* projecting *12 leads*.

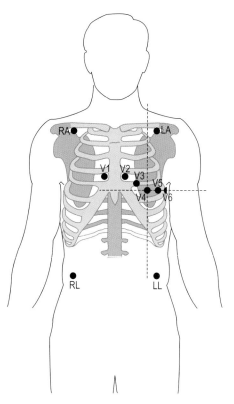

Figure 18.3 Electrode placements

Box 18.1 Electrode placement for an exercise test

V1: fourth intercostal space adjacent to the sternum on the right side

V2: fourth intercostal space adjacent to the sternum on the left side

V3: midway between V2 and V4

V4: fifth intercostal space on the midclavicular line

V5: same horizontal level as V4, on the anterior axillary line

V6: same horizontal level as V4, on the midaxillary line

RA: right subclavicular space, medial to the border of the deltoid muscle

LA: left subclavicular space, medial to the border of the deltoid muscle

RL: above iliac crest on the right anterior axillary line

LL: above iliac crest on the left anterior axillary line

Note: The positions of the electrodes are usually adjusted to avoid breast tissue in women. This involves downward shifting of V3–V6 so that these electrodes are placed under the breast
Source: Kligfield[2]

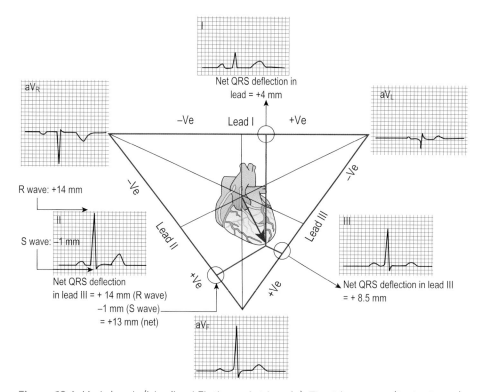

Figure 18.4 Limb leads (idealised Einthoven's triangle). The blue arrow (in the heart) represents the ventricular depolarisation (QRS) vector for this normal ECG; the amplitude and direction are determined by the 'reflections' of leads I, II and III on the three sides of Einthoven's triangle. Each of these three 'reflections' is determined as the difference between the amplitude of the R wave and the amplitude of the Q or S wave (whichever is larger) on the QRS complex. For instance, in the figure above, lead II shows +14 mm for the R wave, 0 mm for Q and −1 mm for S, leaving a net amplitude of +13 mm. This determines the point of perpendicular intersection (black circle) of the orange line with the side of the triangle corresponding to lead II. Orange lines are also drawn perpendicular to the respective sides of the triangle corresponding to leads I and III (as in the figure). The blue arrow − drawn from the centre of the triangle to the common meeting point of all orange vectors − represents the amplitude and direction of the QRS depolarisation vector.

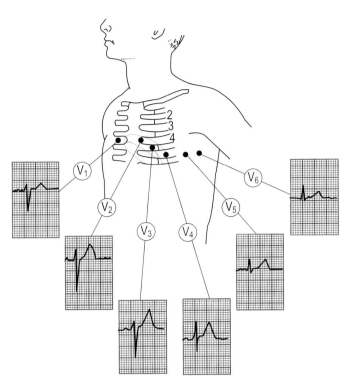

Figure 18.5 Chest leads with an indication of how the traces vary depending on electrode position

---

Note: The 12 leads may also be grouped according to their view of the various surfaces of the heart:

- inferior: leads II, III and aVF
- anterior: leads V3–V4
- lateral: leads I, aVL and V5–V6
- septal (interventricular): leads V1–V2
- posterior: aVR.

Due to this differential orientation/positioning of leads in relation to the heart, the electrical activity occurring during each cardiac cycle will appear differently in each lead. It is important to appreciate that this is because they have a different viewpoint of the *same* electrical activity – not because they are showing different activity.

An electrical signal travelling towards the positive pole of a lead will result in a positive (upward) deflection from the 'isoelectric' baseline, and vice versa. To understand this, look at Figure 18.4 – propagation of the electrical signal from the SA node to the AV node (causing atrial contraction and the P wave on the ECG) is in a direction *away from* the RA electrode (lead aVR) and *towards* the LL electrode (lead aVF). As such, this will cause a *positive* deflection (*upright* P wave) in aVF but a simultaneous *negative* deflection (*downward* P wave) in aVR.

What about the bipolar leads? The same principle applies because these leads also have a positive pole – for lead I it is the LA electrode, and for leads II and III it is the LL electrode. Because the orientation of lead II is usually parallel to the direction of depolarisation (SA node $\rightarrow$ AV node and subsequent vector of ventricular depolarisation; see Figure 18.4), it gives a particularly good view of important components of the conduction pathway and is therefore commonly used as the 'rhythm strip'.

A typical lead II ECG recording is displayed in Figure 18.6. Basic interpretation of the ECG involves examining the magnitude, length and direction of the various deflections/spikes and when they occur in relation to each other. Each of these can be linked to specific components of the electrical conduction pathway, as follows:

- P wave: atrial *de*polarisation (SA node $\rightarrow$ AV node)
- QRS complex: ventricular *de*polarisation (**note:** atrial *re*polarisation is embedded in the QRS and so is not visible on the surface ECG at rest)
- T wave: ventricular *re*polarisation.

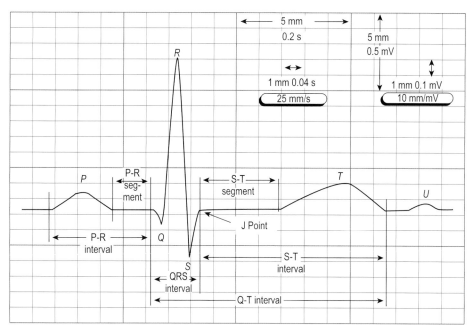

Figure 18.6 Typical ECG recording (lead II)

The presence of positive P waves in lead II is consistent with initiation of depolarisation at the SA node and is therefore used to indicate sinus rhythm. Criteria for a normal ECG are provided in Box 18.2. For the purposes of ECG interpretation in this practical, the PR interval, QRS complex width and QT interval will be calculated from an ECG printout.

Box 18.2 Normal ECG parameters

Pacing the SA node is pacing the heart. This refers to sinus rhythm. Therefore, a 'P' wave normal and present for every 'QRS' complex in a ratio of 1:1.

PR interval between 120 and 200 ms: $<$120 ms may indicate conduction defects such as pre-excitation syndrome; $>$200 ms indicates AV nodal block.

QRS complex is regular with width between 40 and 120 ms, with the most common width being in the range of 40–60 ms. A prolonged QRS complex may indicate conduction defects (particularly bundle branch blocks).

QT interval is between 350 and 400 ms, but is heart rate dependent. Heart rate-corrected QT (QTc) is calculated by the QT/$\sqrt{\text{RR}}$ interval, where the RR interval represents the time between consecutive R waves. QTc should be $\leq$450 ms in men and $\leq$470 ms in women.[7] Prolonged or shortened QT intervals are associated with some ventricular arrhythmias.

Figure 18.7 shows examples of variations in the normal ECG. In a person with a healthy cardiovascular system, variations in the normal ECG may be due to body size and shape (e.g. a tall, slender frame = vertical electrical axis; a short, obese frame = horizontal axis) and rotation of the heart in the chest. Counter-clockwise rotation of the heart causes the left ventricular free wall to be more anterior in the chest and so V3–V4 are positive (e.g. the middle trace in Figure 18.7), and clockwise rotation causes the right ventricular free wall to be more anterior in the chest and so V3–V4 are negative.

An important feature of the ECG, particularly in the context of exercise testing, is the ST segment. This begins at the J point and represents the end of ventricular depolarisation. The position of the ST segment in relation to the isoelectric line, along with T-wave morphology, is central to determining the

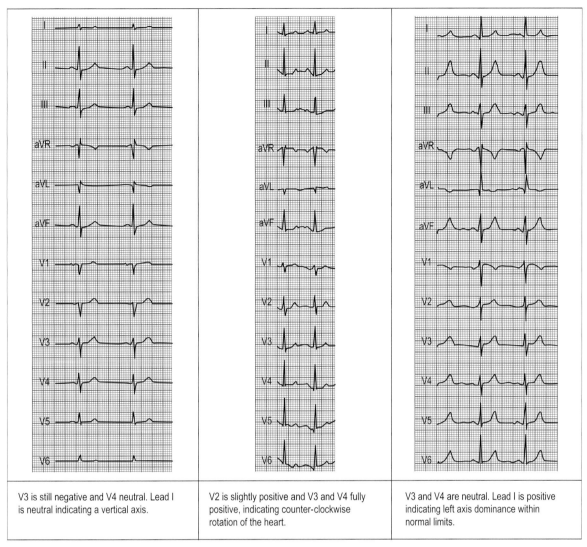

| V3 is still negative and V4 neutral. Lead I is neutral indicating a vertical axis. | V2 is slightly positive and V3 and V4 fully positive, indicating counter-clockwise rotation of the heart. | V3 and V4 are neutral. Lead I is positive indicating left axis dominance within normal limits. |

Figure 18.7 Examples of normal variation in the 12-lead ECG

presence of ischaemia (indicative of CAD) and other abnormalities. Since ST-segment displacement is a fundamental outcome of exercise ECG testing, it has received the most emphasis in this practical and is described in detail in the next section. However, it is important to realise that the range of abnormalities and cardiovascular disorders that may be detected with an ECG (resting and exercise) is extensive. With the additional training that exercise science graduates entering the field of cardiac investigations undertake, it is possible to detect heart axis deviations, changes in chamber size, atrial and ventricular arrhythmias, electrolyte imbalances, drug effects, cardiopulmonary syndromes and numerous other features of the healthy or diseased heart.

USING THE ECG TO DETECT CAD

There are two main clinical manifestations of CAD: angina (chest pain) or an acute myocardial infarction (AMI). Both usually arise from atherosclerosis in the coronary arteries. A lack of angina or history of heart attack *does not exclude* the possibility of CAD. Myocardial ischaemia may occur in the absence of symptoms ('silent ischaemia') or it may be induced only under certain conditions (e.g. during exercise).

ECG evidence of ischaemia

Ischaemia causes changes in the electrical performance of the myocardium, which is then reflected on the surface ECG. The primary manifestation of ischaemia on the ECG is depression of the ST segment (Figure 18.8) – defined as translation of the J point ≥ 1.0 mm below the isoelectric line and extending for 60–80 ms.[1]

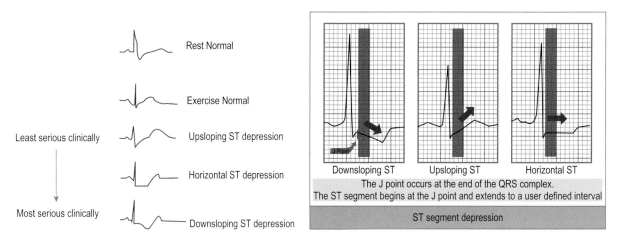

Figure 18.8 ST–segment changes during rest and exercise

In addition to its starting position, the morphology of the ST segment is also meaningful: ST-segment depression can be categorised as upsloping (least significant clinically – sometimes a normal variant that is *not* indicative of ischaemia), horizontal or downsloping (the latter is most significant clinically, indicating that ischaemia is more likely). Remember that ischaemia may be present at rest (usually in more-advanced disease), so the ST segment needs to be examined on the resting ECG and not just during exercise.

The ECG needs to be continually monitored for changes in the ST segment throughout the test. It is also important that people are encouraged to exercise to volitional fatigue (provided there are no indications for termination – Appendix F). Insufficient participant effort may cause a submaximal cardiometabolic response insufficient to elicit ischaemia and associated ST changes even if CAD is present (i.e. a false negative).

In addition to ST-segment depression and morphology, there are many other ECG signs of coronary ischaemia including T-wave inversion, arrhythmias and conduction defects that are sometimes responsible for acute coronary events, even sudden death.

ECG evidence of myocardial infarction

If left untreated, ischaemia may progress to an AMI. It is very difficult to identify those people in whom an AMI is likely to occur. These events are not fully predicted either by the presence or severity of traditional cardiovascular risk factors (e.g. cholesterol levels), or by the severity of coronary artery narrowing (stenosis). This is because of the involvement of other, emerging risk factors and mechanisms (e.g. pro-inflammatory factors) that contribute to the aetiology and pathogenesis of acute coronary events. Diseased arteries may also come in and out of pro-thrombogenic states ('unstable angina'), while coronary arteries may also undergo vasospasm that can cause acute ischaemia and infarctions.

Unfortunately, some AMIs progress to full-wall-thickness infarctions (usually due to lack of urgent medical intervention). These are termed Q infarctions owing to the permanence of deep pathological Q waves on the surface ECG in the region of the necrotic wall (permanent loss of resting membrane potential in that region).

Somewhat confusingly, the manifestation of an AMI on the ECG involves ST elevation. This somewhat paradoxical phenomenon (ST depression and elevation as two separate manifestations of the same disease) is explained by the progression of injury and death of tissue spreading from the endocardium (acute ischaemia and angina) to the epicardium (fully evolved AMI; also known as ST-elevation myocardial infarction (STEMI), Q infarction or full-wall-thickness infarction). The surface ECG electrodes are closest to the epicardium and therefore gradually change their orientations of ST segments as the AMI proceeds. This process takes several hours and explains why urgent thrombolysis or revascularisation are effective only if applied as soon as possible after the onset of the acute event. If the AMI is confined to the endocardium then it is known as non-ST-elevation myocardial infarction (NSTEMI) or non-full wall thickness infarction. The order of progression of ECG changes with myocardial ischaemia and AMI is ST depression (first hour) to ST elevation (first few hours) to deep pathological Q waves (permanent). Fortunately, not all people with ischaemia will necessarily develop an AMI.

EXERCISE PROTOCOL

A treadmill protocol is suggested for exercise stress testing as it is likely to elicit a higher oxygen consumption than other modes (e.g. cycling). There are a number of well-established treadmill protocols for performing exercise ECG tests with pre-set duration, speed and grade at each stage. The most common are the 'Bruce' treadmill protocols (e.g. standard and modified – see Tables 11.4 and 16.2). Although their large and unequal increments in work rate make them less desirable for assessment of cardiorespiratory fitness, they continue to be widely used in clinical settings for exercise ECG. The selection of the protocol depends on the estimated exercise capacity of the participant. For most younger individuals the standard Bruce protocol[8] (featured in the data analysis table) will be appropriate; however, for deconditioned, middle-aged or older participants, the modified Bruce[9] is suggested. As the majority of participants completing this test when using this manual will be younger individuals, the standard Bruce protocol is recommended for this practical.

Activity 18.1 Resting 12-lead ECG

AIM: obtain a resting 12-lead ECG of sufficient quality to enable a medical practitioner to diagnose and identify major components and interpret the trace.

Background

The resting ECG is used to detect potential cardiac abnormalities and to screen for relative (e.g. controlled atrial fibrillation, incomplete conduction defects) and absolute (e.g. uncontrolled atrial fibrillation, left bundle branch block, third-degree AV nodal block) contraindications to exercise. The location of events in the heart may correspond with changes in specific ECG leads with the best view of that region. This is the reason why 12-leads are monitored.

Protocol summary

Place electrodes, generate a good-quality ECG trace, identify the P wave, QRS complex and T wave and measure the PR, QRS and QT intervals.

Protocol

1 Follow the pre-test and test procedures outlined in Appendix B.

2 Ask the participant to lie supine on a comfortable surface (e.g. clinic bed, massage table).

3 If needed, shave hair in an area large enough for each electrode. Be sure to ask the participant for permission prior to shaving.

4 Abrade the skin to remove dead or flaking skin.

5 Cleanse the shaved and/or abraded site with an alcohol wipe.

6 Allow the skin to dry and then apply the electrodes to the prepared area (also refer to Box 18.1).

   a. Place V1 first. To locate the 4th intercostal space, begin by identifying the 1st intercostal space below the right clavicle (the 1st rib is usually hidden behind the clavicle). Then, progressively move your fingers horizontally down each rib and intercostal space (on the immediate right side of the participant's sternum) until you reach the 4th intercostal space.

   b. V2 can then be placed directly opposite V1 on the left side of the sternum, also in the 4th intercostal space.

   c. V4 is placed in the 5th intercostal space of the vertical intersection to the middle of the clavicle (see the Note box below point 6 for placement on women).

d. V3 is placed in a straight line directly between V2 and V4 – in females this position may need to be modified around the sports bra (see the Note box below point 6 for placement on women).

e. Stand side-on to the participant; visually identify the midaxillary line (an imaginary vertical line from the middle of the axilla (armpit) to the ilium along the longitudinal axis of the body) and place V6 in the same horizontal plane as V4.

f. V5 is placed on the anterior axillary line (an imaginary vertical line from the anterior axillary fold (front of armpit)), also in the same horizontal plane as V4.

g. If the participant is having only a resting ECG then the limb electrodes (LA, RA, LL and RL) are placed on the corresponding wrists and ankles. They should be on the inside of the arm/leg just above the wrist/ankle. For participants undergoing an exercise ECG test (see Activity 18.2), the arm limb electrodes (LA, RA) are placed below each clavicle, medial to the border of the deltoid muscle. The leg limb electrodes (LL, RL) can be placed above the iliac crest on the corresponding anterior axillary line. This is usually just above the pants line. If the electrodes are placed on the iliac crest the signal is likely to be poor when the participant is exercising.

> **Note:** The positions of the electrodes are usually adjusted to avoid breast tissue in women. This involves downward shifting of V3–V6 so that these electrodes are placed under the breast.

7 When connecting the cables to the electrodes, minimise cord tangling and ensure the cables do not pull on electrodes.

8 The signal quality of the resting ECG should be verified – artefact or noise in any lead should lead to the inspection of relevant electrodes and cables. Furthermore, the morphology of all leads should be checked to verify that they are appropriately positive or negative. This is done to ensure that cables have not been inadvertently connected to the wrong electrodes.

9 Ensure the cables are not tangled.

10 When the quality of the ECG trace is acceptable, obtain a printout from all 12 leads for 10 seconds.

11 Based on lead II, determine the parameters outlined on the data-recording sheet and give an overall interpretation of the rhythm.

12 Clean and disinfect all equipment (see Appendix A).

Data recording

Participant's name: _____   Date: _____

Age: _____ years   Sex: _____

Considerations:

_____

_____

Parameters:

Heart rate: _____   (60–100 bpm = normal; <60 bpm = bradycardia; >100 bpm = tachycardia)

continued

Data recording *(continued)*

Classification: _____

P wave present and upright in lead II?

_____

(if present, regular and upright in lead II, indicates normal sinus rhythm; if absent or abnormal in shape, orientation or timing, may indicate atrial fibrillation/flutter, or atrial, ventricular or junctional ectopics, or other arrhythmia or conduction defect)

Size/duration: _____

(normal P-wave size <2.5 mm (height) and <120 ms (duration); if heightened, consider atrial enlargement such as in mitral stenosis)

PR interval: _____

(normal $= 120-200$ ms; if prolonged, consider AV block; if shortened, consider pre-excitation)

QRS complex width:

_____

(normal $= 40-120$ ms, with the usual width being $40-60$ ms; ventricular ectopic beats (but not surrounding sinus beats) and partial and complete bundle branch blocks (all beats) have wide QRS complexes)

ST segment — displacement?

_____

(is the J point above (ST elevation), on or below (ST depression) the isoelectric line? If displaced by >1 mm, consider ischaemia or infarction)

Slope: _____

(upsloping, horizontal or downsloping, in order of least to most significant clinically, in the setting of ST depression)

QT interval: _____

(HR dependent; corrected QT (QT / $\sqrt{RR}$ interval) should be ≤ 450 ms (men), ≤ 470 ms (women))[7]

T wave $+$ve or $-$ve:

_____

(should be positive in lead II; T-wave abnormalities (e.g. inversion) may coincide with ST-segment changes)

Interpretation:

_____

_____

_____

_____

_____

_____

Activity 18.2 Exercise ECG

AIM: obtain an exercise 12-lead ECG of sufficient quality to enable a medical practitioner to diagnose and identify major components and interpret the trace.

Background

Exercise is used to increase myocardial oxygen requirements and unmask conditions, such as a limitation in coronary blood flow. The ECG is used to detect these conditions, or other potential abnormalities, while the person is exercising. ST-segment changes during exercise can be difficult to interpret from the ECG if substantive movement artefact occurs. This is a major cause of equivocal or uninterpretable (non-diagnostic) tests. Accordingly, stringent pre-exercise set-up – including skin preparation, electrode placement and cable/belt positioning – is essential.

Protocol summary

The test involves the participant completing the Bruce treadmill protocol while their heart is monitored with a 12-lead ECG, and BP, heart rate and oxygen saturation are measured and recorded every 3 minutes (i.e. at the end of every stage).

Protocol

Pre-test (with participant present)

1 Follow the pre-exercise test procedures outlined in Appendix B.

2 Check Appendix C to ensure there are no contraindications to exercise testing.

3 Skin preparation and electrode application: as per Activity 18.1, with the arm limb electrodes (LA, RA) placed below each clavicle (avoiding the deltoid and pectoral muscles as much as possible), and the leg limb electrodes (LL, RL) placed on the waist (above the iliac crest, on the anterior axillary line).

4 During an exercise ECG, the cables are often connected to a small box-shaped module with a belt, which should be placed and tightened at hip level. When connecting the cables to the electrodes, minimise cord tangling and ensure the cables do not pull on electrodes or interfere with participant's movement or breathing. These steps are important to decrease movement artefact.

5 Attach the pulse oximeter. This will be on either a finger or an earlobe depending on the manufacturer's instructions. It will contain a spring-loaded clamp that will gently pinch either the ear or a finger.

6 Place a chair near the treadmill for the participant to sit on after the test.

7 Resting data to be collected before commencing the exercise test include a 12-lead ECG, heart rate, oxygen saturation and BP. These should be measured in both the supine position and the exercise posture (i.e. standing on a treadmill).

8 Interpretation of the resting ECG is an important final step in determining the presence of any absolute or relative contraindications for exercise. A test may be modified, postponed or cancelled even at this time based on the resting ECG. The resting BP can also be assessed against the absolute and relative contraindications to exercise testing (see Appendix C). It is common to tear off a printout of the supine ECG and have it in close viewing proximity during the test to identify whether any electrical abnormalities have arisen.

9 Further to explaining the nature of the test and its benefits/risks during earlier acquisition of informed consent, the exercise protocol and participant requirements must be emphasised at this point. Remember that inadequate participant effort – whether this is attributed to being unaccustomed to exercise, being anxious about precipitating a cardiac event with exertion, or any other reason – may predispose to a false-negative outcome.

10 Provide treadmill safety precautions to the participant (see Appendix D). An assessment of their ability to walk/jog safely should be conducted prior to starting the test.

11 Provide details of the test, including the protocol, hand signals the participant can use during the test, positioning of the arm during exercise BP measurements (see Practical 3, Cardiovascular health), participant self-reporting of signs/symptoms, explanation of the rating of perceived exertion (RPE) (see Appendix E), test termination and safety (see Appendix F).

Note: There are a number of ECG characteristics representing absolute or relative indications for termination of exercise (see Appendix F). You will need to be familiar with, and always looking for, these ECG characteristics. Test termination criteria for a diagnostic test will be different to those in Appendix F for a non-diagnostic test. However, for the purpose of this practical, and the likelihood that medical supervision will not be readily available, the criteria in Appendix F should be used.

Test

1 Ask the participant to stand on the treadmill and count them in for the start of the treadmill: '3 ... 2 ... 1 ... starting now'.

2 Your primary responsibility during the test is the safety of the participant. A number of changes in ECG morphology may be observed. These may be normal variations related to exercise (e.g. merging of a T wave with the next P wave during sinus tachycardia), or indicative of adverse events (e.g. tachyarrhythmias).

3 During exercise ECG tests for diagnostic purposes, changes in the ST segment represent the primary outcome. The level of the J point with respect to the isoelectric line and slope of the ST segment (upsloping/horizontal/downsloping) must be continually monitored.

4 A 12-lead ECG printout and/or screen shot should be obtained during the final 10 seconds of each stage and also at any time that abnormalities are observed.

5 Additional data to be collected during exercise include the following (see data analysis sheet):

   a BP (final minute of each stage)

   b Heart rate (usually continuous from the ECG machine, record at the end of each stage)

   c RPE (at the end of each stage)

   d Oxygen saturation (O_2sat%) (at the end of each stage).

6 ECG analysis should not distract from monitoring the participant during the test. Signs and/or symptoms indicative of adverse events (with or without ECG changes) need to be scrutinised and recorded (see Appendix F).

7 Encouragement is also essential to ensure the participant remains motivated to continue exercising until volitional exhaustion. However, it should also be made clear that the participant can stop the test at any time they choose.

Recovery

1 As soon as possible after the test, the participant should be seated. As ECG movement artefact/noise at maximal intensity exercise may cause difficulties with interpretation of the ST segment, the superior signal quality facilitated in a seated position – combined with an HR remaining at near-maximal levels – provides a unique opportunity to assess for abnormalities.

2 Participants should be monitored (including ECG, heart rate, BP, oxygen saturation level (O_2sat%) and other signs and symptoms) for a minimum of 5 minutes during post-exercise recovery. This time frame may be extended for as long as may be necessary in case of adverse signs/symptoms, suboptimal heart rate or BP recovery, or intermittent or sustained ECG abnormalities.

3 Usually, the BP will be measured in the first and fifth and/or final minute of recovery. ECG should be constantly monitored with a 10-second printout and/or screen shot at the end of every minute along with a recording of the heart rate, RPE and O_2sat%.

4 Record these values.

5 Clean and disinfect all equipment (see Appendix A).

Data recording

Participant's name: _____   Date: _____

Age: _____ years   Sex: _____

Age-predicted maximal heart rate[a]: _____ bpm

Supine blood pressure: _____ mmHg   Supine heart rate: _____ bpm

Standing blood pressure: _____ mmHg   Standing heart rate: _____ bpm

Stage	Time (mins)	Speed (km/h)	Grade (%)	BP (mmHg)	HR (bpm)	RPE	O_2sat (%)
Pre-test	–	–	–				
1	0–3	2.7	10				
2	3–6	4.0	12				
3	6–9	5.4	14				
4	9–12	6.7	16				
5	12–15	8.0	18				
6	15–18	8.9	20				
7	18–21	9.7	22				
8	21–24	10.5	24				
9	24–27	11.3	26				
10	27–30	12.1	28				
Recovery	0–1						
Recovery	1–2						
Recovery	2–3						
Recovery	3–4						
Recovery	4–5						

ECG changes during exercise: _____ _____

_____

_____

ECG changes during recovery: _____

_____

_____

Additional observations: _____ _____

_____

_____

[a] The formula 220 − age is often used to estimate maximal heart rate. However, the formula used throughout this manual (208 − (0.7 × age)) has been shown to be more accurate.[8]

Interpretation

First, consider the four steps of interpretation outlined in Appendix G. ECG interpretation is a comprehensive topic that will be only briefly addressed in this manual. For further information, books such as the ECG workbook[7] should be used. Figure 18.9 provides some examples of irregular ECG traces.

Atrial flutter: P waves are replaced by saw tooth flutter waves

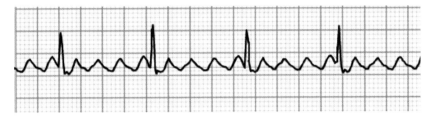

Atrial fibrillation: Note the irregularly irregular tachycardia. P waves absent & replaced by fibrillatory waves

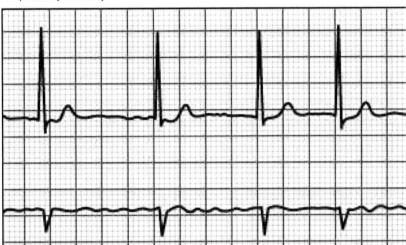

Ventricular bigeminy, in which every other beat is a ventricular ectopic beat. These beats are premature, wider and larger than the sinus beats. The orientation of the ventricular ectopic beats is often, but not always, in the opposite direction to the sinus beats.

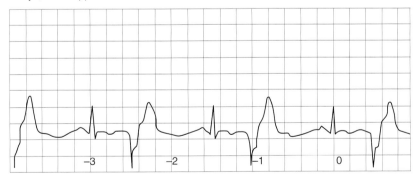

Figure 18.9 Examples of ECG traces representing pathologies

Source: Jayasinghe[7]

continued overpage

Varying morphology of ventricular tachycardi

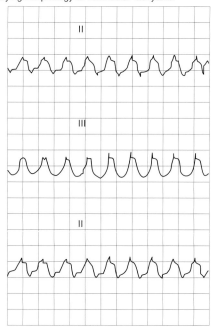

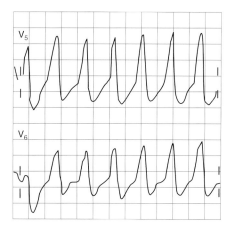

The four images below present different types of heart block: (a) first degree heart block, note the long PR interval; (b) second degree heart block, type 1, note the gradual prolongation of PR interval until one P wave is skipped; (c) second degree heart block, type 2; (d) third degree heart block.

(a) First degree heart block

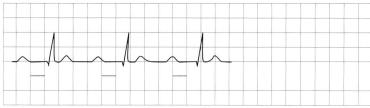

(b) Second degree heart block type 1

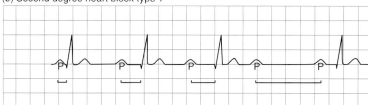

(c) Second degree heart block type 2 3:1

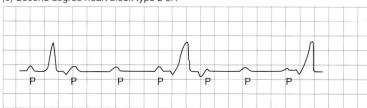

(d) Third degree heart block

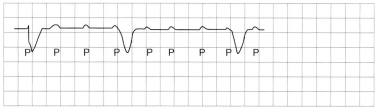

Figure 18.9, cont'd

continued

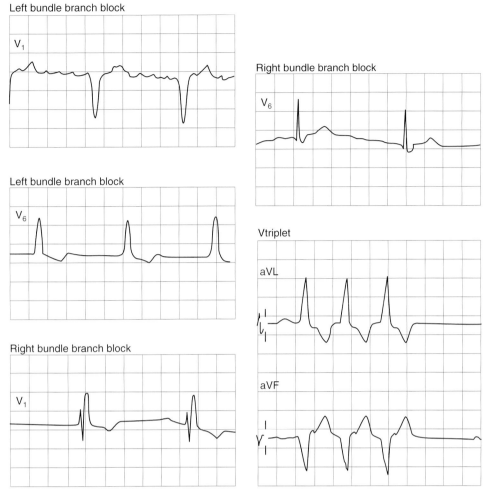

Figure 18.9, cont'd

In addition to 'on the run' ECG interpretation during the test, a post-test review of the rest, exercise (at each stage) and recovery ECGs is essential to ensure valid and thorough interpretation.

In addition to ST-segment changes (magnitude and morphology), other important outcomes include the incidence of any isolated or sustained arrhythmias. These include, but are not limited to, atrial or ventricular ectopics and more-overt abnormalities (e.g. atrial fibrillation, atrial flutter, ventricular tachycardia, ventricular flutter) or conduction defects (e.g. heart blocks or bundle branch blocks). The time of onset, duration and frequency of these abnormalities should be documented.

Other results featured in a typical report include those listed below.

- Signs/symptoms: onset may or may not coincide with ECG abnormalities but should be documented. For example, the work rate at which angina is induced has important implications for people undergoing cardiac rehabilitation.
- Baseline BP (interpreted in Practical 3 Cardiovascular health).
- Baseline heart rate (interpreted in Practical 3).
- Exercise BP: the magnitude of increase in BP during exercise has been shown to have important clinical implications *independent* of the resting BP. A 'hypertensive response to exercise' is usually defined as a maximal exercise BP $\geq$190/105 (women) or $\geq$210/105 (men) (where only one of the systolic or diastolic BP criteria need to be met). Conversely, a blunted BP response to exercise, where systolic BP has small increases,[b] should also be reported. Note that a decrease in systolic BP of 10 mmHg from baseline BP with an increase in work rate, when accompanied

---

[b] This will depend on the individual; however, a young healthy individual usually has a rise in systolic BP of 10–20 mmHg per stage of the Bruce protocol.

by evidence of ischaemia, is an indication to stop the test (see Appendix F). This may reflect an impairment of cardiac output during exercise.

- Exercise heart rate: chronotropism describes the ability of the HR to increase in response to the acute stress imposed by exercise. Chronotropic incompetence is usually defined as an inability to reach 85% of the age-predicted maximal heart rate, or 80% of the heart rate reserve. By considering the resting heart rate, the latter method is likely to be more valid. Certain medications can also blunt the heart rate response to exercise. The best examples of these are beta blockers, implantable pacemakers and calcium channel blockers. Whatever the reason for a diminished heart rate response to exercise, this may substantially reduce the validity (particularly the sensitivity) of the test and the outcomes should be considered in this context.
- Exercise capacity: even without direct measurement of oxygen uptake, the maximal work rate achieved (e.g. METs) remains a powerful predictor of morbidity and mortality in both healthy and clinical populations (see Practical 16, Exercise capacity).

Discussion and feedback

First, consider the three steps of feedback and discussion outlined in Appendix G. The tester should provide education and motivation before, during and after the test. This may include explaining and educating on the health benefits of exercise. Specific feedback may vary considerably owing to the multitude of different reasons for performing an exercise ECG test. For those tests performed for diagnostic purposes, feedback regarding the diagnosis is the responsibility of the medical practitioner, not the exercise professional. Tests performed for other purposes (e.g. to assess the impact of a treatment or the efficacy of cardiac rehabilitation) may allow for feedback based on exercise capacity and work rate corresponding to symptom onset.

The following scenarios are examples of the clinical/practical implications following an exercise ECG test.

- The absence of any adverse signs or symptoms during the exercise test indicates that it is safe for a participant to exercise at any intensity, including maximal and supramaximal intensities.
- The exercise test indicates that the client has improved exercise capacity by 30% as a result of an 8-week phase 3 cardiac rehabilitation program designed and delivered by the exercise professional.
- The participant remained in sinus rhythm throughout exercise and recovery and there were no significant arrhythmias.
- The participant experienced arrhythmias in the form of frequent ectopic beats/tachycardias/conduction defects.
- The participant presented in atrial fibrillation with adequate rate control at rest and during all intensities of exercise used in the exercise test (prescribed medications to achieve rate control include a beta blocker, calcium channel blocker and digoxin).
- There was no electrocardiographic evidence of acute myocardial ischaemia as a result of the exercise.
- There was evidence of horizontal ST depression associated with increasing intensities of exercise that peaked for the inferior leads (-2.9 mm I, -3.3 mm II, -3.2 mm III) and the anteroseptal leads (-2.2 mm V2, -2.4 mm V3). However, these were not associated with adverse signs or symptoms indicative of acute myocardial ischaemia and therefore could be a false-positive finding.
- The participant did not reach 85% of age-predicted maximal heart rate during the exercise test, but this was expected owing to the prescribed medications including a beta blocker and a calcium channel blocker. The implications for this are that care should be taken if prescribing exercise intensity using heart rate methods.
- There was electrocardiographic evidence that may indicate enlargement of part of the participant's heart.

For many of these observations, it will be necessary to communicate these findings to the participant's doctor via a formal letter.

Case studies

Setting: You are working as a cardiac technician in a major hospital cardiac investigations unit.

Case Study 1

Participant: Your next patient is Vishani, a 64-year-old male who was referred to your unit to have his resting ECG taken after an unexplained syncope incident in his home. You conduct the test and the following resting ECG trace is produced:

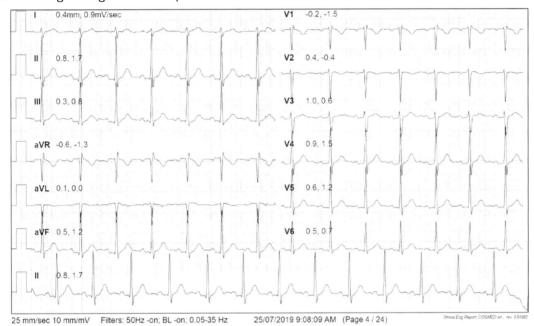

25 mm/sec 10 mm/mV   Filters: 50Hz -on; BL -on; 0.05-35 Hz   25/07/2019 9:08:09 AM (Page 4 / 24)   Stress Ecg Report, COSMED srl , rev 5.51502

Task: Complete the following data table as it relates to Vishani's resting ECG trace.

Parameters:

Heart rate:	(60–100 bpm = normal; <60 bpm = bradycardia; >100 bpm = tachycardia)
Classification:	
P wave present and upright in lead II?	(if present, regular and upright in lead II, indicates normal sinus rhythm; if absent or abnormal in shape, orientation or timing, may indicate atrial fibrillation/flutter, or atrial, ventricular or junctional ectopics, or other arrhythmia or conduction defect)
Size/duration:	(normal P-wave size <2.5 mm (height) and <120 ms (duration); if heightened, consider atrial enlargement such as in mitral stenosis)
PR interval:	(normal = 120–200 ms; if prolonged, consider AV block; if shortened, consider pre-excitation)

continued overpage

Case studies *(continued)*

QRS complex width:	(normal = 40–120 ms, with the usual width being 40–60 ms; ventricular ectopic beats (but not surrounding sinus beats) and partial and complete bundle branch blocks (all beats) have wide QRS complexes)
ST segment — displacement?	(is the J point above (ST elevation), on or below (ST depression) the isoelectric line? If displaced by >1 mm, consider ischaemia or infarction)
Slope:	(upsloping, horizontal or, in order of least to most significant clinically, in the setting of ST segment depression)
QT interval:	(HR dependent; corrected QT (QT/$\sqrt{RR}$ interval) should be ≤450 ms (men), ≤470 ms (women))[7]
T wave +ve or −ve:	(should be positive in lead II; T-wave abnormalities (e.g. inversion) may coincide with ST-segment changes)

Interpretation:

_____

_____

_____

_____

_____

_____

Clarify whether you would recommend the participant is safe to exercise based on this resting ECG trace, and why:

_____

_____

_____

How does your answer compare with the worked example provided in the Answers section (p. XXX)?

_____

_____

Case Study 2

Participant: Theresa, a 55-year-old female, has been referred to your unit by her cardiologist for a stress test after an angiogram revealed blocked coronary arteries. Throughout the test, Theresa

continued

Case studies *(continued)*

indicates she is asymptomatic and keen to continue exercising. Six minutes into the test you take a screenshot of the following ECG trace:

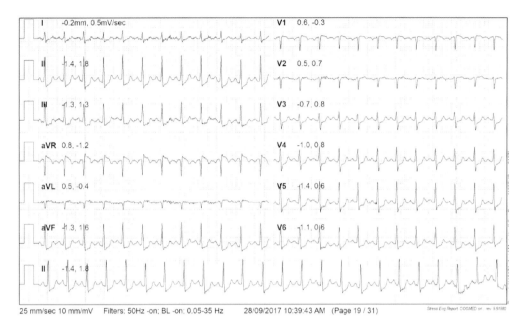

Task: Complete the following data table as it relates to Theresa's ECG trace and determine whether you recommend continuing or prematurely stopping the test based on this rhythm.

Parameters:

Heart rate:	(60–100 bpm = normal; <60 bpm = bradycardia; >100 bpm = tachycardia)
Classification:	
P wave present and upright in lead II?	(if present, regular and upright in lead II, indicates normal sinus rhythm; if absent or abnormal in shape, orientation or timing, may indicate atrial fibrillation/flutter, or atrial, ventricular or junctional ectopics, or other arrhythmia or conduction defect)
Size/duration:	(normal P-wave size <2.5 mm (height) and <120 ms (duration); if heightened, consider atrial enlargement such as in mitral stenosis)
PR interval:	(normal = 120–200 ms; if prolonged, consider AV block; if shortened, consider pre-excitation)
QRS complex width:	(normal = 40–120 ms, with the usual width being 40–60 ms; ventricular ectopic beats (but not surrounding sinus beats) and partial and complete bundle branch blocks (all beats) have wide QRS complexes)
ST segment − displacement?	(is the J point above (ST elevation), on or below (ST depression) the isoelectric line? If displaced by >1 mm, consider ischaemia or infarction)
Slope:	(upsloping, horizontal or downsloping, in order of least to most significant clinically, in the setting of ST segment depression)
QT interval:	(HR dependent; corrected QT (QT/$\sqrt{RR}$ interval) should be ≤450 ms (men), ≤470 ms (women))[7]
T wave +ve or −ve:	(should be positive in lead II; T-wave abnormalities (e.g. inversion) may coincide with ST-segment changes)
	continued overpage

Case studies *(continued)*

Interpretation:

_____

_____

_____

_____

_____

_____

Clarify whether you would recommend continuing or prematurely terminating the stress test, and why:

_____

_____

_____

How does your answer compare to the worked example provided in the Answers section at the end of this manual?

_____

_____

References

[1] Fletcher GF, Balady GJ, Amsterdam EA, Chaitman B, Eckel R, Fleg J, et al. Exercise standards for testing and training: a statement for healthcare professionals from the American Heart Association. Circulation 2001;104:1694–740.

[2] Kligfield P, Lauer MS. Exercise electrocardiogram testing: beyond the ST segment. Circulation 2006;114:2070–82.

[3] Kodama S, Saito K, Tanaka S, Maki M, Yachi Y, Asumi M, et al. Cardiorespiratory fitness as a quantitative predictor of all-cause mortality and cardiovascular events in healthy men and women: a meta-analysis. JAMA 2009;301:2024–35.

[4] Ross R, Blair SN, Arena R, Church TS, Despres J-P, Franklin BA, et al; American Heart Association Physical Activity Committee of the Council on Lifestyle and Cardiometabolic Health; Council on Clinical Cardiology; Council on Epidemiology and Prevention; Council on Cardiovascular and Stroke Nursing; Council on Functional Genomics and Translational Biology; Stroke Council. Importance of assessing cardiorespiratory fitness in clinical practice: a case for fitness as a clinical vital sign: a scientific statement from the American Heart Association. Circulation 2016;134:e653–99.

[5] Martin BJ, Arena R, Haykowsky M, Hauer T, Austford LD, Knudtson M, et al; APPROACH Investigators. Cardiovascular fitness and mortality after contemporary cardiac rehabilitation. Mayo Clin Proc 2013;88:455–63.

[6] Medical Advisory Secretariat. Cardiac magnetic resonance imaging for the diagnosis of coronary artery disease: an evidence-based analysis. Ont Health Technol Assess Ser 2010;10:1–38.

[7] Jayasinghe R. ECG workbook. Chatswood, NSW: Elsevier; 2012.

[8] Bruce RA, Blackman JR, Jones JW, Strait G. Exercise testing in adult normal subjects and cardiovascular patients. Pediatrics 1963;21(Suppl):742–56.

[9] Bruce RA, Kusumi F, Hosmer D. Maximal oxygen intake and nomographic assessment of functional aerobic impairment in cardiovascular disease. Am Heart J 1973;85:546–62.

PRACTICAL 19
DATA ANALYSIS

Jeff Coombes and Dennis Taaffe

LEARNING OBJECTIVES

- Understand the scientific rationale, terminology, purposes, assumptions, limitations and analytical considerations of data analysis
- Identify and explain the common approaches and software required to analyse data
- Perform data collation and basic statistical analysis techniques using computer software
- Develop, statistically test and interpret the results from two hypotheses using a Student's t-test and a correlational analysis

Equipment and other requirements

- Computer with statistical software
- Computer with Microsoft Excel software
- Microsoft Excel spreadsheet containing data to analyse
- Calculator

INTRODUCTION

This practical is designed to provide basic skills to analyse and interpret data using statistical techniques. The preferred approach to complete these tasks is with statistical software (e.g. SPSS, Stata, Prism). However, these programs are expensive and unlikely to be available outside a university. Therefore, this practical has been written predominantly using Excel, with the goal that these skills could be used by practitioners who may wish to complete basic data analyses on their clients. Excel permits the majority of the tasks to be completed, but it takes longer and there are more steps than in statistical software programs. Although most researchers would not use this approach, there is likely to be a pedagogical benefit by using Excel as it is easier to see what is occurring in each step.

We are in an era of 'big data' with large data sets affecting virtually every aspect of our lives. In 2019, the United Nations estimated that 90% of the data in the world had been created in the past 2 years, and it is projected to increase by 40% annually.[1] In exercise and sports science the collection and analysis of data is also extremely prevalent, leading to the creation of new areas of study (e.g. sports analytics) and employment.[2] It is now vital that exercise and sports science practitioners have basic data analytical skills and understand how readily available software applications (e.g. Excel) can assist with analysis.

The practical has been designed to use data from participants (e.g. classmates) who have completed other practicals in this manual. It starts with a single 'sheet' within an Excel spreadsheet. This sheet may contain over 100 variables (Figure 19.1).

	A	B	C	D	E	F	G	H	I	J
1	variable	units	40986XXX	41439XXX	42034XXX	41185XXX	42049XXX	42028XXX	41762XXX	42035XXX
2	Sex	M/F	Male	Female	Male	Male	Female	Male	Male	Female
3	Haematocrit	%	43	40	43	48	48	47	45	50
4	Haemoglobin	g/dL	11.3	14.3	12.5	14.6	13.0	12.5	15.2	11.3
5	Glucose	mmol/L	5.0	4.7	7.0	4.8	4.8	6.2	6.2	4.4
6	Total cholesterol	mmol/L	4.72	2.79	3.32	5.60	4.07	2.68	2.85	3.35
7	HDL cholesterol	mmol/L	1.64	0.98	0.74	2.03	1.47	1.63	0.99	1.98
8	Triglycerides	mmol/L	1.98	1.64	0.93	0.81	0.60	1.59	1.70	0.75
9	LDL cholesterol	mmol/L	2.18	1.05	2.68	3.21	2.33	1.05	1.10	1.03
10	Radial HR	bpm	56	58	60	64	98	60	72	62
11	SBP	mmHg	128	114	123	115	115	110	100	110
12	DBP	mmHg	76	65	73	75	70	70	54	72
13	Pulse pressure	mmHg	66	49	50	40	45	40	46	38
14	Mean arterial pressure	mmHg	98	81	90	88	85	83	69	85
15	Rate pressure product		71.7	66.1	73.8	73.6	112.7	66.0	72.0	68.2
16	Framingham 10-year risk of CHD	%	1	1	2	2	1	1	1	1
17	Height	cm	183	177	182	178	160	185	180	170
18	Mass	kg	72	79	69	77	74	88	73	62
19	BMI	kg/m2	21.5	25.1	20.9	24.3	28.9	25.7	22.5	21.5
20	Waist circumference	cm	74.6	85.7	70.3	78.0	74.5	81.2	78.4	52
21	Gluteal circumference	cm	95.6	102.1	92.1	93.0	108.5	100.6	98	64
22	waist to hip ratio		0.78	0.84	0.76	0.84	0.69	0.80	0.80	0.81
23	waist to height ratio		0.41	0.48	0.39	0.44	0.47	0.44	0.44	0.31
24	Triceps skinfold	mm	4.5	5.8	9.1	6.4	23.4	7.6	6.2	8.0
25	Subscapular skinfold	mm	6.8	9.5	6.5	10.4	20.6	8.3	9.1	12.0
26	Biceps skinfold	mm	2.6	4.0	5.5	4.0	17.8	4.4	2.8	7.0
27	Iliac crest skinfold	mm	8.0	9.6	8.0	12.0	24.5	9.2	9.2	11.0
28	Supraspinale skinfold	mm	6.0	9.1	6.6	6.0	23.2	6.9	5.9	11.0
29	Abdominal skinfold	mm	12.0	13.0	10.5	14.4	25.4	9.8	7.4	7.0
30	Front thigh skinfold	mm	6.5	6.9	13.2	4.6	37.4	7.9	6.4	4.0
31	Medial calf skinfold	mm	4.8	6.2	11.3	6.2	26.4	7.6	4.2	3.0

Original / Sheet2 / Sheet3

Ready   90%

Figure 19.1 'Original' sheet

DEFINITIONS

Coefficient of determination: also known as the R-squared (R^2) value. It is obtained by squaring the r (correlation coefficient) value and reflects the degree to which the model explains all the variability of the response data around its mean. The R^2 value is always between 0 and 1 with a value closer to 1, indicating that the model explains more of the response.

Correlation coefficient: also known as the r value. It measures the strength and direction of a linear relationship between two variables on a scatterplot. The r value is always between $+1$ and -1.

Data: information in a raw or unorganised form that refers to qualitative or quantitative variables.

F-statistic: the test statistic for an F-test.

F-test: used to test if the variances of two populations are equal. This information may be used to inform the use of a t-test.

Hypothesis: an idea or explanation for something that is based on known facts but has not yet been proved.

Non-parametric statistical test: makes no assumptions about the parameters (defining properties) of the population distribution(s) from which the data have been obtained.

Null hypothesis: the hypothesis that there is no significant difference between specified populations (i.e. any observed difference is due to sampling or experimental error).

Parametric statistical test: makes assumptions about the parameters (defining properties) of the population distribution(s) from which the data have been obtained (e.g. that the data are normally distributed). An example is the t-test.

P value: a number between 0 and 1 used in hypothesis testing to represent the significance of a statistical test. The smaller the P value the more likely it is that the null hypothesis can be rejected and the research hypothesis supported (e.g. a P value of 0.05 indicates that it is 5% probable that the difference/relationship is due to chance, or 95% probable that it is not due to chance – and, therefore, the difference/relationship is 'real').

R-squared (R^2) value: also known as the coefficient of determination. It is obtained by squaring the r (correlation coefficient) value and it reflects the degree to which the model explains all the variability of the response data around its mean. The R^2 value is always between 0 and 1, with a value closer to 1 indicating that the model explains more of the response.

r value: also known as the correlation coefficient. It measures the strength and direction of a linear relationship between two variables on a scatter plot. The *r* value is always between $+1$ and -1.

Statistic: a single quantity contained in, or computed from, a set of data.

t-statistic: the test statistic for a t-test.

t-test: used to test whether the means of two populations are equal.

Variable: an element, feature or factor that is liable to vary or change.

Activity 19.1 Data summary table

AIM: construct a data summary table.

Background

A summary table has new data with statistics computed from the original data. These will usually include a measure of the middle value (e.g. mean), the variance (e.g. standard deviation), the range (e.g. maximum and minimum values) and a count of how many individual data points are contributing to these statistics. It is used to visualise and understand the data more easily before perhaps carrying out hypothesis testing. The protocol for this activity is divided into five steps.

Protocol summary

Create a data summary table containing a defined set of variables using data from participants (e.g. classmates) who have completed practicals in this manual.

Protocol

Step 1: data entry

For data entry into a spreadsheet it is easier to have data from a participant in a column (e.g. Figure 19.1), rather than a row. When using Excel, a data entry sheet can be set up that contains validation criteria in a cell that stops the entry of data that falls outside a range. For example, if you were collecting height of a participant and you wanted the data entered in cm units (e.g. 180 cm) then you could set up the cell/s for data entry that allowed only values within a range that was believable (e.g. 140–220 cm). If a person tried to enter a height in metres (e.g. 1.8 m) they would be prompted to re-enter the value to fit within the pre-specified range). Best practice for data entry uses a two-person technique. One person reads out the data from a data sheet and the second person enters it into the spreadsheet. Then, after all data are entered, the second person reads the data of the spreadsheet while the first person checks these against the data on the data sheet.

Step 2: data rearranging

For data analysis it is conventional to have each participant's data in a row. If it has been provided in a column (as suggested above) for data entry, it can be rearranged using the Excel 'Transpose' function.

TRANSPOSING DATA IN EXCEL

1 Select all the cells containing data. These include the variable names and the participant identifiers (e.g. participant numbers). To do this, go to the bottom right-most cell which contains data, click on that cell and drag up and across to the left until all cells are selected.

2 Then select 'Copy' (Figure 19.2).

3 The rearranged (transposed) data will be transferred into a new sheet, 'Sheet 2' (Figure 19.3), which can be renamed by double clicking on 'Sheet 2' and applying the new title: 'Transposed' (Figure 19.4).

4 Click on cell 1A (the most upper-left cell) on the 'Transposed' sheet.

5 Then click on the arrow underneath 'Paste' (Figure 19.5) and select 'Paste special'.

6 From the Paste special menu select 'Values and number formats' and 'Transpose' (Figure 19.6).

7 The sheet should then look similar to Figure 19.7.

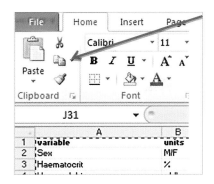

Figure 19.2 Copying the data

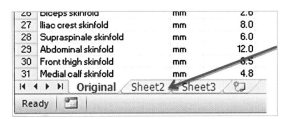

Figure 19.3 Creating a new sheet

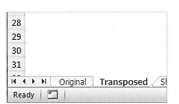

Figure 19.4 Renaming new sheet

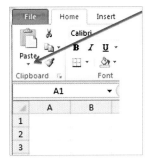

Figure 19.5 Arrow below 'Paste'

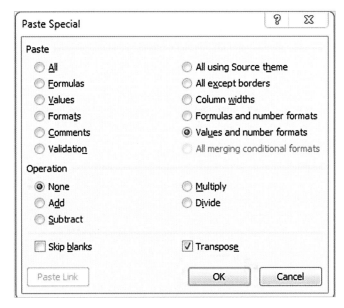

Figure 19.6 Selecting 'Values and number formats' and 'Transpose' on the paste special menu

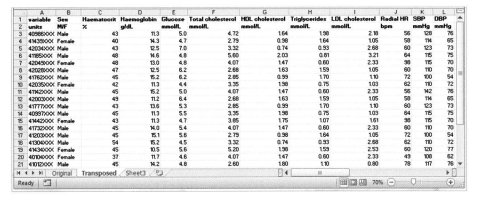

Figure 19.7 Transposed data sheet

Step 3: data checking

Before analysing data, it is important to check that there has not been a mistake during data entry. This part of the analysis process is critical as it helps ensure the integrity of the data, permitting accurate analysis and interpretation.

The main purpose of data checking is to locate any numbers that are incorrect.

Depending on how the data have been entered, there may have already been some data checking. In Excel it is possible to set a range such that any entries outside that range will not be accepted. This is known as *data validation* (explained above in 'Step 1: data entry').

A consistent rule for data checking is that you cannot assume that the datum in question is incorrect as the observation may just represent part of the normal variation. Knowledge of the natural variation of the measure is necessary to check the data.

Another rule of data checking is that you cannot replace a value with one that you think it is meant to be. In the case of 178 metres for a person's height, you cannot assume that someone has missed the decimal place and replace it with 1.78 metres. Therefore, any values that appear incorrect should be checked (e.g. by examining the source data) and re-entered where possible or removed, rather than changed.

In this practical, we will be removing only those values that are clearly outside the normal range for this measure – probably due to a keystroke error. To test for incorrect data, we will generate maximum and minimum values and then, based on knowledge and experience, determine whether a value should be removed. The process of checking for incorrect values should still be done even if the Excel spreadsheet was set up to take only data within certain ranges as there may have been corruption of this feature.

DETERMINING MAXIMUM AND MINIMUM VALUES

1 For minimum values, on the 'Transposed' worksheet go to a row under the last data row and, under the first integer variable (e.g. Haematocrit), type '= MIN(array)'.

> **Note:** Do not type the word 'array'. Array refers to cells from which you are determining the minimum value (e.g. C3:C21). To get these values, after you type the '(' you can click on the first cell and highlight down to the last cell in the array. Then type the ')'.

2 For maximum values, repeat procedures for the minimum values and type '= MAX(array)'.

3 Then fill these rows to the right so that maximum and minimum values are determined for each variable. One way of doing this is to start by highlighting the cell you want to copy and also the adjacent cell/s where it is to be copied; then from the 'Home' menu select 'Fill' (Figure 19.8) then 'Right'.

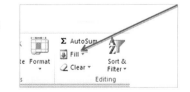

4 The sheet should then look similar to Figure 19.9.

Figure 19.8 Fill on the Home menu

The next step is time consuming and requires that each variable is checked one at a time. You need to complete data checking only on the variables you have been supplied for Activity 19.1. For example, if 'haematocrit' was one of the variables you have been supplied, then in Figure 19.9 look at the minimum and maximum haematocrit values and decide whether 37 and 54 are reasonable for minimum and maximum values. As variables such as pulse pressure, mean arterial pressure and body mass index (BMI) are calculated from other variables, these can be overlooked once the source variables are checked. It is statistical good practice to remove values that are outliers only if you are confident that they are incorrect (e.g. clearly outside a possible physiological or anatomical range). As mentioned above, in this practical we will be removing only those values that are clearly outside the normal range for a measure.

B15 | Female

	A	B	C	D	E	F	G	H	I	J	K	L
1	variable	Sex	Haematocrit	Haemoglobin	Glucose	Total cholesterol	HDL cholesterol	Triglycerides	LDL cholesterol	Radial HR	SBP	DBP
2	units	M/F	%	g/dL	mmol/L	mmol/L	mmol/L	mmol/L	mmol/L	bpm	mmHg	mmHg
3	40986XXX	Male	43	11.3	5.0	4.72	1.64	1.98	2.18	56	128	76
4	41439XXX	Female	40	14.3	4.7	2.79	0.98	1.64	1.05	58	114	65
5	42034XXX	Male	43	12.5	7.0	3.32	0.74	0.93	2.68	60	123	73
6	41185XXX	Male	48	14.6	4.8	5.60	2.03	0.81	3.21	64	115	75
7	42049XXX	Female	48	13.0	4.8	4.07	1.47	0.60	2.33	98	115	70
8	42028XXX	Male	47	12.5	6.2	2.68	1.63	1.59	1.05	60	110	70
9	41762XXX	Male	45	15.2	6.2	2.85	0.99	1.70	1.10	72	100	54
10	42035XXX	Female	42	11.3	4.4	3.35	1.98	0.75	1.03	62	110	72
11	41142XXX	Male	45	15.2	5.0	4.07	1.47	0.60	2.33	56	142	76
12	42003XXX	Male	49	11.2	6.4	2.68	1.63	1.59	1.05	58	114	65
13	41777XXX	Male	43	13.6	5.3	2.85	0.99	1.70	1.10	60	123	73
14	40997XXX	Male	45	11.3	5.5	3.35	1.98	0.75	1.03	64	115	75
15	41442XXX	Female	43	11.3	4.7	3.85	1.75	1.07	1.61	98	115	70
16	41732XXX	Male	45	14.0	5.4	4.07	1.47	0.60	2.33	60	110	70
17	41203XXX	Male	45	15.1	5.6	2.79	0.98	1.64	1.05	72	100	54
18	41304XXX	Male	54	15.2	4.5	3.32	0.74	0.93	2.68	62	110	72
19	41434XXX	Female	45	10.5	5.6	5.20	1.98	1.59	2.53	60	120	77
20	40104XXX	Female	37	11.7	4.6	4.07	1.47	0.60	2.33	49	108	62
21	41012XXX	Male	45	14.2	4.8	2.60	1.80	1.10	0.80	78	117	76
22												
23		Minimum	37	10.5	4.4	2.60	0.74	0.60	0.80	49	100	54
24		Maximum	54	15.2	7.0	5.60	2.03	1.98	3.21	98	142	77

Original | Transposed | Sheet3

Ready 70%

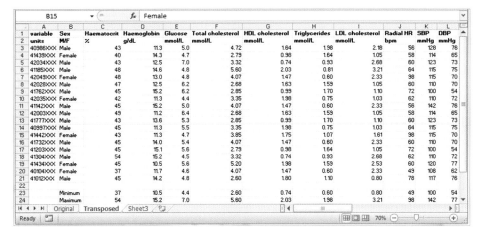

Figure 19.9 Transposed data for minimum and maximum values to enable easier data checking

Step 4: using filters to separate data

For group comparisons we will be comparing males and females. Therefore, it will be helpful to have males and females on separate sheets. To do this we will use the 'Filter' function.

1 On the 'Transposed' sheet select the first row, and then from the 'Home' menu select 'Sort and filter' (Figure 19.10) then 'Filter'.

2 Click on the arrow next to 'Sex' and select a sex (e.g. 'Female').

3 Select all the rows that have been filtered (Figure 19.11).

4 *Copy* these rows.

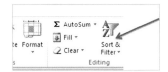

Figure 19.10 Sort & Filter on the Home menu

A1 | variable

	A	B	C	D	E	F	G	H	I	J	K	L
1	variabl	Sex	Haematoci	Haemoglobi	Glucos	Total choleste	HDL choleste	Triglyceride	LDL choleste	Radial H	SBP	DBP
4	41439XXX	Female	40	14.3	4.7	2.79	0.98	1.64	1.05	58	114	65
7	42049XXX	Female	48	13.0	4.8	4.07	1.47	0.60	2.33	98	115	70
10	42035XXX	Female	42	11.3	4.4	3.35	1.98	0.75	1.03	62	110	72
15	41442XXX	Female	43	11.3	4.7	3.85	1.75	1.07	1.61	98	115	70
19	41434XXX	Female	45	10.5	5.6	5.20	1.98	1.59	2.53	60	120	77
20	40104XXX	Female	37	11.7	4.6	4.07	1.47	0.60	2.33	49	108	62

Figure 19.11 Worksheet with filters

5 Create a new sheet. Suggest renaming the sheet 'Females'.

6 *Paste* these rows.

7 Go back to the 'Transposed' worksheet and repeat the process from step 2 to step 6 above for 'Males'.

8 There will now be four sheets: 'Original', 'Transposed', 'Females' and 'Males' (see Figure 19.12).

	A	B	C	D	E	F	G	H	I	J	K	L
1	variable	Sex	Haematocrit	Haemoglobin	Glucose	Total cholesterol	HDL cholesterol	Triglycerides	LDL cholesterol	Radial HR	SBP	DBP
2	40986XXX	Male	43	11.3	5.0	4.72	1.64	1.98	2.18	56	128	76
3	42034XXX	Male	43	12.5	7.0	3.32	0.74	0.93	2.68	60	123	73
4	41185XXX	Male	48	14.6	4.8	5.60	2.03	0.81	3.21	64	115	75
5	42028XXX	Male	47	12.5	6.2	2.68	1.63	1.59	1.05	60	110	70
6	41762XXX	Male	45	15.2	6.2	2.85	0.99	1.70	1.10	72	100	54
7	41142XXX	Male	45	15.2	5.0	4.07	1.47	0.60	2.33	56	142	76
8	42003XXX	Male	49	11.2	6.4	2.68	1.63	1.59	1.05	58	114	65
9	41777XXX	Male	43	13.6	5.3	2.85	0.99	1.70	1.10	60	123	73
10	40997XXX	Male	45	11.3	5.5	3.35	1.98	0.75	1.03	64	115	75
11	41732XXX	Male	45	14.0	5.4	4.07	1.47	0.60	2.33	60	110	70
12	41203XXX	Male	45	15.1	5.6	2.79	0.98	1.64	1.05	72	100	54
13	41304XXX	Male	54	15.2	4.5	3.32	0.74	0.93	2.68	62	110	72
14	41012XXX	Male	45	14.2	4.8	2.60	1.80	1.10	0.80	78	117	76

Original | Transposed | Females | Males

Ready 100%

Figure 19.12 'Males' sheet of the four sheets: 'Original', 'Transposed', 'Females' and 'Males'

Step 5: obtaining summary statistics and assembling them into a table

Summary statistics include participant number (n), a measure of central tendency (e.g. mean), a measure of dispersion (e.g. standard deviation (SD), maximum values and minimum values). The equations for determining these are provided below.

> **Note:** 'Array' refers to the cells being used (e.g. C2:C14).

$$\text{Count } (n): = \text{COUNT(array)}$$
$$\text{Mean}^a: = \text{AVERAGE(array)}$$
$$\text{Standard deviation}^a \text{ (SD)}: = \text{STDEV(array)}$$
$$\text{Maximum (max)}: = \text{MAX(array)}$$
$$\text{Minimum (min)}: = \text{MIN(array)}$$

Excel also allows for an 'Add-in' called 'Data analysis' that provides a summary statistics function. However, due to limited availability on the Macintosh version of Excel and some limitations in the PC version, this will not be used in the following tasks.

The instructor may allocate a list of variables for Activity 19.1 (see Box 19.1). The next goal is to create and complete a 'Summary table' that contains the allocated variables and their summary statistics.

Box 19.1 Allocation variables for activities

For activity 19.1

Haematocrit	LDL cholesterol
Haemoglobin	Radial HR
Glucose	SBP
Total cholesterol	DBP
HDL cholesterol	Pulse pressure
Triglycerides	Mean arterial pressure

For activity 19.2

Height and modified sit and
    reach
Haemoglobin and estimated
    $\dot{V}O_2$max from YMCA cycle test
Total cholesterol and Withers
    equation – body fat

---

1 First create the summary table with column and row headings as shown in Figure 19.13 on a separate sheet. Label this sheet 'Summary tables'.

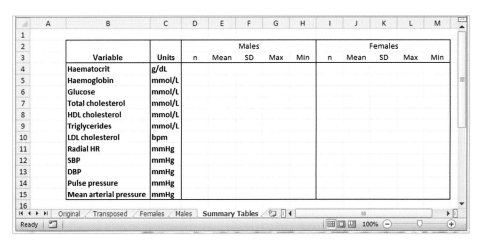

Figure 19.13 'Summary tables' sheet

---

a These should be used only for data that are normally distributed (see 'Checking for normality' later in this practical). If data are not normally distributed then mean is usually replaced with median, and standard deviation is replaced with interquartile range.

2 Place the cursor in the appropriate cell (e.g. start with Males, haematocrit, n, (cell D4 in Figure 19.14)).

Figure 19.14 Completed 'Summary tables' sheet

3 Start typing the first part of the appropriate equation (e.g. for Males, haematocrit, n type '= COUNT('

4 Then go to the appropriate sheet and select the data that are being used (e.g. for Males, haematocrit, n select 'C2:C14')

5 Type ')' and hit *ENTER*.

6 To change the number of decimal places, use the buttons located on the 'Home' menu (Figure 19.15). It is common to generate summary statistics for mean and SD that have the same number of decimal places as the source data (e.g. no decimal places for the mean and SD for haematocrit).

Figure 19.15 Buttons to adjust the decimal places on the 'Home' menu

7 Complete the table by following steps 2–6 above for all variables. The completed table should look similar to Figure 19.14. This table is helpful as it provides all the necessary summary statistics for both groups on the one page.

8 The next step is to create a more simplified summary table, similar to those commonly seen in research articles. The mean and standard deviation are together in the one cell with the '±' symbol separating them and an extra column with the *P* value. This table could be constructed without the need for the previous summary table; however, for teaching purposes the previous table was generated to show the process more easily.

9 Create the table on the right in Figure 19.16 in the 'Summary tables' sheet. Having the variables in the same rows in both tables will make it easier to follow.

Figure 19.16 Second summary table on the right

10 To have the mean and the SD in the same cell use the equation '= (cell)&" ± "&(cell)', where the cell is the location of the number. For example, if the mean was in cell E4 and the SD in F4 then it would be '= (E4)&" ± "&(F4)'. The ± can be found by going to the 'Insert' menu, selecting 'Symbols'

and finding it amongst the options. If you are using Excel on a PC, you may need to paste it into another cell first and then copy and paste it into the formula.

11 If the formula provides values with too many decimal places, use the ROUND function. For example, to return values with two decimal places use '= ROUND(E4,2)&" $\pm$ "&ROUND(F4,2)'. Once you have one cell completed, use the 'Fill down' function, which is located in the drop-down menu next to 'Fill' on the 'Home' menu (Figure 19.17) to fill all cells. You may need to go through and change the number of decimal places it is rounding to for some variables. Then repeat for the other sex.

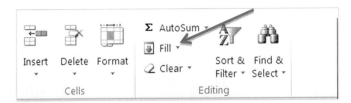

Figure 19.17 Fill-down function

Activity 19.2 Hypothesis testing – comparing means

AIM: to use a t-test to determine whether there is a statistically significant[b] difference between the means of two groups.

Background

This activity is answering the question: Are there significant statistical differences between males and females in the variables used in Activity 19.1? This question has been chosen to explain how to compare means as it is an easy way to separate out the data into two groups. It also leads to interesting applications of anatomical, physiological and exercise physiology knowledge when generating hypotheses. The protocol for this activity is divided into two steps.

Protocol summary

Determine whether there are there statistically significant differences between males and females in the variables used in Activity 19.1.

Protocol

Step 1: determining normality
The first step is to determine whether the data you wish to compare resembles a normal distribution (Figure 19.18). If the data are normally distributed then appropriate parametric statistical tests such as the Student's t-test (referred to simply as the t-test from now) may be used. If it is not normally distributed then you can either: (i) transform the data (e.g. converting each data point to its logarithmic value) and, if the data are now normally distributed, apply a parametric test; or (ii) keep it untransformed and apply non-parametric statistical tests. Non-parametric tests, which are assumption-free statistics, are also used for the analysis of categorical data, such as for ranked scores (e.g. multi-stage sit-up test data that may be from stage 1 to stage 7 for a participant).

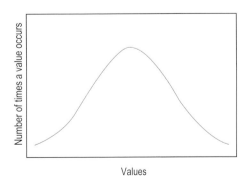

Figure 19.18 Normal distribution

---

b There is a move away from using the term 'statistical significance' because it uses an arbitrary threshold (e.g. $P < 0.05$) to determine significance.[3]

A parametric statistical test (e.g. the t-test) may be used if the data are normally distributed. There are numerous approaches to checking how closely data resemble a normal distribution. In this practical we will use a statistical test called the Kolmogorov–Smirnov test. It is known as a 'goodness of fit' test and basically determines how closely the data fit a theoretical normal distribution. In this example we will use the SPSS statistical software (http://www-01.ibm.com/software/analytics/spss/).

1 Copy and paste your data from the 'Transposed sheet' into an SPSS spreadsheet (Figure 19.19).

	VAR00001	VAR00002	VAR00003	VAR00004	VAR00005	VAR00006	VAR00007	VAR00008	VAR00009	VAR00010	VAR00011	VAR00012
1	43.00	11.30	5.00	4.72	1.64	1.98	2.18	56.00	128.00	76.00	66.00	98.00
2	40.00	14.30	4.70	2.79	.98	1.64	1.05	58.00	114.00	65.00	49.00	81.00
3	43.00	12.50	7.00	3.32	.74	.93	2.68	60.00	123.00	73.00	50.00	90.00
4	48.00	14.60	4.80	5.60	2.03	.81	3.21	64.00	115.00	75.00	40.00	88.00
5	48.00	13.00	4.80	4.07	1.47	.60	2.33	98.00	115.00	70.00	45.00	85.00
6	47.00	12.50	6.20	2.68	1.63	1.59	1.05	60.00	110.00	70.00	40.00	83.00
7	45.00	15.20	6.20	2.85	.99	1.70	1.10	72.00	100.00	54.00	46.00	69.00
8	42.00	11.30	4.40	3.35	1.98	.75	1.03	62.00	110.00	72.00	38.00	85.00
9	45.00	15.20	5.00	4.07	1.47	.60	2.33	56.00	142.00	76.00	66.00	98.00
10	49.00	11.20	6.40	2.68	1.63	1.59	1.05	58.00	114.00	65.00	49.00	81.00
11	43.00	13.60	5.30	2.85	.99	1.70	1.10	60.00	123.00	73.00	50.00	90.00
12	45.00	11.30	5.50	3.35	1.98	.75	1.03	64.00	115.00	75.00	40.00	88.00
13	43.00	11.30	4.70	3.85	1.75	1.07	1.61	98.00	115.00	70.00	45.00	85.00
14	45.00	14.00	5.40	4.07	1.47	.60	2.33	60.00	110.00	70.00	40.00	83.00
15	45.00	15.10	5.60	2.79	.98	1.64	1.05	72.00	100.00	54.00	46.00	69.00
16	54.00	15.20	4.50	3.32	.74	.93	2.68	62.00	110.00	72.00	38.00	85.00
17	45.00	10.50	5.60	5.20	1.98	1.59	2.53	60.00	120.00	77.00	43.00	91.00
18	37.00	11.70	4.60	4.07	1.47	.60	2.33	49.00	108.00	62.00	46.00	77.00
19	45.00	14.20	4.80	2.60	1.80	1.10	.80	78.00	117.00	76.00	41.00	39.00

Data View   Variable View

Figure 19.19 Data pasted into the SPSS 'Data view' sheet

2 Select 'Analyze' then 'Nonparametric tests' and 'Legacy dialogs' then '1-Sample K-S'. The dialog box in Figure 19.20 will appear. If some of the variables are not in the list then this may be because SPSS has classified them not 'numeric' (e.g. 'string'). You will then need to click on the 'variable view' tab in the bottom left of the application window and then change the 'Type' (column 2) of the variable to 'numeric'.

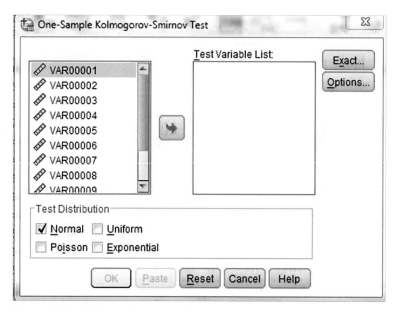

Figure 19.20 Dialogue box for Kolmogorov–Smirnov tests

3 Select all the variables on the left and use the arrow button in the middle to move them into the blank right box. Then click 'OK'. The output will be similar to Figure 19.21.
   To interpret the output, look at the final row; if the value is greater than 0.05, you can assume that the distribution of the variable resembles a normal distribution such that a parametric statistical test

One-Sample Kolmogorov-Smirnov Test		VAR00001	VAR00002	VAR00003	VAR00004	VAR00005	VAR00006	VAR00007	VAR00008	VAR00009	VAR00010	VAR00011	VAR00012
N		19	19	19	19	19	19	19	19	19	19	19	19
Normal Parameters[a,b]	Mean	44.8421	13.0526	5.2895	3.5911	1.4589	1.1668	1.7616	65.6316	115.2105	69.7368	46.2105	82.3684
	Std. Deviation	3.59418	1.65273	.72793	.88728	.43242	.47731	.77322	13.12000	9.58922	6.90283	8.01789	13.00090
Most Extreme Differences	Absolute	.219	.171	.181	.186	.194	.233	.278	.286	.193	.252	.213	.248
	Positive	.219	.171	.181	.186	.177	.164	.278	.286	.193	.146	.213	.148
	Negative	-.149	-.138	-.111	-.132	-.194	-.233	-.190	-.179	-.136	-.252	-.153	-.248
Kolmogorov-Smirnov Z		.956	.747	.788	.811	.847	1.017	1.210	1.248	.841	1.099	.928	1.079
Asymp. Sig. (2-tailed)		.320	.633	.563	.527	.469	.252	.107	.089	.479	.179	.355	.195

a. Test distribution is Normal.
b. Calculated from data.

Figure 19.21 Output for Kolmogorov–Smirnov tests

(e.g. t-test) can be used. If the data are not normally distributed, they either have to be transformed or a non-parametric test should be used. This is outside the scope of this practical and the reader is referred to Berg and Latin[4] for further details.

4 To get a visual representation of the normal distribution histogram for one variable select: Analyse—Descriptive statistics —Explore. Then transfer the variables of interest into the 'Dependent list'. Click on 'Plots' uncheck 'Stem-and-leaf', check 'Histogram' and then 'Continue' and 'OK'. Summary statistics will now be shown as well as the histogram and a boxplot.

Step 2: conduct a t-test[c]

The t-test is the simplest and most appropriate statistical test to compare the means of two samples of parametric data. If you have more than two samples, you use an analysis of variance (ANOVA).

There are essentially two types of t-tests:

1 independent or unpaired t-test – when data from different individuals are compared (e.g. the resting heart rates of males vs females).

2 dependent or paired t-test – when data from the same group of individuals are compared (e.g. comparing the resting heart rates measured on two separate occasions from the same group of males).

Other definitions to be aware of when using t-tests are *one-tailed* vs *two-tailed*. Briefly, if you have a directional hypothesis, for instance a 12-month strength-training program will increase muscle mass, then a one-tailed hypothesis test (in this case the t-test) can be used, which in effect makes it easier to reject the *null hypothesis* (i.e. no difference or no relationship) and accept the alternative hypothesis that it does have an effect. This is because in a one-tailed test the critical value, which is the value that the calculated test statistic has to exceed in order for you to reject the null hypothesis, is smaller as it is derived from only one tail of the sampling distribution. However, as it is commonly believed that all t-tests should be two-tailed (as researchers tend to be conservative in their decision making), you should select this for all the tests in this practical even if you have a directional hypothesis.

The t-test provides a probability or 'P' value. This value represents how probable, or how confident you are, that the observed difference is real. It is common to use a cut-off of $P < 0.05$ when interpreting P values from a t-test. If a t-test returns a P value < 0.05 we can state that it is statistically significant ($P < 0.05$). In other words, we are 95% confident that the difference is real and that it is not a chance finding.

The first step is to use an F-test to determine whether the variances in the two data sets are statistically different (via a P value). The variances refer to the data that are away from the middle value (e.g. mean).

---

c The following statistical tests can be done in SPSS. As mentioned in the Introduction, this practical is using Excel for these tests as it is likely to be more available to practitioners. If using SPSS for the following tests, the check for normality can be obtained during the tests by selecting 'Histogram' and 'Normality plots with tests'.

F-test

To determine the *P* value for an F-test in Excel use the formula '= FTEST(array1,array2)'.

Array 1 is the first data set.

Array 2 is the second data set.

For the arrays you have to go back to the 'Males' and 'Females' worksheets and select the data by dragging the cursor over the required cells.

The steps for calculating the *P* value for the F-test are:

1 Click in the cell where you wish to have the *P* value for the F-test. In the example in Figure 19.22, a separate column has been created for these *P* values (column U).

Variable	Units	Males mean±SD	Females mean±SD	T Test P Value	F Test P Value
Haematocrit	g/dL	46±3	43±4		0.47
Haemoglobin	mmol/L	13.5±1.6	12±1.4		
Glucose	mmol/L	5.5±0.7	4.8±0.4		
Total cholesterol	mmol/L	3.45±0.92	3.89±0.81		
HDL cholesterol	mmol/L	1.39±0.45	1.61±0.38		
Triglycerides	mmol/L	1.22±0.49	1.04±0.48		
LDL cholesterol	bpm	1.74±0.84	1.81±0.68		
Radial HR	mmHg	63±7	71±22		
SBP	mmHg	116±11	114±4		
DBP	mmHg	70±8	69±5		
Pulse pressure	mmHg	47±9	44±4		
Mean arterial press	mmHg	82±16	84±5		

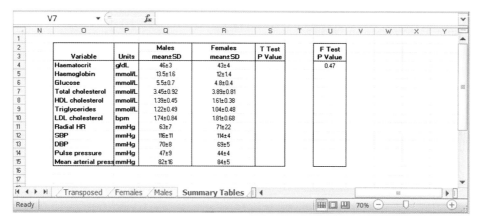

Figure 19.22 The *P* value for the F-test to determine whether the variances in the haematocrit values between males and females are significant

2 Type '= FTEST(,'

3 Click on the sheet (e.g. 'Females').

4 Select the numbers that you wish to compare. This will appear in the formula bar as something like '= FTEST(Females!C2:C7)'. See Figure 19.23.

=FTEST(Females!C2:C7

variable	Sex	Haematocrit	Haemoglobin	Glucose	Total cholesterol	HDL cholesterol	Triglycerides	LDL cholesterol
41439XXX	Female	40	14.3	4.7	2.79	0.98	1.64	1.0
42049XXX	Female	48	13.0	4.8	4.07	1.47	0.60	2.3
42035XXX	Female	42	11.3	4.4	3.35	1.98	0.75	1.0
41442XXX	Female	43	11.3	4.7	3.85	1.75	1.07	1.6
41434XXX	Female	45	10.5	5.6	5.20	1.98	1.59	2.5
40104XXX	Female	37	11.7	4.6	4.07	1.47	0.60	2.3
	Count	6	6	6	6	6	6	

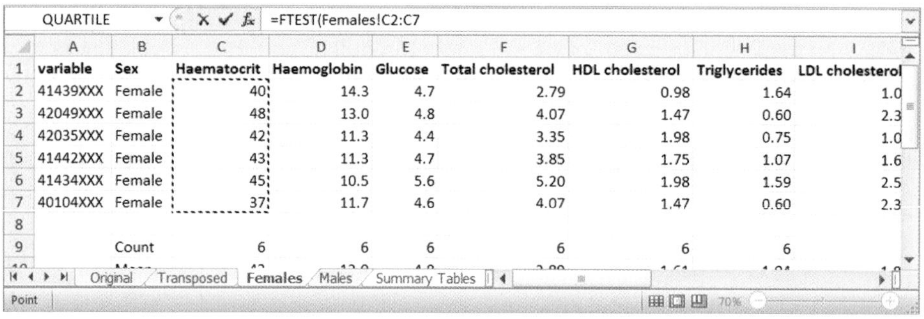

Figure 19.23 The F-test formula appearing in the formula bar after the first array is added

5 Type ','.

6 Click on the other sheet (e.g. 'Males') and select the second set of numbers that you wish to compare. This will appear in the formula bar as something like '= FTEST(Females!C2:C7,Males!C2:C14'. See Figure 19.24.

7 Type ')' then press '*ENTER*'.

8 The cell should now contain the *P* value for the F-test (see Figure 19.22). In this comparison the variance between the haematocrit values of the males and females is not statistically significant

QUARTILE =FTEST(Females!C2:C7,Males!C2:C14)

variable	Sex	Haematocrit	Haemoglobin	Glucose	Total cholesterol	HDL cholesterol	Triglycerides	LDL choleste
40986XXX	Male	43	11.3	5.0	4.72	1.64	1.98	2.
42034XXX	Male	43	12.5	7.0	3.32	0.74	0.93	2.
41185XXX	Male	48	14.6	4.8	5.60	2.03	0.81	3.
42028XXX	Male	47	12.5	6.2	2.68	1.63	1.59	1.
41762XXX	Male	45	15.2	6.2	2.85	0.99	1.70	1.
41142XXX	Male	45	15.2	5.0	4.07	1.47	0.60	2.
42003XXX	Male	49	11.2	6.4	2.68	1.63	1.59	1.
41777XXX	Male	43	13.6	5.3	2.85	0.99	1.70	1.
40997XXX	Male	45	11.3	5.5	3.35	1.98	0.75	1.
41732XXX	Male	45	14.0	5.4	4.07	1.47	0.60	2.
41203XXX	Male	45	15.1	5.6	2.79	0.98	1.64	1.
41304XXX	Male	54	15.2	4.5	3.32	0.74	0.93	2.
41012XXX	Male	45	14.2	4.8	2.60	1.80	1.10	0.

Original Transposed Females Males Summary Tables

Figure 19.24 The F-test formula appearing in the formula bar after the second array is added

(using a threshold of $P < 0.05$). This would mean you would select '2' for the type of t-test (i.e. equal variances). If the value is <0.05 then you would select '3' for the type of t-test (i.e. unequal variances).

9 Complete the *P* values in the table. Unfortunately, the fill down function does not work as the data you need to compare are in columns and you are filling down rows. You will need to enter the individual arrays one by one. The final table is shown in Figure 19.25. Across the measures shown here, there are significant differences ($P < 0.05$) in the variances in systolic blood pressure (SBP) and pulse pressure between males and females. This will affect the type of t-test that will be selected below.

To determine the *P* value for the t-test, use the formula '= TTEST(array1, array2, tails, type)'.

Array 1 is the first data set.

Array 2 is the second data set.

Tails specifies the number of distribution tails. If tails = 1, TTEST uses the one-tailed distribution. If tails = 2, TTEST uses the two-tailed distribution. As mentioned above, you should always use a two-tailed test in the biological sciences, indicating that you should never assume you know which direction a difference will be, even if you have a directional hypothesis.

Type is the kind of t-test to perform. If test = 1, TTEST uses a paired test; if test = 2, TTEST uses a two-sample equal variance test; if test = 3, TTEST uses a two-sample unequal variance test. This was determined above using the F-test.

Variable	Units	Males n	Males Mean	Males SD	Males Max	Males Min	Females n	Females Mean	Females SD	Females Max	Females Min
Haematocrit	g/dL	13	46	3	54	43	6	43	4	48	37
Haemoglobin	mmol/L	13	13.5	1.6	15.2	11.2	6	12.0	1.4	14.3	10.5
Glucose	mmol/L	13	5.5	0.7	7	4.5	6	4.8	0.4	5.6	4.36
Total cholesterol	mmol/L	13	3.45	0.92	5.6	2.6	6	3.89	0.81	5.2	2.79
HDL cholesterol	mmol/L	13	1.39	0.45	2.03	0.74	6	1.61	0.38	1.98	0.98
Triglycerides	mmol/L	13	1.22	0.49	1.98	0.6	6	1.04	0.48	1.64	0.6
LDL cholesterol	bpm	13	1.74	0.84	3.21	0.8	6	1.81	0.68	2.53	1.03
Radial HR	mmHg	13	63	7	78	56	6	71	22	98	49
SBP	mmHg	13	116	11	142	100	6	114	4	120	108
DBP	mmHg	13	70	8	76	54	6	69	5	77	62
Pulse pressure	mmHg	13	47	9	66	38	6	44	4	49	38
Mean arterial pressur	mmHg	13	86	9	98	69	6	84	5	91	77.33

Variable	Units	Males mean±SD	Females mean±SD	T Test P Value	F Test P Value
Haematocrit	g/dL	46±3	43±4		0.47
Haemoglobin	mmol/L	13.5±1.6	12±1.4		0.8182762
Glucose	mmol/L	5.5±0.7	4.8±0.4		0.2212075
Total cholesterol	mmol/L	3.45±0.92	3.89±0.81		0.8336429
HDL cholesterol	mmol/L	1.39±0.45	1.61±0.38		0.7512019
Triglycerides	mmol/L	1.22±0.49	1.04±0.48		0.955185
LDL cholesterol	bpm	1.74±0.84	1.81±0.68		0.6639575
Radial HR	mmHg	63±7	71±22		0.8131988
SBP	mmHg	116±11	114±4		0.0403513
DBP	mmHg	70±8	69±5		0.4117342
Pulse pressure	mmHg	47±9	44±4		0.04954
Mean arterial press	mmHg	86±9	84±5		0.1528522

Transposed Females Males Summary Tables

Figure 19.25 *P* values for all F-tests

For the arrays you have to go back to the 'Males' and 'Females' worksheets and select the data by dragging the cursor over the required cells.

The steps are:

1 Click in the cell where you wish to have the *P* value for the t-test (see Figure 19.25 – cell S4).

2 Type '= TTEST('.

3 Click on the sheet (e.g. 'Females').

4 Select the numbers that you wish to compare. This will appear in the formula bar as something like '= TTEST(Female!C2:C7'. See Figure 19.26.

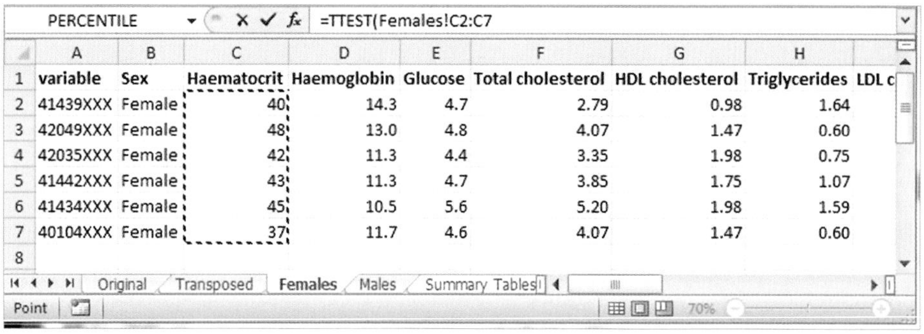

	A	B	C	D	E	F	G	H
1	variable	Sex	Haematocrit	Haemoglobin	Glucose	Total cholesterol	HDL cholesterol	Triglycerides
2	41439XXX	Female	40	14.3	4.7	2.79	0.98	1.64
3	42049XXX	Female	48	13.0	4.8	4.07	1.47	0.60
4	42035XXX	Female	42	11.3	4.4	3.35	1.98	0.75
5	41442XXX	Female	43	11.3	4.7	3.85	1.75	1.07
6	41434XXX	Female	45	10.5	5.6	5.20	1.98	1.59
7	40104XXX	Female	37	11.7	4.6	4.07	1.47	0.60
8								

Figure 19.26 The t-test formula appearing in the formula bar after the first array is added

5 Type ','.

6 Click on the other sheet (e.g. 'Males') and select the second set of numbers that you wish to compare. This will appear in the formula bar as something like '= TTEST(Female!C2:C7,Male! C2:C14'. See Figure 19.27.

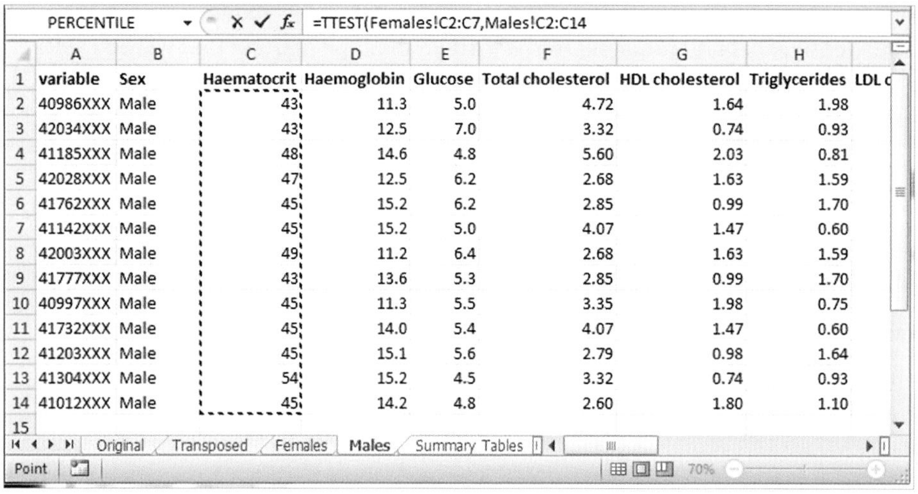

	A	B	C	D	E	F	G	H
1	variable	Sex	Haematocrit	Haemoglobin	Glucose	Total cholesterol	HDL cholesterol	Triglycerides
2	40986XXX	Male	43	11.3	5.0	4.72	1.64	1.98
3	42034XXX	Male	43	12.5	7.0	3.32	0.74	0.93
4	41185XXX	Male	48	14.6	4.8	5.60	2.03	0.81
5	42028XXX	Male	47	12.5	6.2	2.68	1.63	1.59
6	41762XXX	Male	45	15.2	6.2	2.85	0.99	1.70
7	41142XXX	Male	45	15.2	5.0	4.07	1.47	0.60
8	42003XXX	Male	49	11.2	6.4	2.68	1.63	1.59
9	41777XXX	Male	43	13.6	5.3	2.85	0.99	1.70
10	40997XXX	Male	45	11.3	5.5	3.35	1.98	0.75
11	41732XXX	Male	45	14.0	5.4	4.07	1.47	0.60
12	41203XXX	Male	45	15.1	5.6	2.79	0.98	1.64
13	41304XXX	Male	54	15.2	4.5	3.32	0.74	0.93
14	41012XXX	Male	45	14.2	4.8	2.60	1.80	1.10
15								

Figure 19.27 The t-test formula appearing in the formula bar after the second array is added

7 Type ','.

8 Type '2,' as we should use a two-tailed distribution test.

9 Type '2)'as the variances are equal (from the F-test – see previous section on how to obtain and interpret the F-test *P* value).

10 Then press '*ENTER*' (see Figure 19.28).

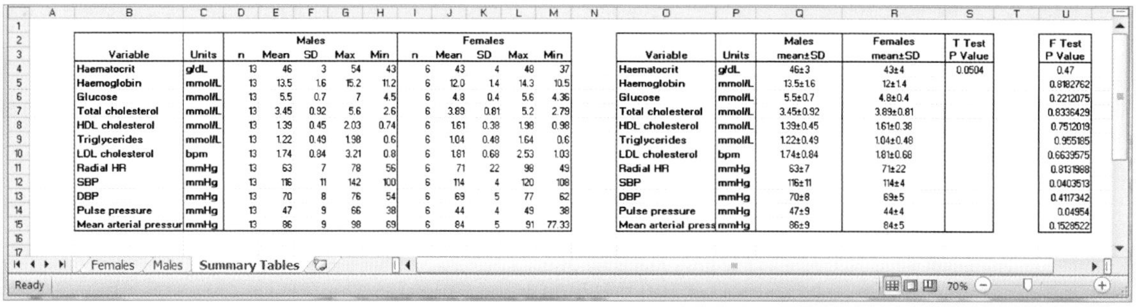

Variable	Units	Males n	Males Mean	Males SD	Males Max	Males Min	Females n	Females Mean	Females SD	Females Max	Females Min
Haematocrit	g/dL	13	46	3	54	43	6	43	4	48	37
Haemoglobin	mmol/L	13	13.5	1.6	15.2	11.2	6	12.0	1.4	14.3	10.5
Glucose	mmol/L	13	5.5	0.7	7	4.5	6	4.8	0.4	5.6	4.36
Total cholesterol	mmol/L	13	3.45	0.92	5.6	2.6	6	3.89	0.81	5.2	2.79
HDL cholesterol	mmol/L	13	1.39	0.45	2.03	0.74	6	1.61	0.38	1.98	0.98
Triglycerides	mmol/L	13	1.22	0.49	1.98	0.6	6	1.04	0.48	1.64	0.6
LDL cholesterol	bpm	13	1.74	0.84	3.21	0.8	6	1.81	0.68	2.53	1.03
Radial HR	mmHg	13	63	7	78	56	6	71	22	98	49
SBP	mmHg	13	116	11	142	100	6	114	4	120	108
DBP	mmHg	13	70	8	76	54	6	69	5	77	62
Pulse pressure	mmHg	13	47	9	66	38	6	44	4	49	38
Mean arterial pressur	mmHg	13	86	9	98	69	6	84	5	91	77.33

Variable	Units	Males mean±SD	Females mean±SD	T Test P Value	F Test P Value
Haematocrit	g/dL	46±3	43±4	0.0504	0.47
Haemoglobin	mmol/L	13.5±1.6	12±1.4		0.8182762
Glucose	mmol/L	5.5±0.7	4.8±0.4		0.2212075
Total cholesterol	mmol/L	3.45±0.92	3.89±0.81		0.8336429
HDL cholesterol	mmol/L	1.39±0.45	1.61±0.38		0.7512019
Triglycerides	mmol/L	1.22±0.49	1.04±0.48		0.955185
LDL cholesterol	bpm	1.74±0.84	1.81±0.68		0.6639575
Radial HR	mmHg	63±7	71±22		0.8131988
SBP	mmHg	116±11	114±4		0.0403513
DBP	mmHg	70±8	69±5		0.4117342
Pulse pressure	mmHg	47±9	44±4		0.04954
Mean arterial press	mmHg	86±9	84±5		0.1528522

Figure 19.28 *P* value for t-test between males and females for haematocrit

Add the P values to the table. Unfortunately, the fill down function does not work as the data you need to compare are in columns and you are filling down rows. You will need to enter the individual arrays one by one. Remember that you select whether the variances are equal based on the F-test. The final table is shown in Figure 19.29. Across these measures there is a significant difference ($P < 0.05$) only in plasma glucose between males and females.

N	O	P	Q	R	S
	Variable	Units	Males mean±SD	Females mean±SD	T Test P Value
	Haematocrit	g/dL	46±3	43±4	0.0504
	Haemoglobin	mmol/L	13.5±1.6	12±1.4	0.0593
	Glucose	mmol/L	5.5±0.7	4.8±0.4	0.0430
	Total cholesterol	mmol/L	3.45±0.92	3.89±0.81	0.3352
	HDL cholesterol	mmol/L	1.39±0.45	1.61±0.38	0.3312
	Triglycerides	mmol/L	1.22±0.49	1.04±0.48	0.4532
	LDL cholesterol	bpm	1.74±0.84	1.81±0.68	0.8494
	Radial HR	mmHg	63±7	71±22	0.2514
	SBP	mmHg	116±11	114±4	0.5381
	DBP	mmHg	70±8	69±5	0.6469
	Pulse pressure	mmHg	47±9	44±4	0.3742
	Mean arterial press	mmHg	86±9	84±5	0.6783

Figure 19.29 P values for all t-tests

Activity 19.3 Hypothesis testing – correlations

AIM: to use a correlation analysis to determine the strength of a relationship between two variables.

Background

A correlation is used to determine the relationship or association between two variables. Specifically, it determines the extent to which two measurement variables 'vary together'. For example, you may wish to determine the relationship between body fat percentage and plasma total cholesterol for all participants in this course.

A correlation coefficient such as the Pearson correlation coefficient – also commonly known as the 'r' value – provides a number that represents the extent of a relationship between two variables. It is commonly accepted that a lower case r is used for this. The value of any correlation coefficient must be between -1 and $+1$ inclusive. When larger values of one variable tend to be associated with larger values of the other, this is a positive correlation. When smaller values of one variable tend to be associated with larger values of the other, this is a negative correlation. As the strength of the association increases, the correlation coefficient (or r value) will get closer to $+1$ or -1. When values of both variables tend to be unrelated, the correlation will be closer to 0. SPSS also calculates a P value for this comparison.

For interpretation, Cohen's levels[5] can be used:

>0.5	Large
0.5 to 0.3	Moderate
0.3 to 0.1	Small
<0.1	Insubstantial.

These also apply to inverse (negative) correlation coefficients (i.e. -0.3 to -0.1 is small).

Another way of interpreting the strength of the relationship is to calculate the coefficient of determination. This is also known as the R-squared (R^2) value. It is commonly accepted to use an upper case 'R' for this. The R^2 value will provide some additional meaning to the correlation coefficient. It represents the amount of variability in one value that can be accounted by the other (shared variability).

To calculate the R^2 value, simply square the r value (e.g. an r value of 0.2 gives you an R^2 value $0.2 \times 0.2 = 0.04$). Excel also allows this to be shown in a figure (e.g. Figure 19.30) by clicking on 'Display R-squared value on chart' in the 'Format Trendline' dialog box (see Figure 19.31). Indeed, to derive the correlation coefficient it may be quicker to get the R^2 value this way and then get the square root ($\sqrt{}$) of the R^2 value to obtain the r value.

After calculating the R^2 value, you convert it to a percentage by multiplying by 100. For example, if the R^2 value was 0.4 we can say that 40% of the variability in y can be accounted for by x.

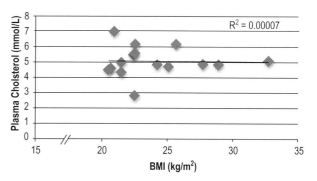

Figure 19.30 Insubstantial relationship between body mass index (BMI) and plasma total cholesterol; R-squared $= 0.00007$ and correlation coefficient (r value) $= \sqrt{0.00007} = 0.0008$

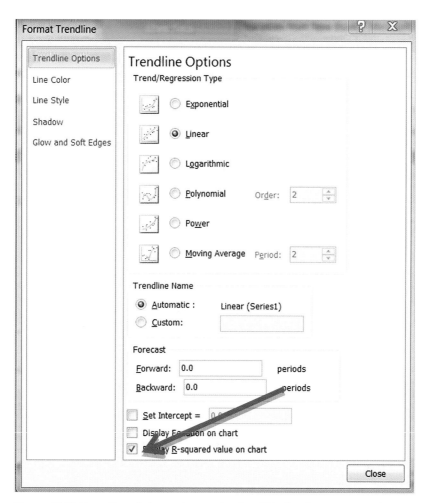

Figure 19.31 Trendline dialogue box: selecting 'Display R-squared value on chart'

Protocol summary

Determine the strength and direction of a relationship between two variables.

Protocol

In some correlations one of the variables may be expected to be influencing or driving the relationship. For example, energy intake would be expected to be influencing body fat percentage. In this situation, energy intake is the independent variable (or input) and the variable that it is influencing the dependent variable (or output): body fat percentage. You should arrange the figure so that the independent variable is on the x (horizontal) axis and the dependent variable is on the y (vertical) axis. Knowledge of the biophysical background will assist in determining whether a variable is going to be independent or dependent.

x axis $\rightarrow$ Independent variable $\rightarrow$ Input

y axis $\rightarrow$ Dependent variable $\rightarrow$ Output

However, for many associations it is unknown whether one variable is independent or dependent and, in this situation, it does not matter which variable is put on which axis. The relationship provided in Figure 19.30 is an example of this situation.

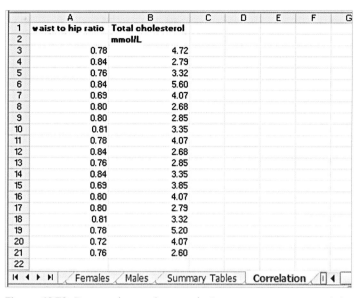

Figure 19.32 Data columns for correlation on a separate worksheet

1 Select the data columns you wish to use and paste them onto a separate worksheet so they are next to each other and label the sheet 'Correlation' (Figure 19.32).

2 Highlight the cells containing data and go to the 'Insert' menu. Then from the Charts section select 'Insert scatter' and select the top left chart (Figure 19.33).

3 To add in the trendline, right-click on one of the data points and select 'Add Trendline …' and select 'Linear'.[d] Also, click on 'Display R-squared value on chart' (see Figure 19.31). Label the axes and re-scale if necessary so that the scatter plot is spread out across the graph area (Figure 19.34). In the example provided R-squared $= 0.02$ and the correlation coefficient (r value) $= \sqrt{0.02} = 0.14 =$ small positive relationship.

The following are examples of a positive relationship (Figure 19.35), a negative relationship (Figure 19.36) and an insubstantial relationship (Figure 19.37) between two variables.

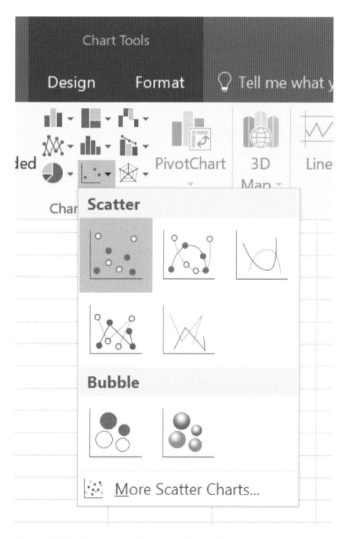

Figure 19.33 'Insert scatter chart' chart tool

---

[d] We assume that the relationship is linear where a scatter plot of the two variables is best represented (line of best fit) by a straight line.

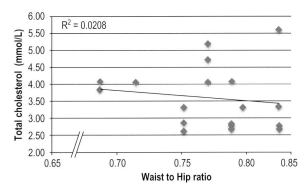

Figure 19.34 Re-scaling the axes to spread data out across the available space

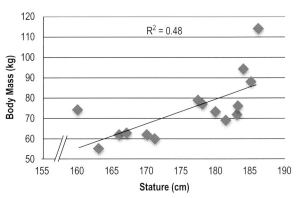

Figure 19.35 The scatter plot indicates a large positive relationship between stature and body mass: R-squared $= 0.48$ and Pearson correlation coefficient (r value) $= \sqrt{0.48} = 0.69$

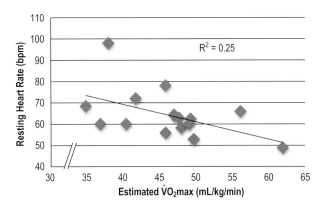

Figure 19.36 The scatter plot indicates a moderate negative relationship between estimated $\dot{V}O_2$max and resting heart rate: R-squared $= 0.25$ and Pearson correlation coefficient (r value) $= \sqrt{0.25} = 0.50$

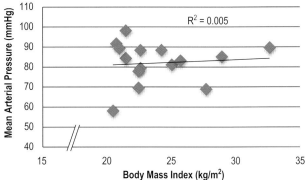

Figure 19.37 The scatter plot indicates an insubstantial relationship between body mass index and mean arterial pressure: R-squared $= 0.005$ and Pearson correlation coefficient (r value) $= \sqrt{0.005} = 0.07$

Activity 19.4 Develop and test hypotheses

AIM: to generate and test hypotheses that address research questions.

Background

One of the first stages in any process that involves data collection (e.g. research) is the generation of a question. In research this is known as the research question. However, generating a question that requires data analysis is not confined to 'research'. For example, you may be working as an Accredited Exercise Physiologist in a musculoskeletal rehabilitation setting and you may have observed something that you wish to investigate further. For example, patients who attend the clinic with a certain injury (injury x that is classified in severity from 1 to 10) appear to have a higher degree of severity of the injury when they have low upper body strength. As mentioned above, one of the first stages in a data collection process is to formulate a question that identifies why you are collecting the data. For the above example the question may be: 'Is there a large positive relationship between injury x and upper body strength in patients attending the clinic?'

If the work were being conducted in a 'research' setting then the next step would be to develop a research hypothesis. For the above example the hypothesis may be: 'There is a large positive relationship between injury x and upper body strength in patients attending the clinic'. In research there is also the null hypothesis, which states that: 'There is no difference, or no relationship (which is assumed to be true unless we can disprove it)'. Therefore, in this example the null hypothesis would be: 'There is no relationship between injury x and upper body strength in patients attending the clinic.'

For this activity you will develop two research questions and corresponding hypotheses. One question/hypothesis will require data to be analysed by comparing means and the other will require a correlational analysis. To develop your questions and hypotheses, it is suggested that you look at your own data and see whether there are any trends that you may be interested in exploring. A question requiring comparison of means might be: 'Do males with a BMI less than or equal to 25 kg/m^2 have a lower predicted $\dot{V}O_2$max compared with males with a BMI greater than 25 kg/m^2?' You might hypothesise that they do. To answer the question/hypothesis you could conduct an independent t-test. To complete this data analysis will require an extra data-filtering step (males with BMI $>$25 kg/m^2 or males with BMI $\leq$25 kg/m^2). In the analysis report you would include a table similar to Figure 19.16 except there would be only one data row.

For the correlation analysis, you notice that your bench press strength is high compared with the rest of the class but your 20-metre sprint time is slow. You would like to know: 'What is the strength of the relationship between bench press strength and 20-metre sprint time?' You hypothesise that there is a large positive relationship. To test the hypothesis, you run the Pearson correlational analysis on these data. For the analysis report you would include the figure that shows this relationship.

Protocol summary

Develop and test two research questions and hypotheses based on the data collected.

Protocol

Comparing means

1 Using data collected in the practicals in this manual, develop a research question that compares the means of two groups.

2 Generate a research hypothesis that addresses this research question.

3 Complete a summary data table containing means, standard deviations and P values that addresses the research question and research hypothesis. See additional instructions below on 'Constructing tables'.

4 State whether the research hypothesis was supported or not.

Correlation

1 Using data collected in the practicals in this manual, develop a research question based on a correlation.

2 Create a research hypothesis that addresses this research question

3 Generate a figure and determine the r value. See additional instructions below on 'Constructing figures'.

4 State whether the research hypothesis was supported or not.

Research question – comparing means:

Research hypothesis – comparing means:

Research question – correlation:

_____

_____

_____

Research hypothesis – correlation:

_____

_____

_____

Constructing tables

When constructing a table, the following features are important (see Figure 19.38 for an example):

Table 1: Comparison of the VO₂max values of males with different BMIs. Values are mean±SD.			
	BMI ≤25 kg/m² (n=21)	BMI >25 kg/m² (n=15)	P Value
VO₂max (mL/kg/min)			

Figure 19.38 Example of a summary table: comparison of the $\dot{V}O_2$max values of males with different BMIs. Values are mean ± SD.

- Caption – a concise title above the table that describes the data presented (e.g. 'Table 1 Comparison of the $\dot{V}O_2$max values of males with different BMIs').

- Column headings.

- Provide information on the number of participants included in the comparisons, which can be reported as '($n =$)' after or under the column headings.

- The row will have the name of the variable (e.g. $\dot{V}O_2$max) and measurement units (e.g. mL/kg/min).

- Indicate that the values presented are the mean and standard deviation. This can either be written as '(Values are mean ± SD)' at the end of the title or in the footnotes directly after the table.

Constructing figures

Many of the screen-captured figures in this practical are graphs. When constructing graphs, the following features are important (see Figure 19.39 for an example):

- Caption – a concise title below the figure that describes the graph (e.g. 'Figure 1 Large positive relationship between hand grip strength and vertical jump height').

- Axes – add the appropriate axes labels with units and change the scale so that the data are equally distributed along the axes.

- Adjust the size of the font of the axes labels and units (usually increase) so they are easily read.

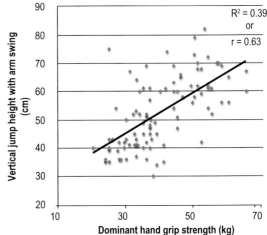

Figure 1: Large positive relationship between hand grip strength and vertical jump height

Figure 19.39 Example of a summary figure.

Case studies

Case Study 1
RESEARCH QUESTION

Is there a difference between the ages of people who had a positive exercise stress test and individuals who did not have a positive stress test?

RESEARCH HYPOTHESIS

People who have had a positive exercise stress test will be older than individuals who did not have a positive stress test.

ANALYSIS

You complete the data analysis by first calculating the group means and standard deviations. You then use an independent t-test to see whether there is a statistically significant difference between the means. A table is prepared with the summary statistics and the t-test P value (Table 19.1).

TABLE 19.1 Summary table for Case study 1: comparison of the ages of people who had a positive exercise stress test with individuals who did not have a positive exercise stress test			
Variable	Positive stress test ($n = 12$)	Did not have a positive stress test ($n = 832$)	P Value
Age (years)	74 ± 7	57 ± 6	0.0004

INTERPRETATION

The table shows that people who had a positive exercise stress test were, on average, 17 years older than individuals who did not have a positive stress test. This difference was statistically significant ($P = 0.0004$).

Case Study 2
RESEARCH QUESTION

Is there a relationship between the 20 m sprint time measured just before the start of the season and the average total sprint distance collected during each game?

RESEARCH HYPOTHESIS

There will be a strong negative relationship between the 20 m sprint time and the average total sprint distance from each game. This would indicate that faster runners just before the start of the season cover more distance sprinting in games during the season.

continued overpage

ANALYSIS

You complete the data analysis by first preparing a scatter plot (Figure 19.40). The 20 m sprint time is on the y-axis as this is the independent variable (i.e. the sprint distance run during a game is thought to be dependent on the 20 m sprint time measured just before the start of the season). You then determine the r value for the relationship.

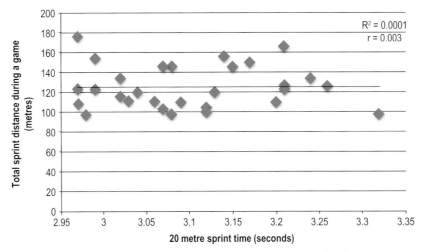

Figure 19.40 Summary figure for Case study 2: insubstantial relationship between the 20 m sprint time. measured just before the start of the season and average total sprint distance during each game during the season.

INTERPRETATION

The figure shows an insubstantial relationship between the 20 m sprint time measured just before the start of the season and the average total sprint distance from each game. This indicates that players who were faster in the pre-season have not completed more distance sprinting during each game.

References

[1] United Nations. Big data for sustainable development. New York: UN; 2019. https://www.un.org/en/global-issues/big-data-for-sustainable-development.
[2] Wasserman EB, Herzog MM, Collins CL, Morris SN, Marshall SW. Fundamentals of sports analytics. Clin Sports Med 2018;37:387–400.
[3] Amrhein V, Greenland S, McShane B. Scientists rise up against statistical significance. Nature 2019;567:305–7.
[4] Berg KE, Latin RW. Essentials of research methods in health, physical education, exercise science, and recreation. Baltimore, MD: Lippincott Williams & Wilkins; 2008.
[5] Cohen J. Statistical power analysis for the behavioral sciences. Hillsdale, NJ: Lawrence Erlbaum; 1988.

APPENDIX A
LABORATORY SAFETY, CLEANING AND DISINFECTING

Equipment and other requirements

- Non-latex gloves of appropriate size (S, M, L)
- Paper towels
- Antimicrobial soap or alcohol-based/antiseptic rubs
- Cleaning solution (e.g. Sonidet)
- Disinfecting solution (e.g. Viraclean)
- Alcohol wipes
- Cleaning solution container/s
- Breathing tube solution container/s
- Spray bottle
- Sink
- Drying cabinet
- Biohazardous waste containers
- Hanging rack
- Sharps container
- Lab coat
- Safety glasses
- First aid kit

Occupational health and safety
All Australian universities and healthcare centres (such as hospitals) have strict occupational health and safety guidelines. The institution-specific guidelines should be read before participating in practical sessions. In addition, your institution may have an associated safety declaration form that will need to be completed before someone is permitted to participate. A risk assessment should be conducted by the instructor for all activities, including chemicals or biological material that are to be used during practical classes.

Emergencies
It is important to become familiar with the emergency/evacuation procedures for your workplace. This includes the location of:
- emergency exits and alarm buttons
- meeting points
- firefighting hoses and extinguishers
- first aid kits
- defibrillators
- safety showers
- eye wash stations
- telephones and procedures to call for help if required.

Personal protective equipment

You should arrive 'ready to participate' for all practical sessions detailed. From a safety perspective, this may require wearing appropriate exercise clothing and covered footwear (exercise shoes) during practical classes. Thongs, open-weave shoes, sandals and so forth are not appropriate footwear. Long hair should be tied back to avoid injury.

In addition to these standard safety precautions, there are additional precautions that must be adhered to when completing specific technical skills. These will be detailed at the start of the appropriate practicals. For example, the blood analysis practical requires wearing the following personal protective equipment (PPE):

- lab coat
- approved safety glasses
- gloves.
  Safety glasses should remain on the face throughout the practical, not lifted and rested on top of the head.

Preparation for class

It is recommended that you prepare for each class by following the pre-exercise test procedures outlined in Appendix B. This will increase the validity of your results from each test, as well as reduce the risk of an untoward event. You should inform your instructor if you have any existing medical conditions or injuries that may limit your ability to exercise safely. Similarly, if you know that you will have difficulties with a specific skill or session (e.g. if you have an aversion to needles or feel faint when having blood collected), then you should discuss this with the instructor before the session. Please note that food and drink must not be consumed in laboratories.

FIRST AID

The likelihood of a participant experiencing an adverse event while exercising (e.g. chest pain, dyspnoea (shortness of breath) or dizziness) is quite low. Although extremely rare, serious complications such as myocardial infarction are also possible during some of the more demanding exercise protocols. Should complications arise, an individual with first aid training, including cardiopulmonary resuscitation (CPR), should be on hand. It is recommended that you complete courses in administering first aid and CPR before taking part in the practicals. At a minimum, the instructor should have completed first aid and CPR courses to enable them to deal with an untoward event occurring within the teaching laboratory.

PROCEDURE FOR FIRST AID IN CASE OF INJURY, ILLNESS OR CHEMICAL/BIOLOGICAL SPILL

- At the start of the first session, familiarise yourself with the safety facilities of the teaching laboratory, including the location of emergency equipment and call buttons, first aid kits and ice packs.
- First aid should be administered by a person who has completed first aid training.
- Immediately report all exposure to chemicals, injuries and illnesses, no matter how small, to the instructor.
- Non-injury causing incidents, such as spills, electrical faults or damage to equipment, must also be reported to the instructor.

Eye injuries

- Eye injuries are always serious, whether caused by chemical or mechanical injury, or a splash by biological material.
- Chemical or biological treatment requires immediate and prolonged flushing with water (20 minutes minimum) at the eye wash station (preferable) or under a tap.
- Eyelids should be held open during flushing.
- Medical advice should be obtained for an eye injury.
- The material safety data sheet (MSDS) for the chemical involved should accompany the student if it is necessary to seek medical treatment.

Chemical or biological spills on skin

- Thoroughly wash the affected area with copious quantities of water.
- Remove contaminated clothes.
- Consult a MSDS to determine appropriate first aid. The MSDS for the chemical involved should accompany the student if it is necessary to seek medical treatment.

Ingestion (swallowing)

- Do *not* induce vomiting.
- Seek medical advice or contact a poisons information centre.

Sharps injuries
- Wash the wound and encourage bleeding.
- Seek medical advice.

Unwell or dizzy
- If a student is feeling unwell or dizzy when participating in an experiment, encourage them to stop the activity immediately and sit or lie down.

Incident reporting

Should any injury, illness or incident occur during participation in the teaching laboratory, it is important to report it to the instructor immediately. Incidents that don't cause injury, such as spills, must also be reported. Please also ensure that any broken or faulty equipment is reported to the instructor so that it can be repaired to avoid any adverse events occurring during subsequent and/or inadvertent use.

It is likely that your institution will require documentation of all injuries, illnesses and incidents. It is recommended that these documents be completed as soon as possible to ensure accurate reporting.

HAND WASHING

Hand washing is a component of what is referred to as *standard precautions* in healthcare settings. These are infection control practices that all individuals involved in healthcare settings should use to reduce the risk of transmission of microorganisms, thereby protecting both the healthcare worker and the participants from contact with infective agents. Hand washing is used in conjunction with the appropriate use of protective gloves (for example, gloves should be used in addition to hand washing for points 2 and 3 below). The World Health Organization (WHO) has released the 5 moments of hand hygiene[1] which have been identified as the critical times when hand washing should occur:

1. before touching a participant (e.g. shaking hands, clinical examination, measuring skinfolds)
2. before doing a procedure (e.g. lancet of finger for blood collection)
3. after a procedure or body fluid exposure risk (e.g. after blood sample collection)
4. after touching a participant (e.g. shaking hands, clinical examination, measuring skinfolds)
5. after touching a participant's surroundings (e.g. when leaving after finishing a consult in which you have touched any object in the participant's surroundings even if the participant has not been touched).

It is good practice to start adhering to the 5 moments of hand hygiene within the practical sessions so that the process becomes a habit. Either antimicrobial soap (that is rinsed under running water) or alcohol-based/antiseptic rubs (that do not need to be washed off) should be made available to you.

CLEANING AND DISINFECTION

The practicals described within this textbook involve the use of multiple pieces of exercise equipment (e.g. bicycle ergometers) and associated items to assist with participant monitoring and data collection (e.g. heart rate monitors). These items will be shared between participants and thereby carry a risk of contamination that may be transferred between users. Therefore, all of the equipment that you use when testing must be adequately cleaned or disinfected following use.

Cleaning refers to the removal of all adherent visible material from the surfaces, crevices, joints and lumens of instruments, and is normally accomplished using water with detergents or enzymatic products.[2] Bacteriostatic detergents (e.g. Sonidet) stops bacteria from reproducing. These detergents are *cleaners*, not *disinfectants*, and are intended for use in the cleaning of non-critical medical devices.[3]

Disinfecting is a more meticulous thermal or chemical process that removes or kills the majority of microorganisms (e.g. bacteria, fungi, viruses) with the exception of high numbers of bacterial spores.[2] A hospital grade *disinfectant* (e.g. Viraclean) kills numerous common bacteria (i.e. is bactericidal) and viruses. It is intended for use in the disinfecting of non-critical and semi-critical medical devices.[4] There are other hospital grade *disinfectants* (e.g. Milton) that are even more meticulous, involving the complete destruction of all forms of microorganism, including bacteria (i.e. is bactericidal), viruses, fungi and spores.[2] It can be used for the disinfection of non-critical and semi-critical medical devices, as well as various other items. To be effective, disinfection and sterilisation processes must be preceded by fastidious mechanical or manual cleaning to remove all foreign material.[2]

Non-critical, semi-critical and critical medical devices

Most of the equipment described in the following practicals is classed as *non-critical medical devices*, which means it either does not come into direct contact with the participant or comes into contact with intact skin only.[2] Examples of such equipment include heart rate monitors and watches, stethoscopes and blood pressure cuffs. The cleaning and disinfecting of such devices is very important to prevent transfer of common microorganisms that can survive on these surfaces for long periods (e.g. methicillin-resistant *Staphylococcus aureus*, *Escherichia coli*).

Equipment that is categorised as *semi-critical* or *critical medical devices* has also been described in the practicals. Semi-critical devices are those that come in contact with mucous membranes or non-intact skin but do not actually penetrate with normal use. These include the mouthpieces of breathing apparatus used for measuring $\dot{V}O_2max$ (which contact mucous membranes) and blood analysers (which contact non-intact skin). These items must be diligently disinfected after every use. Viruses such as Epstein–Barr virus (glandular fever) can be transmitted from the saliva of infected individuals if disinfecting is inadequate. Use of critical medical devices that penetrate the skin (e.g. lancets for blood collection) is limited in the practicals in this manual.

The critical medical devices described will be single use only and must be discarded into a sharps container immediately after use. Although these are used only once, they directly penetrate skin and thus carry a greater risk of infection. It is therefore important to disinfect the skin with alcohol wipes and allow it to dry before puncturing so that the risk of infection is reduced.

Preparation of detergents and disinfectant solutions

There are many different types of detergent, disinfectant and sterilisation solutions that are used across various institutions. Below we have provided protocols for the preparation and use of detergents (i.e. Sonidet) and disinfectant/sterilisation (i.e. Viraclean and Milton) solutions commonly used within hospitals and universities around Australia. In facilities where these specific solutions are not available/used, follow the manufacturer's guidelines for the preparation of detergent and disinfectant solutions.

SONIDET PREPARATION

1 Put on a pair of gloves.
2 Using a measuring cup, measure 5 mL of Sonidet per 1 L of water into a container marked 'Sonidet'.
3 Dilute with the appropriate volume of cold tap water. When diluted correctly, Sonidet should be a clear odourless liquid detergent.[3] If the solution is still yellow after it has been diluted, then too much Sonidet has been added.
4 Sonidet solution should be changed when it becomes cloudy (indicates excessive fouling) or if it has been in use for $\geq$24 hours.[3]
5 It should be rinsed off cleaned equipment so that no residue remains.[3]

VIRACLEAN PREPARATION

1 Put on a pair of gloves.
2 Viraclean solution is not diluted when used so it should maintain a pink colour.[4]
3 Pour enough 100% Viraclean into a container marked 'Viraclean' to ensure the items being disinfected are totally submerged.
4 The required exposure time is 10 minutes.[5]
5 Viraclean should be changed after every use.
6 It should be rinsed off disinfected equipment so that so that no residue remains.

MILTON PREPARATION

1 Put on a pair of gloves.
2 A laboratory coat is also recommended as Milton solution is dilute (2%) sodium hypochlorite solution (bleach) and may damage or bleach clothes on contact.
3 Use a small measuring cup to measure 6.25 mL of Milton solution per 1 L of water.[6] Milton solution is recommended for disinfecting $\dot{V}O_2$ breathing tubes.
4 The required exposure time is 30 minutes (however, the solution remains sterile for 24 hours).[6]
5 It does not need to be rinsed off disinfected equipment before the equipment is used again.[7]

Cleaning and disinfecting of stethoscope earpieces, heart rate monitor straps and chest transmitters

1 Put on a pair of gloves.
2 Rinse excessive sweat off the heart rate monitor strap under cold tap water.
3 Place the heart rate monitor strap and stethoscope earpieces in the prepared Sonidet solution.
4 Gently agitate the solution until the equipment is clean and then rinse under cold tap water.
5 Place the heart rate monitor strap, stethoscope earpieces as well as the heart rate transmitter into prepared Viraclean solution for disinfecting and agitate briefly. Leave to stand for 10 minutes.

> **Note:** Certain heart rate transmitter models should not be placed in solutions but rather gently disinfected with alcohol wipes. Please check the cleaning and disinfecting instructions for your transmitters prior to submerging in solution.

6 After 10 minutes, remove items from Viraclean and rinse under cold tap water.
7 Hang the heart rate monitor chest strap and transmitter on a drying rack and place the stethoscope earpieces on a clean paper towel to dry.
8 Discard solutions unless there is the potential that others may use the Sonidet solution within the next 24 hours.

Cleaning and disinfecting of mouthpiece, nose clip and breathing tubes used in $\dot{V}O_2max$, lactate threshold and maximally accumulated oxygen deficit (MAOD) testing

MOUTHPIECE AND NOSE CLIP
1 Put on a pair of gloves.
2 Separate the mouthpiece components in the sink.
3 Rinse excessive saliva from the mouthpiece under cold tap water.
4 Place the mouthpiece and nose clip into prepared Sonidet solution. Gently agitate until clean and then rinse under cold tap water.
5 Place the mouthpiece and nose clip into prepared Viraclean solution for disinfecting and agitate briefly. Leave to stand for 10 minutes.
6 After 10 minutes, remove items from Viraclean and rinse under cold tap water.

> **Note:** This step is especially important for the mouthpiece to avoid it 'tasting' like disinfection solution for the next participant.

7 Allow the mouthpiece and nose clip to dry, preferably in a drying cabinet at 65°C–75°C to reduce the risk of re-contamination during assembly of the mouthpiece.[2]
8 Discard solutions unless there is the potential that others may use the Sonidet solution within the next 24 hours.

CLEANING AND DISINFECTING OF BREATHING TUBES
1 Put on a pair of gloves.
2 Rinse excessive saliva from the breathing tube under cold tap water.
3 Place the breathing tube into prepared Sonidet solution. Gently agitate until clean and then rinse under cold tap water.
4 Place the breathing tube into prepared Milton solution for disinfecting and agitate briefly. Leave to stand for 30 minutes.
5 After 30 minutes, remove the breathing tube from the Milton solution.

> **Note:** Breathing tubes do not need to be rinsed.

6 Place the breathing tube on a hanging rack to dry.
7 Discard solutions unless there is the potential that others may use the solution within the next 24 hours.

> **Note:** You are responsible for cleaning and disinfecting all of the equipment you use. You should not leave your equipment soaking for others to finish. Leaving equipment in cleaning solution also has the potential to reduce the lifespan of the equipment.

Disinfection of general teaching laboratory equipment (e.g. treadmills, mats, bikes, heart rate watches, sphygmomanometers)

1 Put on a pair of gloves.
2 Use 100% undiluted Viraclean in a spray bottle.
3 Spray and wipe down with paper towel all surfaces that may have come in contact with bodily fluids (e.g. secretions such as sweat and saliva).
4 Discard paper towel into a clinical waste bin.

WASTE DISPOSAL

It is particularly important that all waste be disposed of in the appropriate manner under health and safety guidelines.

- All sharps must be disposed of in a designated (puncture proof) medical/clinical sharps container. If you have used a sharp instrument then it is your responsibility to ensure it is properly disposed of. Do not leave sharp instruments sitting on a bench top where another individual may come into contact with them.
- All clinical waste that carries any risk of contamination (e.g. paper towels, gloves, wrapping foil from analyser chips) must be disposed of in the biohazardous waste container.

References

[1] Hand Hygiene Australia. 5 moments for hand hygiene. Melbourne, Vic: HHA; 2009. https://www.hha.org.au/hand-hygiene/5-moments-for-hand-hygiene.

[2] Queensland Health. Disinfection and sterilisation. Infection control guidelines. Brisbane, Qld: Queensland Health; 2010. https://citeseerx.ist.psu.edu/viewdoc/download;jsessionid=81AD1EE6EA8CD8328080EB617DF62548?doi=10.1.1.170.1772&rep=rep1&type=pdf.

[3] Whiteley Medical. Sonident technical bulletin. North Sydney, NSW: Whiteley Medical; 2011. https://www.whiteley.com.au/documents/technical-bulletin/SONIDET-TB2-July2011.pdf.

[4] Whiteley Medical. Viraclean technical bulletin. North Sydney, NSW: Whiteley Medical; 2019. https://www.whiteley.com.au/documents/brochures/Viraclean%20brochure%20April%202020%20final.pdf.

[5] Whiteley Medical. Material safety data sheet: Viraclean. North Sydney, NSW: Whiteley Medical; 2016. https://www.whiteley.com.au/documents/msds/Viraclean-12.pdf.

[6] Milton Pharmaceutical Ltd. Milton 2% – for clinical use dilution chart. Bournemouth, Dorset: Milton Pharmaceutical; 2018. https://www.coventryrugbyccg.nhs.uk/mf.ashx?ID=7b7ca1cf-dfa8-4593-a13a-a48d38a0adb8.

[7] Chemwatch. Milton material safety data sheet. Laverton North, Vic: Milton Pharmaceutical Australia; 2011. https://www.ebosonline.com.au/images/product/documents/Antibacterial%20Solution%202011%20-%20PC55123,%20PC55139.pdf.

APPENDIX B
PRE-EXERCISE TEST PROCEDURES

PRIOR TO THE DAY OF TESTING

1 Participants should be provided with the following pre-test instructions, recognising that these may need to be amended according to the specific test requirements:
   a Avoid significant exertion or exercise prior to testing that is likely to influence the test results (e.g. for maximal tests, no strenuous exercise 24 hours prior to the test).
   b Refrain from heavy meals, alcohol, caffeine and tobacco products for 3 hours prior to testing.
      i. For maximal aerobic tests (e.g. lactate threshold, $\dot{V}O_2max$, MAOD) it is recommended that a high-carbohydrate meal is consumed 2–4 hours prior to testing.
   c Arrive for testing in a euhydrated state.
   d Wear appropriate clothing including footwear. For most exercise tests this includes light clothing that doesn't restrict movement and comfortable enclosed footwear suitable for exercise. Women should wear a supportive sports bra or equivalent. Specific tests require additional requirements, including:
      i. For anthropometry tests, minimal clothing that allows access to the skin on the upper thigh, stomach and upper back is required. Thin material shorts (i.e. bike shorts) will improve the accuracy of circumference measurements.
      ii. For ECG testing, women may wish to bring a loose-fitting, short-sleeved shirt that buttons down the front, as access to the skin on the chest is required.
   e Bring a water bottle and towel.
   f Continue use of aids (cane, walker, etc.) during tests where appropriate.
   g Continue medication/s as usual.

> **Note:** For diagnostic tests, participants may be asked by the doctor not to take their medications prior to the test.

2 Ask whether the participant has previously completed this test and, if so, whether they have a copy of the results for standardisation of testing procedures. It would be beneficial to obtain the past results as this may influence the details provided to ensure that the participant understands the requirements of the test and the feedback can be modified accordingly. This would also allow comparisons between the results to determine whether there have been changes over time, rather than a cross-sectional comparison to the normative data.
3 The benefits, risks and discomforts of the test should be explained to the participant with sufficient time for them to consider their involvement in this test (i.e. at least 12 hours prior to testing).
4 For all tests involving exercise, maximal effort (e.g. pulmonary function), invasive procedures (e.g. blood collection) or potentially sensitive information (e.g. anthropometry), the participant should provide signed informed consent. This acknowledges that they are aware of the requirements, benefits, risks and discomforts of the test. A combined participant information and informed consent form (Box B.1) can be used for this purpose.
5 The participant should be risk stratified using the Adult Pre-exercise Screening System (APSS) (see Practical 6, Pre-exercise health screening) and assessed for contraindications to exercise (see Appendix C). In addition, determining the participant's health history through medical records (where appropriate) and/or interview will assist in determining whether the participant has any 'red flags' or contraindications prior to testing. This would allow for medical supervision to be organised, if required.
6 Ask the participant whether they have any questions.

Box B.1 Combined participant information and informed consent form

PARTICIPANT INFORMATION AND INFORMED CONSENT FORM
Measurement of lactate threshold
Purpose of the test
The sampling of blood (for the analysis of lactate) during progressive exercise to fatigue can allow researchers to identify a 'break-point', where a non-linear increase in blood lactate concentrations (relative to workload) occurs. This break-point has been termed the *lactate threshold* and is often used by sports scientists to determine whether there has been a change in aerobic fitness of an athlete in response to a training program.

Requirements
1 To make sure the test provides the most accurate values, it is requested that you adhere to the following instructions:

   a Avoid significant exertion or exercise on the day of testing.

   b Refrain from heavy meals, alcohol, caffeine and tobacco products for 3 hours prior to testing.

   c Arrive for testing in a euhydrated state.

   d Wear lightweight/loose clothing and appropriate footwear.

2 The test will require you to undergo/complete the following:

   a Measurement of body mass.

   b Exercise at increasing intensities until you are unable to continue exercising. This will take around 15 minutes.

3 While exercising you will provide around six small blood samples via finger or ear prick.

4 While exercising your heart rate and rating of perceived exertion will be monitored.

Possible risks or discomforts
During the exercise test you will be exercising at a very high intensity. When people exercise at this level, the risk of a cardiac event (e.g. heart attack or stroke) increases. However, this increased risk is very low (1 in 15,000). Exercising at a high intensity may also lead to feeling unwell or dizzy. Every effort will be made to minimise these occurrences. First aid, emergency equipment and trained personnel are available to deal with these situations if they arise. A small amount of pain is associated with the finger/ear prick and as with any breach of the skin, there is a very minor risk of infection. Sterile equipment and occupational health and safety procedures will be used to minimise these risks. Any personal information collected will be kept strictly confidential.

Expected benefits from testing
This test allows the determination of your lactate threshold, which is a strong predictor of performance in endurance activities. This may assist in understanding the effects of your recent training and/or be used for future comparisons.

Stopping the test
You are free to stop the test at any point, if you so desire.

I have read this information sheet carefully and fully understand the test procedures that I will perform and their risks and discomforts.

I have had the opportunity to ask questions and they have been answered to my satisfaction.

Box B.1 Combined participant information and informed consent form *(continued)*

I confirm that I am physically and mentally capable of undertaking the activities in which I will involve myself.

I consent to participate in this test.

| Participant's name | Signature | Date |

| Witness, parent or guardian name | Signature | Date |

ON THE DAY OF TESTING BEFORE THE PARTICIPANT ARRIVES

1 Have all data collection forms ready for completion.
2 Collect and arrange all equipment to optimise efficiency and accuracy during the test.
3 If comparing with previous or future tests, standardise environmental conditions.

ON THE DAY OF TESTING WHEN THE PARTICIPANT ARRIVES

1 Orientate the client by first explaining the procedures and purpose of the test.
2 Reiterate the benefits, risks and discomforts of the test.
3 Ask the participant whether they have any questions.
4 Request the participant to provide signed informed consent.
5 Check that pre-test instructions have been followed. Where the pre-test instructions have not been followed, the tester should use their clinical judgment to determine how much this may influence the accuracy and validity of the results. The tester will then need to decide whether to conduct the test, whether there is a way to reduce the impact of the pre-test deviation on the test result, or whether to reschedule testing for another day.

Assessment of hydration status

There are many tests contained within this manual that can be influenced by hydration status. If a participant is dehydrated, this could reduce the validity of the test (e.g. percentage body fat via bioelectrical impedance analysis), decrease the cognitive capacity of the participant to complete the test (e.g. functional measures) or increase the physiological strain of the participant during the test (e.g. during extended endurance tests such as the lactate threshold test). Therefore, it is often important to determine whether a participant is dehydrated before starting an exercise test so as to optimise safety and validity.

Hydration status can be assessed using a variety of different techniques. Several methods rely on the collection of body fluids such as urine (e.g. urine output, urine specific gravity, urine osmolality and urine colour), blood (e.g. plasma osmolarity and plasma volume), saliva (e.g. saliva osmolality and total protein), tears (e.g. tear osmolarity), or any bodily fluid (e.g. isotope dilution).[1,2] Other measures of hydration require devices (e.g. bioelectrical impedance), self-report (e.g. morning thirst perception)[3] or rely on changes over time (e.g. change in body mass). The decision of which measure of hydration status to use is often limited by the resources, cost, safety, acceptability, time and expertise required to conduct and analyse the results. As many experts argue that there is no 'gold-standard' technique and one can never be achieved, the tester should consider the sensitivity and accuracy with which hydration status needs to be measured, together with the cost, technical and time requirements involved.

Where a one-off measure to differentiate dehydration from euhydration is required, collection of a participant's first urination of the morning for analysis via urine specific gravity or urine osmolality has been suggested to be sufficiently simple, inexpensive and sensitive to be used as a sole source of hydration assessment.[4,5] Where a more accurate determination of hydration status is required, multiple tests of hydration status using different techniques is recommended (e.g. total body water via isotope dilution, plasma osmolality and urine specific gravity). This is because they reflect different types of dehydration.

For example, urine can be more sensitive to acute changes in fluid status so may be more appropriate for athletes who frequently experience acute post-exercise dehydration.[6] In contrast, blood markers can be more suitable to identify more chronic levels of dehydration.

Stretching

Depending on the test and the participant, it may be recommended to include some stretching exercises between the aerobic warm-up and exercise test. For most flexibility tests, it is recommended that adequate stretches be included for the areas being tested to ensure the participant is achieving a maximum ROM during testing. Participants completing maximal tests or neuromuscular strength, power and strength endurance tests may prefer to stretch prior to completing the test. However, evidence for the effects of static stretching on safety (injury during the test) and exercise performance are controversial.[7] Furthermore, whilst stretching is generally safe for most individuals, there are certain populations where stretching may be considered a relative contraindication (see Box C.1).[8]

References

[1] Oppliger RA, Bartok C. Hydration testing of athletes. Sports Med 2002;32:959–71.

[2] Armstrong LE. Assessing hydration status: the elusive gold standard. J Am Coll Nutr 2007;26:575S–84S.

[3] Armstrong LE, Ganio MS, Klau JF, Johnson EC, Casa DJ, Maresh CM. Novel hydration assessment techniques employing thirst and a water intake challenge in healthy men. Appl Physiol Nutr Metab 2014;39:138–44.

[4] Cheuvront SN, Sawka MN. Hydration assessment of athletes. Bradenton, FL: Gatorade Sports Science Institute; 2006. https://www.gssiweb.org/sports-science-exchange/article/sse-97-hydration-assessment-of-athletes.

[5] Baron S, Courbebaisse M, Lepicard EM, Friedlander G. Assessment of hydration status in a large population. Br J Nutr 2015;113:147–58.

[6] Bak A, Tsiami A, Greene C. Methods of assessment of hydration status and their usefulness in detecting dehydration in the elderly. Curr Res Nutr Food Sci 2017;5:2.

[7] Simic L, Sarabon N, Markovic G. Does pre-exercise static stretching inhibit maximal muscular performance? A meta-analytical review. Scand J Med Sci Sports 2013;23:131–48.

[8] Imagama S, Hasegawa Y, Wakao N, Hirano K, Muramoto A, Ishiguro N. Impact of spinal alignment and back muscle strength on shoulder range of motion in middle-aged and elderly people in a prospective cohort study. Eur Spine J. 2014;23:1414–19.

APPENDIX C
CONTRAINDICATIONS TO EXERCISE TESTING

It is not always appropriate to conduct exercise tests, even if they are submaximal. It is important to compare the benefits gained from the test with the risks to make this decision. Box C.1 provides absolute and relative contraindications to exercise testing that will assist in decision making.

Absolute and relative contraindications to exercise testing balance the risk of the test with the potential benefit of the information derived from the test. Assessment of this balance requires knowledge of the purpose of the test for the participant and what symptom or sign end points will be for the individual test.

Performing a pre-exercise screening and careful review of a participant's medical history will help identify potential contraindications.

Box C.1 Contraindications to exercise testing

ABSOLUTE CONTRAINDICATIONS
- Acute myocardial infarction (MI), within 2 days
- Ongoing unstable angina
- Uncontrolled cardiac arrhythmia with haemodynamic compromise
- Active endocarditis
- Symptomatic severe aortic stenosis
- Decompensated heart failure
- Acute pulmonary embolism, pulmonary infarction or deep vein thrombosis
- Acute myocarditis or pericarditis
- Acute aortic dissection
- Physical disability that precludes safe and adequate testing

RELATIVE CONTRAINDICATIONS
- Known obstructive left main coronary artery stenosis
- Moderate-to-severe aortic stenosis with uncertain relation to symptoms
- Tachyarrhythmia with uncontrolled ventricular rates
- Acquired advanced or complete heart block
- Hypertrophic obstructive cardiomyopathy with severe resting gradient
- Recent stroke or transient ischaemic attack
- Mental impairment with limited ability to cooperate
- Resting hypertension with systolic or diastolic blood pressures >200/110 mmHg
- Uncorrected medical conditions, such as significant anaemia, important electrolyte imbalance and hyperthyroidism

Source: Exercise standards for testing and training: a scientific statement by the American Heart Association[1]

ABSOLUTE CONTRAINDICATIONS

An absolute contraindication is a reason or criterion that makes it inadvisable to conduct or continue the test. Undertaking or continuing the test could place the participant at a higher risk of an untoward event (e.g. injury or medical condition) occurring as a result of the test. Participants with absolute contraindications should not perform exercise tests until such conditions are stabilised or adequately treated.

RELATIVE CONTRAINDICATIONS

A relative contraindication is a reason or criterion that needs to be considered in deciding whether to conduct, modify or continue the test. Factors such as the risk versus benefit, qualifications, knowledge and experience of the tester and access to medical support may need to be considered. Participants with relative contraindications should not perform exercise tests until the risks and benefits are carefully assessed. In certain situations (e.g. the participant is having a diagnostic exercise stress test following a cardiac event), the condition may be the indication (and not a contraindication) for the test.

Reference

[1] Fletcher GF, Ades PA, Kligfield P, Arena R, Balady GJ, Bittner VA, et al; American Heart Association Exercise, Cardiac Rehabilitation, and Prevention Committee of the Council on Clinical Cardiology, Council on Nutrition, Physical Activity and Metabolism, Council on Cardiovascular and Stroke Nursing, and Council on Epidemiology and Prevention. Exercise standards for testing and training: a scientific statement from the American Heart Association. Circulation 2013;128: 873–934.

APPENDIX D
TREADMILL SAFETY

Treadmills are one of the most commonly used pieces of equipment for conducting aerobic exercise tests, and they are also one of the most dangerous. The following precautions will help to reduce the risk of injury when testing a participant on a treadmill.

TREADMILL LOCATION

The treadmill should be placed so that there is no possibility that a person who falls while on the treadmill could become trapped between the treadmill and something behind it (e.g. another piece of equipment). A minimum clearance of 0.5 m on each side of the treadmill and 2.0 m behind a treadmill is recommended.

SAFETY FEATURES

It is important that the tester operating the treadmill is aware of the safety features of the treadmill (e.g. safety stop button, tether with a key/magnetic clip). Instruct the participant on the safety features of the treadmill prior to starting the test and establish a non-verbal sign that the participant can use to tell the tester to stop the treadmill (e.g. one hand in the air making a stop sign).

TREADMILL OPERATION

Commonly used recreational treadmills now have multiple features. The tester should take the time to familiarise themselves with the different functions and understand the purpose of all the buttons. This includes whether the treadmill can be programmed and how quickly/slowly the treadmill changes speed/grade within a program or when buttons (e.g. stop button) are pressed.

Starting the treadmill
With the treadmill belt stationary, ask the participant to walk to the front of the treadmill, hold the handrail and straddle the belt. Ensure that no part of the participants' foot is in contact with the belt. Start the treadmill and increase its speed until it reaches a speed that will allow the participant to start walking comfortably. Ask the participant to continue holding the handrail and carefully step on the belt and start walking when they are ready. Once the participant has achieved a normal walking pace, ask them to safely remove their hands from the handrail.

Handrails
For all treadmill exercise tests it is important that the participant uses the handrails sparingly other than when starting and stopping the belt. For a person unaccustomed to walking on a treadmill, encourage the participant to practise walking on the treadmill prior to conducting the test. Cues such as 'stand up tall', 'step out in front of you' and 'take longer strides' may help to correct unnatural walking techniques. Participants learning how to walk on a treadmill should hold on to the handrails until their walking technique has normalised, but should then be encouraged to let go as soon as they feel comfortable. Older and/or frail individuals, people with poor balance, poor balance confidence or gait dysfunction may need to maintain some contact with the handrails during the test. In these situations, encourage the participant to touch the handrails as lightly as safely possible (e.g. just with their fingertips).

Eyes
Instruct the participant to keep their eyes looking forwards, especially if the person is veering off to the side. It is common for people who are unaccustomed to a treadmill to look at their feet while exercising.

Positioning
Instruct the participant to stay in the centre of the belt – both from left to right and from front to back. If the participant is too close to the front of the belt, their foot can catch on the motor cover and trip.

If too far down the belt the participant may come off the back of the treadmill. As the participant becomes fatigued, they will usually shift towards the back of the treadmill. The tester should gently place their arm on the participant's back if they are getting too close to the end of the treadmill, and ask them to try to move forwards.

Test completion

When the participant gives a verbal or non-verbal (e.g. one hand in the air making a stop sign) instruction to stop/slow the treadmill, the tester should tell the participant to grab the handrail with both hands whilst the tester presses the stop button or reduces the speed/grade of the treadmill. The type of test (e.g. maximal vs submaximal) will dictate how the treadmill is stopped or slowed down. For exhausted participants who look to be struggling to keep up with the belt on completion of a maximal test, the tester should place their own hand on top of one of the participant's hands with some pressure whilst hitting the stop button to ensure the participant remains holding the handrail until the treadmill comes to a complete stop. The participant may also press the stop button to stop/slow the treadmill. A participant should *never* step off a moving treadmill.

Exiting the treadmill

When the treadmill comes to a complete stop once the participant completes a test, they may feel dizzy or have 'jelly legs'. The tester should be in close proximity as the participant steps off the treadmill, ready to provide support if indicated.

APPENDIX E
BORG RATING OF PERCEIVED EXERTION (RPE) SCALE

INSTRUCTIONS

- Have the scale in full view at all times
- Make the participant aware of what RPE stands for and that this is an 'all-over' integrated rating which incorporates both peripheral muscular and central cardiorespiratory sensations.
- Focus the participant's attention on the verbal descriptors of the scale as much as on the numerical values.
- Anchor the top and bottom ratings to previously experienced sensations of 'no exertion at all' and 'extremely hard/maximal exertion'.
- Allow the participant to understand that there is no right or wrong rating; it represents how hard the participant felt they were working at the time of providing the rating.

RPE SCALE

6
7 VERY, VERY LIGHT
8
9 VERY LIGHT
10
11 FAIRLY LIGHT
12
13 SOMEWHAT HARD
14
15 HARD
16
17 VERY HARD
18
19 VERY, VERY HARD
20

APPENDIX F
INDICATIONS FOR STOPPING AN EXERCISE TEST

One of the main factors determining whether to stop an exercise test is whether the test is diagnostic or non-diagnostic.

A diagnostic exercise test is performed to diagnose a medical condition (e.g. coronary artery disease by an exercise stress test). Therefore, it is important that the cardiovascular system is adequately stressed to uncover any underlying pathology. For this reason a participant may be asked to continue exercising after relative indications to stop the test have occurred. Non-diagnostic tests include submaximal and maximal exercise tests where the main aim is to assess cardiorespiratory fitness and/or exercise capacity.

During all exercise tests, there is a need to always remain vigilant and monitor the participant closely. It is important to be well prepared to respond appropriately to adverse events. Box F.1 provides absolute and relative indications for stopping an exercise test.

Box F.1 Indications for stopping an exercise test

ABSOLUTE INDICATIONS

- ST-segment elevation (>1.0 mm) in leads without pre-existing Q waves because of prior MI (other than aVR, aVL and V1)
- Drop in systolic blood pressure >10 mmHg, despite an increase in workload, when accompanied by any other evidence of ischaemia
- Moderate-to-severe angina
- Central nervous system symptoms (e.g. ataxia, dizziness, near syncope)
- Signs of poor perfusion (cyanosis or pallor)
- Sustained ventricular tachycardia (VT) or other arrhythmia, including second- or third-degree atrioventricular (AV) block, that interferes with normal maintenance of cardiac output during exercise
- Technical difficulties in monitoring the ECG or systolic blood pressure
- The subject's request to stop

RELATIVE INDICATIONS

- Marked ST displacement (horizontal or downsloping of >2 mm, measured 60–80 ms after the J point (the end of the QRS complex)) in a patient with suspected ischaemia
- Drop in systolic blood pressure >10 mmHg (persistently below baseline) despite an increase in workload, in the absence of other evidence of ischaemia
- Increasing chest pain
- Fatigue, shortness of breath, wheezing, leg cramps or claudication
- Arrhythmias other than sustained VT, including multifocal ectopy, ventricular triplets, supraventricular tachycardia, and bradyarrhythmias that have the potential to become more complex or to interfere with haemodynamic stability
- Exaggerated hypertensive response (systolic blood pressure >250 mmHg or diastolic blood pressure >115 mmHg)
- Development of bundle branch block that cannot immediately be distinguished from VT

aVL = augmented voltage left, aVR = augmented voltage right, MI = myocardial infarction, V1 = chest lead 1
Source: Exercise standards for testing and training: a scientific statement by the American Heart Association[1]

Reference

[1] Fletcher GF, Ades PA, Kligfield P, Arena R, Balady GJ, Bittner VA, et al; American Heart Association Exercise, Cardiac Rehabilitation, and Prevention Committee of the Council on Clinical Cardiology, Council on Nutrition, Physical Activity and Metabolism, Council on Cardiovascular and Stroke Nursing, and Council on Epidemiology and Prevention. Exercise standards for testing and training: a scientific statement from the American Heart Association. Circulation 2013;128: 873–934.

APPENDIX G
INTERPRETATION, FEEDBACK AND DISCUSSION

INTRODUCTION

The ability of an exercise professional to follow a protocol that generates accurate, reliable and valid test results is usually only part of the overall task. In most situations the tester will be required to interpret the data and provide feedback to the participant. Furthermore, there should be an opportunity for the participant to discuss the feedback with the tester in the context of the practical and/or clinical implications. Interpretation, feedback and discussion of the test and test results are generally more challenging than conducting the test. Numerous additional factors may arise during these processes that may require the practitioner to think quickly to respond in an appropriate and timely manner. The following sections provide a number of steps to assist the tester in correctly interpreting the test results and providing quality feedback, and suggestions on how a discussion with the participant can be optimised. Most practicals contained within this manual include activities to practise these skills.

Participants usually expect to be provided with feedback immediately after a health and fitness test or testing session. This scenario of immediate verbal feedback will be used in the following discussion. It should be noted that there would also be situations where the tester will have more time to provide feedback to the participant in person and/or in a written form. For example, in many corporate health settings, different components of a health assessment may be conducted on separate occasions; the practitioner may then be required to collate all the data and provide both a written report and verbal feedback for the individual and the company.

DATA SHEET

In clinical research a great deal of emphasis is placed on the data sheet that contains the participant's information and test results. In research, the data sheet is called a *case report form* or *CRF* with guidelines on how they should be used.[1] With the advent of technology there has been greater use of electronic data collection forms, but most of the principles are still the same. To start with, it is vital that the data sheet is treated with the strictest of confidence. After it has been used to gather information on the participant, it should be filed in a locked cabinet or room. If stored on a computer, it should be password protected.

Other useful tips on completing the data form from the use of CRFs include:
- Always use a black or blue pen for data recording on the data sheet (not a red pen or pencil).
- Do *not* use any type of correction fluid (e.g. white-out). If a mistake is made, draw a single line through the incorrect entry, place the correct answer near the mistake, and initial and date the correction as shown below.

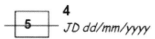

- Write down the value on the data sheet as soon as it has been collected (e.g. blood pressure during an exercise test). Relying on memory at the end of the test can be problematic.

INTERPRETATION

In this context, interpretation is referred to as the process of understanding the test results prior to providing feedback. In simple terms, interpretation is what is done before starting to talk to the participant or writing the report about the test results. The following steps should be used as a guide during this phase.

Step 1. Consider whether the test has provided meaningful results (i.e. should some or all of the test results be <u>accepted</u>)?

This will be based on issues such as:
- Was the protocol followed correctly?
- Does the data collected during the test appear accurate?
- When the data is compared with reference values, does it still appear accurate?

These questions will often need to be answered by the tester in a short space of time and this can place significant stress on less-experienced testers. At the end of this process the tester needs to decide whether the test, or part of the test, will be accepted and what specific feedback regarding the test results can be provided to the participant.

Step 2. How do the test results compare with reference values?

In Step 1 the reference values may have been looked at to decide whether the results are meaningful. In every situation it is essential that the reference data used for the comparison is appropriate for the individual being tested.

Finding appropriate reference data can often be difficult. In this manual, reference data tables for the described tests have been provided where possible. The majority of these data have been collected on individuals similar to the expected users of this manual (i.e. Australian men and women, 18–30 years of age). Where the reference data provided within this manual is not relevant, or is inappropriate to enable comparisons to the participant, the references provided at the end of the practical may be helpful to source additional reference data. If the plan is to provide immediate feedback to the participant then the appropriate reference tables should be sourced prior to testing and be available to make comparisons on completion of testing.

Step 3. Identify any health concerns (e.g. red flags)

In a number of testing situations, measures may be made that indicate poor health (e.g. high blood pressure). The term 'red flag' is used to describe a warning sign that suggests referral to a health professional may be warranted. In appropriate practicals, the criteria for red flags are provided.

Step 4. Prepare for the feedback

Where verbal feedback is to be provided to the participant, then a plan of what is going to be said and the order in which it will be delivered should have been decided at the end of the interpretation phase, before starting to discuss the feedback with the participant.

FEEDBACK

Feedback is defined as a process where information is provided (fed back) with the aim of modifying a future action or behaviour, if needed.[2] Important elements of feedback in the exercise and sport science context are: (1) establishing a positive working relationship with the participant and (2) ensuring the feedback is constructive. The definition of feedback is important as it separates the first component of explaining the test results with the second element of relating how the test result could be improved (if needed) or maintained and the clinical and/or practical implications. This section will deal primarily with verbal feedback and it is suggested to further divide this feedback regarding a test into three steps – **e**xplain the test; **s**tate the result/s; **c**an the results be maintained or improved? – which can be given the acronym *ESC*:

Step 1. Explain the test

Details about the test should have been explained to the participant prior to testing, however it is useful to re-state these when providing feedback. Why the participant is having the test conducted should have also been determined. This will help to provide feedback that is relevant to their circumstances. Where measures are being made as part of a fitness test, knowing what the participant's health/fitness goals are will help to contextualise the test explanation. For example, if providing feedback on blood pressure and the participant indicates their wish to '*improve their health*', you could to use the world 'health' when providing feedback on these values – that is, '*As part of the fitness test we measured your resting blood pressure as this is an important indicator of the overall health of your cardiovascular system.*'

During this step it may be appropriate to point out the accuracy, validity and limitations of the test. This may not need to be done in all situations. For example, when conducting a fitness test that has multiple components, it may not be necessary to explain the accuracy, validity and limitations of each test. If it is considered appropriate to discuss the limitations of a test, then it is important to avoid being too negative about the test. After all, the participant may have just completed some relatively hard exercise and they should not hear that the test might not be that accurate or valid. A good example is the submaximal test for estimating cardiorespiratory fitness. If the protocol is followed, and assumptions met, the test can provide valid VO_2max predictions. However, most practitioners have experienced situations where the test does not provide a meaningful value and sometimes indicate a lack of trust in the test when providing feedback. The following is an example of how you might start feedback on results from a submaximal cardiorespiratory fitness to improve a participant's perception of the usefulness of the test and the accuracy and validity of the data.

'You completed a submaximal fitness test which provides an estimate of your aerobic fitness. The test has some limitations but as we have closely followed the protocol we have an accurate result ...'

Step 2. State the result/s including qualitative wording

It is important that the tester provides the participant with their test result (e.g. value) and states how that compares with reference values. Following a test the participant may be provided with a lot of numbers. During a typical fitness test the person could be told that:

'Your resting heart rate is 72 bpm, blood pressure is 130 over 90 mmHg, BMI is 29 kg/m², body fat percentage is 27%, grip strength is 45 kg, flexibility is 12 cm and your estimated VO_2max is 32 mL/kg/min.'

Providing feedback in this manner would not be effective communication. The participant is unlikely to be able to take in and remember all these numbers. Therefore, it is vital that written feedback is also provided that contains these data. Where the reference data include a large range within a specific percentile category, it is suggested that the tester narrow the reference data range to within 10%. For example, if a 62-year-old female participant reached -7.5 cm on the back scratch test, then this would place them between the 25th percentile and the at-risk categories for loss of functional mobility, according to Table 9.4. However, a result near the 25th percentile would probably result in a very different action plan compared with a result near the 'at risk' category. Therefore, for the example above, the tester should quickly be able to calculate that the participant's back scratch result places them between the 15th and 25th percentile relative to their sex. More important (and more memorable) to the individual will be the qualitative words (e.g. categories such as 'above average') that should be used in addition to the numerical data.

This stage of the feedback is where any health implications of the data should be conveyed. For example, low cardiorespiratory (aerobic) fitness, overweight or obesity and low muscular strength all have important health implications. If any test results are a 'red flag', a discussion regarding referral to the appropriate health professional (usually the participant's general practitioner) should occur. However, as explored further in the next step, care needs to be taken to maintain a constructive environment during this part of the feedback process.

Step 3. Can the results be maintained or improved?

This is generally the hardest part of the feedback stages. Can the test result/s be improved? Does the participant want/need improvement/s? A good understanding of exercise and sport science should help in answering the first question; understanding the reason why the person is having the test conducted will help answer the second.

It may be useful to suggest monitoring of any areas of concern with follow-up testing planned for set times in the future. However, it is essential to know what the expected time frames are for changing exercise test parameters (e.g. how long would it take to lose a certain amount of fat/body mass/waist circumference?).

This stage of feedback can also allow an opportunity to reflect on the constructive aspects of the process. Undergoing exercise and health tests can often be a very negative experience for the participant. For some individuals, explaining that their health or fitness is in a poor state may be what is needed to encourage them to start changing their behaviour. However, psychology research has shown that creating a constructive, supportive environment is more likely to be beneficial for behaviour change in the majority of people.[3] This doesn't mean that poor test results should not be conveyed to the participant. The goal is to do it in such a way that promotes a constructive feel about the whole process – for example:

'Your body fat percentage and BMI places you in the obese category and your aerobic fitness is very low for someone of your age and sex. We know that being unfit and overweight increases your risk of diseases such as heart disease and diabetes. It is great that we now know what these values are because I can write you an individualised program that will improve your fitness and assist you to reduce your body mass. We can also re-measure these values in a few months to see how much you are improving.'

Effective communication

Effective communication between a practitioner and participant improves outcomes.[4] Throughout a test it is important to communicate to the participant using words and phrases they can understand.

Assessing a person's level of understanding is best done by asking open-ended questions at the start of the test (i.e. questions starting with how, what or why) – for example, '*What do you know about the tests you are doing today?*'

A question similar to this should generate a response, leading to a discussion which will enable identification of the participant's literacy and health literacy levels (i.e. the ability to read, understand and use healthcare information to make decisions and follow instructions for treatment). This information will enable the use of terminology and explanations during the session that are appropriate to the participant. These questions should also include an assessment of whether the participant has any anxiety about the tests. If this becomes apparent then every effort should be made to lessen these feelings.

To improve communication, a useful skill is *active listening*. It is a structured way of listening and responding to others that improves mutual understanding.[5] It requires the tester to feed back what they hear to the participant. This can be done by re-stating or paraphrasing what they have heard in their own words – for example, '*So, what I am hearing is that you would like to improve your upper body strength?*'

Other important considerations

- Establish a physical environment that promotes good communication (e.g. private, opportunity to both sit down).
- Do not allow external factors to distract attention from the participant.
- Make appropriate eye contact early in the session.
- Be aware of attempts to minimise problems arising from differences in language and culture.
- Seek to understand the participant's expectations from the session.
- If the participant has hearing and/or cognitive impairments, ensure instructions are explained slowly, clearly and at a volume that provides the participant with the best chance of understanding the directions and questions.
- Be sensitive and/or empathetic if the participant is sharing medical information. This is expanded on in the following section 'Addressing distress'.
- A participant who is having a number of tests at the same time (e.g. fitness test) may feel overwhelmed by all the information. Providing some of the feedback in writing may help in this situation.
- Try not to speak in a condescending tone or overly simplify what is being said too much.
- Provide continuous opportunities for questions.

Being clear and concise, without using complicated medical or scientific terminology, is the best approach to effective communication in most situations.

Addressing distress

As practitioners you may interact with people who are distressed. Distress can manifest as:

- impatience
- anger
- tearfulness
- feeling down/depressed
- feeling fearful/anxious
- hypervigilance/increased startle response
- lack of reactivity – 'flat' affect
- decreased motivation
- increased fatigue
- poor concentration/short term memory deficits.

You should aim to make every interaction with a participant as positive as possible. Be aware of your own reactions and aim to stay calm and respond in a manner that is caring and respectful. It is important not to misrepresent your role – your job is not to make the person feel better, but simply to respond in a way that is respectful, calm and concerned and provides them with an opportunity to link to support. A useful acronym to remember in these situations is LARK (listen, acknowledge, reassure and know):

Listen: the single most impactful communication technique. Show genuine interest/care in your body language and tone of voice (stopping what you are doing, turning towards and focusing on the person, embody a sense of calm and compassion in your tone of voice).

Acknowledge: let them know you hear what they are saying by reflecting back what you hear/observe and especially the emotion behind what they are saying. Help the person to feel understood, that you appreciate their situation is difficult, for example:

'*That sounds really frustrating for you.*'
'*That is really tough / difficult / stressful.*'

'You're dealing with a lot.'
'Things are really difficult for you at the moment.'

Reassure: in your response let them know it is normal to be feeling overwhelmed at times. It is important to let them know that – although it is not your role – you can put them in touch with someone who can help them. For example:

'It's OK to feel like this.'
'It's common for people to feel overwhelmed at times during their cancer journey.'
'You don't have to do this alone – I know services that can help.'
'There are people who can help you with that.'
'I can direct you to support services.'

Know: know what services you can link to and provide details/offer to connect: Lifeline provides 24-hour telephone support for people experiencing a personal crisis and suicide prevention services.

Helpful hint: If the person starts to talk in depth about reasons behind their distress, it is OK (and often appropriate) to politely interrupt and advise that you will link the person to someone who is better able to assist. By letting the person go into details about their concerns, you are giving the impression that you are the person who is best placed to assist, for example: *'It sounds like you are going through a really hard time. Although I am not trained to help, I know there is specialist support here in Brisbane and I can provide you with details of the service if you would like.'*

Manage your own responses

It is common for us with our own backgrounds and personalities – when faced with other people's strong emotions – to sometimes feel overwhelmed. Be aware of what strong emotions you find difficult (e.g. anger, overwhelming sadness and anxiety). Know your automatic response (usually a way of avoiding your own discomfort) – for example, ignore, distract, be quick to reassure and tell them it will all get better, etc.

Each person is unique in the reasons behind their sadness/anxiety/anger. If you feel upset or uneasy after an encounter with a participant, make a deliberate effort to seek peer support. If you still feel uneasy or find that you are continuing to ruminate about that person and their situation, make a time to speak with your supervisor. Always notify a supervisor if a participant mentions suicide or self-harm.

DISCUSSION

When providing feedback, it is important to gain an understanding of the participant's thoughts, feelings and concerns and then respond to these empathetically. The participant should be encouraged to ask questions and discuss the test/test results throughout the whole process (see 'Effective communication' above). The tester should make a statement at the start of the session to encourage the participant to ask questions or make comments throughout to ensure they fully understand the results. In addition, it is important to allow time at the end of the session for the participant to ask any remaining questions about any of the results or regarding their health concerns.

Considering the range of tests that are conducted in exercise and sport science settings, the questions could cover a wide theoretical range. It is likely that some questions will fall outside of the tester's knowledge. In these situations it is vital that guesses are not made. If the guessed answer is incorrect, this can lead to the participant adopting a behaviour that is unnecessary or a belief that is wrong. The tester should state that *'I am sorry I don't know'* and, if possible, *'I will find out and get back to you with the answer.'* Examples where this is common is when a participant has a medical condition, or is taking a drug or supplement, and they question whether this has affected one of the test results. Unless the tester is certain of the answer, they should not guess. In these situations it may be suggested that the person discuss this with their general practitioner.

References

[1] Bellary S, Krishnankutty B, Latha MS. Basics of case report form designing in clinical research. Perspect Clin Res 2014;5:159–66.
[2] Thomas JD, Arnold RM. Giving feedback. J Palliat Med 2011;14:233–9.
[3] Sarkany D, Deitte L. Providing feedback: practical skills and strategies. Acad Radiol 2017;24:740–6.
[4] Riedl D, Schussler G. The influence of doctor–patient communication on health outcomes: a systematic review. Z Psychosom Med Psychother 2017;63:131–50.
[5] Papanikitas AN. Listening is key, but ask the right questions. BMJ 2017;358:j3515.

CASE STUDY ANSWERS

PRACTICAL 1 TEST ACCURACY, RELIABILITY AND VALIDITY

Case study 1

Was the room air or tank 1 calibration successful or unsuccessful? The readings after adjustment for the calibration of room air differed by 0.01% and 0.01% for the O_2 and CO_2 analysers respectively (absolute values). As these values are less than 0.03 (O_2) and 0.02 (CO_2) (absolute), the calibration was considered successful.

What action would you take based on the room air or tank 1 calibration? No action is required as the calibration was successful. Therefore, you should continue on to the gas tank calibration.

Was tank 2 calibration successful or unsuccessful? The readings after adjustment for the calibration of tank 2 differed by 0.01% and 0.0% for the O_2 and CO_2 analysers respectively (absolute values). As these values are less than 0.03 (O_2) and 0.02 (CO_2) (absolute), the calibration was considered successful.

What action would you take, based on tank 2 calibration? No action is required as the calibration was successful. Therefore, you should continue on to the flow/volume calibration.

Was the flow/volume rate calibration successful or unsuccessful? The reading after adjustment for the calibration of the flow/volume rate was 0.009 L = 0.3% (relative). As this is <1%, the calibration was considered successful.

What action would you take, based on the flow/volume rate calibration? No action is required as the calibration was successful.

Was the O_2 and/or CO_2 analyser drift from pre- to post-exercise acceptable? The drift from pre- to post-test in the O_2 and CO_2 analysers were 0% and 0.12% respectively (absolute values). The O_2 analyser drift was acceptable; however, the CO_2 analyser drift was unacceptable (i.e. $\geq$0.1% absolute drift).

What action would you take, based on the O_2 and/or CO_2 analyser drift from pre- to post-exercise? As the CO_2 analyser drift was unacceptable, the respiratory exchange ratio (RER) will be invalid. Therefore, the RER and $\dot{V}CO_2$ should not be reported or used for the calculation of training prescription/intensity zones. As the participant's coach requested the test to inform subsequent training prescription, you should request that the athlete return to the laboratory on a later date to repeat the test. To identify why the drift occurred, check that all connections are tightly sealed and the tubing and inspired air line is intact. If no issues are clearly visible, report the issue to the lab technician and/or contact the manufacturer for advice and potential servicing. Make a comment within the database where the test data are stored to indicate any issues and actions taken. Before scheduling the repeat test with the athlete, conduct a further set of calibrations to determine whether this was a one-off issue or if there is an underlying cause that needs to be addressed.

Case study 2
Treadmill speed measurements

Tape #1 to #2 = 1.1 m
Tape #2 to #3 = 0.9 m
Tape #3 to #1 = 0.5 m
Total treadmill belt length (sum of the 3 distances above) = *2.5 m*

	With participant walking/running on treadmill	
	5 km/h	**15 km/h**
Treadmill speed	30 revs/46 s	30 revs/16 s
Treadmill speed	*0.65* revs/s	*1.88* revs/s
Revolutions per min	*39.1* revs/min	*112.5* revs/min
Distance covered in 1 min	*97.8* m/min	*281.3* m/min
		continued overpage

	With participant walking/running on treadmill	
	5 km/h	**15 km/h**
Treadmill speed	_0.0978_ km/min	_0.2813_ km/min
Treadmill speed	_5.9_ km/h	_16.9_ km/h
% error between displayed and real speed	_15.3_ %	_11.2_ %

Speed percentage error at 5 km/h acceptable? _NO_
Speed percentage error at 15 km/h acceptable? _NO_
Therefore, a calibration curve and equation of the line for speed are required for this treadmill.

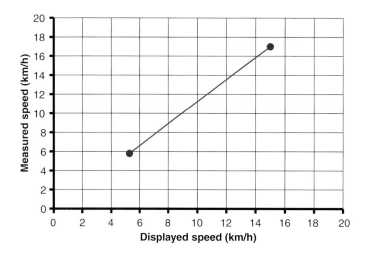

The equation of the line using $y = mx + c$
where $x1 = $ _5.0_; $y1 = $ _5.9_; $x2 = $ _15.0_; $y2 = $ _16.9_
$$m = (y2 - y1) / (x2 - x1)$$
$$m = (16.9 - 5.9) / 15.0 - 5.0)$$
$$= 1.1$$
Then substituting one of the points' coordinates for y (e.g. $y1 = 5.9$) and x (e.g. $x1 = 5.0$) in the problem:
$$5.9 = 1.1 \times 5.0 + c$$
$$5.9 = 5.5 + c$$
$$c = 0.4$$
Therefore, the equation of the line is $y = $ _1.1x + 0.4_.

Treadmill grade measurements

		5%	**15%**
If using a 1 m long spirit level			
Distance between treadmill and bottom end of the spirit level		5.0 cm	14.9 cm
Treadmill grade		_5.0_%	_14.9_%
% error between displayed and real grade		_0_%	_0.7_%

Grade percentage error at 5% acceptable?   _YES_
Grade percentage error at 15% acceptable?   _YES_
Therefore, a calibration curve and equation of the line for % grade is not required for this treadmill.

Interpretation

Compared with the predetermined criteria of $<1\%$, the treadmill speed was deemed unacceptable, particularly at the lower speeds. In contrast, the treadmill grade was deemed acceptable. You decide to repeat the treadmill speed verification to confirm the results. If the percentage error results remain unacceptable, you should discuss the following action options with your supervisor:

- Determine whether there is another treadmill available and, if so, complete treadmill speed and grade verification on it to determine whether its percentage error is acceptable, and use this treadmill instead.
- Determine whether it is feasible, with consideration of the time, warranty period and subsequent costs, to send the treadmill back to the manufacturer for calibration.
- If another treadmill is not available, and it is not feasible to have the treadmill calibrated, repeat the treadmill speed verification at additional speeds (i.e. 5.0, 7.5, 10.0, 12.5, 15.0 km/h) to create another calibration curve. This curve should have greater accuracy because of the increased number of data points than the two-point calibration curve above. In this case, use the calibration curve to adjust the displayed speed to the actual speed for each participant.

PRACTICAL 2 BLOOD ANALYSIS

Case study 1

Variable	Value	Appropriate value or range	Classification (e.g. 'low')
Haematocrit (%)	42	Normal $= 40 - 52$	Normal
Haemoglobin (g/dL)	13.6	Normal $= 13.0 - 18.0$	Normal
Glucose (mmol/L)	6.7	Normal $= 3.0 - 5.4$	Impaired fasting glucose
Total cholesterol (mmol/L)	4.52	Desirable $= <5.17$	Desirable
HDL cholesterol (mmol/L)	1.34	High $= \geq 1.55$	Less than high
Triglycerides (mmol/L)	2.15	Normal $= <1.69$	Borderline high
LDL cholesterol (mmol/L)	2.75	Optimal $= <2.58$	Near optimal

Interpretation

Two of these values (glucose and triglycerides) are outside of the normal ranges (red flags). The other values are normal/desirable/near optimal.

Discussion and feedback

First, determine whether the employee has seen his doctor recently and whether he has had any of these values measured previously. Also, confirm when he last consumed food/drinks. If he indicates that there have been no previous reports of abnormal blood values, the main goal will be to provide feedback that leads to him seeing a doctor, especially regarding the blood glucose value. This feedback should contain the mandatory statements informing the person that these measures are for screening purposes only and are not diagnostic. Positive messages can be conveyed regarding the values that are appropriate, and this could stimulate a discussion around healthy eating and exercise to educate the employee about the impact that these lifestyle factors have on these values and the diseases they are measured to detect. Then the importance of the abnormal blood glucose value should be stated. Feedback mentioning diseases and conditions associated with high blood glucose such as kidney disease and blindness is appropriate. The word 'diabetes' can be used and it may be helpful to show where on the reference chart his value (if validated) places him. The elevated triglyceride value should also be stated with an explanation of why this is a concern by mentioning heart disease and stroke. It should be pointed out that the LDL cholesterol is just slightly above optimal. In summary, in this situation there must be appropriate health messages to attempt to stimulate action to seek a medical follow-up. There should be important messages regarding the benefits that regular exercise and good nutrition will have on lowering these values.

Case study 2

Variable	Value	Appropriate value or range	Classification (e.g. 'low')
Haematocrit (%)	34	Normal = 36−48	Low
Haemoglobin (g/dL)	11.1	Normal = 11.5−16.5	Low
Glucose (mmol/L)	4.5	Normal = 3.0−5.4	Normal
Total cholesterol (mmol/L)	3.56	Desirable = <5.17	Desirable
HDL cholesterol (mmol/L)	1.62	High = ≥1.55	High
Triglycerides (mmol/L)	1.45	Normal = <1.69	Normal
LDL cholesterol (mmol/L)	2.14	Optimal = <2.58	Optimal

Interpretation

Two of these values (haematocrit and haemoglobin) are outside of the normal ranges (red flags). The other values are normal/desirable/optimal/high (HDL cholesterol).

Discussion and feedback

First, determine whether the employee has seen her doctor recently and whether she has had any of these values measured previously. Also, confirm when she last consumed food/drinks. If she indicates that there have been no previous reports of abnormal blood values, the main goal will be to provide feedback that results in her seeing a doctor about the measures. This feedback should contain the mandatory statements informing the person that these measures are for screening purposes only and are not diagnostic. Positive messages can be conveyed regarding the blood lipids (especially the HDL cholesterol) and glucose results and this could stimulate a discussion around healthy eating and exercise to educate the employee about the impact that these lifestyle factors have on these values and the diseases they are measured to detect. The low haematocrit and haemoglobin values could lead to questions assessing whether she has been unusually tired or lethargic recently and factors that influence these values. In summary, in this situation there must be appropriate health messages to attempt to stimulate action to seek a medical follow-up.

PRACTICAL 3 CARDIOVASCULAR HEALTH

Case study 1
What questions would you ask Kelly and what feedback would you provide?

The heart rate is normal, SBP is in the high-normal category and DBP is in the grade 1 mild hypertension category. Therefore, using the higher category, her blood pressure is categorised as mild hypertension. You would first provide the values and say that the heart rate is normal and the blood pressure is in the mild hypertension category. It would be appropriate to show the blood pressure categorisation table and how the diastolic pressure of 92 mmHg is the reason for the mild hypertension category. You would then acknowledge her answer to the blood pressure question in the APSS but check that this is correct (ask again: has she ever been told that she has high blood pressure?). You need to inform Kelly that this single measure in this range is not a diagnosis of high blood pressure and that this can only be made by a doctor and you would wait until two separate readings in this category would prompt seeking medical follow-up. Mentioning the common occurrence of white coat hypertension should be included along with education that high blood pressure is a risk factor for CVD. Finally, you should suggest that you could take the measure again when she is next at the centre.

Case study 2
What questions would you ask Michael and what feedback would you provide?

The heart rate is normal, SBP is in the grade 1 mild hypertension category and DBP is in the grade 2 moderate hypertension category. Therefore, using the higher category, his blood pressure is categorised as moderate hypertension. Your feedback and questioning would be similar to case study 1, but with the recommendation rather than a suggestion that Michael sees his doctor about his blood pressure. You write a letter to the doctor providing details on the measures and ask Michael to let you know the outcome.

Case study 3
What questions would you ask Emma and what feedback would you provide?

The heart rate is low and based on the systolic value being less than 90 mmHg, the blood pressure could be defined as low (although low blood pressure is not a category in the guidelines). You would first provide the values and say that they are both low. At this point it would be good to reassure that low blood pressure generally does not indicate a problem and ask whether Emma gets lightheaded or dizzy, perhaps when getting up quickly. You should check to see whether Emma has been told previously that she has low blood pressure. If there appears to be no corresponding manifestations of the low blood pressure then you can reassure Emma that having low blood pressure without any symptoms should be nothing to worry about. For feedback on the heart rate, you should wait for completion of the cardiorespiratory fitness test to see whether the likely explanation for the low heart rate is due to a good aerobic capacity.

Case study 4
What questions would you ask Sandie and what feedback would you provide?

This equates to a 25%–29% (high) risk of CVD in the next 5 years. Stopping smoking would decrease Sandie's risk to between 16% and 19%. Lowering blood pressure and cholesterol levels could further decrease the risk to 5%–9%, which is a low risk. A discussion of these modifiable risk factors would be appropriate in this context with questions regarding her lifestyle. This would focus on exercise, diet and adherence to medications that Sandie may be taking for her blood pressure, cholesterol and diabetes.

PRACTICAL 4 PHYSIQUE ASSESSMENT

Case study 1

After 3 months of training, Matthew's body mass decreased 1.4 kg and his sum of 7 skinfolds decreased by 12 mm. According to Table 4.6, a reduction in body mass combined with a reduction in skinfold thickness suggests a certain amount of fat loss, with a potential loss of lean mass. It is not possible to determine with certainty whether lean mass was lost, without conducting a more comprehensive assessment of body composition such as DXA or BOD POD, which will differentiate between the two types of tissue.[1]

To increase power-to-weight ratio, you can suggest to the coach that, although challenging to achieve simultaneously, Matthew's body composition could be optimised through an increase in lean mass and/or a reduction in fat mass. The increased lean mass will provide the capacity to generate greater force and power during rowing and thus increase the power-to-weight ratio. You can inform the coach that, if there is a reduction in fat mass and increase in lean mass, the skinfold thickness should reduce during this period, but the body mass may remain stable owing to the shift between lean and fat mass proportions. Body composition will continue to be monitored over time, to allow the sport science and medicine team to further refine training and/or diet, so as to get the athlete closer to their body composition goal.

Optimising an athlete's body composition will require the input of other relevant professionals in your team, namely the strength and conditioning coach and the sports dietitian. The strength and conditioning coach would work with the rowing coach to develop a strength-training program that focuses on enhancing strength in part by increasing muscle mass; the sports dietitian would be responsible for developing an eating plan for Matthew that supports muscle growth while remaining focused on optimising fuelling and recovery of training.

In an elite sport setting it is accepted practice to work in a multidisciplinary manner with other practitioners, where each practitioner provides services within their scope of practice. This will ensure that the athletes and coaches receive the expertise and knowledge from relevant professionals in each field to obtain the best outcomes.

Case study 2

According to Table 4.1, Marcus' BMI of 30.4 kg/m^2 classifies him as obese, his waist circumference places him at moderate risk and, when combined with BMI, he is placed at high risk for obesity-related diseases. Additionally, the WHR ratio also places Marcus in the high-risk category for obesity-related diseases (see Table 4.4).

When designing the exercise program for Marcus, it is important to consider his baseline physical activity levels and, if he is currently inactive, the potential physical restrictions that his body mass may place on his range of motion, his cardiovascular capacity, potential risk of joint pain and his moderate risk of an adverse event (refer to Practical 6 for risk stratification). Therefore, it would be advised to ensure SMART goals with Marcus that are progressive in nature and begin at an appropriate intensity and duration, taking into consideration his preferred activities to enhance exercise adherence.

Case study 3

You would start by first checking with Jerry to confirm what he did in the lead-up to each test to ensure that that he followed all pre-testing procedures. Given the potential for body composition to be influenced by diet, hydration, clothing etc., data should be interpreted with caution if pre-testing procedures were not accurately followed. Once you are confident of the pre-testing conditions, ensure that you check the report and the website of where Jerry's scans were taken to determine whether inter- and/or intra-tester reliability values are available (see Practical 1, Test accuracy, reliability and validity). This will ensure that you are able to provide feedback on the validity of the data, and a meaningful explanation to Jerry, considering the four steps of interpretation and the three steps of feedback and discussion outlined in Appendix G.

Jerry's body mass was 99.2 kg according to the DXA scan, and 98.0 kg according to the BOD POD. His fat mass was 17.5 kg according to the DXA, which relative to his height placed him in the 14th percentile compared with age-matched control, meaning 86% of men his age have more fat mass than Jerry. In comparison, his fat mass from the BOD POD was 17.2 kg. Jerry's lean mass plus bone mineral content was 81.7 kg according to the DXA, which relative to his height placed him in the 91st percentile compared with age-matched control. In comparison, his fat-free mass from the BOD POD was 80.8 kg. For percentage body fat, Jerry's result according to the DXA was 17.7%, placing him in the 2nd percentile compared with age-matched control, meaning 98% of men his age have a greater percentage body fat than Jerry. In comparison, according to the BOD POD, Jerry's body fat was 17.5%, placing him in the 'moderately lean' body fat rating for men, meaning his fat levels are generally acceptable for good health.

Explain to Jerry that, although there were fairly similar results between the DXA and BOD POD results for fat mass, fat-free mass and % fat, longitudinal tracking of his progress over the next 6 months will be important for tracking changes in body composition. To help interpret longitudinal changes in body composition, appreciation of test–retest reliability or precision of measurement is necessary (see Practical 1, Test accuracy, reliability and validity). The International Society for Clinical Densitometry advocate this should be established across a minimum of 20 volunteers, and ideally performed on individuals with physique traits that are reflective of the population typically assessed.[2] Recent research has confirmed that, although an absolute estimate of body composition change is required, both DXA and BOD POD have similar precision error, far superior to BIA.[3] Although raw surface anthropometry data does not provide an absolute measure of body composition change, it has the best precision of all physique assessment techniques, and thus can be used on a more regular basis to help further personalise interventions for clients.[4]

References

[1] Slater GJ, Duthie GM, Pyne DB, Hopkins WG. Validation of a skinfold based index for tracking proportional changes in lean mass. Br J Sports Med 2006;40:208–13.

[2] Hangartner TN, Warner S, Braillon P, Jankowski L, Shepherd J. The official positions of the international society for clinical densitometry: acquisition of dual-energy x-ray absorptiometry body composition and considerations regarding analysis and repeatability of measures. J Clin Densitom 2013;16:520–36.

[3] Kerr A, Slater GJ, Byrne N. Impact of food and fluid intake on technical and biological measurement error in body composition assessment methods in athletes. Br J Nutr 2017;117:591–601.

[4] Orphanidou C, McCargar L, Birmingham CL, Mathieson J, Goldner E. Accuracy of subcutaneous fat measurement: Comparison of skinfold calipers, ultrasound, and computed tomography. J Am Diet Assoc 1994;94:855–8.

PRACTICAL 5 PHYSICAL ACTIVITY

Case study 1

CONTINUOUS SCORE

Vigorous: __4__ days per week (Q1) $\times$ __1 h__ time (Q2) = __240__ (min) $\times$ 8] = __1920__ MET-minutes/week

or from interviewer probe question = _____ (min) $\times$ 8) = _____ MET-minutes/week

Moderate: __3__ days per week (Q3) $\times$ __30 min__ time (Q4) = __90__ (min) $\times$ 4.4) = __396__ MET-minutes/week

or from interviewer probe question = _____ (min) $\times$ 4.4] = _____ MET-minutes/week

Walking: __3__ days per week (Q5) $\times$ __20 min__ time (Q6) = __60__ (min) $\times$ 3] = __180__ MET-minutes/week

or from interviewer probe question = _____ (min) $\times$ 3] = _____ MET-minutes/week

Total MET-minutes per week] = vigorous + moderate + walking = __2496__ MET-minutes/week

Participant meeting the 500 MET-minutes per week guideline? (circle): (YES)/NO

Categorical assessment (circle): (High)/ Moderate / Low

Interpretation

Based on his responses, Mohammed has a high level of physical activity and is completing more than double the MET-minutes per week guidelines.

Discussion and feedback

First determine the activities that are leading to Mohammed achieving the high levels of physical activity. This behaviour should be reinforced with positive feedback. He should be informed that doing *more* than the 500–1000 MET-minutes per week should lead to greater health benefits than those obtained from meeting the minimum physical activity guidelines.

Case study 2
Accuracy

1 Smartphone and app combination

$$\text{Percentage error} = 100 - \left[\frac{1178 \times 100\%}{1150} \right]$$

$$\text{Percentage error} = 2.4\%$$

2 Wearable device and app combination

$$\text{Percentage error} = 100 - \left[\frac{1162 \times 100\%}{1150} \right]$$

$$\text{Percentage error} = 1.0\%$$

Interpretation

The percentage error between the first approach (smartphone and app) and the real measure of step count is 2.4%, whereas the second approach (wearable device and app) is 1%. This indicates that the second approach is more accurate to measure step count. In a research setting, understanding the accuracy of these approaches would be useful when analysing data from them for a study.

Agreement between the two approaches

1 Steps

$$\text{Percentage difference} = \left[\frac{\text{largest measure} - \text{smallest measure}}{\text{smallest measure}} \right] \times 100$$

$$\text{Percentage difference} = \left[\frac{1178 - 1162}{1162} \right] \times 100$$

$$\text{Percentage difference} = 1.4\%$$

2 Distance

$$\text{Percentage difference} = \left[\frac{\text{largest measure} - \text{smallest measure}}{\text{smallest measure}} \right] \times 100$$

$$\text{Percentage difference} = \left[\frac{840 - 830}{830} \right] \times 100$$

$$\text{Percentage difference} = 1.2\%$$

3 Energy expenditure

$$\text{Percentage difference} = \left[\frac{\text{largest measure} - \text{smallest measure}}{\text{smallest measure}} \right] \times 100$$

$$\text{Percentage difference} = \left[\frac{282 - 206}{206} \right] \times 100$$

$$\text{Percentage difference} = 36.9\%$$

Interpretation

The agreement between the two approaches for measuring steps and distance is very good, and similar (1.4% and 1.2% respectively). The agreement for energy expenditure is very poor at 36.9%. This indicates that the two approaches should not be used together in the same research study to measure energy expenditure.

PRACTICAL 6 PRE-EXERCISE HEALTH SCREENING

Case study 1
Based on the 'yes' answer to question 2 in stage 1 of the APSS, you ask Rosa the following question:
'Would you please tell me more about the chest pains you have experienced during exercise?'

Rosa tells you that she gets pain in her chest and left shoulder when increasing her exercise intensity. Based on this information you need to ask Rosa to see her GP as soon as possible and before starting to exercise at your centre. You should write a letter to her GP outlining her exercise intentions and what she has told you regarding her chest pain, and request guidance from the doctor. She should not be permitted to exercise until guidance has been obtained from her GP.

Case study 2
You ask Jedda the following question:
'Would you please tell me more about the exercise that you are currently doing?'

Jedda tells you that he has been training with a personal trainer three times per week. He wears a heart rate monitor during the sessions and is completing 90 minutes of moderate-intensity and 30 minutes of vigorous-intensity exercise per week. Based on this detail, you confirm Jedda's weighted physical activity is 150 min/week. Based on this information and Figure 1 in the APSS (see Figure 6.1), he can continue with this exercise. His BMI of 30 places him in the obese category and his waist circumference confirms that this body mass is a cardiovascular disease risk factor. This information should assist with a discussion regarding weight loss being a goal of his exercise prescription.

Case study 3
You ask Maria the following question:
'Would you please tell me more about the exercise that you are currently doing?'

Maria tells you that she goes for two 30-minute walks per week with her husband. You wish to know more about the intensity she selected and ask her:
'Are you able to carry out a conversation with your husband when walking?'

She tells you she is able to talk easily when walking. Based on this information, Maria's weighted physical activity is 60 min/week. From Figure 1 in the APSS (see Figure 6.1) she can continue with her current low-intensity physical activity. She has three cardiovascular disease risk factors: family history, body composition (BMI of 32.0 kg/m^2 places her in the obese category, with her waist circumference confirming that this body mass is problematic) and high blood pressure. As a result of her risk factors, more care should be taken progressing her physical activity levels.

PRACTICAL 7 NEUROMUSCULAR STRENGTH, POWER AND STRENGTH ENDURANCE

Case study 1
The athlete's vertical jump, reactive strength and 3RM leg press performances placed her in the 'poor' categories. With these performance ratings, there is certainly scope for improvement for this basketball player.

From discussions regarding her current training habits, you discover that she places a high focus on skill maintenance and improvement, although she currently doesn't partake in any formal resistance training. Overall body strength and power are attributes of successful basketball players owing to the physicality of play and to reduce the instances of non-contact injuries. Successful play will demand a high level of lower body power development, for bursts of acceleration away from the opposition, and to aid jump performance for shooting. It is well documented that the capacity to express high levels of lower body power are related to overall muscular strength.[1] To work on improving lower body power, it would firstly be appropriate to consider further lower body strength testing to identify a training load that can then be incorporated into a resistance training regime to target the development of lower body strength.[2] The first priority of this athlete would be to increase lower body strength prior to targeting the development of power.[3] It is likely that increasing lower body strength, with exercises such as back squats, will result in improvements in performance in both the vertical jump and the reactive strength tests. As the athlete's strength increases, more focus can be placed on basketball-specific agility and plyometric drills, such as countermovement drop jumps incorporating rapid changes in direction. A periodised resistance program that integrates both strength and power development and exercises such as the back squat and power clean would be an effective strategy for increasing lower body strength.[3]

Case study 2
Although minimising muscle asymmetry between limbs should be considered important, it is not uncommon for deficits such as those the coach identified to exist. It is appropriate to identify those players with a greater degree of asymmetry, and consider incorporating targeted strength-training interventions to address these deficiencies to reduce knee injury risk.[4,5] For any athlete with greater than 2.2% asymmetry in the peak force and RFD achieved between the right and left leg during these

tests, ensure that you first contextualise the data.[4] It is not uncommon to see a greater asymmetry, especially in an athlete returning from a lower limb injury such as an anterior cruciate ligament injury. When an athlete is returning from injury, it is not uncommon for the peak force developed to increase more quickly than the RFD. When working with athletes who display these asymmetries, targeted strength-training interventions should be developed to first increase strength and then target the RFD. This can be done with specific unilateral training interventions, such as single-leg squats to target strength and unilateral plyometrics to target the development of explosive strength (e.g. RFD).

Case study 3

You choose the grip strength test as it has good prognostic validity, is safe, easy to administer and requires minimal equipment. Testing reveals the following results:

Dominant hand: *Best* = 12 kg   Non-dominant hand: *Best* = 10 kg

Rating: *Poor*

Interpretation

The client was assessed as having poor grip strength for a woman of her age.

Discussion and feedback

Provide the client with the grip strength measure and her corresponding rating relative to her age and sex. Focus on the positives, yet remain realistic, when providing feedback. Clarify that a poor performance on the grip strength test indicates insufficient muscle strength and future difficulty rising from the floor after sustaining a fall. Furthermore, the combination of poor strength and osteoporosis puts the client at an increased risk for sustaining a fracture (commonly at the hip, lumbar spine or wrist). Completing additional tests (such as balance and balance confidence tests described in Practical 15) will provide further clarification of the client's falls risk. Reassure her that her strength can be improved by targeted muscle strengthening exercises. Ask the client if she would prefer to exercise in the gym or with her husband at home and explain that you could design a home or gym program depending on her preference. Ask the client if she has any questions about the tests, her test result or the exercises.

References

[1] Haff GG, Nimphius S. Training principles for power. Strength Cond J 2012;34:2–12.
[2] Haff GG. Strength-isometric and dynamic testing. In: Comfort P, Jones PA, McMahon JJ, eds. Performance assessment in strength and conditioning. New York, NY: Routledge, Taylor Francis; 2019, p. 166–92.
[3] Haff GG. Periodization and power integration. In: McGuigan M, ed. Developing power. Champaign, IL: Human Kinetics; 2017, p. 33–62.
[4] Jordan MJ, Aagaard P, Herzog W. Lower limb asymmetry in mechanical muscle function: A comparison between ski racers with and without ACL reconstruction. Scand J Med Sci Sports 2015;25:e301–9.
[5] Jordan MJ, Aagaard P, Herzog W. Rapid hamstrings/quadriceps strength in ACL-reconstructed elite Alpine ski racers. Med Sci Sports Exerc 2015;47:109–19.

PRACTICAL 8 STATIC AND DYNAMIC POSTURE

None.

PRACTICAL 9 FLEXIBILITY

Case study 1
PRIORITY TEST 1

The Beighton Scoring System is suggested as one of the flexibility tests to prioritise in the testing battery owing to the observed hyperextension of the swimmer's knees and elbows.

Beighton test	Is the 18-year-old female swimming client able to:		Score
1	Place hands flat on the floor with straight legs	No	0
2	Hyperextend left knee (bending knee backwards >0° extension)	Yes	1
3	Hyperextend right knee (bending knee backwards >0° extension)	Yes	1
4	Hyperextend left elbow (bending elbow backwards >0° extension)	Yes	1

continued overpage

Beighton test	Is the 18-year-old female swimming client able to:		Score
5	Hyperextend right elbow (bending elbow backwards $>0°$ extension)	Yes	1
6	Touch the left thumb to the forearm	Yes	1
7	Touch the right thumb to the forearm	Yes	1
8	Bend left little finger backwards past 90°	No	0
9	Bend right little finger backwards past 90°	No	0

Data analysis

Sum of Beighton Scoring System test: 6/9

Interpretation

A score of 6/9 on the Beighton Scoring System indicates that the client is considered to have excessive ROM throughout the body, commonly known as hypermobility.[1]

Discussion and feedback

Provide the athlete with the individual scores on the Beighton Scoring System together with the total value, indicating that by scoring 'yes' on 6/9 tests she is considered to have hypermobility. It would be appropriate to highlight how common hypermobility is in elite athlete populations, particularly swimmers,[2] and that with individualised training and frequent ROM screening she will be better able to manage her career. You need to inform her that this is a generic hypermobility test and that more-specific ROM measures will need to be performed to allow safe prescription of flexibility exercises. General stretching would be a relative contraindication in this case and should be performed only when a specific joint ROM deficit has been detected. The team doctor and coach should also be notified.

PRIORITY TEST 2

Shoulder flexion was chosen as the second priority test owing to the diving issues identified by the coach, potentially indicating a reduction in shoulder flexion.

Data recording and analysis

Joint	Action	Rom (°)	Functional ROM (°)	'Normal' end feels	Recorded ROM (°)	Interpretation
Shoulder	Flexion	0–180	Eating: 35 Drinking: 45 Combing hair: 110	SL and LL: muscular	150	Seated shoulder flexion on inclinometer 150° bilaterally, muscular end feel (latissimus dorsi) Functional ROM activities should not be affected
LL = long lever; SL = short lever						

Interpretation

The client was assessed as having reduced shoulder flexion, with a seated shoulder flexion on inclinometer of 150° bilaterally. The end feel was muscular, specifically the latissimus dorsi. However, the shoulder flexion ROM was sufficient to enable functional ROM movements of eating, drinking and combing the hair.

Discussion and feedback

Provide the athlete with the shoulder flexion score together with the expected range, indicating that they have a ROM of 150°, which is a 30° reduction in shoulder flexion (normal 180°). It would be appropriate to highlight how shoulder flexion is important for swimming performance and for reducing shoulder pain,[3] and that with individualised training and frequent ROM screening she will be better able to manage her career. As the swimmer's shoulder flexion was limited by muscular end feel in the latissimus dorsi, stretching of this muscle is recommended. The team doctor and coach should also be notified.

Case study 2
PRIORITY TEST

The standard sit and reach test was chosen as it is an efficient, functional test that is similar to the movement of picking something up off the floor.

Objective data

Trial 1: − 18 cm	Trial 2: − 15 cm	Trial 3: − 14 cm
Best: − 14 cm	Best + 35 cm: 21 cm	Rating: poor

Subjective data

It was necessary to consistently remind the client to keep his knees straight (180°) as they kept bending (to approximately 160°) during the testing, causing the tests to be invalid and therefore needing to be re-administered to achieve three trials with correct technique. He reported tightness in his low back and thighs, but no pain.

Interpretation

A score of 21 cm on the standard sit and reach protocol indicates that the client is considered to have poor low back, gluteal, hip and/or hamstring flexibility (average = 29.9–39.6 cm).

Discussion and feedback

You would first provide the client with the individual scores on the standard sit and reach protocol and then the total value, indicating that with a best score of 21 cm he is considered to have poor ROM. It would be appropriate to highlight that, because of his results, his job, the recent commencement of his exercise program and the fact that flexibility decreases with age, he should incorporate stretches into his gym program. Due to the subjective information you observed during testing (consistent knee flexion) and the fact that tightness was reported in his low back and posterior thighs, you recommend a standing hamstring stretch and a four-point kneel lower back stretch in accordance with the American College of Sports Medicine guidelines.[4]

References

[1] Grahame R, Bird HA, Child A. The revised (Brighton 1998) criteria for the diagnosis of benign joint hypermobility syndrome (BJHS). J Rheumatol 2000;27:1777–9.

[2] Zemek MJ, Magee DJ. Comparison of glenohumeral joint laxity in elite and recreational swimmers. Clin J Sport Med 1996;6:40–7.

[3] Tate A, Turner GN, Knab SE, Jorgensen C, Strittmatter A, Michener LA. Risk factors associated with shoulder pain and disability across the lifespan of competitive swimmers. J Athl Train 2012;47:149–58.

[4] American College of Sports Medicine. ACSM's guidelines for exercise testing and prescription, 10th ed. Baltimore, MD: Lippincott, Williams and Wilkins; 2018.

PRACTICAL 10 $\dot{V}O_2$ MAX

Case study

Stage	Time (min: s)	Work Rate (watts)	$V_E{}^a$ (L/min)	F_EO_2 (fraction)	F_ECO_2 (fraction)	HR (bmp)	RPE (6–20)	Metabolic System $\dot{V}O_2$ (mL/ kg/min)	Calculated[b] $\dot{V}O_2$ (mL/ kg/min)
1	0:30	25	14.37	0.1598	0.0399			12.1	
	1:00		15.95	0.1587	0.0390	72	6	13.8	
2	1:30	50	22.12	0.1606	0.0397			18.3	
	2:00		21.36	0.1602	0.0395	90	6	17.9	
3	2:30	75	29.43	0.1723	0.0338			18.2	
	3:00		28.65	0.1609	0.0376	103	7	23.8	

continued overpage

Stage	Time (min: s)	Work Rate (watts)	$V_E{}^a$ (L/min)	F_EO_2 (fraction)	F_ECO_2 (fraction)	HR (bmp)	RPE (6–20)	Metabolic System $\dot{V}O_2$ (mL/ kg/min)	Calculated[b] $\dot{V}O_2$ (mL/ kg/min)
4	3:30	100	33.04	0.1631	0.0401			25.7	
	4:00		34.88	0.1637	0.0403	119	7	26.7	
5	4:30	125	35.28	0.1648	0.0399			26.3	
	5:00		37.91	0.1663	0.0409	131	9	27.0	
6	5:30	150	46.06	0.1670	0.0408			32.2	
	6:00		46.80	0.1687	0.0404	148	11	31.2	
7	6:30	175	54.11	0.1677	0.0416			37.0	
	7:00		58.94	0.1708	0.0401	163	13	36.9	
8	7:30	200	68.13	0.1715	0.0391			42.0	
	8:00		68.92	0.1729	0.0386	174	15	40.7	
9	8:30	225	78.44	0.1734	0.0381			45.6	
	9:00		86.07	0.1759	0.0371	185	17	46.1	

[a] Depending on the system and the position of the flow-measuring device (e.g. this will be V_E if the flow colume is collected on the expited side)
[b] Calculate $\dot{V}O_2$ manually for the last two completed 30-second intervals

Maximum heart rate = _185_ bpm
Maximum work rate = _225_ watts
Plateau criteria: <150 mL/min/body mass = <2.5 mL/kg/min
Circle: $\dot{V}O_2$max or (V̇O₂peak) = 45.9 mL/kg/min

For an endurance athlete the $\dot{V}O_2$max value is most useful to compare with values obtained from previous or future tests. For this athlete the injury has led to a very large loss in cardiorespiratory fitness and these values should be conveyed to the athlete and coach. The feedback should be provided with your knowledge that it is expected that once training resumes she should be able to eventually return to her previous fitness. The current relatively low value for this athlete would have implications for the coach in regards to the volume of training that should be prescribed and the speed of progression.

PRACTICAL 11 SUBMAXIMAL TESTING FOR CARDIORESPIRATORY FITNESS
Case study 1

$\dot{V}O_2$ at 2nd last work rate: $\underline{1.76} \times [\underline{125} \times \underline{6.12/80}] + 3.5 = \underline{20.3}$ mL/kg/min

$\dot{V}O_2$ at last work rate: $\underline{1.76} \times [[\underline{150} \times \underline{6.12/80}] + 3.5 = \underline{23.7}$ mL/kg/min

$$\text{Slope (m)} = \frac{(\dot{V}O_2 \text{ at last work rate} - \dot{V}O_2 \text{ at 2nd last work rate})}{(\text{final heart rate at last work rate} - \text{final heart rate 2nd last work rate})}$$

$$= \frac{23.7 - 20.3}{137 - 119}$$

$$= 0.189$$

Estimated $\dot{V}O_2$max (mL/kg/min) $= m(\text{HRmax} - \text{final heart rate at last work rate})$

$+ \dot{V}O_2$ at last work rate

$= 0.189 (192 - 137) + 23.7$

$= \underline{33.2}$ mL/kg/min

Percentile calculation: Step 1. *33.2 – 25.5 = 7.7* mL/kg/min
Step 2. *34.7 – 25.5 = 9.2* mL/kg/min
Step 3. *7.7/9.2 = 0.84*
Step 4. *25–5 = 20*
Step 5. $0.84 \times 20 = 16.8$
Step 6. $5 + 16.8 = 21.8$

Percentile: *22nd*   Rating: *Poor*

Discussion and feedback

The test has indicated Matthew has a poor level of cardiorespiratory fitness. The feedback should focus on this, presenting the associated health implications. Given that he is a medical student a more detailed discussion of the association between cardiorespiratory fitness and cardio-metabolic diseases would be appropriate. A discussion of how this value can be improved should include providing an understanding of how the eight-week exercise training program will improve his $\dot{V}O_2max$.

Case study 2

$\dot{V}O_2$ at 2nd last stage: $45.1 \times [0.17 + (0.10 \times 0.79)] + 3.5 = 14.7$ mL/kg/min

$\dot{V}O_2$ at last stage: $66.8 \times [0.17 + (0.12 \times 0.79)] + 3.5 = 21.2$ mL/kg/min

$$\text{Slope (m)} = \frac{\left(\dot{V}O_2 \text{ at last stage} - \dot{V}O_2 \text{ at 2nd last stage}\right)}{\left(\text{final heart rate at last stage} - \text{final heart rate at 2nd last stage}\right)}$$

$$= \frac{(21.2 - 14.7)}{(150 - 102)}$$

$$= 0.135$$

$$\text{Estimated } \dot{V}O_2max \text{ (mL/kg/min)} = m(HRmax - \text{final heart rate at last stage})$$

$$+ \dot{V}O_2 \text{ at last stage}$$

$$= 0.135 (178 - 150) + 21.2$$

$$= 25.0 \text{ mL/kg/min}$$

Percentile calculation: Step 1. *25 – 22.1 = 2.9* mL/kg/min
Step 2. *26.7 – 22.1 = 4.6* mL/kg/min
Step 3. 2.9/4.6 = 0.63
Step 4. *50 – 25 = 25*
Step 5. $0.63 \times 25 = 15.8$
Step 6. $25 + 15.8 = 40.8$

Percentile: *41st*   Rating: *Below average*

Case study 3

$\dot{V}O_2$ at stage 1 *17.3*
$\dot{V}O_2$ at stage 2 *21.9*
$\dot{V}O_2$ at stage 3 *26.5*
$\dot{V}O_2$ at stage 4 *31.0*

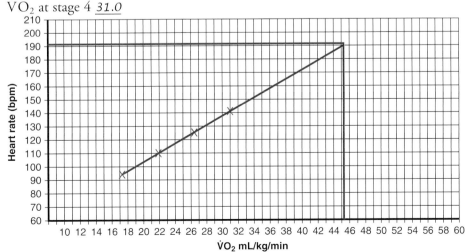

Estimated $\dot{V}O_2max$: *45* mL/kg/min

Given the proximity of the value to the 95th percentile (45.2 mL/kg/min) calculating the exact percentile would not be necessary.

Percentile: *95th*   Rating: *Superior*

PRACTICAL 12 LACTATE THRESHOLD

Case study

1 Maximum/peak work rate: $\underline{294}$ W Maximum/peak HR = $\underline{198}$ bpm

Analysis

2 Circle: (Valid) or Invalid $\dot{V}O_2$max/peak test
   Plateau criteria: < 150 mL/min/body mass = < $\underline{2.11}$ mL/kg/min
   Circle: ($\dot{V}O_2$max) or $\dot{V}O_2$peak = $\underline{62.82}$ mL/kg/min

3 Lactate and HR against work rate plot.

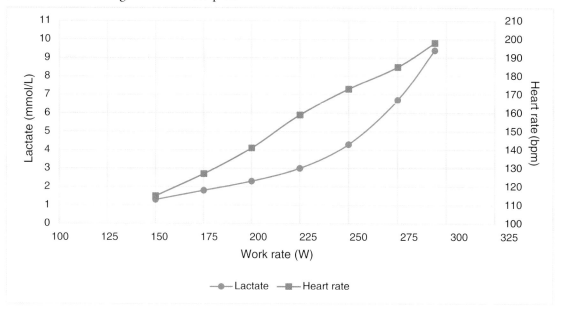

4 $\dot{V}O_2$ and HR against work rate plot.

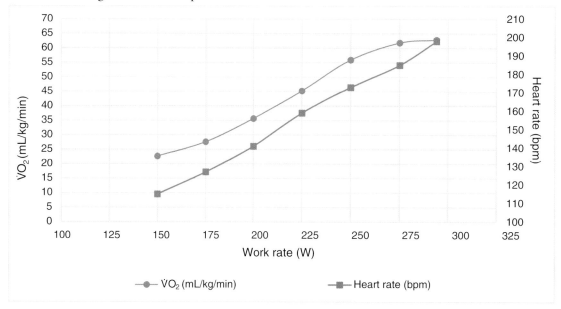

5 Record the HR, work rate and percentage $\dot{V}O_2$max for each lactate parameter.
   a 2 mmol/L: Work rate = $\underline{185}$ W $\dot{V}O_2$max = $\underline{49.3}$%   HR = $\underline{120}$ bpm
   b LT1 = $\underline{1.7}$ mmoL/L   Work rate = $\underline{165}$ W $\dot{V}O_2$max = $\underline{40.6}$%   HR = $\underline{115}$ bpm
   c LT2 = $\underline{2.3}$ mmoL/L   Work rate = $\underline{200}$ W $\dot{V}O_2$max = $\underline{56.7}$%   HR = $\underline{123}$ bpm
   d 4 mmol/L: Work rate = $\underline{245}$ W $\dot{V}O_2$max = $\underline{87.6}$%   HR = $\underline{140}$ bpm

6 Use peak HR to calculate the heart rates corresponding to the five 'aerobic' training zones described in Table 12.5.
   L1: $\underline{129}$ bpm   to $\underline{149}$ bpm
   L2: $\underline{149}$ bpm   to $\underline{158}$ bpm
   L3: $\underline{158}$ bpm   to $\underline{168}$ bpm
   L4: $\underline{168}$ bpm   to $\underline{182}$ bpm
   L5: $\underline{182}$ bpm   to $\underline{198}$ bpm

Discussion and feedback:

You would first give a brief explanation to the coach on the significance of the LT2 with respect to aerobic and anaerobic training. You can then explain the athlete's LT2 results to the coach, in particular, the $\dot{V}O_2$ (mL/kg/min) and percentage $\dot{V}O_2$max at LT2, and how that relates to their current training status, considering the four steps of interpretation and the three steps of feedback and discussion outlined in Appendix G. If the results are not within the expected range for this athlete's training status (i.e. national team), then you can provide suggestions on how to increase $\dot{V}O_2$max or improve the percentage $\dot{V}O_2$max at LT2. In order to guide the athlete's training, you can explain the five training intensity zones, and the corresponding HR, RPE and power values, which can be used to prescribe and monitor training intensity. When you suggest particular training methods to the coach, explain the intensities using these easily measurable parameters, and how the coach can utilise them to achieve the desired physiological outcomes.

PRACTICAL 13 HIGH-INTENSITY EXERCISE

Case study 1

1 Peak power (W) = force (kp) $\times$ distance / time (s)
$$= [(\underline{\quad} \times 9.81) \times (\underline{\quad}rev \times 6\ m)] / 5\ s$$
$$= [(\underline{4.6} \times 9.81) \times (\underline{10} \times 6)] / 5$$
$$= \underline{541.5}\ W$$
   Percentile (according to Table 13.1) = 85th–90th percentile.

2 Relative peak power (W/kg) = peak power (W) / body mass (kg)
$$= \underline{541.5} / \underline{61.2}$$
$$= \underline{8.8}\ W/kg$$
   Percentile (according to Table 13.1) = 80th percentile.

3 Total work (J) = force (kp) $\times$ total distance (m)
$$= (\underline{\quad} \times 9.81) \times [\underline{\quad}\ rev + \underline{\quad}\ rev + \underline{\quad}\ rev + \underline{\quad}\ rev + \underline{\quad}\ rev + \underline{\quad}\ rev) \times 6\ m)]$$
$$= (\underline{4.6} \times 9.81) \times [(\underline{10} + \underline{8} + \underline{7} + \underline{6} + \underline{5} + \underline{4}) \times 6]$$
$$= \underline{10,830.2}\ J$$

4 Mean power (W) = total work (J) / 30 s
$$= \underline{10,830.2} / 30$$
$$= \underline{361.0}$$
$$= \underline{361.0}\ W$$
   Percentile (according to Table 13.2) = 35th percentile.

5 Relative mean power = mean power (W) / body mass (kg)
$$= \underline{361.0} / \underline{61.2}$$
$$= \underline{5.90}\ W/kg$$
   Percentile (according to Table 13.2) = 25th percentile.

6 Fatigue index (%) = [peak power (W) $-$ lowest power (W)] / peak power (W) $\times$ 100

> **Note:** Lowest power (W) in the final 5-second interval = force (kp) $\times$ distance / time (s)
> $$= [(\underline{\quad} \times 9.81) \times (\underline{\quad}rev \times 6\ m)] / 5\ s$$
> $$= [(\underline{4.6} \times 9.81) \times (\underline{4} \times 6)] / 5$$
> $$= \underline{216.6}\ W$$

   Fatigue index (%) = [($\underline{541.5} - \underline{216.6}$) / $\underline{541.5}$] $\times$ 100
$$= \underline{60.0}\%$$
   Percentile (according to Table 13.3) = $\le \underline{5th}$ percentile.

   The client achieved in the 85th–90th percentile for peak power and 80th percentile for relative peak power. She was classified in the 35th and 20th–25th percentile for mean power and relative mean power, respectively, but <5th percentile for the fatigue index. Therefore, she is ineligible for inclusion in the cycling team. The results demonstrate that, although this client has excellent acceleration (as demonstrated by the excellent peak power result), she has a poor anaerobic capacity (as demonstrated by the poor mean power and very poor fatigue index results).

Discussion

Discussion of these results following completion of the test should involve an explanation of the difference between peak power, mean power and fatigue index, providing her values and how they compare with normative data. The client should be provided with examples of how she could train to improve her speed-endurance and resistance to fatigue e.g. by including a number of maximal sprints lasting 20–40 seconds, with 'incomplete' recovery periods between each sprint into her training regime.

Case study 2
Interpretation

Testing day 1

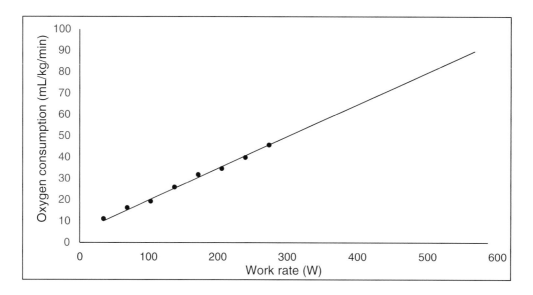

Construction of the linear relationship between oxygen consumption and work rate, with the y-intercept at 5 mL/kg/min determined from the eight submaximal intensities outputs on a cycle ergometer; regression analysis was used to establish a linear relationship that can be extrapolated to supramaximal power outputs.

Two points that lie on, or are very close to, the line are randomly selected; these are:

Point A: $\dot{V}O_2 = 26.02$ mL/kg/min   Power $= 140$ W
Point B: $\dot{V}O_2max = 45.86$ mL/kg/min   Power $= 280$ W

1 Calculate $\Delta\dot{V}O_2max$:
   $\Delta\dot{V}O_2max$ (mL/kg/min) $= 45.86 - 26.02$
   $\Delta\dot{V}O_2max = 19.84$

2 Calculate Δ work rate:
   Δwork rate (W) $= 280 - 140$
   Δwork rate $= 140$ W

3 Calculate m (slope):
   $m = \dot{V}O_2max / \Delta$Work rate
   $m = 19.84 / 140$
   $m = 0.142$

Substitute the slope (m) to establish the linear regression equation:

$\dot{V}O_2 = m \times$ work rate $+ c$
$\dot{V}O_2 = 0.142 \times$ work rate $+ 5$

This is the linear regression equation.

Testing day 2

Now we can calculate the work rate that corresponds to 115% $\dot{V}O_2max$:

$$\text{Work rate (W)} = \frac{[(1.15 \times \dot{V}O_2max) - 5]}{\text{slope}}$$

$$= \frac{[(1.15 \times 44.96) - 5]}{0.142} = \frac{(51.70 - 5)}{0.142}$$

$$= \frac{46.70}{0.142}$$

$$= 329 \text{ W}$$

Testing day 3

1 Calculate accumulated $\dot{V}O_2$:
   Accumulated $\dot{V}O_2 = 2.5 + 5.5 + 11.5 + 16.5 + 19.5 + 21.0 + 22.45 + 22.45$
   Accumulated $\dot{V}O_2 = 121.4$ mL/kg
2 Calculate accumulated $\dot{V}O_2$Demand:
   Accumulated $\dot{V}O_2$Demand $= 2.5 + 25.85 + 25.85 + 25.85 + 25.85 + 25.85 + 25.85 + 25.85 =$
   183.45 mL/kg
3 Calculate accumulated $\dot{V}O_2$Deficit:
   Accumulated $\dot{V}O_2$Deficit $= 183.45 - 121.4$ mL/kg
   $\qquad\qquad\qquad\qquad = 62.05$ mL/kg
   Accumulated $\dot{V}O_2$Deficit $\times 0.9^a = 55.85$ mL/kg

$$\frac{\text{Accumulated } \dot{V}O_2\text{Deficit} \times \text{body mass (78 kg)}}{1000} = 4.36 \text{ L}$$

This is the MAOD.

Classification (according to Table 13.6) – this client's MAOD is excellent compared with other untrained males; however, when his result is compared with that of trained male cyclists, his MAOD score is very poor.

Case study 3
Interpretation

Classification of 5 m sprint time (according to Table 13.7) = excellent
Classification of 10 m sprint time (according to Table 13.7) = good
Classification of 20 m sprint time (according to Table 13.7) = poor
Estimating peak running velocity:
   Calculate average velocity from 10 m to 20 m gates:
      Average velocity $= (d_r - d_i) / (t_r - t_i)$
      Average velocity $= (20 - 10) / (3.82 - 2.10)$
      Average velocity $= 10/1.72$
      Average velocity $= 5.81$ m/s
Classification of average velocity from 10 to 20 m (according to Table 13.7): very poor
Estimating average acceleration:
   Step 1: calculate the velocity at the 5 m mark; that is, average velocity from 0 to 10 m:
      Average velocity $= (d_r - d_i) / (t_r - t_i)$
      Average velocity $= (10 - 0) / (2.10 - 0)$
      Average velocity $= 10/2.10$
      Average velocity $= 4.76$ m/s
   Step 2: calculate average acceleration from 0 to 5 m:
      Average acceleration $= (v_r - v_i)/(t_r - t_i)$
      Average acceleration $= (4.76 - 0)/(1.19 - 0)$
      Average acceleration $= 4.76/1.19$
      Average acceleration $= 4.0$ m/s^2
Classification of average acceleration from 0 to 5 m (according to Table 13.7) = Excellent

---

^{a} Typically, this value is reduced by 9% to correct for reductions in the O_2 stores of the body.

Kerry's 5 m sprint time is excellent, as is her average acceleration over 5 m. However, her average velocity is poor, which is a result of her slower sprint time between 10 m and 20 m. This test indicates that, over short distances requiring sharp bursts of acceleration, Kerry is very quick; however, her ability to reach maximal speed (i.e. 20 m) is not well developed. Over the pre-season training, Kerry's focus should be on improving her maximal speed through bouts of repeated sprints, and working on her technique (i.e. her body position and leg drive).

Case study 4
Interpretation

1 Best total sprint time (s) = best sprint time $\times$ number of sprints performed = $4.80 \times 6 = 28.8$ s.
2 Calculation of sprint performance decrement:
   Decrement = [1 − (best total sprint time / total sprint time)] $\times$ 100
   Decrement = [1 − (28.80 / 30.56)] $\times$ 100
   Decrement = [1 − 0.942] $\times$ 100
   Decrement = $0.058 \times$ 100
   Decrement = 5.8%
Classification (according to Table 13.10) = $Average$

The athlete's sprint performance decrement is average compared with the norms for other male athletes, albeit from a different test. It is evident that the athlete has not regained their full sprinting ability following knee surgery, therefore it would not be recommended for the athlete to begin competing yet. Further work in rehabilitation to increase the lower body strength and explosive leg power would be recommended, along with high-intensity exercise sessions that include multiple short, repeated sprints.

PRACTICAL 14 NUTRITION

Case study 1
1 Predicted BMR using Table 14.2: $(0.034 \times 60) + 3.538 = 5.578$ MJ/day
2 Physical activity level for light activity is 1.6
3 Estimated energy expenditure/requirements = BMR $\times$ physical activity level
$$5.578 \times 1.6 = 8.925 \text{ MJ/day}$$
$$\times 1000 = 8925 \text{ kJ/day}$$
Based on this calculation you inform your friend that she would need to reduce her energy intake from 10,000 kJ/day to lose weight.

Case study 2
With a score of 2 from the quiz, it is clear that you need to provide assistance to Ruth. You should attempt to gain more information regarding her eating habits. Ask her to complete a typical 3-day food diary and assess this against the Australian Dietary Guidelines (see Table 14.1). With this additional information you could then make specific recommendations around her nutrition. This could start with a basic counselling session and first determining whether her health literacy is sufficient for her to know why she should consider changing her food habits. Advice should also be provided on how she might improve her fruit and vegetable intake and general choices of meats and grain foods. Additional information on lifestyle modification counselling would also be indicated. If you discover that Ruth has a chronic disease or another limiting dietary factor, or that you do not have the level of knowledge or skill to adequately provide specific advice, then referral to a dietitian is necessary.

Case study 3
1 You need to clarify a number of specifics regarding his diet diary including the amounts and types of most of the foods reported. This will require going through the individual entries with him. You might use food props or known portion sizes to increase the accuracy of this information.
2 It is important to probe with further questions to determine the following:
   a Is this diet representative of your typical diet?
   b What are other typical breakfast, snack, lunch and drink options?
   c Is this your normal alcohol intake?
   d Do you take any dietary supplements?

3 After obtaining more information, you enter the foods into FoodWorks (Figure CS14.1) and complete relevant parts of the data-recording sheet (Figure CS14.2) using outputs from FoodWorks (Figures CS14.3–14.5). The recording sheet includes the interpretation and feedback you would provide to Bruce.

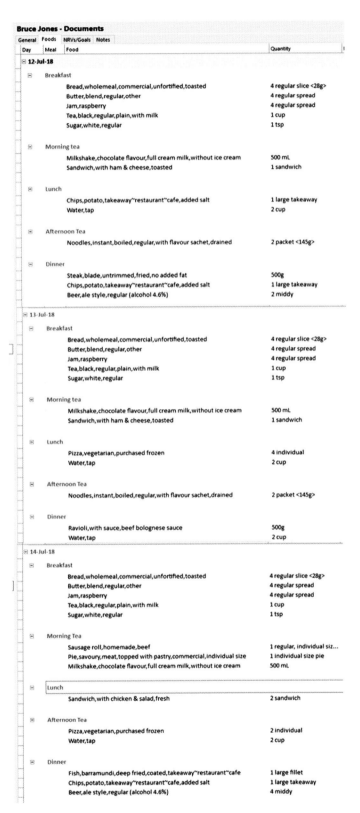

Figure CS14.1 Three-day diet diary for Case study 2 worked example entered into FoodWorks

Used with permission from Xyris software

Name: _Bruce Jones_

Age Group (circle) Male: 9-13 yr 14-18 yr (19-30 yr) 31-50 yr 51-70 yr > 70 yr		
Female*: 9-13 yr 14-18 yr 19-30 yr 31-50 yr 51-70 yr > 70 yr		
Activities 4 and 10: Energy Requirement and Intake		
	Daily Estimated Energy Requirement (EER) in kJ	**Your actual intake based on the diet diary analysis (kJ)**
From Schofield equations (Activity 4)	$BMR = (0.063 \times 92) + 2.896 = 8.692\ MJ = 8,692\ kJ$ $8,692\ kJ \times 1.6 = 13,907\ kJ$	
From Foodworks® (Activity 10)	13,907 kJ	19,201 kJ

* Not pregnant or lactating

Activities 5 and 10: Nutrient Reference Values			
Macronutrients and related	**Range or target based on AMDR or NRVs (Activity 5)**	**Equivalent in g/mg for your EER (use EER from Foodworks® - Activity 10)**	**Your intake in g/mg from Foodworks® (Activity 10)**
Total fat	20-35% of total energy intake	20% of 13,907=2,781kJ/37.7=74 g 35% of 13,907=4,867kJ/37.7=129 g	178 g
Saturated fat & trans fat	< 10% of total energy intake	10% of 13,907=1,391kJ/37.7=37 g	69.8 g
Long chain n-3 PUFA	0.2% of total energy intake	0.2% of 13,907=27.8kJ/37.7=0.74 g	0.26 g
Total carbohydrate	45-65% of total energy intake	45% of 13,907=6,258kJ/16.7=375 g 65% of 13,907=9,040kJ/16.7=541 g	499 g
Protein	15-25% of total energy intake	15% of 13,907=2,086kJ/16.7=125 g 25% of 13,907=3,477kJ/16.7=208 g	189 g
Dietary Fibre	AI = 30g, SDT = min 38g		48.4 g

Vitamins	**Daily NRV (add value where applicable) – provide units**				**Your daily intake (provide units)**
	RDI	**AI**	**SDT**	**UL**	
Vitamin A (retinol equivalents)	900 µg		min.1500µg	3000 µg	901 µg
Thiamin (B1)	1.2 mg				2.3 mg
Riboflavin (B2)	1.3 mg				2.4 mg
Niacin (B3) (Niacin equivalents)	16 mg			35 mg as nicotinic acid	80.8 mg
Pyridoxine (B6)	1.3 mg			50 mg	1.9 mg
Cobalamin (B12)	2.4 µg				9.0 µg
Total Folate (Dietary Folate equivalents)	400 µg		min. 300 µg	1000 µg as folic acid	683 µg
Vitamin C	45 mg		min.220 mg		56.7 mg
Vitamin E		10 mg	min. 19 mg	300 mg	15.6 mg

Figure CS14.2 Completed data-recording sheet for Case study 2 worked example

Minerals	Daily NRV (add value where applicable)				Your daily intake
	RDI	AI	SDT	UL	
Calcium	1000 mg			2500 mg	1502 mg
Iodine	150 µg			1100 µg	378 µg
Iron	8 mg			45 mg	20.1 mg
Magnesium	400 mg			350 mg as a supplement	577 mg
Potassium		3800 mg	min. 4700mg		6060 mg
Sodium		460-920 mg	max. 2000mg		5171 mg
Zinc	14 mg			40 mg	23.4 mg

Activities 6 and 10: Food Groups		
Food group	Recommended number of serves (Activity 6)	Number of serves in your diet from Foodworks® analysis (Activity 10)
Vegetables and legumes/beans	6	17.1
Fruit	2	0.1
Bread /grain and cereals	6	13.3
Lean meat, poultry, fish, eggs, nuts and seeds, legumes/beans	3	3.6
Milk, yoghurt, cheese and/or alternatives	2.5	3.4

Activities 7 and 10: Alcohol		
	Guideline for Alcohol (Activities 7 and 8)	Your intake from Foodworks® analysis (Activity 10) and how this was distributed over 3 days
Alcohol (in standard drinks/day)	≤ 2.0 and no more than 4 standard drinks on a single occasion	2.1 Consumed over two days only, therefore on both these days the guidelines for alcohol was exceeded.

Figure CS14.2 Cont'd

Activities 10 and 11: Diet Diary Validity

Your Energy Intake (EI) from Foodworks® (Activity 10)	Your EER from Foodworks® (Activity 10)	EI:EER bias cut-offs	Your EI:EER and state any bias (e.g. 'under-reporter')
19,201 kJ	13,907 kJ	'Under-reporters' < 0.76 'Over-reporters' >1.24	1.38 Indicating 'over-reporting'

Question. If this was valid data what would the expected outcome on your body mass be over time?

Bruce would be putting on weight. Eating an extra 5300 kJ/day would result in the addition of extra kilogram of fat each week (using 37,000 kJ = 1 kg of fat).

Activity 12: Interpretation, feedback and discussion

Looking at the diet analysis, provide feedback by pointing out 4 positives and 4 points of improvement. Is there any reason to refer to a dietitian?

Four positive points about the diet

1. *Wholemeal bread rather than white bread*
2. *Meeting the serves/day recommendation for the 'Lean meat, poultry, fish, eggs, nuts and seeds, legumes/beans' category with the foods coming from a different sources (red meat and fish)*
3. *Meeting the serves/day recommendation for the 'Milk, yoghurt, cheese and/or alternatives' category although this is mainly due to large chocolate milk drinks*
4. *Meeting the RDIs and AIs for most nutrients*

Four improvements that you could make to the diet

1. *Need to decrease the overall energy intake by limiting foods such as chips, pies, pizza and beer*
2. *Need more variety in diet with same foods being eaten each day (e.g. breakfast and morning tea)*
3. *Although the serves/day recommendation is being met for the 'Vegetables and legumes/beans' category this is due to the high intake of potatoes (chips). More variety is needed for vegetable intake and there is hardly any fruit being consumed.*
4. *Alcohol intake needs to be reduced*

Additional Comments: *This case study is a good example of when it is important to look at more than just the nutrient RDI's and AI's. Focussing on the foods that are being consumed will provide the most information to give feedback to Bruce to decrease his energy intake and meet his weight loss goals. A discussion that focusses on whether his current situation (e.g. new job) is leading to these nutrition behaviours would be a good starting point.*

Figure CS14.2 Cont'd

General

Weight	3800.7 g

Macro-Nutrients

Energy	19201.1 kJ
Protein	189 g
Total fat	178 g
Saturated fat	66.4 g
Trans Fatty Acids	3.4 g
Polyunsaturated	39.8 g
Monounsaturate	58.9 g
Cholesterol	418.7 mg
Carbohydrate	498.9 g
Sugars	116.1 g
Starch	371.8 g
Water	2815.2 g
Alcohol	20.7 g
Dietary fibre	48.4 g
Ash	32.8 g

Vitamins

Thiamin	2.306 mg
Riboflavin	2.363 mg
Niacin	46.553 mg
Niacin equival	80.768 mg
Vitamin C	56.693 mg
Vitamin E	15.592 mg
Tocopherol, al	14.697 mg
Vitamin B6 (by a	1.902 mg
Vitamin B12	8.976 µg
Total folate	683.372 µg
Folic acid	418.003 µg
Folate food	265.514 µg
Folate,total D	963.959 µg
Total vitamin	901.300 µg
Retinol	592.102 µg
Beta caroter	1887.263 µg
Beta caroter	1606.797 µg

Minerals

Sodium	5171.352 mg
Potassium	6059.814 mg
Magnesium	576.982 mg
Calcium	1501.824 mg
Phosphorus	2895.123 mg
Iron	20.067 mg
Zinc	23.443 mg
Selenium	143.620 µg
Iodine	378.169 µg

Figure CS14.3 NRV summaries for Case study 2 worked example using output from FoodWorks
Used with permission from Xyris software

Food Groups

GRAINS	13.28 serve
- Refined	8.83 serve
- Wholegrains	4.46 serve
· Wholegrains pe	33.6 %
FRUIT	0.11 serve
- Citrus, melons &	0 serve
- Other fruit	0.11 serve
- Fruit juice	0 serve
· Fruit juice percent	0 %
VEGETABLES	17.09 serve
- Dark green ve	0.10 serve
- Red & orange	0.64 serve
- Tomatoes	0.47 serve
- Other red &	0.17 serve
- Starchy vege	15.37 serve
- Potatoes	15.37 serve
- Other starchy v	0 serve
· Starchy vegetal	89.9 %
- Legumes	0 serve
- Other vegeta	0.98 serve

PROTEIN FOOD	3.64 serve
- Red meats	2.83 serve
- Poultry	0.16 serve
- Eggs	0.01 serve
- Processed me	0.24 serve
- Organ meats	0 serve
- Seafood high in	0 serve
- Seafood low	0.37 serve
- Nuts & seeds	0.03 serve
- Legumes	0 serve
- Soy products	0 serve
DAIRY	3.40 serve
- Milk	1.66 serve
- Cheese	1.73 serve
- Yoghurt	0 serve
- Milk alternatives	0 serve
OIL EQUIVALENTS	18.2 tsp
SOLID FAT EQUIVAL	20 tsp
ADDED SUGARS	15.5 tsp
· kJ from added	1038.8 kJ
· kJ from added su	5.4 %
ALCOHOLIC DRIN	2.07 sd
UNCLASSIFIED V	51.80 g
· Unclassified weig	1.4 %
UNCLASSIFIED	308.35 kJ

Figure CS14.4 Food groups' summaries for Case study 2 worked example using output from FoodWorks
Used with permission from Xyris software

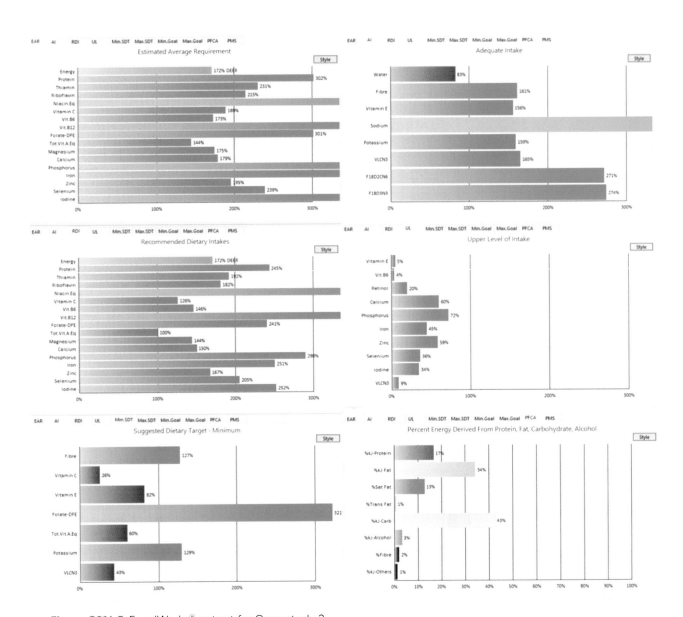

Figure CS14.5 FoodWorks® output for Case study 2
Used with permission from Xyris software

PRACTICAL 15 FUNCTIONAL MEASURES
Case study 1

Balance is the most important functional measure that you would test. You decide to take this man through a physical performance battery. Testing reveals the following results.	
Side-by-side stand score	
If held <10 s	_4.2_ s
Held for 10 s	☐ 0 points
Not held for 10 s	☐ 0 points
Not attempted	☐ 0 points
	continued

Semi-tandem stand score	
If held <10 s	☐ 1 point
Held for 10 s	☐ 1 point
Not held for 10 s	☐ 1 points
Not attempted	X 0 points
If participant did not attempt a test or failed, circle why.	
Participant not able to understand instructions	☐
Participant refused	X
Not attempted, tester felt unsafe	☐
Not attempted, participant felt unsafe	☐
Participant could not hold the position unassisted	☐
Participant tried but was unable to finish the test	☐
Other (specify): _____	☐
Tandem stand score:	
If held <10 s:	_____._____ s
Held for 10 s:	☐ 2 points
Held for 3 to 9.99 s:	☐ 1 point
Held for $<$ than 3 s:	☐ 0 points
Not attempted	X 0 points
If participant did not attempt test or failed to complete the test, circle why.	
Participant not able to understand instructions	☐
Participant refused	X
Not attempted, tester felt unsafe	☐
Not attempted, participant felt unsafe	☐
Participant could not hold the position unassisted	☐
Participant tried but was unable to finish the test	☐
Other (specify): _____	☐
For 3 m walk	
If the participant was unable to do the walk	☐ 0 points
If time is 6.5 s or more	X 1 point
If time is 4.7 to 6.5 s	☐ 2 points
If time is 3.6 to 4.7 s	☐ 3 points
If time is less than 3.6 s	☐ 4 points

continued overpage

Single chair stand score	
Safe to stand without help	X Yes ☐ No
Participant stood without using arms	X Go to repeated chair rise test
Repeated chair stand score	
Safe to stand five times	X Yes ☐ No
Time to complete 5 stands	18.1 s
Participant unable to complete five chair stands	☐ 0 points
Participant completes stands in $>$60 s	☐ 0 points
If time is 16.7 s or more	X 1 point
If time is 13.7 to 16.7 s	☐ 2 points
If time is 11.2 to 13.7 s	☐ 3 points
If time is $<$11.2 s	☐ 4 points
Scoring for the physical performance battery	
Total balance test score	0 point
Usual walk speed test score	1 points
Chair stand test score	1 points
Total score	**2 points** (sum of points above)

Data analysis

Balance test duration = _4.2 s_
Rating: High risk of persistent and severe functional limitation, hospitalisation and mortality.
Physical performance battery score: _0_
$$\text{Usual walk speed} = \text{distance covered (m)/time taken (s)}$$
$$= \underline{3\ m}/\underline{6.6\ s}$$
$$= \underline{0.45\ m/s}$$
Percentile: 18th percentile
Rating: High risk of persistent and severe functional limitation, hospitalisation and mortality.
Physical performance battery score: _1_
Chair stand test duration = _26.1 s_
Percentile: _<10th percentile_
Rating: High risk of persistent and severe functional limitation, hospitalisation and mortality.
Physical performance battery score: _1_

Interpretation

The client was assessed as having poor balance, slow usual walk speed (18th percentile) and reduced leg power (10th percentile). Each of these results places the client in a high risk of persistent and severe functional limitation, hospitalisation and mortality.

Discussion and feedback

Provide the client with the individual scores on each test comprised within the physical performance battery. It would be appropriate to highlight that balance, leg strength and power are very important for maintaining his independence and for preventing falls. Reassure the client that all three components (balance, leg strength and power and walking speed) can be improved by targeted exercises. In line with his results and his goals, retraining his balance would be the target of his program and this can be achieved through simple balance-retraining exercises as well as leg muscle-strengthening exercises. Focus on the positives yet remain realistic when providing feedback. As this man lives alone and may have limited socialisation, you could refer him to a GP or psychologist or suggest he attend group exercise classes for social interaction, if this is feasible for him. Alternatively, explain to the client that you could design a home program for him if this is his preference. Ask the client whether he has any questions about the tests, his results or the exercises.

Case study 2

Power is the most important functional measure that you would test. You decide to take this woman through the floor rise to standing test. Testing reveals the following results.

Floor rise to standing test:

Best = <u>4.65</u> s

Interpretation

Based on Table 15.4, the client was assessed as having a poor floor rise to standing result for a woman of her age.

Discussion and feedback

Provide the client with the floor rise to standing score and her corresponding rating relative to her age and sex. Focus on the positives yet remain realistic when providing feedback. Clarify that a poor performance on the floor rise to standing test may indicate insufficient muscle strength and future difficulty in rising from the floor after sustaining a fall. Furthermore, the combination of poor leg strength and osteoporosis puts the client at an increased risk for sustaining a fracture (commonly at the hip, lumbar spine or wrist). Reassure her that leg strength can be improved by targeted exercises. Inform the client that muscle-strengthening would be the target of her program. Ask the client if she would prefer to exercise in the gym or with her husband at home and explain that you could design a home or gym program depending on her preference. Ask the client whether she has any questions about the tests, her test result or the exercises.

PRACTICAL 16 EXERCISE CAPACITY

Case study 1

Although this value is in the 'good' category, as an elite footballer this value needs to be higher as Australian Rules Football requires excellent endurance. You would ask the player whether she has been tested previously using the MSRT and what values she obtained. You should then find out how much aerobic training she has completed recently. Based on her answers, you would explain why it is important to increase her score and provide training recommendations that aim to improve her endurance. The feedback would need to include information regarding her score and the expectations for improvement. A re-test visit should be scheduled in 4–6 weeks to monitor progress.

Case study 2

Category: 11 minutes 20 seconds = 11.33 minutes; from Table 16.3 this is classified as 'Average'. The last stage completed (increment 34) was at 4.1 km/h and 15.4%
Calculation: 4.1 km/h = 4.1 × 16.7 = 68.5 m/min

$$\dot{V}O_2max = speed \times [0.17 + (grade \times 0.79)] + 3.5$$
$$= 68.5 \times [0.17 + (0.154 \times 0.79)] + 3.5$$
$$= 23.5 \text{ mL/kg/min}$$
$$= 6.7 \text{ METs}$$

The feedback provided should include the time (11 minutes and 20 seconds), MET value (6.7 METs) and the category of the result (average), indicating that this is between 41% and 60% for females of her age. You should discuss the importance of exercise capacity for general health and lowering risks of diseases such as cardiovascular disease and diabetes. Goal setting to improve the score can also be included, as well as providing exercise training recommendations.

Case study 3

Category: below average.
You would first tell the client the distance they covered (520 m) and that this is 'below average' for females of her age. The feedback should focus on how exercise training will be able to improve this value, and that this will lead to improved general health and lower risk of cardiovascular disease. You should remember that, as she is a client with a diagnosed medical condition, you might also have to provide feedback regarding her exercise capacity to her general practitioner.

Case study 4

Category: 3 minutes and 40 seconds = _220_ seconds = _Good_

Feedback should include the time and category, with recognition that this exercise capacity should result in good general health and a lower risk of cardiovascular disease. Discussion should focus on how to maintain/improve this capacity.

PRACTICAL 17 PULMONARY FUNCTION

Case study 1

What additional questions would you ask the client?

Can she remember having her lung function tested before and, if yes, what the findings were? Obtain further information such as whether she is a smoker or was raised in a house with a smoker, and any family history of anyone having lung disease (e.g. asthma or COPD).

What are her predicted FVC, FEV_1 and FEV_1/FVC values?

FVC

Participant's best FVC result = 3.78 L

Predicted FVC (L)[a] = (height constant × height) + (age constant × age) + constant
$\quad = (\underline{0.0491} \times \underline{167}) + (-0.0216 \times \underline{34}) + -\underline{3.590}$
$\quad = \underline{3.88}\,L$

Difference between participant's best FVC result vs predicted FVC: _100 mL lower than predicted_

Comparison of participant's best FVC result (absolute values) vs predicted FVC:

$\downarrow\downarrow$	$\downarrow$	$\overset{\longleftrightarrow}{\text{(circled)}}$	$\uparrow$	$\uparrow\uparrow$

$$\text{Percent (\%) predicted FVC} = \frac{\text{Best FVC result} \times 100}{\text{Predicted FVC result}}$$
$$= 97.4\%$$

Comparison of participant's best FVC result (relative values) vs predicted FVC:

$\downarrow\downarrow$	$\downarrow$	$\overset{\longleftrightarrow}{\text{(circled)}}$	$\uparrow$	$\uparrow\uparrow$

FEV_1

Participant's best FEV_1 result = 2.47 L

Predicted FEV_1 (L)[a] = (height constant × height) + (age constant × age) + constant
$\quad = (\underline{0.0342} \times \underline{167}) + (-\underline{0.0255} \times \underline{34}) + -\underline{1.578}$
$\quad = \underline{3.27}\,L$

Difference between participant's best FEV_1 result vs predicted FEV_1: _800 mL lower than predicted_

Comparison of participant's best FEV_1 result (absolute values) vs predicted FEV_1 (please circle) – refer to the 'Interpreting and classifying abnormal values' section for guidance:

$\downarrow\downarrow$	$\overset{\downarrow}{\text{(circled)}}$	$\longleftrightarrow$	$\uparrow$	$\uparrow\uparrow$

$$\text{Percent (\%) predicted } FEV_1 = \frac{\text{Best } FEV_1 \text{ result} \times 100}{\text{Predicted } FEV_1 \text{ result}}$$
$$= \underline{75.5\%}$$

Comparison of participant's best FEV_1 result (relative values) vs predicted FEV_1:

$\downarrow\downarrow$	$\overset{\downarrow}{\text{(circled)}}$	$\longleftrightarrow$	$\uparrow$	$\uparrow\uparrow$

continued

FEV$_1$/FVC

$$\text{Participant's best FEV}_1/\text{FVC result} = \frac{\text{FEV}_1}{\text{FVC}}$$
$$= \frac{2.47}{3.78}$$
$$= \underline{65.3\%}$$

$$\text{Predicted FEV}_1/\text{FVC} = \frac{\text{Predicted FEV}_1^a}{\text{Predicted FVC}^a}$$
$$= \frac{3.27}{3.88}$$
$$= \underline{84.3\%}$$

Difference between participant's best FEV$_1$/FVC result vs predicted FEV$_1$/FVC: *19% lower than predicted*

Comparison of participant's best FEV$_1$/FVC result (relative values) vs predicted FEV$_1$/FVC:

$\downarrow\downarrow$　　　($\downarrow$)　　　$\leftrightarrow$　　　$\uparrow$　　　$\uparrow\uparrow$

Classification of spirometric values (according to Table 17.2)

- ☒ 'Normal'
- ☐ Obstructive disorder
- ☐ Restrictive disorder
- ☐ Mixed disorder

^{a} From Table 17.1

Her predicted FVC and FEV$_1$ are 3.88 L and 3.27 L, respectively.

Discussion and feedback

You would first provide both her actual values and the predicted values and explain that the FEV$_1$ appears quite a bit lower than the predicted value for a female her age and height. However, the FVC is almost equivalent to the expected volume for a female of her age and height. It would be appropriate to explain to her that the FEV$_1$ represents how quickly a person can move air through the smaller airways while the FVC represents the total volume of air that a person is able to move with each breath. You should then explain that this single result is not a diagnosis and that you recommend she see her GP to have some more specific tests done. You would be happy to send the results to her GP.

Case study 2

What additional factors would you consider in trying to decide how to manage this patient?

Although organising pulmonary function testing may be very useful for this man, it is also important to first determine whether it is appropriate. Keep in mind that respiratory function testing can put a large amount of stress on the chest wall and internal structures and may be contraindicated in this patient for several reasons (e.g. recent thoracic surgery, possible pneumothorax/myocardial infarction/pulmonary embolism/angina/severe hypertension (systolic >200 mmHg, diastolic >120 mmHg) or client discomfort). Although it is not your job to determine whether he has any of these conditions, you should still seek to determine his current functional capacity to help guide your clinical management. You should find out information about when the surgery was, how his recovery has been to date, whether he has been cleared to exercise by his doctor, whether he has any pain or discomfort and whether he has done pulmonary function testing before and what the results were.

What are his predicted FEV_1 and FVC values?

FVC

Participant's best FVC result = 3.17 L

Predicted FVC $(L)^a$ = (height constant $\times$ height) + (age constant $\times$ age) + constant
$$= (0.0600 \times \underline{183}) + (-0.0214 \times \underline{51}) + - \underline{4.65}0$$
$$= \underline{5.23}\,L$$

Difference between participant's best FVC result vs. predicted FVC: *2.06 L lower than predicted*

Comparison of participant's best FVC result (absolute values) vs. predicted FVC:

$\downarrow\downarrow$ ⬭$\downarrow$ $\leftrightarrow$ $\uparrow$ $\uparrow\uparrow$

Percent (%) predicted FVC $= \dfrac{\text{Best FVC result} = 100}{\text{Predicted FVC result}}$
$$= \underline{60.6}\,\%$$

Comparison of participant's best FVC result (relative values) vs. predicted FVC:

$\downarrow\downarrow$ ⬭$\downarrow$ $\leftrightarrow$ $\uparrow$ $\uparrow\uparrow$

FEV_1

Participant's best FEV_1 result = 3.02 L

Predicted FEV_1 $(L)^*$ = (height constant $\times$ height) + (age constant $\times$ age) + constant
$$= (0.0414 \times \underline{183}) + (-0.0244 \times \underline{51}) + - \underline{2.190}$$
$$= \underline{4.14}\,L$$

Difference between participant's best FEV_1 result vs. predicted FEV_1: *1.12 L lower than predicted*

Comparison of participant's best FEV_1 result (absolute values) vs. predicted FEV_1 (please circle) – refer to the 'Interpreting and classifying abnormal values' section for guidance:

$\downarrow\downarrow$ ⬭$\downarrow$ $\leftrightarrow$ $\uparrow$ $\uparrow\uparrow$

Percent (%) predicted $FEV_1 = \dfrac{\text{Best FEV}_1\text{result} \times 100}{\text{Predicted FEV}_1\text{ result}}$
$$= \underline{72.9}\,\%$$

Comparison of participant's best FEV_1 result (relative values) vs. predicted FEV_1:

$\downarrow\downarrow$ ⬭$\downarrow$ $\leftrightarrow$ $\uparrow$ $\uparrow\uparrow$

FEV_1/FVC

Participant's best FEV_1/FVC result $= \dfrac{FEV_1}{FVC}$
$$= \dfrac{3.02}{3.17}$$
$$= \underline{95.3}\%$$

Predicted FEV_1/FVC $= \dfrac{\text{Predicted FEV}_1{}^a}{\text{Predicted FVC}^a}$
$$= \dfrac{4.14}{5.23}$$
$$= \underline{79.2}\%$$

continued

Difference between participant's best FEV_1/FVC result vs. predicted FEV_1/FVC:

15.9% higher than predicted

Comparison of participant's best FEV_1/FVC result (relative values) vs. predicted FEV_1/FVC:

$\downarrow\downarrow$	$\downarrow$	$\leftrightarrow$	$\uparrow$ (circled)	$\uparrow\uparrow$

Classification of spirometric values (according to Table 17.2)

- ☐ 'Normal'
- ☐ Obstructive disorder
- ☒ Restrictive disorder
- ☐ Mixed disorder

ªFrom Table 17.1

Discussion and feedback

You would first provide both his actual values and the predicted values and explain that both the FEV_1 and FVC are low for a man his age and height, and his FEV_1/FVC is higher than normal. It would be appropriate to explain to him that the FEV_1 represents how quickly you can move air through the smaller airways while the FVC represents the total volume of air that you are able to move with each breath. You should then explain that this single result is not a diagnosis (especially in the context of this patient who has had extensive trauma to the chest wall during surgery) and that you will refer him to his GP to have some more-specific tests done. You would be happy to send the results to his GP.

Case study 3

Interpretation

Jane does not show signs of exercise-induced bronchoconstriction. However, a clue is given by the observation that her 'wheeze' occurs during inspiration only. Combined with the observed signs of an extrathoracic 'variable' upper airways obstruction, these findings together provide circumstantial evidence of a condition called 'inspiratory stridor', a symptom of vocal cord dysfunction which is commonly observed in athletes, and is often mistaken for asthma.

Discussion and feedback

You would first provide both Jane's actual and predicted values and explain that her baseline pulmonary function appears within the normal range for her age and height. You would then explain that her pulmonary function tests after exercise did not change in a direction that would raise major suspicion of asthma. It would be appropriate to then disclaim that, although other tests are needed to completely rule out the possibility of asthma, it may be that she is experiencing inspiratory stridor during exercise, a symptom of vocal cord dysfunction that is commonly mistaken for asthma in athletes. You should then explain that these tests are not a diagnosis and that you recommend her to see her GP to have some more-specific tests done to explore the possibility of an extrathoracic 'variable' upper airways obstruction.

PRACTICAL 18 RESTING AND EXERCISE ELECTROCARDIOGRAPHY (ECG)

Case study 1

Heart rate: _78_ bpm
Classification: _normal_
P wave present and upright in lead II? _Yes_
Size/duration: _1 mm/ 80 ms_
PR interval: _160 ms_
QRS complex width: _80 ms_
ST segment – displacement? _nil displacement_
Slope: _N/A_
QT interval: _410 ms_
T wave +ve or − ve: _positive_
Interpretation: _normal sinus rhythm_
Clarify whether you would recommend the participant is safe to exercise based on this resting ECG trace, and why: _safe to exercise as normal sinus rhythm and normal resting heart rate_

Case study 2

Heart rate: _144_ bpm

Classification: _tachycardia_

P wave present and upright in lead II? _present_

Size/duration: _1 mm_/ _80 ms_

PR interval: _120 ms_

QRS complex width: _40 ms_

ST segment − displacement? _inferior/anterior/lateral depression_

Slope: _horizontal_

QT interval: _434 ms_

T wave +ve or −ve: _positive_

Interpretation: _sinus tachycardia with significant ST depression_

Clarify whether you would recommend continuing or prematurely terminating the stress test, and why: _Stop the test due to significant ST depression indicating ischaemic changes. The patient may require further investigation and should be referred on to a cardiologist._

PRACTICAL 19 DATA ANALYSIS

Worked examples are provided in the Practical.

ABBREVIATIONS

ABC-S	Activities-specific Balance Confidence Scale
ACSM	American College of Sports Medicine
ADLs	activities of daily living
AEP	Accredited Exercise Physiologist
AFL	Australian Football League
AI	adequate intake
AMDR	acceptable macronutrient distribution range
AMI	acute myocardial infarction
ANOVA	analysis of variance
ANS	autonomic nervous system
APD	Accredited Practising Dietitian
APSS	Adult Pre-exercise Screening System
AROM	active range of motion
ASIS	anterior superior iliac spine
ATP	adenosine triphosphate
AV	atrioventricular
BIA	bioelectrical impedance analysis
BJHS	benign joint hypermobility syndrome
BMI	body mass index
BMR	basal metabolic rate
BMS	Ballistic Measurement System
BoS	base of support
BP	blood pressure
bpm	beats per minute
BSU	Ball State University
BTPS	body temperature and pressure saturated
CABG	coronary artery bypass graft
CAD	coronary artery disease
CHD	coronary heart disease

CMJ	countermovement vertical jump
COPD	chronic obstructive pulmonary disease
CPET	cardiopulmonary exercise test
CPR	cardiopulmonary resuscitation
CRF	case report form
CT	computed tomography
CV	cross-validation, coefficient of variation
CVD	cardiovascular disease
DAA	Dietitians Association of Australia
DBP	diastolic blood pressure
DXA	dual-energy x-ray absorptiometry
EAR	estimated average requirement
ECG	electrocardiogram
EER	estimated energy requirement
EI	energy intake
ERV	expiratory reserve volume
ESSA	Exercise and Sports Science Australia
FA	Fitness Australia
FFM	fat-free mass
FM	fat mass
FRC	functional residual capacity
FRIEND	Fitness Registry and the Importance of Exercise National Database
FSANZ	Food Standards Australia New Zealand
FVC	forced vital capacity
GP	general practitioner
GPS	global positioning system
GXT	graded exercise test
HbA_{1c}	glycated haemoglobin
HDL	high-density lipoprotein
HITT	high-intensity interval training
IAT	individual anaerobic threshold
ICC	intraclass correlation coefficient
ICO	index of central obesity
IHD	ischaemic heart disease

IPAQ	International Physical Activity Questionnaire
IRV	inspiratory reserve volume
ISAK	International Society for the Advancement of Kinanthropometry
ISO	International Organization for Standardization
kpm	kilopond metres
LDCW	long-distance corridor walk
LDL	low-density lipoprotein
LLN	lower limit of normal
LT	lactate transition
MAOD	maximal accumulated oxygen deficit
MAP	mean arterial pressure
MEP	maximal expiratory pressure
MET	metabolic equivalent
MI	myocardial infarction
MIP	maximal inspiratory pressure
MLSS	maximal lactate steady state
MRI	magnetic resonance imaging
MSDS	material safety data sheet
MSRT	multi-stage shuttle run test
6MWT	6-minute walk test
NRV	nutrient reference value
NSSQA	National Sport Science Quality Assurance
NSTEMI	non-ST elevation myocardial infarction
NVDPA	National Vascular Disease Prevention Alliance
OBLA	onset of blood lactate accumulation
OR	odds ratio
OUES	oxygen uptake efficiency slope
PAL	physical activity level
PCr	phosphocreatine
PEFR	peak expiratory flow rate
PIFR	peak inspiratory flow rate
PNF	proprioceptive neuromuscular facilitation
PP	pulse pressure
PROM	passive range of motion

PSIS	posterior superior iliac spine
RCPA	Royal College of Pathologists of Australasia
RDI	recommended dietary intake
RER	respiratory exchange ratio
RFD	rate of force development
RM	repetition maximum
RMR	resting metabolic rate
ROM	range of motion
RPE	rating of perceived exertion
rpm	revolutions per minute
RPP	rate pressure product
RR	relative risk
RSA	repeat sprint ability
RV	residual volume
SA	sinoatrial
SBP	systolic blood pressure
SD	standard deviation
SDT	suggested dietary target
SEM	standard error of the measurement
SMA	Sports Medicine Australia
STA	soft tissue approximation
STEMI	ST elevation myocardial infarction
STPD	standard temperature pressure dry
TC	total cholesterol
TE	typical error
TEM	technical error of the measurement
TLC	total lung capacity
UAO	upper airways obstruction
UL	upper level
VAT	visceral adipose tissue
VC	vital capacity
vLDL	very-low-density lipoprotein
WHR	waist-to-hip ratio

Index

Page numbers followed by 'f' indicate figures, 't' indicate tables, and 'b' indicate boxes.